PROGRESS IN BRAIN RESEARCH

VOLUME 48

MATURATION OF THE NERVOUS SYSTEM

Recent volumes in PROGRESS IN BRAIN RESEARCH

Volume 47: Hypertension and Brain Mechanisms, W. De Jong, A.P. Provoost and A.P. Shapiro (Eds.) — 1977

Volume 46: Membrane Morphology of the Vertebrate Nervous System. A Study with Freeze-etch Technique, C. Sandri, J.M. Van Buren and K. Akert — 1977

Volume 45: Perspectives in Brain Research, M.A. Corner and D.F. Swaab (Eds.) — 1976

Volume 44: Understanding the Stretch Reflex, H. Homma (Ed.) — 1976.

PROGRESS IN BRAIN RESEARCH

VOLUME 48

MATURATION

OF THE NERVOUS SYSTEM

Proceedings of the 10th International Summer School of Brain Research, Organized by the Netherlands Central Institute for Brain Research, Amsterdam, and held at the Royal Netherlands Academy of Arts and Sciences, Amsterdam, The Netherlands on July 11–15, 1977

EDITED BY

M. A. CORNER

R. E. BAKER

N. E. VAN DE POLL

D. F. SWAAB

AND

H. B. M. UYLINGS

Netherlands Central Institute for Brain Research,
IJdijk 28, Amsterdam (The Netherlands)

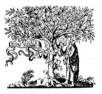

ELSEVIER SCIENTIFIC PUBLISHING COMPANY

AMSTERDAM/NEW YORK/OXFORD

1978

PUBLISHED BY:
ELSEVIER/NORTH-HOLLAND BIOMEDICAL PRESS
335 JAN VAN GALENSTRAAT, P.O. BOX 211
AMSTERDAM, THE NETHERLANDS

SOLE DISTRIBUTORS FOR THE U.S.A. AND CANADA:
ELSEVIER NORTH-HOLLAND INC.
52 VANDERBILT AVENUE
NEW YORK, N.Y. 10017, U.S.A.

ISBN 0-444-80036-0

Library of Congress Cataloging in Publication Data

International Summer School of Brain Research, 10th,
    Amsterdam, Netherlands, 1977.
    Maturation of the nervous system.

    (Progress in brain research; v. 48)
    Includes bibliographical references and index.
    1. Developmental neurology—Congresses. I. Corner, M.A. II.
Amsterdam. Nederlands Centraal Instituut voor Hersenonderzoek. III.
Title. IV. Series. [DNLM: 1. Nervous system—Embryology—Congresses.
2. Nervous system—Growth and development—Congresses. 3. Syn-
apses—Congresses. 4. Genetics—Congresses. 5. Receptors, Sensory—
Congresses. 6. Environment—Congresses. 7. Hormones—Physiology
—Congresses. 8. Behavior—Physiology—Congresses. W1 PR667J v. 48/
WL101.3 I61 1977m]
QP376.P7 vol. 48   [QP363.5]   612'.82'08s   78-2638
ISBN 0-444-80036-0   [599'.01'88]

WITH 169 ILLUSTRATIONS AND 38 TABLES

PRINTED IN THE NETHERLANDS

List of Contributors

J. ADRIEN, CHU-Pitié Salpétrière, Dept. of Physiology, Paris, France.

R.E. BAKER, Netherlands Institute for Brain Research, Amsterdam, The Netherlands.

J. BALSAMO, University of Wisconsin, Dept. of Zoology, Madison, Wisc., U.S.A.

M. BERRY, University of Birmingham, Department of Anatomy, Birmingham, Great Britain.

A. BJÖRKLUND, University of Lund, Dept. of Ophthalmology, Lund, Sweden.

N. BLEICHRODT, Free University of Amsterdam, Dept. of Industrial and Organizational Psychology and Test Development, Amsterdam, The Netherlands.

T.V.P. BLISS, National Institute for Medical Research, Dept. of Developmental Biology, London, Great Britain.

V. BOELI EVERTS, University Hospital Groningen, Dept. of Developmental Neurology, Groningen, The Netherlands.

G.J. BOER, Netherlands Institute for Brain Research, Amsterdam, The Netherlands.

K. BOER, Netherlands Institute for Brain Research, Amsterdam, The Netherlands.

B. BOHUS, University of Utrecht, Rudolf Magnus Institute for Pharmacology, Utrecht, The Netherlands.

S. BORGES, University of Birmingham, Department of Anatomy, Birmingham, Great Britain.

P. BRADLEY, University of Birmingham, Department of Anatomy, Birmingham, Great Britain.

J.-P. CHANGEUX, Institut Pasteur, Dept. of Molecular Biology, Paris, France.

M.A. CORNER, Netherlands Institute for Brain Research, Amsterdam, The Netherlands.

J.P.C. de BRUIN, Netherlands Institute for Brain Research, Amsterdam, The Netherlands.

C.J. de GROOT, University Hospital Groningen, Dept. of Developmental Neurology, Groningen, The Netherlands.

D. de WIED, University of Utrecht, Rudolf Magnus Institute for Pharmacology, Utrecht, The Netherlands.

R. DJOKOMOELJANTO, Diponegoro University, Dept. of Medicine, Semarang, Indonesia.

J. DOGTEROM, Netherlands Institute for Brain Research, Amsterdam, The Netherlands.

R.F. DREWETT, University of Durham, Dept. of Psychology, Durham, Great Britain.

T.V. DUNWIDDIE, University of California, Dept. of Psychobiology, Irvine, Calif., U.S.A.

C. GALL, University of California, Dept. of Psychobiology, Irvine, Calif., U.S.A.

F.A. HOMMES, University Hospital Groningen, Dept. of Developmental Neurology, Groningen, The Netherlands.

J. HOOISMA, Medical Biological Laboratory TNO, Rijswijk, The Netherlands.

J.K.S. JANSEN, University of Oslo, Dept. of Physiology, Oslo, Norway.

D. KUFFLER, University of Oslo, Dept. of Physiology, Oslo, Norway.

K. KUIJPERS, Netherlands Institute for Brain Research, Amsterdam, The Netherlands.

J. LILIEN, University of Wisconsin, Dept. of Zoology, Madison, Wisc., U.S.A.

G. LYNCH, University of California, Dept. of Psychobiology, Irvine, Calif., U.S.A.

T. MAGCHIELSE, Medical Biological Laboratory TNO, Rijswijk, The Netherlands.

B. McEWEN, The Rockefeller University, New York, N.Y., U.S.A.

E. MEETER, Medical Biological Laboratory TNO, Rijswijk, The Netherlands.

E. MEISAMI, University of Tehran, Institute of Biochemistry and Biophysics, Tehran, Iran.

K. MIKOSHIBA, Institut Pasteur, Dept. of Molecular Biology, Paris, France.

J.G. PARNAVELAS, University College London, Dept. of Anatomy, London, Great Britain.

A. QUERIDO, University of Leiden, Dept. of Medicine, Leiden, The Netherlands.

J. SEDLÁČEK, Charles University, Research Lab. of Psychiatry, Prague, Czechoslovakia.

D.W. SLAAF, Medical Biological Laboratory TNO, Rijswijk, The Netherlands.

C. SOTELO, Centre Médico-Chirurgical Foch, Lab. of Neuromorphology, Suresnes, France.

U. STENEVI, University of Lund, Dept. of Histology, Lund, Sweden.

W.F. STEVENS, Medical Biological Laboratory TNO, Rijswijk, The Netherlands.

R.V. STIRLING, National Institute for Medical Research, Dept. of Developmental Biology, London, Great Britain.

D.F. SWAAB, Netherlands Institute for Brain Research, Amsterdam, The Netherlands.

W. THOMPSON, University of Oslo, Department. of Physiology, Oslo, Norway.

B.C.L. TOUWEN, University Hospital Groningen, Dept. of Developmental Neurology, Groningen, The Netherlands.

J.L. VALATX, Université Claude Bernard, Dept. of Experimental Medicine, Lyon, France.

N.E. van de POLL, Netherlands Institute for Brain Research, Amsterdam, The Netherlands.

H. van DIS, Municipal University of Amsterdam, Dept. of Clinical Psychology, Amsterdam, The Netherlands.

F.W. van LEEUWEN, Netherlands Institute for Brain Research, Amsterdam, The Netherlands.

H.G. van OYEN, Netherlands Institute for Brain Research, Amsterdam, The Netherlands.

W.A.M. VELTMAN, Netherlands Institute for Brain Research, Amsterdam, The Netherlands.

M. VISSER, University Hospital Amsterdam, Wilhelmina Gasthuis, Dept. of Obstetrics and Gynaecology, Amsterdam, The Netherlands.

G. VRENSEN, The Netherlands Ophthalmic Research Institute, Wilhelmina Gasthuis, Amsterdam, The Netherlands.

J. ZIMMER, University of Aarhus, Institute of Anatomy-B, Aarhus, Denmark.

Introduction

'Maturation of the Nervous System' was the theme of the 10th in a series of International Summer Schools organized by the Netherlands Institute for Brain Research in Amsterdam. It had been noted at our previous meeting, devoted to 'Perspectives in Brain Research' (see *Progress in Brain Research, Vol. 45*, edited by M.A. Corner and D.F. Swaab), that a wide variety of developmental questions kept popping up even in those contributions which were not explicitly concerned with ontogenetic problems. We also commented at that time that the maturation and adaptation of the nervous system is sure to become one of the more active research areas in coming years. It therefore seemed appropriate to choose this as the general topic for our subsequent Summer School which, in keeping with tradition, was held during the Summer of 1977 at the Academy of Sciences building in the center of Amsterdam.

The theme of nervous system maturation was all the more appropriate at the present time, since the Brain Research Institute had just completed a thoroughgoing process of reorganization, as recommended by a ministerial evaluation committee under the direction of Prof. H.B.G. Casimir (President of the Royal Dutch Academy of Sciences). The themes of neural *maturation* (and the myriad factors regulating and influencing it) and of *adaptation* to environmental challenges were already heavily represented in various projects, and therefore became a logical choice for a more concentrated research effort. The 'maturational' facet of this 'central theme' is reflected here in a number of contributions written by institute staff members. The 'adaptational' facet, i.e. short- and long-term neuronal plasticity in all its forms, is planned for the Summer School which is to be held in 1979.

As regards the present volume, the material is presented under six headings, each containing four or five papers. Most of these give a broad treatment of some particular field in developmental neuroscience, but a few more specialized reports have been included as well. Portions of the discussions held at the Summer School were felt to provide important clarifications of certain points, and have therefore been published following the appropriate papers. In addition, we are grateful to Dr. Sedláček and to Drs. Stirling and Bliss for making available to us papers which they were unable to present at the meeting itself. While trying to be as comprehensive as was feasible, we recognize the impossibility of covering in a single volume more than a fraction of the exciting research developments which would have fallen under the chosen title. We opted instead for choosing *clusters* of related topics, reflecting those fields which currently appear to be the most active.

One such cluster is, of course, the problem of *specificity in synaptic innervation patterns*. The neuromuscular junction still constitutes the most convenient model system for studying basic mechanisms in synaptogenesis, and a review of the work of three highly active European groups is presented in the first section. Section two deals both with the central nervous system (where, for a change, the visual system is *under*-represented, in the interests of a wider survey) and with the primary afferent nerve connections, where we are fortunate to have one of the few groups working in this area present a comprehensive and up-to-date treatment of the subject. The large question of *determinants of neuronal development* has been split into parts dealing with, respectively, intrinsic (i.e. organismic) and extrinsic (i.e. environmental) factors. The former section handles normal development as well as the effects of genetic alterations, whereas the latter section emphasizes (arbitrarily, to be sure) those effects of the environment which are mediated via stimulation of sensory receptors. In addition to the attention necessarily given here to the visual system, we have been able to include some recent work on the subject of olfactory influences in development. The visual studies presented are heavily biased towards morphological approaches, with the justification that this side of the picture is perhaps less well known than are the often reviewed neurophysiological and behavioral dimensions.

Hormones too, of course, are important determinants of neurogenesis, and in fact often serve as intervening variables in genetic and environmental influences such as those described in sections III and IV. Reflecting the current level of activity in this field, an entire section has been devoted to *hormonal effects upon nervous system maturation*. The book closes with a section on the *early development of behavior*, with emphasis upon the underlying neuronal mechanisms. This is still a very young field of research, and the coverage is of necessity devoted largely to the regulation of sleep and wakefulness (especially the former). It will hopefully be evident from the presented papers, however, where some good opportunities for future research lie in this important area.

Acknowledgements

We are pleased to acknowledge the generous financial support given to the Summer School by all of the following:

Aemstelstad B.V.

Babajeff, Algemene Im- en Export

Beckman Instruments B.V.

Beyer & Eggelaar B.V., Metaalindustrie

Brunschwig Chemie B.V.

Elmekanic B.V.

Emergo B.V., Industrie- en Handelsonder-
neming

European Training Programme in Brain and
Behaviour Research

Hope Farms B.V.

C.H. van den Houten Fund

IBRO Education Program

IBM Nederland N.V., Scientific Programs

A. de Jong B.V., Technische Handelsonder-
neming

Van Oortmerssen, Wetenschappelijke
Instrumenten B.V.

Organon Nederland B.V.

Philips Duphar B.V.

Schering Nederland B.V.

Shell Nederland B.V.

Society for the Advancement of Physics
and the Healing Arts

P.M. Tamson B.V.

Zuid-Holland, v/h B. Höfelt B.V.

Dr. Saal van Zwanenberg Foundation

The Editors would also like to acknowledge the following publishers, and all of the authors involved, for their cooperation in allowing the reproduction of figures originally appearing in their own publications.

Ankho Press, for two figures used in the article by R.E. Baker (from *Brain Res. Bull.*, 2, 1977); Cold Spring Harbor Laboratories, for one figure in the article by R.E. Baker (from *Cold Spr. Harb. Symp. quant. Biol.*, 40, 1976); Ciba Foundation, for two figures in the article by D.F. Swaab et al. (from *The Fetus and Birth*, J. Knight and M. O'Connor, Eds., 1977); New York Academy of Sciences, for one figure in the article by D.F. Swaab et al. (from *Ann. N.Y. Acad. Sci.*, 55, 1952); Endocrine Society, for two figures in the article by B.S. McEwen (from *Endocrinology*, 94, 1974); British Endocrinology Society, for one figure in the article by B.S. McEwen (from *J. Endocr.*, 72, 1977); Wiley Interscience, for one figure in the article by B.S. McEwen (from *Biological Determinants of Sexual Behavior*, J. Hutchinson, Ed., 1977) and one figure in the article by R.E. Baker (from *Develop. Psychobiol.*, 10, 1977); MacMillan Journals Ltd., for one figure from the article by J.P. Changeux and K. Mikoshiba (from *Nature (Lond.)*, 264, 1976); World Health Organization, for one figure in the article by A. Querido et al. (from *WHO Chronicle*, 1974); Charles C. Thomas and Co., for one figure in the article by A. Querido et al. (from *Pediatrics*, 19, 1957); Marine Biological Laboratory, Woods Hole, for two figures in the article by M.A. Corner (from *Biol. Bull.*, 145, 1973); Pergamon Press for three figures in the article by M.A. Corner (from *Progr. Neurobiol.*, 8, 1977).

Finally, we are deeply indebted to Mr. J. Overdijk for the taping of the discussions, and for attending to the other technical details during the Summer School, and to Miss J. Sels for painstakingly transcribing the taped material and typing the final versions. She also took care of the innumerable organizational details without which neither the book nor the meeting would have been possible.

Contents

SECTION I

FORMATION OF
NEUROMUSCULAR SYNAPSES

The Formation and Maintenance of Synaptic Connections as Illustrated by Studies of the Neuromuscular Junction

J.K.S. JANSEN, W. THOMPSON and D.P. KUFFLER

Department of Physiology, University of Oslo, Oslo (Norway)

INTRODUCTION

To understand the functioning of the nervous system we have to know the ground rules for how synaptic connections between neurons are formed and maintained. Today our insights are at best fragmentary. An experimental approach to the problem in the brain itself is a difficult task, both on account of the large number of neurons which interact, and on account of the intricate structure of the neuropil. In the peripheral nervous system the situation is much simpler and it may turn out to be a good strategy to examine peripheral tissues first and then determine the extent to which the rules established here also apply to synapse formation in the brain.

In this account we shall review some observations on the innervation of skeletal muscle, which has been a useful preparation for the study of formation of synapses. There are several reasons for this. The functions of muscles are well known and convenient to monitor. The physiology of synaptic transmission at the neuromuscular end-plate has been examined extensively. All the synapses in a muscle are equal, and the normal pattern of innervation is simple: one axon terminal and end-plate for each muscle fiber. Finally, skeletal muscle offers a number of experimental advantages. It survives well in vitro, it differentiates and is easily maintained in culture, and its organization and geometry make it favorable for the application of powerful histological and physiological techniques.

Most of our information still consists of observations obtained by experimental manipulations of adult muscle. Some of this is of interest in itself and some of it may also apply to the initial formation of synapses during development. At present there are no established mechanistic explanations for the phenomena which we describe. They do, however, illustrate and characterize the type of processes involved, and in some cases they restrict the number of potential mechanisms.

The following account is mainly based on experiments performed in our own laboratory. Other observations are included only when they are closely related to our own points of view. We have made no attempt to make a comprehensive review since several other recent reviews cover more or less the same ground from different perspectives (Purves, 1976; Harris, 1974; Fambrough, 1976). Nor are we making any claims for the originality of the interpretations presented. Most of them, we believe, are more or less current among the colleagues working in this field. Our intent, then, is only to give an account of what we consider to be the most interesting aspects of a rapidly developing field.

EXPERIMENTAL OBSERVATIONS

The stimulus for synapse formation

Formation of functional synapses requires a competent presynaptic neuron and an adequate target. For skeletal muscle the competence of the presynaptic axon largely appears to be its ability to release acetylcholine (ACh) at its terminals. Thus, in vertebrates, all motor neurons can innervate any skeletal muscle under the appropriate experimental conditions. Furthermore, skeletal muscle can be innervated by cholinergic preganglionic sympathetic neurons (Langley and Anderson, 1904) and by preganglionic vagal axons (Landmesser, 1971). On the other hand, adrenergic postganglionic sympathetic neurons will not form synapses in skeletal muscle under comparable conditions (Langley and Anderson, 1904). A major feature of the potential target for motor neurons appears to be the presence of available ACh receptors in its plasma membrane. Motor axons will, therefore, readily innervate denervated skeletal muscle, and even a denervated sympathetic ganglion (Langley and Anderson, 1904).

However, in order to accept innervation the muscle has to be in a particular 'receptive state'. As long as a muscle is innervated and active, a foreign motor nerve implanted into the muscle is unable to form any new synapses (Elsberg, 1917). Once the muscle is denervated by section of its original nerve, the foreign motor axons are activated and form functional synapses within 3–4 days (Fex and Thesleff, 1967). However, actual denervation is not required to induce the receptive state in the muscle. A comparable period of paralysis appears to be equally effective. Prolonged inactivity of the muscle without surgical denervation has been achieved by local treatment with botulinum toxin (Fex et al., 1966), and by a reversible block of nerve impulse conduction after implantation of a cuff containing a local anesthetic (Jansen et al., 1973). In both cases implanted foreign motor nerves will innervate the muscle. These observations suggest that the receptive state of the muscle is induced by inactivity, and this deduction is supported by the converse experiment. It was possible to entirely prevent synapse formation by the foreign nerve in the denervated muscle by keeping it active during the relevant period. This was achieved by direct electrical stimulation of the muscle through implanted electrodes (Frank et al., 1975). Accordingly, we believe that inactive muscle activates neighboring motor axons to form terminal structures and synapses. This mechanism may also explain the refusal of normal muscle to become hyper-innervated.

The signal from inactive muscle to the nerves is unknown. The experiments with implanted foreign nerves are complicated and it is, therefore, difficult to speculate about the nature of the signal. Such nerve implant experiments require that the foreign nerve is cut and transplanted to another muscle. Axonal section in itself is a stimulus to sprouting (Ramón y Cajal, 1959), and the implanted axons grow extensively even in innervated active muscle. The detailed relationship between the muscle fibers and the axonal processes is therefore difficult to ascertain at the time when formation of new synapses is induced by section of the original nerve.

Experiments involving *partial* denervation of the muscle are simpler to interpret. This procedure activates the remaining motor axons to sprout and innervate the denervated muscle fibers (Edds, 1953). In this situation the stimulus to sprout acts upon intact motor neurons and, again, it probably originates in the denervated muscle fibers. Brown and Ironton (1977a), for instance, have shown that sprouting is induced in innervated muscle after block of impulses in the muscle nerve, and that such sprouting can be prevented by direct stimulation of the muscle. In this case, therefore, the signal for sprouting from the inactive muscle fibers appears to act at a distance on motor axons or terminals of neighboring innervated muscle fibers. Hence, it is difficult to escape the conclusion that the signal for sprouting is a diffusible substance released from inactive muscle fibers. Presumably this is the same substance that induces synapse formation by foreign nerves implanted into a denervated muscle. However, as will be argued later, it is unlikely that the presence of this substance alone is sufficient for the establishment of functional synapses. Additional changes in the surface membrane of the target are probably also required.

The extent of the peripheral field of innervation of motor neurons

The sizes of the motor units, that is the number of muscle fibers innervated by each motor neuron, vary in a characteristic way between different muscles. In certain muscles, such as the rat soleus, the motor units are rather uniform in size; they vary only by about a factor of two (Close, 1967). In others, such as the gastrocnemius, some motor units are some ten times larger than the smallest ones. Different sized motor units are innervated by motor neurons with distinct functional properties, the larger ones by so-called *phasic* and the smaller ones by *tonic* motor neurons (see Burke and Edgerton, 1975). It appears reasonable that the extent of terminal arborizations that a motor neuron can establish and maintain is restricted by the capacity of the metabolic machinery of the cell body. Such a limit to the capacity of a neuron to form functional terminals can be demonstrated in partially denervated muscles, and it achieves prominence in the present connection as one of the factors which determines whether or not synapses are formed. In a partially denervated muscle the remaining intact motor axons sprout and innervate a certain number of the denervated muscle fibers. As is reasonable, this number depends upon the number of remaining motor axons in the muscle. In the rat soleus each of these will sprout to innervate up to four times their normal number of muscle fibers. With seven or more motor axons remaining (i.e. $\frac{1}{4}$ of the normal number), the muscle will therefore become fully innervated by the sprouting axons. With any smaller number of remaining motor axons only some of the muscle fibers are innervated by the sprouts, while the rest atrophy and eventually disappear. With one to seven remaining motor axons, the number of surviving innervated muscle fibers increases proportionally with the number of remaining axons (Thompson and Jansen, 1977). This point means that, even with a small number of remaining axons, each axon will sprout to no more than about four times its normal size, even though there may still be a large number of denervated muscle fibers as potential targets in the muscle. This can be regarded as the limit to the extent of the peripheral field of innervation which a motor neuron can establish under favorable conditions.

Similar observations have recently been obtained after partial denervation of the extensor digitorum longus (EDL) muscle in mice. In this muscle the sizes of motor units are distributed over a wide range, but the limit to their expansion during sprouting still appears to be about five-fold for all classes of motor units (Brown and Ironton, 1978).

THE SELECTIVITY OF NEUROMUSCULAR CONNECTIONS

In addition to the more general factors considered above, there are at least two different kinds of selectivity which contribute to the refinement of the pattern of innervation of muscle. The first is the preference for innervation of a specific site on the muscle fiber. The second is a preference for a specific type of motor neuron.

Site of synapse

As mentioned, most vertebrate skeletal muscle fibers are innervated by a single motor axon. The end-plate is usually located approximately in the middle of the muscle fiber. This pattern has been reasonably explained by Bennett and Pettigrew (1974a). The muscle fibers are very short when initially innervated. They grow in length by adding new sarcomeres at both ends, while the end-plate of the fiber remains at the center. However, different patterns of distribution of end-plates exist as well. The fast muscle fibers of the body wall of the hagfish are innervated by single motor axons. Their end-plates are placed at the very end of the muscle fibers (Alnæs et al., 1964). In this case we do not have any developmental observations explaining the pattern. Presumably the end-plate is formed at the site first encountered by the motor axon and subsequently moves along with the growing end of the muscle fiber.

Still other muscle fibers are innervated by several motor axons. Such 'distributed innervation' occurs in all slow muscle fibers which are activated without an intervening muscle fiber action potential, but it is also found in some fast muscles such as the frog sartorius (Katz and Kuffler, 1941). The general rule in these cases is that the synaptic regions are evenly distributed along the length of the muscle fiber (Bennett and Pettigrew, 1974b; Gordon et al., 1974). The distance between neighboring synaptic sites seems to be a characteristic of each type of muscle. This feature of the pattern of innervation of muscle is better considered in a subsequent section, after a discussion of some of the factors which control the maintenance of synapses in muscle.

The synaptic site originally established during development appears to be a preferred target for motor axon terminals reinnervating a denervated muscle (Gutman and Young, 1944; Bennett et al., 1973; Frank et al., 1975). Recently, the phenomenon has been studied in remarkable detail with refined techniques in the cutaneous pectoris muscle of the frog (Letinsky et al., 1976). The regenerating axon terminals were found to reoccupy the original synaptic gutter with amazing precision.

Part of the explanation for this precise reinnervation of the original end-plate region is probably that the regenerating axon terminals are guided to this region of the muscle fibers by the degenerated remains of the distal stump of the motor nerve (Ramón y Cajal, 1959). This, however, is certainly not the full explanation. For instance, there are reports of reinnervation of the original end-plate site even when the central end of the nerve has been deliberately displaced to prevent contact with the distal stump (Bennett et al., 1973). Similarly, we have seen foreign nerves transplanted to the rat soleus muscle establish most of their synapses in the original end-plate region, even when the nerves have been transplanted well outside the end-plate region (unpublished observation). It is difficult or impossible, however, to rule out axonal guidance entirely in these cases, since it is not known to what extent the regenerating motor axons may encounter intra-muscular nerve branches. Unequivocal evidence for special membrane properties at the denervated end-plate has, however, been obtained in other types of experiments.

When the superficial fibular nerve is transplanted to the proximal region of the rat soleus muscle, and the muscle denervated, all the foreign synapses are formed in the region of the implant, entirely removed from the original end-plate band. This synapse formation on virgin regions of the muscle can be entirely prevented by direct electrical stimulation of the muscle during the period of synapse formation. In contrast, similar electrical stimulation of the muscle has no effect on reinnervation of the muscle by the original nerve, which reaches the original end-plate sites (Frank et al., 1975). This stability of the factor which permits synapse formation at the original end-plate site is clearly a property induced at that site by the earlier contact with the motor axon. It is not a property of that particular region of the muscle per se, and it is not a property of the original nerve, as distinct from a foreign motor nerve. This was demonstrated by reinnervation of ectopic end-plate sites on muscle fibers that were kept normally active by their regenerated original nerves (Frank et al., 1975).

There is, however, a clear limit to the persistence of the factor allowing reinnervation of a previously innervated site. This was demonstrated by comparing the success of reinnervation of the original site at different times after the foreign innervation of the muscle had been established (Frank et al., 1975). At the earliest times of about one week (after a crush of the original nerve), virtually all muscle fibers which were innervated by the foreign nerve were also reinnervated by the original nerve. With longer delays of reinnervation (obtained by repeated crushes, simple nerve section, or resection of a segment of the nerve), a progressively smaller fraction of the muscle fibers with foreign innervation were reinnervated by the original nerve. This reduced efficiency of reinnervation appears to be due to a loss of a required 'innervation factor' at the old end-plate site. The alternative, i.e. that it is due to some presynaptic deficiency due to delayed regrowth, is ruled out by the finding that reinnervation is virtually complete even after nerve resection in the absence of foreign nerve innervation of the muscle.

The simplest, tentative, interpretation of these observations is obtained by analogy with the behavior of the ACh receptor (see Lømo and Westgaard, 1976, for summary). In normal muscle the receptor is present only at the end-plate region and in a form which is resistant to muscle activity. In paralyzed muscle extra-junctional receptors appear over the entire surface of the muscle fibers. The extra-junctional receptors are rapidly eliminated by activity while ectopic innervation induces the formation of receptors resistant to activity (Frank et al., 1975). Accordingly, the postulated membrane innervation factor and the ACh receptor behave in surprisingly similar ways.

These findings supported the appealing suggestion that perhaps the ACh receptor itself was the required membrane innervation factor (Katz and Miledi, 1964). However, several recent observations have made this suggestion less attractive. For instance, the denervated original end-plate sites of cross-innervated muscle lose most of their receptivity while still retaining their ACh receptors (Frank et al., 1975). In fact the presence of ectopic innervation appears to protect the ACh receptors at the denervated original site (Frank et al., 1975), while simultaneously reducing its receptivity to reinnervation. Furthermore, the application of drugs that bind specifically to the ACh receptor does not prevent formation of new synapses either in organ culture (Cohen, 1972; Kidokoro et al., 1976) or in vivo (Jansen and Van Essen, 1976).

While these observations are open to the objection that the drugs may bind to a region of the receptor different from that required for receptivity to nerves, they demonstrate that synapses can form even though all postsynaptic effects of the transmitter are blocked. In this respect they recall the 'autapses' formed in cell cultures of sympathetic neurons (Landis, 1976; Furshpan et al., 1976). The recent finding of Marshall et al. (1977) also suggests that the ACh receptors are not directly required for synapse formation on muscle. They find that synapse formation is induced by the remaining basement membrane of the end-plate region after necrosis of the muscle fiber itself. This suggests that the relevant factor is one or more of the constituents of the basement membrane of the end-plate region. However, in view of the striking similarity between the ACh receptor and the innervation factor, it is tempting to consider analogous or parallel regulatory mechanisms for the two substances (see Lømo and Slater, 1977).

Preference for specific motor neurons

There are striking differences among animal species in the degree of selectivity of motor neurons for a particular muscle. In adult mammals the degree of selectivity is small. Most experiments suggest that a skeletal muscle can be innervated as efficiently by a foreign motor nerve as by its own. Moreover, in the rat soleus, established foreign innervation will, as was mentioned, eventually prevent reinnervation by the original nerve (Frank et al., 1975). It is, however, difficult to obtain an experimental situation which ensures equal possibilities for innervation by the original and a foreign nerve in a competitive situation. In an attempt to give both nerves equal opportunities for innervating the rat soleus, Weiss and Hoag (1946) found no preference for the original nerve. More recent experiments suggest that there may be differences among muscles in this respect. Hoh (1975) has reported that, while the rat soleus muscle readily accepts innervation by the EDL nerve, the cross-innervation of the EDL muscle by the soleus nerve is much less efficient. However, in such experiments it is difficult to entirely exclude trivial mechanical factors such as the length of nerves or their blood supply. After reinnervation of cat muscle spindles, on the other hand, Brown and Butler (1976) found that the fusimotor fibers consistently had the same type of effect on all the muscle spindles that they innervated. Since the fusimotor effects are determined by the type of intrafusal muscle fiber that the motor nerve activates, this clearly suggests some preference of muscle fibers for a particular type of motor nerve fiber.

Similarly, in lower vertebrates there are clear illustrations of a preference for the original nerve in a situation of competitive reinnervation. This has been demonstrated for fin muscles in the fish (Sperry and Arora, 1965; Mark, 1965). In the salamander, Grimm (1971) found essentially correct reinnervation of the forelimb even after deliberate displacement of the major nerve trunks. A notable example of selectivity has been demonstrated during rein-nervation of a frog muscle which contains both twitch and slow muscle fibers (Schmidt and Stephani, 1976). The two types of muscle fibers are innervated by different classes of axons which can be recognized from their impulse conduction velocities. After nerve section the slow muscle fibers are first innervated by the thicker motor axons which normally innervate the twitch muscle fibers. However, the more slowly regenerating thin motor axons are able to replace the fast axons when they eventually reach their targets.

Among invertebrates, muscles are often innervated by a single or just a few motor neurons, and equally clear examples of selective reinnervation have been reported (Pearson and Bradley, 1972; Young, 1972). In the leech, it is even clear that some regenerating motor neurons must grow through extensive regions of foreign denervated muscle without making functional synapses, before reinnervating their original target (Van Essen and Jansen, 1977). These observations suggest that some muscles contain labels which ensure a relative, or even absolute, preference for their original motor neurons. A potential complication of this inter-pretation is the possibility of specific guidance by the remaining distal nerve stumps. This objection is relevant to all the examples discussed, and its importance is so far unknown.

The initial formation of neuromuscular junctions

The account so far has dealt with re-establishment of innervation in denervated mature muscle. The initial innervation during embryological development presents additional problems. In vertebrates the first neuromuscular junctions are formed half to two-thirds of the way through embryological development with appreciable difference in timing in dif-ferent species (Hamburger, 1970). The limb buds are well developed at this time, and the actual formation of neuromuscular junctions is preceded by a stage when the motor axons are growing from the primitive motor neuron to the yet undifferentiated anlage of their target muscle. To a surprising degree, the appropriate motor axons tend to be present at the correct sites even before any functional connections have been made (Landmesser and Morris, 1975). The nature of the process guiding the growing axons to their prospective targets is at present unknown.

In the rat diaphragm the first functional neuromuscular junctions are formed on early myotubes when they are about 300 μm long (Bennett and Pettigrew, 1974a). It is commonly assumed that this is associated with the development of specific molecules or molecular configurations in the plasma membrane of the myotubes, and that these are acting as recognizable structures which trigger the formation of synapses. For technical reasons the details of the earliest synapse formation during embryogenesis have been difficult to study. However, one remarkable feature is well established. During the earliest stages several different motor axons form functional synaptic connections with each muscle fiber (Redfern, 1970; Bennett and Pettigrew, 1974a). In the newborn rat soleus, each muscle fiber is innervated by about five different motor axons. All these have their terminal arborizations within one circumscribed end-plate region (Brown et al., 1976), which is much smaller than the length of the myotube at the time of the first innervation. It is as if this particular region has been an especially attractive target for the motor nerve fibers in the neighborhood. Alternatively, it could be that the first axon to establish contact serves to attract the others. Neither can it be excluded by the present observations that the earliest synapses are formed randomly over the surface of the myotube, only to migrate subsequently to the final end-plate region of the muscle fiber.

In tissue culture, the experimental conditions can be better controlled, and these culture systems offer great promise for the more detailed study of the mechanisms of early synapse formation. After the first demonstrations that neuromuscular junctions can be formed in vitro (see Crain, 1976, for review), a central question in these studies has been whether the synapses are formed at predetermined spots on the surface of the myotubes. As yet, our possibilities for mapping the distribution of the various components of the plasma membrane are limited, and most of the current interest has been focused on the possible association between the distribution of acetylcholine receptors and the sites where synapses are formed. The regular association between the presence of ACh receptors and synapse formation in adult muscle (see above) has made this an attractive idea. In addition the presence of the appropriate receptors postsynaptically is obviously a requirement for the formation of a functional synapse. Isolated myotubes and myofibers in culture have ACh receptors distributed over their entire surface membrane. Characteristically, however, the receptors are not evenly distributed but appear in much higher densities in small regions of the membrane, termed 'hot spots' (Fischbach and Cohen, 1973; Sytkowski et al., 1973). Direct observation of early synapse formation in culture has now demonstrated that the synapses are not preferentially formed at pre-existing hot spots (Anderson et al., 1977; Frank and Fischbach, 1977). Very soon, however, ACh receptors accumulate at the point of contact. At the same time pre-existing hot spots in the neighborhood tend to disappear. Quite possibly the ACh receptors can move in the membrane and are attracted and trapped by the nerve terminal (Anderson and Cohen, 1977).

ELIMINATION OF REDUNDANT INNERVATION

We have thus far considered some events associated with synapse formation. However, synapses are also lost from muscle fibers, both during normal maturation and in certain experimental situations.

Normal maturation

The demonstration of the initial polyneuronal innervation of mammalian skeletal muscle (Redfern 1970; Bennett and Pettigrew, 1974a; Bagust et al., 1973) raised the question of how the adult pattern of innervation is established during early maturation. A priori there are two possibilities. Either there might be an initial surplus of motor neurons that degenerate and die leaving behind just the number required to innervate the muscle. Alternatively, there might be an appropriate reduction in the number of terminal branches from a constant number of motor neurons. In the rat soleus muscle the mature pattern of innervation is established within three weeks after birth. Over this period the number of motor neurons innervating the muscle remains constant while the average size of the motor units (a measure of the extent of terminal axonal branching) is reduced by about 80%. Consequently, the elimination of the polyneuronal innervation is fully explained by the reduction in the peripheral field of innervation of the average motor neuron (Brown et al., 1976).

In order to speculate about the mechanism of this process, it is useful to first consider the end result of the maturation, i.e. one motor axon innervating each muscle fiber. This indicates that the elimination is not entirely random and suggests a process of competitive interaction among the group of axons which initially innervate each muscle fiber. If one of the terminals for some reason obtains a competitive advantage, the others could be increasingly handicapped and eventually inactivated. This view has been tested experimentally. By partial denervation of a muscle at birth it is possible to eliminate the majority of the potentially competing motor axons. The prediction was that this should delay the elimination of polyneuronal innervation and permit the remaining motor units to retain their neonatal large size. The outcome of the experiment was only a moderate delay in the elimination of polyneuronal innervation.

The remaining motor units eventually reduced their size almost to the extent that they do in normal muscle (Brown et al., 1976). This reduction in size of motor units in partially denervated muscle took place at the expense of leaving large numbers of muscle fibers without any innervation. These muscle fibers atrophied and eventually disappeared. Since the muscle fibers belonging to a particular motor unit are scattered randomly over the entire cross-section of the muscle, it is clear that many muscle fibers lost their last motor axon (Thompson and Jansen, 1977). Accordingly, a competitive interaction between the motor nerve terminals on a particular muscle fiber cannot fully explain the reduction in motor unit size and the elimination of polyneuronal innervation which takes place during early maturation. It is rather as if most of the reduction in terminal arborization of the motor neurons is due to their inherent properties, or to some external signal which is independent of the state of innervation of the muscle.

There is, however, an alternative explanation of the finding that a large number of muscle fibers atrophy and appear to disapper in the muscles that were partially denervated just after birth. If the extensive polyneuronal innervation of the newborn muscles were required for trophic maintenance of the muscle fibers, then many muscle fibers might die after partial denervation even though they had retained some of their motor innervation. The size of the remaining motor units would then be determined by the number of muscle fibers that happened to survive and not by a limit to the number of muscle fibers that a motor neuron could innervate. This possibility is difficult to exclude rigorously, but it appears unlikely on considering reasonable distributions of remaining end-plates in the partially denervated muscles (Thompson and Jansen, 1977). In muscles with only two axons remaining after denervation, it is likely that some muscle fibers survive even though they are initially left with only a single motor axon. On the other hand, in muscles with 10–15 remaining axons it is likely that some muscle fibers are lost in spite of being polyneuronally innervated initially.

Accepting that the early reduction in motor unit size is at least partly due to an inherent property of the motor neurons, the next question is whether this non-competitive process alone can explain the early postnatal maturation of the pattern of innervation. A non-competitive process would imply that a substantial number of muscle fibers became transiently denervated during the maturation process and then subsequently reinnervated by sprouts from neighboring intact motor axons. Muscles have, therefore, been carefully examined for the presence of an appreciable number of denervated muscle fibers during the relevant period (Brown et al., 1976). By microelectrode recording of synaptic activity, inactive fibers were found only occasionally. The incidence of such fibers was no higher than in fully mature muscle where their occasional occurrence is explained by a shift in the location of the end-plate band. Therefore, in order to explain the establishment of the final pattern of muscle innervation, we have to postulate that a second process involving a competitive interaction between axon terminals also contributes to the maturation, making it possible to keep the muscle innervated continuously, and ensuring that eventually each end-plate is innervated by only a single axon. There is some justification of this suggestion in the demonstration of such competitive interactions in other experimental situations (see later).

A further point to consider is what happens morphologically to the axon terminals that are eliminated during maturation. They could degenerate and disappear, they could be retracted from the end-plates, or they could remain morphologically intact but functionally inactivated. In suitable histological preparations it is possible to demonstrate that each end-plate is supplied by several preterminal axons in newborn animals, whereas there is only one axon to each end-plate in mature muscle (Bennett and Pettigrew, 1974a; Brown et al., 1976). There is even a reasonable agreement between the functional maturation and the time of disappearance of the extra preterminal axons (Riley, 1976). This excludes the possibility of inactivated, morphologically intact terminals. A study of the ultrastructure of the end-plates during the relevant period failed to reveal any signs of degenerating axon terminals. Therefore, it was suggested that the elimination is brought about by retraction of terminal branches from the end-plates and back into the parent axons (Korneliussen and Jansen, 1977).

Elimination of end-plates at separate sites

In the newborn animal all the terminals of the five or so axons which innervate a given muscle fiber are all located within one circumscribed end-plate region (Brown et al., 1976). The diameter of this end-plate region is of the order of one muscle fiber diameter. Accordingly, the various terminals of the immature end-plate are very closely spaced. It is therefore possible that the interaction which leads to elimination is acting only over very small distances, and it is questionable whether end-plates that are spatially separate on a muscle fiber can be eliminated. Our best information in this connection has been obtained by implanting foreign nerves onto the soleus muscle of rats. The foreign nerve innervates the muscle at ectopic sites after section of the original nerve. Initially, many muscle fibers are innervated by several different axons. The individual end-plates are often situated at separate sites on the muscle fibers, as demonstrated both functionally by the existence of separate sites for recording focal end-plate potentials, and histologically by the presence of separate end-plate regions staining for ACh esterase. With time (2−3 weeks) there is a sharp reduction in the frequency of muscle fibers innervated by more than a single foreign axon, and in very young rats there was also a significant reduction in the frequency of closely spaced esterase-stained end-plates on individual muscle fibers (Brown et al., 1976).

In a separate set of experiments two foreign nerves were transplanted to the soleus muscle of young adult rats (Kuffler et al., 1977). The region where each of the two nerves formed their end-plates was largely determined by the site of implantation of the nerves. With the two nerves transplanted to closely neighboring regions, many muscle fibers were initially innervated by both nerves at separate but fairly close sites. At late times after synapse formation, the great majority of the muscle fibers in such muscles were innervated by only one or the other of the two nerves. Presumably, the second input had been inactivated or eliminated. In contrast, if the end-plates of the two nerves were separated by 10 mm or more along the length of the muscle fibers, the frequency of doubly innervated fibers was as high at late as at early times. These observations indicate that end-plates can interact in a way which leads to the inactivation of one of them, even if they are located separately on the muscle fiber. However, there appears to be a limited distance over which this interaction is effective. One of a pair of close (<2 mm) end-plates is inactivated, while distant (>10 mm) end-plates can both survive and remain functional for prolonged periods.

The final question to consider is what happens morphologically to the close end-plates which are eliminated. This was examined in muscles with close transplants at a time when the majority of the muscle fibers were functionally connected only to a single motor axon. In such muscles there were still many muscle fibers with two or more esterase-stained end-plates. These end-plate sites were examined electron microscopically. One of the end-plates on a muscle fiber always contained the normal presynaptic terminal, as well as postsynaptic specializations. Also, the second end-plate showed typical postsynaptic structures, with synaptic clefts, end-plate esterase and the usual end-plate sarcoplasm. A substantial fraction, however, were without presynaptic terminals. In some cases the postsynaptic site was covered with satellite cells. In others there were still preterminal axons surrounded by Schwann cell cytoplasm but no region where the axon came in synaptic contact with the postsynaptic membrane. These 'empty' end-plate sites were interpreted as the remains of synapses which had been functional during the initial period of synapse formation. Subsequently, the presynaptic terminal had been removed as a result of the interaction with the other end-plate on the same fiber (Kuffler et al., 1977). There were never any signs of degenerating axons in this material. This suggests that the elimination of these synapses is also brought about by retraction of the axon terminal, as suggested for the elimination of synapses during early postnatal development.

GENERAL CONSIDERATIONS

The perinatal polyneuronal innervation

It is curious that the extensive hyperinnervation of mammalian skeletal muscle should develop so consistently, only to be completely eliminated over the first two or three weeks after birth. From the point of view of control of muscle contraction it is certainly only a complication, since it increases the average size of the motor units about five-fold, and since the effect of activating a particular motor neuron will depend heavily on which of the others are already active. The significance of the hyperinnervation is probably to be sought in some other context. Perhaps it is useful only to ensure that the target tissue is initially fully innervated during development. This, however, is far from convincing, since motor axons in a partially denervated muscle have a remarkable ability to sprout and seek out any denervated muscle fiber.

The maturation of the pattern of innervation of the muscle is not a simple process. One part of its seems to be due to an inherent tendency of motor neurons to reduce the extent of their terminal arborizations over the relevant period. For instance, it could be that each motor neuron has a limited capacity to support synaptic membrane and, as the terminals at each end-plate are growing, the number that a motor neuron can maintain is reduced. Alternatively, during the initial phase of innervation of muscle the motor neurons could be stimulated by some external signals. This stimulus would fall during early post-natal development to a level which permits the motor neuron to maintain a number of terminals which is just in excess of that required to innervate the muscle fully. This external signal is not produced by the muscle. At least it is independent of the state of innervation of the muscle, as we saw in the case of partially denervated newborn muscles. In these, the number of innervated fibers was determined by the number of remaining motor neurons, not by the degree of denervation of the muscle.

Although our understanding of these mechanisms is at best fragmentary, the phenomenon is of considerable general interest. It is now becoming clear that a comparable early hyperinnervation and subsequent elimination of redundant terminals is also taking place during the initial innervation of the submandibular ganglion (Lichtman, 1977). Similarly, Crepel et al. (1976) have reported that cerebellar Purkinje cells at birth are innervated by several climbing fibers, while the mature pattern is only one climbing fiber to each Purkinje cell. Similarly, there is a substantial loss of synapses on motor neurons in the early post-natal period (Ronnevi and Conradi, 1974). The initial, transient hyperinnervation may turn out to be a regular feature of the developing nervous system. In any case, it will be important to know in which systems it does occur.

Competitive interactions between synapses

As long as the actual mechanism of the process is unknown, the term competition is used in an entirely loose sense. It signifies the eventual inactivation or elimination of one terminal on account of the existence of another. A great deal of interest attaches to this type of process, particularly if the competitive advantage is associated with some sort of functional or adaptive advantage. A notable example is the change in eye dominance of cortical neurons following mononuclear deprivation (Wiesel and Hubel, 1963). In other connections one can imagine this type of process contributing to the precision and specificity of the wiring of the nervous system.

A competitive component appears to be required to explain the final pattern of innervation of skeletal muscles. With the information available, we can restrict the potential mechanisms involved in the competitive interactions between these synapses. The advantageous property is not one which is permanently and uniformly distributed over the entire motor neuron. A potentially important factor such as level of activity is thus excluded. If activity had been an important factor, we would expect the end result of the competition to be one or a few large motor units innervating the muscle, while other less active ones would be eliminated completely. On the contrary, we find that the number of motor units remains constant, and that they all attain approximately the same size. Since one surviving axon terminal is the required end result, some sort of selection of the survivor by the muscle fiber appears to be the simplest explanation. The preferred feature cannot simply be ability to activate the muscle fiber, since this is shared by most or all of the interacting axon terminals.

The best clue to what determines the outcome of the competition is probably obtained by consideration of the distribution of sizes of motor units in the immature muscles. At birth there is a large degree of scatter in motor unit sizes. Some are ten times larger than the smallest, which appear to have already reached their final size. The reduction in size during maturation predominantly affects the large motor units so that the final distribution of sizes is rather narrow. Presumably an extended size is a competitive handicap during maturation. We shall see that this is an attractive possibility also for other examples of competitive interactions.

After partial denervation of a muscle, the remaining axons sprout and innervate the denervated fibers. At a later stage the original axons regenerate and reoccupy some of the lost territory at the expense of their expanded neighbors. This sequence has been examined in several different cases in amphibia (Cass et al., 1973; Haimann et al., 1976; Bennett and Raftos, 1977; Harris et al., 1977). As the original nerve regains its lost territory, the size and efficiency of the foreign synapses are progressively reduced (Yip and Dennis, 1976). Bennett and Raftos (1977) also report that the sprouting axons are appreciably slower than the regenerating original axons in forming end-plates of a certain size and efficiency. They attribute this to a selective preference of muscle fibers for their original innervation. An alternative suggestion is that the competitive disadvantage of the sprouted axons is due to their enlarged field of innervation.

In this type of experiment on axolotls the re-establishment of the expanded territory of the sprouted nerve after a second section of its original nerve is much quicker than was the rate of sprouting into virgin territory. A possible explanation of this is that the sprouted synapses remain in a functionally repressed form after their muscle fibers have been reclaimed by the original nerve (Cass et al., 1973). The second section of the original nerve should then lead to their rapid reactivation. A recent report by Harris et al. (1977) demonstrates special properties of the spontaneous transmitter release of such repressed end-plates. The frequency of release is less than at normal end-plates and it is not activated by increased external potassium or by addition of lanthanum. The interpretation of these experiments presented by the authors rests on the time course of the complicated series of events. A possibility which brings these findings more in line with those discussed previously in this paper is that the 'repressed' end-plates are in fact retracted, or in the process of being retracted. The rapid re-expansion of the axons during the second episode of sprouting could be due to nerve pathways which were laid down during the initial sprouting. In any case morphological observations are required to substantiate claims of functional repression of synapses that remain morphologically intact (Cass et al., 1973).

The possibility of overexpansion representing a competitive disadvantage for sprouted motor neurons is supported by experiments on the peroneus tertius muscle of mice (Brown and Ironton, 1977). After partial denervation the muscle is fully innervated by sprouting of the remaining axons. Nevertheless, upon regeneration the original axons reclaim part of the muscle, while the sprouted axons are retracted. This is interesting as an example of hyperinnervation of fully innervated and active muscle fibers. Both the sprouted and the returning original terminals establish their contact with the muscle fiber at the original end-plate site. Apparently this region retains its receptivity in spite of the activity and the presence of the sprouted terminal. Similar results have been obtained for the rat soleus (Thompson, 1978).

An analogous situation has been described in the reinnervation of rat EDL muscle after nerve section (McArdle, 1975). Many polyinnervated muscle fibers are found shortly after reformation of the synapses. Over the next several weeks the redundant innervation is eliminated. All these synapses are again located at the original end-plate site, and the competitive advantage of the survivors could be related to the extent of their peripheral fields. This example also brings out a curious difference between rat and frog muscle. In the latter there is a three-fold increased frequency in polyneuronal innervation after reinnervation by the original nerve (Rotschenker and McMahan, 1976). All the regenerated synapses are at the original site. In doubly innervated fibers the two axon terminals are running side by side in the same postsynaptic gutter. However, in contrast to the behavior of rat neuromuscular junctions, the experimental hyperinnervation of frog muscle fibers appeared to be stable, and to be maintained for long periods. Such well documented differences between species emphasizes the hazards of generalizations in the description of neuromuscular interactions at this stage.

There are also well documented cases of competitive interaction between end-plates at separate sites on a muscle fiber. In the rat (see above) this appears to be limited to a restricted region, perhaps 3–4 mm, along a muscle fiber. In the frog, Grinnell et al. (1977) have comparable evidence on the transplanted sartorius muscle innervated by two foreign nerves. A spatially restricted process is appealing to explain the regular spacing of normal distributed innervation. If the extent of the process varies in different types of muscle the various patterns of innervation of fast and slow skeletal muscle fibers are readily accounted for.

To end this discussion properly we would like to present a general scheme which would place the extensive amount of experimental observations firmly in a consistent and coherent picture. Unfortunately, this appears to be premature. There are still apparent contradictions in the basic observations. Eventually these will turn out to be due either to differences between species or to differences in experimental conditions. At present, all we can do is to outline a scheme which possibly accounts for most of the established behavior. It really is not much more than an indication of present ways of thinking about the problems.

A parsimonious view is that there is an 'innervation factor' produced by the muscle fibers. The rate of production of the substance is increased in inactive muscle and it is released from the fiber surface or basement membrane in sufficient amounts to activate neighboring motor axons to sprout. By its presence at the surface of the muscle fiber, the substance is responsible for the receptive state of the fiber. Once a synapse is formed the substance is changed locally to a more stable, activity resistant form which remains localized and permits innervation of this region even on active muscle fibers. The maintenance of the presynaptic terminals depends on a steady supply and uptake of the substance. In denervated, inactive fibers the supply is sufficient for the establishment of synapses at closely neighboring sites. With the onset of muscle activity its production is reduced to limiting amounts, thereby representing the basis for the competitive interaction between end-plates. Overexpanded motor neurons require more of the substance and are therefore handicapped in the competition. In the fully active muscle fiber the rate of production of the substance is sufficiently low to explain the refusal of such fibers to be hyperinnervated.

Such a scheme represents little more than a summary of observations which require explanation. Certainly more complicated schemes with more postulated factors are perhaps more likely. Different substances for the function of local and of diffusible factors may well be the case. Diamond et al. (1976) have, for instance, suggested an antagonistic substance from nerves to counteract a trophic substance from the target tissue, to explain sprouting. The existing evidence does not justify a critical discussion of the various possibilities. The only safe conclusion appears to be that the neuromuscular interactions are still a rewarding field of enquiry, and their study may eventually contribute significantly to our understanding of the formation and maintenance of synapses.

REFERENCES

Alnæs,. E., Jansen, J.K.S. and Rudjord, T. (1964) Spontaneous junctional activity of fast and slow parietal muscle fibres of the hagfish, *Acta physiol, scand.*, 60: 240–255.

16

Anderson, M.J. and Cohen, M.W. (1977) Nerve-induced and spontaneous redistribution of acetylcholine receptors on cultured muscle cells, *J. Physiol. (Lond.)*, 268: 757–773.

Anderson, M.J., Cohen, M.W. and Zorychta, E. (1977) Effects of innervation on the distribution of acetylcholine receptors on cultured muscle cells, *J. Physiol. (Lond.)*, 268: 731–756.

Bagust, J., Lewis, D.M. and Westerman, R.A. (1973) Polyneuronal innervation of kitten skeletal muscle, *J. Physiol. (Lond.)*, 229: 241–255.

Bennett, M.R., McLachlan, E.M. and Taylor, R.S. (1973) The formation of synapses in reinnervated mammalian striated muscle, *J. Physiol. (Lond.)*, 233: 481–500.

Bennett, M.R. and Pettigrew, A.G. (1974a) The formation of synapses in striated muscle during development, *J. Physiol. (Lond.)*, 241: 515–545.

Bennett, M.R. and Pettigrew, A.G. (1974b) The formation of synapses in reinnervated and cross-innervated striated muscle during development, *J. Physiol. (Lond.)*, 241: 547–573.

Bennett, M.R. and Raftos, J. (1977) The formation and regression of synapses during the reinnervation of axolotl striated muscle. *J. Physiol. (Lond.)*, 265: 261–295.

Brown, M.C. and Butler, R.G. (1976) Regeneration of afferent fibres to muscle spindles after nerve injury in adult cats, *J. Physiol. (Lond.)*, 260: 253–266.

Brown, M.C. and Ironton, R. (1977a) Motor neurone sprouting by prolonged tetrodotoxin block of nerve action potentials, *Nature (Lond.)*, in press.

Brown, M.C. and Ironton, R. (1977b) Suppression of motor nerve terminal sprouting in partially denervated muscles, *J. Physiol. (Lond.)*, in press.

Brown, M.C. and Ironton, R. (1978) The sprouting capacity of motoneurones in partially denervated mouse muscles, and the effects of subsequent re-innervation, *J. Physiol. (Lond.)*, in press.

Brown, M.C., Jansen, J.K.S. and Van Essen, D. (1976) Polyneuronal innervation of skeletal muscle in new-born rats and its elimination during maturation, *J. Physiol. (Lond.)*, 261: 387–422.

Burke, R.E. and Edgerton, V.R. (1975) Motor unit properties and selective involvement in movement, *Exercise Sport Sci. Rev.*, 3: 31–81.

Cass, D.T., Sutton, T.J. and Mark, R.F. (1973) Competition between nerves for functional connexions with axolotl muscles, *Nature (Lond.)*, 243: 201–203.

Close, R. (1967) Properties of motor units in fast and slow skeletal muscles of the rat, *J. Physiol. (Lond.)*, 193: 45–55.

Cohen, M.W. (1972) The development of neuromuscular connexions in the presence of D-tubocurarine, *Brain Res.*, 41: 457–463.

Crain, S.M. (1976) *Neurophysiologic Studies in Tissue Culture*, Raven Press, New York.

Crepel, F., Mariani, J. and Delhaye-Bouchaud, N. (1976) Evidence for a multiple innervation of Purkinje cells by climbing fibers in the immature rat cerebellum, *J. Neurobiol.*, 7: 567–578.

Diamond, J., Cooper, E., Turner, C. and MacIntyre, L. (1976) Trophic regulation of nerve sprouting, *Science*, 193: 371–377.

Edds, M.V., Jr. (1953) Collateral nerve regeneration, *Quart. Rev. Biol.*, 28: 260–276.

Elsberg, C.A. (1917) Experiments on motor nerve regeneration and the direct neurotization of paralyzed muscles by their own and by foreign nerves, *Science*, 45: 318–320.

Fambrough, D.M. (1976) Specificity of nerve muscle interactions. In *Neuronal Recognition*, S.H. Barondes (Ed.), Plenum Press, New York, pp. 25–67.

Fex, S., Sonesson, B., Thesleff, S. and Zelená, J. (1966) Nerve implants in botulinum poisoned mammalian muscle, *J. Physiol. (Lond.)*, 184: 872–882.

Fex, S. and Thesleff, S. (1967) The time required for innervation of denervated muscle by nerve implants, *Life Sci.*, 6: 635–639.

Fischbach, G.D. and Cohen, S.A. (1973) The distribution of acetylcholine sensitivity over reinnervated and innervated muscle fibers grown in cell culture, *Develop. Biol.*, 31: 147–162.

Frank, E., Gautvik, K. and Sommerschild, H. (1975) Cholinergic receptors at denervated mammalian motor end-plates, *Acta physiol. scand.*, 95: 66–76.

Frank, E., Jansen, J.K.S., Lømo, T. and Westgaard, R.H. (1975) The interaction between foreign and original motor nerves innervating the soleus muscle of rats, *J. Physiol. (Lond.)*, 247: 725–743.

Furshpan, E.J., MacLeish, P.R., O'Lague, P.H. and Potter, D.D. (1976) Chemical transmission between rat sympathetic neurons and cardiac myocytes developing in microcultures: evidence for cholinergic, adrenergic, and dual-function neurons, *Proc. nat. Acad. Sci. (Wash.)*, 73: 4225–4229.

Gordon, T., Perry, R., Tuffery, A.R. and Vrobvá, G. (1974) Possible mechanisms determining synapse formation in developing skeletal muscles of the chick, *Cell Tiss. Res.*, 155: 13–25.

Grimm, L.M. (1971) An evaluation of myotypic respecification in axolotls, *J. exp. Zoöl.*, 178: 479–496.

Grinnell, A.D. Rheuben, M.B. and Letinsky, M.S. (1977) Mutual repression of synaptic efficacy by pairs of foreign nerves innervating frog skeletal muscle, *Nature (Lond.)*, 265: 368–370.

Gutmann, E. and Young, J.Z. (1944) The reinnervation of muscle after various periods of atrophy, *J. Anat. (Lond.)*, 78: 15–43.

Haimann, C., Mallart, A. and Zilber Gachelin (1976) Competition between motor nerves in the establishment of neuromuscular junction in striated muscles of *Xenopus laevis, Neurosci. Lett.*, 3: 15–20.

Hamburger, V. (1970) Embryonic motility in vertebrates. In *The Neurosciences*, F.O. Schmitt (Ed.), Rockefeller Univ. Press, pp. 141–151.

Harris, A.J. (1974) Inductive functions of the nervous system, *Ann. Rev. Physiol.*, 36: 251–305.

Harris, A.J., Ziskind, L. and Wigston, D. (1977) Spontaneous release of transmitter from 'repressed' nerve terminals in axolotl muscle, *Nature (Lond.)*, 268: 265–267.

Hoh, J.F.Y. (1975) Selective and non-selective reinnervation of fast-twitch and slow-twitch rat skeletal muscle, *J. Physiol. (Lond.)*, 251: 791–803.

Jansen, J.K.S., Lømo, T., Nicolaysen, K. and Westgaard, R.H. (1973) Hyperinnervation of skeletal muscle fibers: dependence on muscle activity, *Science*, 181: 559–561.

Jansen, J.K.S. and Van Essen, D.C. (1975) Re-innervation of rat skeletal muscle in the presence of α-bungarotoxin, *J. Physiol. (Lond.)*, 250: 651–667.

Katz, B. and Kuffler, S.W. (1941) Multiple motor innervation of the frog sartorius muscle, *J. Neurophysiol.*, 4: 209–223.

Katz, B. and Miledi, R. (1964) The development of acetylcholine sensitivity in nerve-free segments of skeletal muscle, *J. Physiol. (Lond.)*, 170: 389–396.

Kidokoro, Y., Heinemann, S., Schubert, D., Brandt, B.L. and Klier, F.G. (1976) Synapse formation and neurotrophic effects on muscle cell lines, *Cold Spr. Harb. Symp. quant. Biol.*, 40: 373–388.

Korneliussen, H. and Jansen, J.K.S. (1976) Morphological aspects of the elimination of polyneuronal innervation of skeletal muscle fibres in newborn rats, *J. Neurocytol.*, 5: 591–604.

Kuffler, D., Thompson, W. and Jansen, J.K.S. (1977) The elimination of synapses in multiply-innervated skeletal muscle fibres of the rat: dependence on distance between end-plates, *Brain Res.*, 138: 353–358.

Landis, S.C. (1976) Rat sympathetic neurons and cardiac myocytes developing in microcultures: correlation of the fine structure of endings with neurotransmitter function in single neurons, *Proc. nat. Acad. Sci. (Wash.)*, 73: 4220–4224.

Landmesser, L. (1971) Contractile and electrical responses of vagus-innervated frog sartorius fibres, *J. Physiol. (Lond.)*, 213: 707–725.

Landmesser, L. and Morris, D.G. (1975) The development of functional innervation in the hind limb of chick embryo, *J. Physiol. (Lond.)*, 249: 301–326.

Langley, J.N. and Anderson, H.K. (1904) The union of different kinds of nerve fibres, *J. Physiol. (Lond.)*, 31: 365–391.

Letinsky, M.S., Fischbeck, K.H. and McMahan, U.J. (1976) Precision of reinnervation of original postsynaptic sites in frog muscle after a nerve crush, *J. Neurocytol.*, 5: 691–718.

Lichtman, J. (1977) The reorganization of synaptic connections in the rat submandibular ganglion during postnatal development, *J. Physiol. (Lond.)*, 273: 155–177.

Lømo, T. and Slater, C.R. (1978) Control of acetylcholine sensitivity and synapse formation by muscle activity, *J. Physiol. (Lond.)*, in press.

Lømo, T. and Westgaard, R.H. (1976) Control of ACH sensitivity in rat muscle fibres, *Cold Spr. Harb. Symp. quant. Biol.*, 40: 263–274.

Mark, R.F. (1965) Fin movement after regeneration of neuromuscular connections: an investigation of myotypic specificity, *Exp. Neurol.*, 12: 292–302.

Marshall, L.M., Sanes, J.R. and McMahan, U.J. (1977) Reinnervation of original synaptic sites on muscle fiber basement membrane after disruption of the muscle cells, *Proc. nat. Acad. Sci. (Wash.)*, in press.

McArdle, J.J. (1975) Complex end-plate potentials at regenerating neuromuscular junction of the rat, *Exp. Neurol.*, 49: 629–638.

Pearson, K.G. and Bradley, A.B. (1972) Specific regeneration of excitatory motoneurones to leg muscles in the cockroach, *Brain Res.*, 47: 492–496.

Purves, D. (1976) Long-term regulation in the vertebrate peripheral nervous system, *Int. Rev. Physiol.*, 10: 125–177.

Ramón y Cajal, S. (1959) *Degeneration and Regeneration of the Nervous System*, Hafner Publ., New York.

18

Redfern, P.A. (1970) Neuromuscular transmission in newborn rats, *J. Physiol. (Lond.)*, 209: 701–709.

Riley, D.A. (1976) Multiple axon branches innervating single endplates of kitten soleus myofibres, *Brain Res.*, 110: 158–161.

Ronnevi, L.-O. and Conradi, S. (1974) Ultrastructural evidence for spontaneous elimination of synaptic terminals on spinal motoneurons in the kitten, *Brain Res.*, 80: 335–339.

Rotshenker, S. and McMahan, U.J. (1976) Altered patterns of innervation in frog muscle after denervation, *J. Neurocytol.*, 5: 719–730.

Schmidt, H. and Stefani, E. (1976) Re-innervation of twitch and slow muscle fibres of the frog after crushing the motor nerves, *J. Physiol. (Lond.)*, 258: 99–123.

Sperry, R.W. and Arora, H.L. (1965) Selectivity in regeneration of the oculomotor nerve on the cichlid fish, *Astronotus ocellotus. J. Embryol. exp. Morph.*, 14: 307–317.

Sytkowski, A.J., Vogel, Z. and Nirenberg, M.W. (1973) Development of acetylcholine receptor clusters on cultured muscle cells, *Proc. nat. Acad. Sci. (Wash.)*, 70: 270–274.

Thompson, W. (1978) Reinnervation of partially denervated rat soleus muscle, *Acta physiol. scand.*, in press.

Thompson, W. and Jansen, J.K.S. (1977) The extent of sprouting of remaining motor units in partly denervated immature and mature rat soleus muscle, *Neuroscience*, 2: 523–536.

Van Essen, D.C. and Jansen, J.K.S. (1977) The specificity of re-innervation by identified sensory and motor neurons in the leech, *J. comp. Neurol.*, 171: 433–454.

Weiss, P. and Hoag, A. (1946) Competitive reinnervation of rat muscles by their own and foreign nerves, *J. Neurophysiol.*, 9: 413–418.

Wiesel, T.N. and Hubel, D.H. (1963) Effects of visual deprivation on morphology and physiology of cells in the cat's lateral geniculate body, *J. Neurophysiol.*, 26: 978–993.

Yip, J.W. and Dennis, M.J. (1976) Suppression of transmission of foreign synapses in adult newt muscles involves reduction in quantal content, *Nature (Lond.)*, 260: 350–352.

Young, D. (1972) Specific re-innervation of limbs transplanted in the cockroach, *J. exp. Biol.*, 57: 305–316.

DISCUSSION

ZIMMER: Is there any preference where an end-plate will normally be formed along a muscle fiber? Is it on the distal part or is it in the middle of the fiber? And when you implant two nerves and find that one is suppressed, is the non-suppressed nerve the one that finds its way to where an end-plate would have normally formed?

JANSEN: In normal mammalian skeletal muscle the end-plates are usually located in the middle of the muscle fibers. In many cases this original end-plate site is preferentially innervated by the regenerating motor axons, for instance after nerve section. In our experiments on the soleus muscle of rat, the foreign nerves make their end-plates on virgin regions of the muscle fibers, outside the original end-plate zone. Just where these ectopic end-plates are formed is largely determined by the site of implantation of the foreign nerve. With two foreign nerves implanted we find that the connection from one or the other can become functionally suppressed with time. In the individual case we cannot tell which of the two axons will lose in the competition, but we do know that both the suppressed end-plate and the surviving end-plate are ectopically located, i.e. outside the original end-plate region.

CHANGEUX: I wonder if you could make an extract of your nerve-muscle preparation where you know a competition is going on between two terminal fields, and induce a loss of innervation in a preparation where you have only one nerve-muscle, in order to study the nature of the competition?

JANSEN: We have tried a simple version of it. To see whether we could influence the time-course of the elimination of synapses in newborn animals we have in some cases denervated all the other muscles of the lower leg, except the soleus. In other cases we have transplanted a second soleus muscle alongside our intact experimental muscle. In neither case did we find an appreciable effect on the time-course of elimination of the extra-innervation.

PARNAVELAS: I did not quite catch what was the evidence that this multiple innervation is not due to branching of the same axon. Also, the reduction of fibers which you observed: does this occur progressively or all of a sudden, i.e. within a few days do you observe a loss of all the extra-fibers? Do you think, by the way, that there is any adaptive value in this loss of nerve fibers?

JANSEN: The reduction in innervation occurs from the time the animal is born, continuously over the first two or three weeks. How do we know that all the innervation we see is not due to branches of the same axons? If this were so, then a cross-section of the nerve distal to the point of stimulation should contain 5 times as many fibers as it does proximal to the site of branching. This is not the case. Furthermore, we can follow the nerve all the way to the ventral root, to where it emerges from the spinal cord, and then stimulate at that point. If we do this we still get the same pattern of innervation of the muscle. As regards the possible adaptive value of the early hyperinnervation, unfortunately we do not have any appealing views on this question

DE GROOT: Did you rely on electrophysiological measurements? How is the myelination in those immature motor nerves in the newborn animal? For I can imagine that, when you increase your stimulus, you will get cross-talk between the different axons *in* the nerve terminal. That means you will get a larger average size of the motor units, not because they are innervated by more axons but simply because the isolating effect of the myelin is not present at that time. I am not sure about the peripheral nervous system, but centrally the myelination occurs only much later.

JANSEN: There are certainly complications in the type of experiment where you stimulate a group of nerve fibers electrically. In nerve-muscle preparations one can sometimes see cross-talk such as the so-called 'back response'. This is due to ephaptic activation of axons by the electrical activity in the muscle. It can be seen, for instance, as an antidromic signal in non-stimulated axons. There is no evidence that this takes place in the neonatal muscles, however. The myelination of the nerves occurs during the first week. At birth there is very little myelin in the motor nerves, but it is quite well developed after a week. The polyneuronal innervation lasts for at least another week.

Neurotransmission and Specificity of Innervation in Mixed Culture of Embryonic Ciliary Ganglia and Skeletal Muscle Cells

WILLEM F. STEVENS, DIRK W. SLAAF*, JACOB HOOISMA, TOM MAGCHIELSE and E. MEETER

Medical Biological Laboratory TNO, Rijswijk, (The Netherlands)

INTRODUCTION

Tissue culture was introduced into electrophysiology about 20 years ago when Crain (1954), in cooperation with Peterson and Murray, recorded from spinal ganglia and, much later, from small fragments of cerebral cortex and spinal cord in culture (see Crain, 1976). Shortly thereafter, together with Corner (1965), he carried out an investigation of the development of bioelectric phenomena in 'presumptive neuromuscular frog tissues'. Since that time, the formation of the neuromuscular junction has been studied extensively in various combinations of mammalian tissues, which have demonstrated that in tissue culture: (1) neuromuscular junctions are formed if embryonic spinal cord and skeletal muscle tissue are brought together; (2) the formation of such neuromuscular junctions is not prevented by a block of electrical events in the junctions due to the presence of D-tubocurarine or Xylocaine; (3) spinal cord explants exert a neurotrophic influence on the morphology of surrounding muscle cells; and (4) functional neuromuscular junctions can be formed between cells from different mammalian species and between mammalian and avian cells.

The study of the formation and the maintenance of the neuromuscular junction at the monocellular level became possible by the work of Fischbach (1970, 1972), who demonstrated that individual spinal cord cells obtained by dissociation of embryonic chick spinal cord were able to form functional junctions with chick muscle fibers in culture. It was shown that electrical stimulation of individual spinal cord cells in such mixed cultures evoked end-plate potentials (e.p.p.'s) in innervated muscle fibers (for a comprehensive review, see Nelson, 1975).

In this paper experiments will be discussed in which synapse formation and neurotransmission have been studied in tissue culture, using the ciliary ganglion of the chick embryo as a source of neurons. This ganglion was chosen because it contains only two types of cholinergic neurons (Marwitt et al., 1971), which in vivo form nicotinic neuromuscular junctions with the sphincter iridis and with the ciliary body of the chick, both composed of striated muscle fibers. In mixed cultures of ciliary ganglion plus skeletal muscle cells, functional nicotinic neuromuscular junctions are formed (Hooisma et al., 1975; Betz, 1976). Finally, some recent findings on the specificity of innervation by ciliary ganglia of mammalian and avian origin will be described.

---

* Present address: Biophysics Department, State University of Limburg, Maastricht, The Netherlands.

INNERVATION BY THE CILIARY GANGLION

Embryonic chick muscle cells and ciliary ganglia were co-cultivated in a modified Eagle's minimum essential medium with horse serum (15%) and freshly prepared chick embryo extract (5%) (Slaaf, 1977). Fusion of myoblasts was observed within one day after plating of the cells, and long multinucleated muscle fibers with cross striation over their entire surface had developed after four days. These fibers contracted spontaneously as well as after electrical stimulation. Ciliary ganglia were allowed to settle on muscle cells that usually had been in culture for 2–6 days. The growth of processes from the ganglion started within a few hours and after one day a corona of neurites surrounded the ganglion. Although the neurites usually ran parallel with the myotubes, many of them were found coursing across, or on top of, the muscle fibers, and often seemed to end upon them (Fig. 1).

Intracellular recording from muscle fibers situated in the vicinity of the ganglion revealed that about 90% of the visibly innervated myotubes were also innervated functionally. End-plate potentials having amplitudes of up to 20 mV could be recorded from these tubes (Fig. 2), the functional innervation being established within 24 hr after introduction of the ganglia (Hooisma et al., 1975). This has been confirmed by Fischbach (personal communication), and by Obata and Tanaka (1977) who found that e.p.p.'s are generated as soon as the growing tip of the neurite reaches a myotube. End-plate potentials could also be elicited by extracellular stimulation of a neurite which runs from a ciliary ganglion to a muscle fiber. Repeated stimulation of such a neurite with graded stimuli evoked e.p.p.'s in an all-or-none pattern (Fig. 3). By extracellular stimulation of several neurites which ended on the same myotube, it could be demonstrated that myotubes in the vicinity of the ganglion were often multiply innervated (Slaaf, 1977). This explains why e.p.p.'s of similar amplitudes in the same fiber often differ so much in their time course (Fig. 2). End-plate potentials could also be evoked by stimulation of the cholinoceptive neurons in the ganglion by microionto-phoretic application of acetylcholine (ACh) on the ganglion. Pulses of ACh on the ganglion caused contractions of one or a few muscle fibers in the vicinity of the ganglion, from which e.p.p.'s could be recorded during and shortly after the ACh pulse. The generation of these evoked potentials was reversibly abolished by blocking nerve impulse conduction with tetrodotoxin (TTX). The generation of e.p.p.'s could be blocked by D-tubocurarine (0.1–1 μg/ml) and, at a much higher concentration (100 μg/ml), also by atropine.

Taken together, these data show that in mixed cultures of the ciliary ganglion and skeletal muscle cells, stimulation of the neurons within the ganglion gives rise to action potentials which are conducted through the neurite, and which stimulate the nerve endings to release ACh. The interaction of the neurotransmitter with the postsynaptic receptor leads to the generation of e.p.p.'s and to contractions in many of the muscle fibers. Apparently functional motor innervation develops in the mixed culture of ciliary ganglion and muscle cells. The electrophysiological and pharmacological properties of this preparation are such as to justify its use as a model system for the study of innervation and of long term interactions in the neuromuscular system.

NEUROMUSCULAR TRANSMISSION IN TISSUE CULTURE

An important question to be answered in the study of the neuromuscular transmission in tissue culture is whether spontaneous e.p.p.'s are generated by spontaneous release of transmitter at the neuromuscular junction, or are due to action potentials which are generated

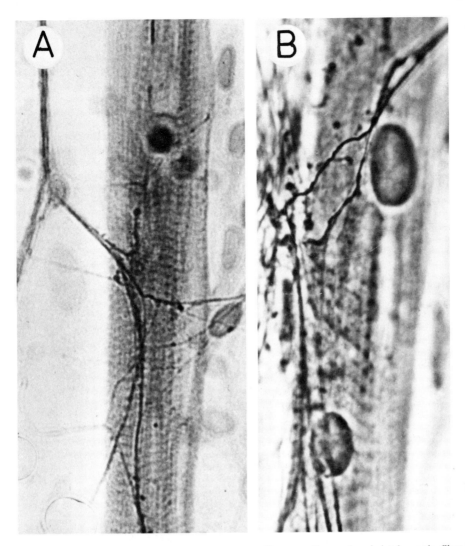

Fig. 1. Neuromuscular connections formed between a ciliary ganglion and a skeletal muscle fiber in culture. A: innervated cross-striated myotube. Neurites coming from the ciliary ganglion seem to make small beads where they contact a myotube. Ciliary ganglion and muscle cells 1 and 6 days in vitro, respectively. B: innervated myotube with cross-striations and nuclei. In the central part, neurites coming from upper right show varicosities where they contact the myotube. Same preparation as in A. A and B: Bielschowsky silver impregnation, phase contrast lens 40 × and 100 × oil, respectively. Total magnification A, 600 ×; B, 1200 ×.

spontaneously in the perikaryon and conducted to the nerve terminal (Robbins and Yonezawa, 1971; Fischbach, 1970, 1972; Hooisma et al., 1975; Obata, 1977). These alternatives can be distinguished by studying the effect of a blockade of impulse conduction by TTX on the generation of the e.p.p.'s .

Fischbach (1972) and Hooisma et al. (1977) observed in their preparation of *spinal cord* neurons and skeletal muscle cells that only small potentials were generated in the presence of TTX, probably being miniature end-plate potentials (m.e.p.p.'s). Consequently, the larger amplitude potentials which were observed in the absence of TTX must have been evoked

24

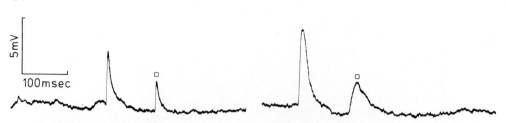

Fig. 2. Spontaneous end-plate potentials. The traces represent the membrane resting potential and show various spontaneous end-plate potentials occurring in the same cell. End-plate potentials of approximately the same amplitude, □, differ markedly in time course.

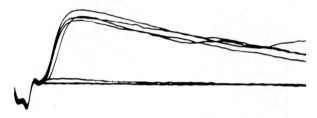

Fig. 3. Extracellular stimulation. Traces recorded from a muscle fiber after extracellular stimulation of a ciliary ganglion neurite which contacted the fiber. Graded stimulus intensity changes resulted in abrupt potential transient changes. Ciliary ganglion and muscle cell 2 and 5 days in vitro, respectively. $V_m = -75$ mV.

by action potentials originating from the neuronal perikaryon. However, a report on the formation of functional neuromuscular junctions between the *ciliary ganglion* and skeletal muscle fibers in tissue culture (Slaaf, 1977) describes large e.p.p.'s which persist in the presence of TTX. Only in a few of his experiments (Table I) did Slaaf observe an obvious elimination of large e.p.p.'s after blocking nerve impulse conduction with TTX (as in the experiment of Fig. 4). This indicates that in most of these young synapses the generation of e.p.p.'s was not controlled by axonal activity of the neurons, but rather occurred spontaneously at the terminals. Our present data suggest that in older cultures of ciliary ganglion and muscle, the perikaryon starts to play a more important role, but additional experiments are required to establish this point.

An elevated Mg^{2+}/Ca^{2+} ratio in the bath fluid reduces the quantum content of the e.p.p. and thus its amplitude, but leaves the size of the quantum essentially unaffected. Under these circumstances, the m.e.p.p. amplitude decreases only slightly, due to a reduction in post-synaptic sensitivity. Although the quantum content of the e.p.p.'s could not be measured in the cultured innervated muscle fibers, because of multiplicity of the innervation, it could be demonstrated that a 40-fold increase of the Mg^{2+}/Ca^{2+} ratio in the bath caused a two-fold reduction in the amplitude of the TTX-resistant e.p.p.'s (Table II). This reduction of TTX-resistant spontaneous e.p.p.'s to a raised ionic ratio is exemplified in Fig. 4. The change (by a factor of 2) could be a consequence of the same phenomenon which causes the slight change in amplitude of the m.e.p.p.'s in vivo. Alternatively, it could be due to a multi-quantal nature of the TTX-resistant spontaneous e.p.p.'s. Spontaneous release of ACh in multi-quantal amounts by the nerve terminals might, in fact, be a special feature of the ciliary neuron, since Pilar (1969) and Pilar and Vaughan (1969) observed TTX-resistant large e.p.p.'s in their isolated iris nerve-muscle preparations from the adult pigeon.

TABLE I

EFFECT OF TETRODOTOXIN ON THE GENERATION OF SPONTANEOUS END-PLATE POTENTIALS IN CHICK MUSCLE FIBERS INNERVATED BY CHICK CILIARY GANGLION, CULTURED TOGETHER FOR VARIOUS NUMBERS OF DAYS

Days in vitro		Effect of tetrodotoxin (1 µg/ml)		
Ciliary ganglion	Muscle cells*	Effect	$\dfrac{Frequency_{TTX}}{Frequency_{control}}$	Maximum amplitude [§] of end-plate potential in presence of TTX (mV)
1	6	−	1	10
1	6	−	1	7
2	5	−	1	8
2	4	+	1	$15 \rightarrow 7$
2	6	−	1	8
2	5	−	1	10
2	5	−	1	11
3	4	+	1/4	$16 \rightarrow 6$
4	4	−	1	6
5	4	+	1/2	$7 \rightarrow 4$
6	3	+	1	$16 \rightarrow 4$
9	3	+	1/3	$10 \rightarrow 3$
9	2	−	1	10

* At the time of explantation of the ciliary ganglion. + = effect of TTX on either the maximum amplitude or the frequency of the end-plate potentials. − = no effect.
[§] One figure indicates no effect of TTX, if two figures are given they refer to maximum amplitude before and during TTX treatment, respectively.

SPECIFICITY OF INNERVATION IN TISSUE CULTURE

The method of tissue culture offers the opportunity of cultivating muscle cells together with neurons that originate from different regions of the nervous system, or which differ in neuropharmacological properties. Data from the former type of experiments have been reported by Obata (1977), who could find no specificity of innervation in mixed cultures of pectoral or thigh muscle fibers together with spinal cord neurons taken from either the cervical, brachial or lumbar level. It is known, however, that not all types of neurons are able to form functional junctions with other cells in culture. Dorsal root ganglion cells and neurons in cortex explants, for instance, visibly contact cultured muscle cells but make no functional synapses (Fischbach et al., 1973; Obata and Tanaka, 1977; Hooisma, 1977). Moreover, a remarkable degree of regional specificity has been observed in mixed cultures of dorsal root ganglia together with various neural explants. Thus, neurites of the dorsal root ganglion form synaptic connections preferentially with neurons in the dorsal horn region of the spinal cord, and also with the dorsal column nuclei of the medulla (Crain and Peterson, 1975; Peterson and Crain, 1975).

In our study of the specificity of innervation, two questions have been posed: (1) are neurons which in vivo form exclusively muscarinic neuromuscular junctions with *smooth* muscle cells able to synapse at all with *striated* muscle fibers in culture; and (2) if they do, what type of ACh receptor is involved. The mammalian ciliary ganglion, like that in birds, is a parasympathetic ganglion in the nervous pathway from the Edinger-Westphal nucleus to

26

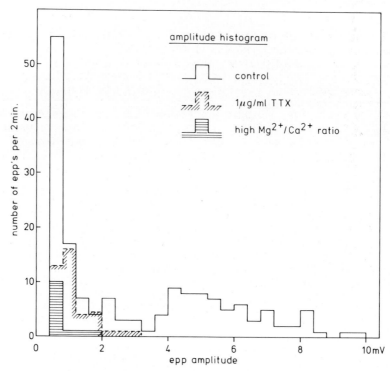

Fig. 4. The effects of tetrodotoxin (TTX) and of a change in the ratio of the Mg^{2+} and Ca^{2+} concentrations on the amplitude of the spontaneous end-plate potentials in a muscle cell innervated by a ciliary ganglion. The figure shows a histogram of the control situation, in which distinct peaks can be seen for neurally evoked end-plate potentials (>3 mV) and spontaneous end-plate potentials (<3 mV). In the presence of TTX, the neurally evoked end-plate potentials have disappeared. A high Mg^{2+}/Ca^{2+} ratio in the perfusion fluid (see legend Table II) affects the amplitude distribution of the spontaneous end-plate potentials. Ciliary ganglion and muscle cells 9 and 12 days in vitro, respectively. $V_m = -70$ mV.

TABLE II

COMPARISON OF THE EFFECTS OF TETRODOTOXIN AND HIGH Mg^{2+}/Ca^{2+} ON THE GENERATION OF SPONTANEOUS END-PLATE POTENTIALS

Chick muscle cells cultivated for 4–6 days, and subsequently grown together with the ciliary ganglion for another 2–9 days.

Maximum amplitude in control situation (mV)	Maximum amplitude in presence of TTX (1 μg/ml) (mV)	Maximum amplitude in Mg^{2+}/Ca^{2+} * (mV)
8	8	4
10	3	1.8
6	6	4
7	4	1.6

* The Mg^{2+}/Ca^{2+} ratio was raised by a factor of 40, the final concentrations were 4.9 mM Mg^{2+} and 0.45 mM Ca^{2+}.

the muscle fibers of the sphincter iridis and the ciliary body (Kerr, 1973). In mammals this ganglion forms exclusively muscarinic cholinergic junctions with these muscles (Westheimer, 1974). The present results showed that functional neuromuscular junctions were formed in mixed cultures of ciliary ganglia of the newborn rabbit with chick skeletal muscle cells. The original predestination to innervate smooth muscle thus did not prevent these neurons from innervating striated muscle cells. Moreover, the sensitivities of these junctions to D-tubo-curarine and atropine are similar to those of the normal (nicotinic) junctions formed between the *chick* ciliary ganglion and skeletal muscle fibers. Neurotransmission was 100-times more sensitive to blockage by D-tubocurarine than by atropine. The pharmacological properties of the ACh receptors in these junctions is apparently dictated by the muscle and not by the neuron.

Landmesser (1972) observed that vagus neurons are able to form functional neuro-muscular junctions in vivo with denervated diaphragm. Patterson and Chun (1977) demonstrated that sympathetic neurons can be raised to become either noradrenergic or cholinergic, depending on the culture conditions; they can even be induced to make use of more than one transmitter at their myoneuronal connections (Furshpan et al. 1976). More-over, the micro-environment determines whether autonomic neuroblasts from the neural crest will differentiate to become either adrenergic or cholinergic cells (Le Douarin et al., 1975). The fact that dorsal root ganglion neurons and those from embryonic cerebral cortex never develop functional end-plates with muscle fibers suggests that perhaps only autonomic neurons possess this plasticity. Another possibility is that all neurons have the same plasticity, but only during well-defined periods in their embryonic development, which do not coincide in various types of neurons. Whatever the case may be, until more is known about these mechanisms it is unjustified to assume that a neurotransmitter (or a type of junction normally used by a neuron in vivo) will also be used if the neuron is confronted with another target or micro-environment in experimental specificity studies.

Specific neuromuscular junctions may be the result of an initial random and profuse synaptogenesis, followed by selective degradation of superfluous synapses by some com-petition mechanism (see Changeux and Mikoshiba and Jansen et al., this volume). Perhaps the amount of bioelectric activity plays a decisive role in this competition between synapses. It would be most interesting to study the specificity of innervation by neurons in tissue culture when their long-term electrical activity is manipulated at will, and competition thus controlled experimentally!

SUMMARY

(1) In tissue culture, the chick ciliary ganglion forms functional junctions with skeletal muscle cells within 24 hours.

(2) Stimulation of neurons in the ganglion leads to the generation of end-plate potentials in the muscle fibers they innervate and to contractions of these fibers.

(3) The neuromuscular junctions are of the *nicotinic* type, i.e., they are much more sensitive to D-tubocurarine than to atropine.

(4) The results suggest that most of the spontaneously occurring end-plate potentials are not under control of the perikaryon, but are generated locally at the neuromuscular junction.

(5) Reduction of the amplitude of these end-plate potentials by an increase of the Mg^{2+}/Ca^{2+} ratio in the bath suggests that some of these potentials are multi-quantal in nature.

(6) Rabbit ciliary ganglion neurons which form *muscarinic* neuromuscular junctions with smooth muscle in vivo form functional *nicotinic* junctions with skeletal muscle fibers in culture.

28

ACKNOWLEDGEMENTS

The very stimulating discussions with Drs. D. de Wied and T.D. Kernell are gratefully acknowledged. Our thanks are due to Mrs M. Remmelts, Richard van Ruler and André Beijersbergen van Henegouwen for excellent technical assistance. This work was supported in part by the Foundation Promeso, by the Jan Dekker Foundation and the Dr. Ludgardine Bouwman Foundation.

REFERENCES

Betz, W. (1976) The formation of synapses between chick embryo skeletal muscle and ciliary ganglia grown in vitro, *J. Physiol. (Lond.)*, 254: 63–73.

Corner, M.A. and Crain, S.M. (1965) Spontaneous contractions and bioelectric activity after differentiation in culture of presumptive neuromuscular tissues of the early frog, *Experientia (Basel)*, 21: 422–424.

Crain, S.M. (1954) Action potentials in tissue cultures of chick embryo spinal ganglia, *Anat. Rec.*, 118: 292.

Crain, S.M. (1976) *Neurophysiologic Studies in Tissue Culture*, Raven Press, New York.

Crain, S.M. and Peterson, E.R. (1975) Development of specific sensory-evoked synaptic networks in fetal mouse cord-brainstem cultures, *Science*, 188: 275–278.

Douarin, N.M. le, Renaud, D., Teillet, M.A. and Douarin, G.H. le (1975) Cholinergic differentiation of presumptive adrenergic neuroblasts in interspecific chimeras after heterotopic transplantations, *Proc. nat. Acad. Sci. (Wash.)*, 72: 728–732.

Fischbach, G.D. (1970) Synaptic potentials recorded in cell cultures of nerve and muscle, *Science*, 169: 1331–1333.

Fischbach, G.D. (1972) Synapse formation between dissociated nerve and muscle cells in low density cultures, *Develop. Biol.*, 28: 407–429.

Fischbach, G.D., Fambrough, D. and Nelson, P.G. (1973) A discussion of neuron and muscle cell cultures, *Fed. Proc.*, 32: 1636–1642.

Furshpan, E.J., MacLeish, P.R., O'Lague, P.H. and Potter, D.D. (1976) Chemical transmission between rat sympathetic neurons and cardiac myocytes developing in microcultures: evidence for cholinergic, adrenergic and dual-function neurons, *Proc. nat. Acad. Sci. (Wash.)*, 73: 4225–4229.

Hooisma, J., Slaaf, D.W., Meeter, E. and Stevens, W.F. (1975) The innervation of chick striated muscle fibres by the chick ciliary ganglion in tissue culture, *Brain Res.*, 85: 79–85.

Hooisma, J., Slaaf, D.W., Meeter, E. and Stevens, W.F. (1977) Some electrophysiological properties of synapses formed between mouse spinal cord and chick muscle fibers in tissue culture, *Arzneimittelforsch.*, 27: 454–455.

Hooisma, J. (1977) *Innervation and Trophic Support of Muscle Cells in Tissue Culture*, Doctoral dissertation, State University of Utrecht.

Kerr, A.W.S. (1973) The head and neck. In *A Companion to Medical Studies*, P. Passmore and J.S. Robson (Eds.), Oxford Univ. Press, ch. 21.

Landmesser, L. (1972) Pharmacological properties, cholinesterase activity and anatomy of nerve-muscle junctions in vagus-innervated frog sartorius, *J. Physiol. (Lond.)*, 220: 243–256.

Marwitt, R., Pilar, G., and Weakly, J.N. (1971) Characterization of two ganglion cell populations in avian ciliary ganglia, *Brain Res.*, 25: 317–334.

Nelson, P.G. (1975) Nerve and muscle cells in culture, *Physiol. Rev.*, 55: 1–61.

Obata, K. (1977) Development of neuromuscular transmission in culture with a variety of neurons and in the presence of cholinergic substances and tetrodotoxin, *Brain Res.*, 119: 141–153.

Obata, K. and Tanaka, H. (1977) Contact and transmission between nerve and muscle in culture. In *Proc. Int. Congr. Physiol. Sci., Vol. 13*, Paris, p. 558.

Patterson, P.H. and Chun, L.L.Y. (1977) The induction of acetylcholine synthesis in primary cultures of dissociated rat sympathetic neurons. I. Effects of conditioned medium. *Develop. Biol.*, 56: 263–280.

Peterson, E.R. and Crain, S.M. (1975) Selective growth of neurites from isolated fetal mouse dorsal root ganglia toward specific CNS target tissues. In *Soc. Neurosci. 5th Annu. Meet.*, New York, p. 783.

Pilar, G. (1969) Effect of tetrodotoxin on spontaneous potentials at pigeon iris neuromuscular junctions, *Europ. J. Pharmacol.*, 6: 129–137.

Pilar, G. and Vaughan, P.C. (1969) Electrophysiological investigations of the pigeon iris neuromuscular junctions, *Comp. Biochem. Physiol.*, 29: 51–72.

Robbins, N. and Yonezawa, T. (1971) Physiological studies during formation and development of rat neuromuscular junctions in tissue culture, *J. gen. Physiol.*, 58: 467–481.

Slaaf, D.W. (1977) *Electrophysiological Characterization of Striated Muscle Cells Innervated by Ciliary Neurons in Tissue Culture*, Doctoral dissertation, State University of Utrecht.

Westheimer, G. (1974) The eye. In *Medical Physiology*, V.B. Mountcastle (Ed.), Mosby, St. Louis, pp. 440–457.

Neurotrophic Influences in Tissue Culture

WILLEM F. STEVENS, JACOB HOOISMA, DIRK W. SLAAF* and E. MEETER

Medical Biological Laboratory TNO, Rijswijk (The Netherlands)

INTRODUCTION

The development and survival of cultured muscle cells can be enhanced either by co-cultivation with spinal cord tissue or by addition of extracts of nervous tissue to the culture medium (Crain and Peterson, 1974; Paul and Powell, 1974; Engelhardt et al., 1976; Oh et al., 1972; Oh, 1975, 1976). The mechanism of this supportive or 'neurotrophic' influence is still under debate (Drachman, 1976). Either the neurally evoked muscle activity, the release of the transmitter acetylcholine (ACh) or the influence of an as yet unidentified trophic substance are held responsible. The tissue culture technique has great advantages for a comparative investigation of the trophic effects of neural material on muscle fibers since various types of tissue can be combined at will. The lack of a quantitative method for the estimation of trophic effects on morphology, however, has severely limited its usefulness thus far. The present paper presents preliminary data obtained with a method which allows scoring of the 'quality' of the morphology of muscle fibers, under the influence of tissue extracts or neural explants.

TROPHIC EFFECT OF TISSUE EXTRACTS

Recently Hooisma (1977) introduced a semi-quantitative estimation of the morphological quality of muscle cells grown in culture. The method is based on an evaluation of four morphological properties of muscle fibers in a culture dish: the number of fibers, the quality of their cross-striation, their thickness and the absence of vacuoles. Each of these properties was rated on a scale from 0 to 4, with 4 indicating an optimal result (Table I). With this method, the effect of embryo extract was studied on muscle cells that had been cultured for two days in tissue culture medium containing embryo extract, and subsequently grown either in the absence or in the continued presence of extract.

In cultures of chick muscle cells cultivated for 5 days in the absence of embryo extract, flat vacuolized multi-nuclear cells with no, or only faint, cross-striations were observed. Conversely, in media containing embryo extract, many thick cross-striated fibers developed within 5 days (Fig. 1). The results of the semi-quantitative evaluation of the morphology during 27 days is shown in Figs. 2 and 3. For all 4 parameters, the extract-treated cultures were

---

* Present address: Biophysics Department, State University of Limburg, Maastricht, The Netherlands.

TABLE I

CRITERIA FOR SCORING THE MORPHOLOGICAL PROPERTIES OF MUSCLE FIBERS

Score	Cross-striation	Score	Thickness
0	no striation	0	fibers thin like fibroblasts
1	a few fibers faintly striated	1	a few fibers are clearly thicker
2	more fibers, more clearly striated	2	no fibroblast-like fibers
3	good striation in many fibers	3	some fibers with pronounced phase boundaries
4	most fibers show good striation	4	many fibers with marked phase boundaries

Score	Number of vacuoles	Score	Total number of fibers
0	no fibers without vacuoles	0	hardly any fibers present
1	a few without vacuoles	1	18–20 fibers per mm^2
2	about 50% of the fibers with vacuoles	2	better than '1' but no full culture
3	fibers with vacuoles easy to find	3	a full culture
4	fibers with vacuoles rare	4	fibers densely packed

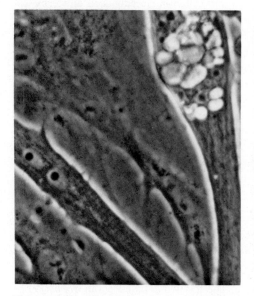 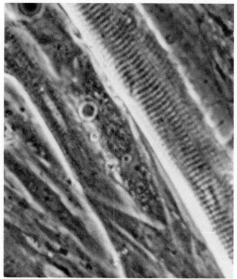

Fig. 1. Muscle cells obtained by trypsin dissociation of leg muscles from 11-day-old chick embyro, cultured for 5 days in a modified Eagle's minimum essential medium, with 15% horse serum in the absence (left) and in the presence (right) of 5% freshly prepared embryo extract.

scored significantly higher than the controls. For most parameters this difference increased as time went on, as a result of gradual deterioration of the control cultures. When extracts from different parts of the embryo were compared, it appeared (Table II) that extracts from head plus spinal cord ('brain extract') as well as extracts from the remainder of the body ('body extract') were both active, whereas liver extracts had no effect.

Few data are presently available regarding the properties of the active factor in brain or body extracts. The activity of the factor is only slightly reduced by heating at 70 °C (30 min), and gel filtration studies suggest a molecular weight between 20,000 and 60,000 daltons. Oh (1975, 1976) isolated a trophic factor from chick brain which was absent in decapitated chick embryos. This factor accelerated the synthesis of acetylcholinesterase, concomitant

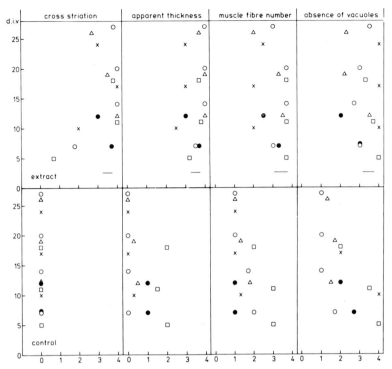

Fig. 2. The effect of chick embryo extract on the morphology of chick muscle fibers in culture. Abscissa: mean score of the 4 morphological parameters. Ordinate: days in vitro (d.i.v.). Top: morphological properties of muscle fibers in experimental cultures in medium containing embryo extract. Bottom: morphological properties of muscle fibers in control cultures, i.e. in medium without embryo extract from the second day of cultivation onwards. Symbols: ○, ●, □ and △, mean of three cultures; ✕, mean of 2 cultures. Bar = 2 ✕ S.E.M.

TABLE II

EFFECT OF EXTRACTS OF VARIOUS EMBRYONIC TISSUES ON CULTURED MUSCLE CELLS

Each number in the table represents the mean score of 4–6 muscle cell cultures for a morphological property. These values represent the differences between mean scores for the extract treated cultures and the corresponding controls. Muscle cell culture medium supplemented with 5% extract, prepared from various embryonic tissues.

Extract	Protein (mg/ml)	Cross-striation	Thickness	Number of muscle fibers	Absence of vacuoles
Brain extract	3.8	2.5*	1.3*	0.1	0.3
Body extract	4.3	2.8*	1.7*	0.4	0.1
Liver extract	5.3	0.3	0.5	0.3	0.3

* Significant at at least $P_2 < 0.05$.

with the appearance of cross-striations in cultured muscle cells. Moreover, there was a prolongation of muscle fiber survival in vitro from two weeks (control) to eight weeks. The factor has a molecular weight of 3×10^5 daltons, and is destroyed at 60 °C (30 min). Extracts of adult motor axons had similar long-term effects. This factor, and the one to be described in the present report, do not seem to be identical, but further purification of the active components is required to establish this point.

TROPHIC INFLUENCE OF NEURAL EXPLANTS

When spinal cord slices were explanted on top of chick muscle cells cultured in medium containing embryo extract, no trophic influence of the explants was observed. If, however, the supply of embryo extract was discontinued after two days, i.e. at the time when the neural tissue was explanted, those fibers lying in a zone concentric with an explant thrived as if extract was still present, while more distant fibers deteriorated rapidly. Clearly, embryo extract by its own trophic influence masks the trophic action of an explant. Following these observations, it became our standard practice to allow the muscle cells to proliferate and fuse for two days in the presence of embyro extract, and then to discontinue the supply of extract when neural explants were placed upon the muscle fibers. Control cultures received no explants.

Explants from chick spinal cord, ciliary ganglia and sympathetic ganglia were tested, since it is known that neurons from these three types of explants form functional neuromuscular junctions (Crain et al., 1970; Hooisma et al., 1975; Nurse and O'Lague, 1975). The trophic influence of these three tissues appeared to differ considerably: spinal cord had a strong positive effect on all four morphological parameters scored, while the ciliary ganglion only improved fiber thickness and delayed vacuolization, and the sympathetic ganglia appeared to have no effect whatsoever.

In heterologous combinations of chick muscle cells with mouse spinal neurons, spinal cord explants exerted a trophic influence which was no less effective than that exerted by chick spinal cord (Fig. 4). Dorsal root ganglia, which did not produce functional neuromuscular junctions (as demonstrated by the absence of end-plate potentials in the muscle fibers), were without any trophic effect. Mouse cerebral cortex explants, on the other hand, exerted a significant trophic influence, although they too did not form functional neuromuscular junctions.

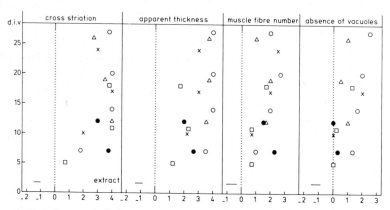

Fig. 3. The relative influence of chick embryo extract on the morphology of chick muscle fibers in culture. The values in the graph were calculated from those presented in Fig. 2. Abscissa: differences between the mean scores of experimental and control cultures estimated on the same day in culture. Further details as in Fig. 2.

MECHANISM OF TROPHIC INFLUENCE

The question was then raised whether the favorable influence of neurons upon muscle fibers might simply be caused by the substantial increase in contractile activity that is brought about by innervation. It is known that prolonged neuromuscular block in tissue culture by addition of D-tubocurarine to the medium does not prevent the formation of neuromuscular junctions (Crain and Peterson, 1971; Cohen, 1972). Spinal cord explants were therefore grown on muscle cells in the continuous presence of a blocking concentration of D-tubocurarine. As expected, when the curare was washed away after some days, those neuromuscular junctions which had developed immediately manifested themselves in the form of lively spontaneous contractions in the muscle fibers. Morphologically, the curarized muscle fibers did not differ from the non-curarized controls (Hooisma, 1977), which demonstrates that the increased electrical and contractile activity of the fibers which is normally brought about by innervation was not responsible for the trophic effects observed. It also refutes the idea that the trophic effect was exerted by an interaction of ACh with its receptors on the muscle fibers.

It has been shown for spinal cord explants that trophic support of muscle fibers in tissue culture is correlated with innervation (Robbins and Yonezawa, 1971; Hooisma, 1977). The ciliary ganglion, however, which very efficiently forms functional junctions (Obata, 1977; Slaaf, 1977), exerts only a moderate trophic influence, whereas cerebral cortex (which makes no functional junctions at all) has an approximately equal effect. Moreover, Harris et al. (1971) have observed that close cellular contact between neuroblastoma cells and muscle fibers, without the occurrence of any electrical activity at these sites, exerted a trophic influence which is expressed in an alteration of the distribution of ACh sensitivity along the fibers. It seems that functional innervation per se is not always sufficient for trophic action (but is no prerequisite either), and that a close proximity between neurons and muscle fibers is sufficient for stimulating muscle fiber maturation, provided the neuron releases the correct trophic substance(s).

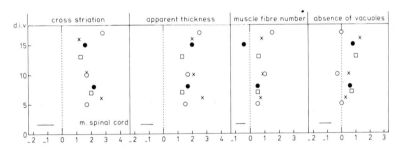

Fig. 4. The relative influence of spinal cord explants of mouse embryos on the morphology of chick muscle fibers. Muscle cells were cultured for two days in the presence of embryo extract, and thereafter without embryo extract. In the experimental cultures, spinal cord explants were added after 48 hr. Abscissa: differences of the mean score of various morphological properties for mixed cultures and the corresponding control cultures (without explants) both rated at the same day in culture. Ordinate: days in vitro (d.i.v.) Symbols: ○, ✗ and □, mean of 3 cultures; ●, mean of 4 cultures. Bar = 2 × S.E.M. of all experimental and control cultures.

If impulse transmission is not necessary for trophic action, the question arises whether simple diffusion of a trophic factor from an explant to the surrounding muscle fibers might be the explanation for the concentric zone of well developed fibers. This would require a stable, radially oriented, gradient of trophic agent around an explant. Those familiar with the actual practice of tissue culture will not easily be convinced of the likelihood of such stable gradients.

TABLE III

TROPHIC INFLUENCES ON ELECTRICAL PROPERTIES OF MUSCLE FIBERS IN TISSUE CULTURE

Parameter	Experimental condition	Observation[†]	Reference
Resting membrane potential	Spinal cord explant	no effect	Engelhardt et al. (1976)
	Spinal cord conditioned medium	no effect	Engelhardt et al. (1977b)
	Embryonic brain extract	no effect	Hooisma (1977)
	Ciliary ganglion	no effect	Hoosima et al. (1975)
Input resistance (MΩ)	Spinal cord conditioned medium	$5.1 \rightarrow 2.5$*	Engelhardt et al. (1977b)
	Embryonic extract	$4.8 \rightarrow 2.8$	Hooisma (1977)
	Spinal cord explant	$5.1 \rightarrow 1.2$	Engelhardt et al. (1977b)
Membrane resistance (KΩ/cm²)	Spinal cord explant	$3.1 \rightarrow 1.4$	Engelhardt et al. (1977a)
Maximum rate of rise of action potentials (V/sec)	Spinal cord extract	$504 \rightarrow 673$**,***	Hasegawa and Kuromi (1977)
Maximum rate of rise of action potentials in the presence of TTX	Spinal cord extract	$64\% \rightarrow 27\%$**,***,§	Hasegawa and Kuromi (1977)

[†] Control versus experimental conditon.
* Liver conditioned medium produced no effect.
** Observed in mouse extensor digitorum longus muscle in organ culture.
*** Extracts of non-nervous tissue ineffective.
§ Expressed as percentage of the values obtained in the same muscle fibers in the absence of TTX.

TROPHIC SUPPORT AND ELECTRICAL PROPERTIES

Various properties of the muscle fiber membrane are influenced in vivo by innervation: denervation lowers the resting membrane potential (Redfern and Thesleff, 1971), raises the specific membrane resistance (Albuquerque and McIsaac, 1970), and leads to the appearance of slow action potentials that are resistant to tetrodotoxin (TTX) (Redfern and Thesleff, 1971). These changes are reversed by re-innervation. In cultured muscle fibers, on the other hand, the resting potential is affected neither by the presence of embryo extract nor by innervation. The input resistance and the membrane resistance, however, are lowered by embryo extract as well as by innervation (see Table III). Moreover, Hasegawa and Kuromi (1977) observed the disappearance of slow TTX-resistant action potentials in embryo extract-treated organ cultures.

The ACh sensitivity of a non-innervated muscle fiber in vivo is evenly distributed over its membrane. Following innervation, the sensitivity becomes localized at the neuromuscular junction, whereas the extra-junctional membrane loses most of its ACh sensitivity (Axelsson and Thesleff, 1959). Junctional and extra-junctional ACh sensitivity have been measured in tissue culture (Table IV), and it appears that the extra-junctional sensitivity is changed neither by innervation (Fischbach and Cohen, 1973) nor by exposure to embryo extract (Hoosima, 1977), but can be lowered by electrical field stimulation (Cohen and Fischbach, 1973; also see Shainberg and Burstein, 1976). Increased ACh sensitivity is found at sites where nerve processes of neuroblastoma cells contact muscle cells, however, although no neurotransmission takes place at these sites (Harris et al., 1971). This trophic effect is not blocked either by inhibitors of ACh synthesis or by blockade of the ACh receptors (Steinbach et al., 1973). Recently, Cohen and Fischbach (1977) and Slaaf (1977) demonstrated the induction of sites of high ACh sensitivity on muscle fibers innervated by neurons from the spinal cord or the ciliary ganglion.

TABLE IV

TROPHIC INFLUENCES ON THE DISTRIBUTION OF THE ACh SENSITIVITY OF MUSCLE FIBERS IN TISSUE CULTURE

Parameter	Experimental condition	Result [§]	Reference
General ACh sensitivity mV/nC	Electrical stimulation	$200 \rightarrow 10$*	Cohen and Fischbach (1973)
	Innervation by spinal cord	no effect	Fischbach and Cohen (1973)
	Embryonic brain extract	no effect	Hooisma (1977)
ACh sensitivity at synapse	Neuroblastoma cell contact	enhanced	Harris et al. (1971)
	Innervation by spinal cord	enhanced	Cohen and Fischbach (1977)
	Innervation by ciliary ganglion	enhanced	Slaaf (1977)

* Control muscle fibers inactivated by tetrodotoxin or lidocaine.
[§] Control versus experimental condition.

The unambiguous demonstration of neurally induced hypersensitive loci on cultured muscle fibers has been hampered by the circumstance that cultured, non-innervated, fibers develop 'hot spots' with a high density of ACh receptors (Hartzell and Fambrough, 1973; Sytkowski et al., 1973; Prives et al., 1976). For reasons yet unknown, non-innervated muscle cells cultivated in our laboratory develop no such hot spots (Table V). Careful mapping of the ACh sensitivity at 326 positions along the length of 51 muscle fibers revealed local variations in sensitivity that never deviated more than three-fold from the average

TABLE V

LOCALIZED ACh SENSITIVITY (mV/nC) OF MUSCLE CELL MEMBRANE IN TISSUE CULTURE

Muscle cells: 7–14 days in culture; ciliary ganglion: 2–9 days in culture; spinal cord: 6–9 days in culture.

Areas with high ACh sensitivity	Non-innervated	Innervated	
		Ciliary ganglion	Spinal cord
Occurrence	no 'hot spots'	present	present
Number		14	5
Relative ACh sensitivity*		4.1–36.4	4.3–8.1
Membrane area tested	81,000 μm^2	35,000 μm^2	19,000 μm^2

* Maximum ACh sensitivity of the hypersensitive locus, divided by the averaged general sensitivity of the muscle cell membrane.

sensitivity found in the fiber studies, although between fibers the general sensitivity of fibers varied between 29 and 670 mV/nC (Slaaf, 1977). In contrast, fibers innervated by explanted ciliary ganglia and spinal cord explants showed no alteration in general sensitivity but instead carried sharply defined loci of 10–15 μm in diameter, where the sensitivity for iontophoretically applied ACh was 4–36 times higher than that of the surrounding membrane (Table V). These electrophysiological observations have been confirmed by autoradiography of cultures in which the ACh receptors were labeled with $[^{125}I]\alpha$-bungarotoxin (kindly supplied by Dr. Z. Vogel, Rehovoth, Israel). It was found in non-innervated muscle fibers that there were hardly any clusters of silver grains. If spinal cord fragments had been explanted on the muscle fibers, however, many clusters of α-bungarotoxin-binding sites were observed surrounding the explants, but not on more distantly situated muscle fibers.

It can be concluded that both maturation of neuromuscular junctions and neurotrophic maintenance of striated muscle fibers take place in tissue culture, and that currently available morphological, histological and electrophysiological techniques are suitable for studying these phenomena. It may be expected that this approach will rapidly further our understanding of the mechanisms underlying neuromuscular maturation and neurotrophic support.

SUMMARY

(1) The trophic influence of chick spinal cord explants on cultured skeletal muscle cells was quantified and compared with the effects of neural tissue extracts, and with the effects of other chick and mouse explanted tissues.

(2) The trophic influence was not diminished if D-tubocurarine was continuously present in the cultivation medium, suggesting that neither neurally induced activity in the muscle fibers nor acetylcholine itself mediates the trophic effect. Arguments are presented for the concept of a humoral neurotrophic agent, which is transferred to the muscle fibers by direct cellular communication.

(3) A survey is given of trophic effects on electrophysiological properties of cultured muscle cells.

(4) Muscle cells are described which are devoid of clusters of ACh receptors ('hot spots') but in which, after innervation, sharply defined loci become induced which are hypersensitive to ACh.

ACKNOWLEDGEMENTS

The authors wish to acknowledge Drs. T.D. Kernell and D. de Wied for their continuous interest. Expert technical assistance was given by Annelies van der Plaats-van Herk, Bert Bierman and Ton van der Laaken. The work was supported in part by the Foundation Promeso, and the Foundation for Medical Research FUNGO, which is subsidized by the Netherlands Organization for the Advancement of Pure Research (ZWO).

REFERENCES

Albuquerque, E.X. and McIsaac, R.J. (1970) Fast and slow mammalian muscles after denervation, *Exp. Neurol.*, 26: 183–202.

Axelsson, J. and Thesleff, S. (1959) A study of supersensitivity in denervated mammalian skeletal muscle, *J. Physiol. (Lond.)*, 147: 178–193.

Cohen, M.W. (1972) The development of neuromuscular connexions in the presence of D-tubocurarine, *Brain Res.*, 41: 457–463.

Cohen, S.A. and Fischbach, G.D. (1973) Regulation of muscle acetylcholine sensitivity by muscle activity in cell culture, *Science*, 181: 76–78.

Cohen, S.A. and Fischbach, G.D. (1977) Cluster of acetylcholine receptors located at identified nerve-muscle synapses in vitro, *Develop. Biol.*, 59: 24–38.

Crain, S.M., Alfei, L. and Peterson, E.R. (1970) Neuromuscular transmission in cultures of adult human and rodent skeletal muscle after innervation in vitro by fetal rodent spinal cord, *J. Neurobiol.*, 1: 471–489.

Crain, S.M. and Peterson, E.R. (1971) Development of paired explants of fetal spinal cord and adult skeletal muscle during chronic exposure to curare and hemicholinium, *In vitro*, 6: 373.

Crain, S.M. and Peterson, E.R. (1974) Development of neural connections in culture, *Ann. N.Y. Acad. Sci.*, 228: 6–35.

Drachman, D.B. (1976) Trophic interactions between nerves and muscles: the role of cholinergic transmission (including usage) and other factors. In *Biology of Cholinergic Function*, M. Goldberg and I. Hanin (Eds.), Raven Press, New York, pp. 161–187.

Engelhardt, J.K., Ishikawa, K., Lisbin, S.J. and Mori, J. (1976) Neurotrophic effects on passive electrical properties of cultured chick skeletal muscle, *Brain Res.*, 110: 170–174.

Engelhardt, J.K., Ishikawa, K., Mori, J. and Shimabukuro, Y. (1977a) Passive electrical properties of cultured chick skeletal muscle: neurotrophic effect on sample distribution. *Brain Res.*, 126: 172–175.

Engelhardt, J.K., Ishikawa, K., Mori, J. and Shimabukuro, Y. (1977b) Neurotrophic effects on the electrical properties of cultured muscle produced by conditioned medium from spinal cord explants, *Brain Res.*, 128: 243–248.

Fischbach, G.D. and Cohen, S.A. (1973) The distribution of acetylcholine sensitivity over un-innervated and innervated muscle fibers grown in cell culture, *Develop. Biol.*, 31: 147–162.

Harris, A.J., Heinemann, S., Schubert, D. and Tarakis, H. (1971) Trophic interaction between cloned tissue culture lines of nerve and muscle, *Nature (Lond.)*, 231: 296–301.

Hartzell, H.C., and Fambrough, D.M. (1973) Acetylcholine receptor production and incorporation into membranes of developing muscle fibres. *Develop. Biol.* 30: 153–165.

Hasegawa, S. and Kuromi, H. (1977) Effects of spinal cord and other tissue extracts on resting and action potentials of organ cultured mouse skeletal muscle, *Brain Res.*, 119: 133–140.

Hooisma, J., Slaaf, D.W., Meeter, E. and Stevens, W.F. (1975) The innervation of chick striated muscle fibres by the chick ciliary ganglion in tissue culture, *Brain Res.*, 85: 79–85.

Hooisma, J. (1977) *Innervation and Trophic Support of Muscle Cells in Tissue Culture*. Doctoral dissertation, State University of Utrecht.

Nurse, C.A. and O'Lague, P.H. (1975) Formation of cholinergic synapses between dissociated sympathetic neurons and skeletal myotubes of the rat in cell culture, *Proc. nat. Acad. Sci. (Wash.)*, 72: 1955–1959.

Obata, K. (1977) Development of neuromuscular transmission in culture with a variety of neurons and in the presence of cholinergic substances and tetrodotoxin, *Brain Res.*, 119: 141–153.

Oh, T.H. (1975) Neurotrophic effects: characterization of the nerve extract that stimulates muscle development in culture, *Exp. Neurol.*, 46: 432–438.

Oh, T.H. (1976) Neurotrophic effects of sciatic nerve extracts on muscle development in culture, *Exp. Neurol.*, 50: 376–386.

Oh, T.H., Johnson, D.D. and Kim, S.U. (1972) Neurotrophic effect on isolated chick embryo muscle in culture, *Science*, 178: 1298–1300.

Paul, C.V. and Powell, J.A. (1974) Organ culture studies of coupled fetal cord and adult muscle from normal and dystrophic mice, *J. neurol. Sci.*, 21: 365–379.

Prives, J., Silman, I. and Amsterdam, A. (1976) Appearance and disappearance of acetylcholine receptor during differentiation of chick skeletal muscle in vitro, *Cell*, 7: 543–550.

Redfern, P. and Thesleff, S. (1971) Action potential generation in denervated rat skeletal muscle. 1. Quantitative aspects, *Acta physiol. scand.*, 81: 557–564.

Robbins, N. and Yonezawa, T. (1971) Physiological studies during formation and development of rat neuromuscular junctions in tissue culture, *J. gen. Physiol.*, 58: 467–481.

Shainberg, A. and Burstein, M. (1976) Decrease of acetylcholine receptor synthesis in muscle cultures by electrical stimulation, *Nature (Lond.)*, 264: 368–369.

Slaaf, D.W. (1977) *Electrophysiological Characterization of Striated Muscle Cells Innervated by Ciliary Neurons in Tissue Culture*. Doctoral dissertation, State University of Utrecht.

Steinbach, J.H., Harris, A.J., Patrick, J., Schubert, D. and Heinemann, S. (1973) Nerve-muscle interaction in vitro: role of acetylcholine, *J. gen. Physiol.*, 62: 255–270.

Sytkowski, A.J., Vogel, Z. and Nirenberg, M.W. (1973) Development of acetylcholine receptor clusters on cultured muscle cells, *Proc. nat. Acad. Sci. (Wash.)*, 70: 270–274.

DISCUSSION

CHANGEUX: I wonder if it is not possible to create conditions where you would see 'hot spots' in the absence of nerves? Your cultures do not have them in the absence of innervation, so my question is: can you change the conditions so that hot spots are formed?

STEVENS: Those experiments are presently under investigation.

CHANGEUX: You mentioned at the EMBO meeting last year in St. Odile that the membrane potentials of the muscle fibers are unusually high in your cultures. Could this explain the absence of hot spots in these preparations?

STEVENS: There are several possibilities to explain the differences between our results and those of other laboratories. For instance, the resting membrane potentials which we observe are usually in the neighborhood of -80 mV, whereas other laboratories find membrane potentials of the muscle fibers around -50 to -60 mV. The membrane potential of -80 mV is established very early in our cultures (in fact, as soon as we can impale the muscle fibers). Other workers have observed a slower development of the resting potential, during 5–6 days, to the final value of -60 mV. Also, in our hands cross-striation develops faster: we observe beautiful cross-striations as early as 5 days in culture, while most other laboratories describe them only at about days 7–10. Thus, there is a difference in the kinetics of myogenesis and, since it has been described that the hot spots disappear with prolonged cultivation, it could be that they start to disappear shortly after their synthesis in our cultures, so that they escape detection. So far we have no good explanation for why we have no hot spots, but it does make the system much more suitable for the study of synapse formation!

Genetic and 'Epigenetic' Factors Regulating Synapse Formation in Vertebrate Cerebellum and Neuromuscular Junction

JEAN-PIERRE CHANGEUX and KATSUHIKO MIKOSHIBA

Institut Pasteur, 75015 Paris (France)

Among the complex sequence of events which take place during the development of the nervous system one may distinguish (a) the setting out of cell bodies (neuronal somas and glial cells) through cell proliferation, migration and differentiation, and (b) the establishment of the highly organized and complex network of interneuronal connections. Molecular biologists interested in the nervous system have been primarily concerned with its genetic determinism: are there enough genes in the DNA to code for the 100,000 billion synapses of the human brain? Fewer than one million structural genes are present to do the job, so that one has to imagine mechanisms capable of creating complexity from a limited number of genetic determinants. Step (a) above is a matter of embryonic development and may result from the combination of a small number of genes expressing themselves in a sequential manner. Step (b) is a fundamental characteristic of the nervous system, and is of a higher order of complexity.

Several categories of mechanisms which could create order and diversity in the development of synaptic connections from a relatively small number of structural determinants have been proposed in the past. These models differ chiefly in the role assigned to the activity of the system (Fig. 1). According to the *preformist* attitude this role may be neglected. The growing nerve fibers bear chemical labels complementary to those present on the target neurons, the selectivity of the assembly between pre- and post-synaptic partners depending entirely upon the 'affinity' between cell surfaces ('*Chemo-affinity hypothesis*': Sperry, 1963; Gaze, 1970; Prestige and Willshaw, 1975) or differential growth of the nerve terminals ('*Timing hypothesis*') might be instrumental in establishing order within a developing nerve system (Jacobson, 1969; Levinthal et al., 1975).

Alternatively, activity might contribute to the specification of the developing network, either by tracing pathways in a completely random network (*empirist* attitude) or by stabilizing an already specified synaptic organization ('*functional verification*' hypothesis: Wiesel and Hubel, 1974). As a compromise between these two extreme views, the '*selective stabilization hypothesis*' (Changeux et al., 1973; Changeux and Danchin, 1976), proposes that the genetic program directs the proper interaction between main categories of neurons but that, at *a critical stage of development*, a 'limited redundancy' in connectivity exists. The activity of the developing network, spontaneous in the embryo and/or evoked after birth, would bring additional order by reducing this redundancy and stabilizing selectively some of the labile contacts.

As a mechanism it was further postulated that the first synaptic contacts to form may exist under at least three states: labile (L), stable (S) and regressed (D), the growth process

44

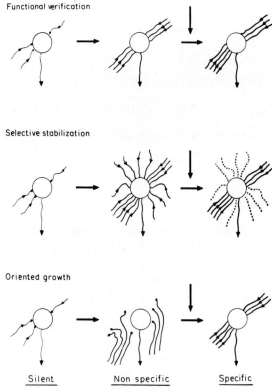

Functional verification

Selective stabilization

Oriented growth

Silent   Non specific   Specific

Fig. 1. Hypotheses regarding the effect of functional activity on the specification of a neuronal network. The three possibilities considered deal with *changes in connectivity*, but alternative (or additional) mechanisms may take place such as *changes of efficacy* of excitatory and/or inhibitory synapses, *growth of new sets of connections* and so on (adapted from Changeux and Danchin, 1976). The vertical arrow indicates the onset of spontaneous or evoked activity.

being viewed as the emergence of the labile state (Not → L). The labile and stable states would transmit nerve impulses, but the regressed one obviously would not.

The labile state may either become stabilized (L → S) or regress (L → D), this regression being irreversible. An essential statement of the theory (Changeux et al., 1973) is that the transitions of the labile state of the synapse (L → S and L → D) are regulated by the total activity of the postsynaptic cell, including the activity of the considered synapse. Accordingly, the precocious activity of the developing network would 'stabilize selectively' particular synapses among the many equivalent contacts which emerge during growth and thereby create diversity and specificity (in a concomitant manner the non-stabilized contacts will regress). As a consequence, a 'critical period' exists in the development of a nerve terminal, during which it requires a given pattern of activity to become stable.

The major advantage of this selective stabilization hypothesis is that it affords an economy of genes. Some of the genes which dictate, for instance, the general rules of growth, the stability properties of the immature synapses (postulate-1), the regulation of their stability by the activity of the immature synapse (postulate-2), the integrative properties of the postsynaptic neuron, may indeed be shared by different categories of neurons, or even be common to all neurons. The set of genes involved (the genetic envelope) could, therefore, be smaller than would be the case if each synapse were determined individually.

In summary, according to these views, synapse formation would involve at least two distinct processes: (1) a *recognition* between cell surfaces, and (2) a *stabilization* of pre-formed labile contacts. The first would not require activity, and therefore would be entirely under strict genetic determinism; the second on the other hand, would be coupled to the activity of the network, and thus be an '*epi*genetic' phenomenon.

THE FIRST STEP OF SYNAPSE FORMATION: THE 'RECOGNITION' BETWEEN CELL SURFACES

As has already been mentioned, the establishment of the first contacts between the exploratory nerve fibers and their target cell may take place even if these contacts are not functional. It was therefore postulated that the selectivity of this initial step primarily relies on processes of cell surface recognition. Few biochemical investigations have yet been devoted to this subject, primarily due to difficulties in obtaining large enough quantities of relevant material.

In this respect, the vertebrate cerebellum appears to be a particularly convenient structure, since it is made up of only a small number of cell types (5 classes of neurons) repeated a large number of times, yielding both chemical homogeneity and richness. In the field of central neuronal biochemistry, therefore, the cerebellum could play a role similar to that of fish electric organs in the study of the neuromuscular synapse. Moreover, the electrical activity of single neurons, or even single categories of synapses, can be recorded by juxta- or intra-cellular recordings upon stimulation of the afferent pathways (Eccles et al., 1967), or by iontophoretic applications of various categories of effectors (Yamamoto, personal communication). The cerebellum also has a rather unique position in brain physiology since, in the adult, its functional circuitry is almost completely understood down to the synaptic level (Eccles et al., 1967). This is illustrated by Fig. 2, taken from the early but still entirely valid work of Ramón y Cajal (1911). The two main categories of neurons, the Purkinje cells

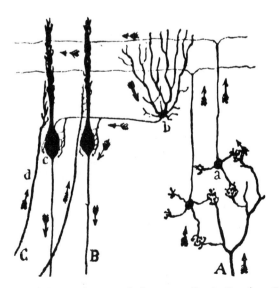

Fig. 2. Functional circuitry of the vertebrate cerebellum according to Ramón y Cajal (1911). A, mossy fiber; B, Purkinje cell axon; C, climbing fiber; a, granule cell; b, basket cell; c, Purkinje cell.

and the granule cells, receive the two principal cerebellar inputs (the climbing fibers and the mossy fibers) while there exists only a single efferent pathway for the whole cerebellum: the axons of the Purkinje cells. In addition, inhibitory interneurons (Golgi, basket and stellate cells) are branched, in parallel, between the granule and the Purkinje cells.

Another advantage offered by the cerebellum is (in the mouse) the existence of a number of mapped gene mutations which cause well-defined lesions of its anatomical organisation, and therefore of its physiology as well (Fig. 3; for reviews see Sidman, 1974; Rakic, 1976; Sotelo, 1975). For instance, in 'nervous' and 'Purkinje cell degeneration' (PCD) mouse mutants, the lesion affects the Purkinje cells, which are almost completely absent in the adult. In the '*weaver*' mutant it is the granule cells which are missing. In '*staggerer*', the major deficit concerns one category of synaptic contact: the synapse between the parallel fibers and the spines of the Purkinje cell dendrites. Also, in '*reeler*' a severe perturbation results from an incomplete migration of the Purkinje cells to their normal position in the cerebellar cortex. In addition, phenocopies of some of these mutations exist. For instance, the lack of granule cells caused by the 'weaver' mutation may also be induced in several mammals by drug injection, virus infection or X-irradiation (for review see Sotelo, 1975; Mariani et al., 1977).

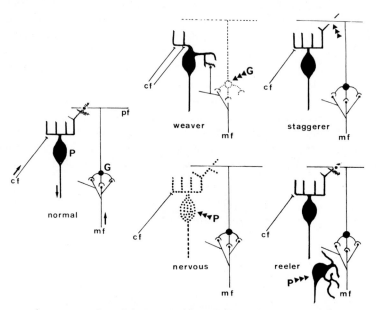

Fig. 3. Diagrammatic representation of the connectivity of the cerebellum from the homozygous mutant mice: weaver, staggerer, nervous and reeler. P, Purkinje cell; G, granule cell; mf, mossy fiber; cf, climbing fiber; pf, parallel fiber (axons of granule cells). → indicates the direction of propagation of the nerve impulse; ▶▶▶ indicates the site of the lesion.

The 'staggerer' (*sg*) mutation is particularly relevant to the problem of synapse formation, since in the homozygous *sg/sg* mouse the parallel fiber-Purkinje cell spine synapses do not form (Sax et al., 1968; Landis, 1974; Sidman, 1974; Sotelo and Changeux, 1974; Hirano and Dembitzer, 1975), even though the two neuronal partners — the granule and the Purkinje cells — are both present and functional. Ultrastructural studies reveal that specialized adhesion zones or attachment plates are numerous between the smooth surface of the Purkinje cell dendrites at the immature nonsynaptic segment of the parallel fiber. Such attachment plates, which have been considered as a first morphological sign of synaptic contact, fail to evolve into typical synaptic contacts in the *sg/sg* animals (with some exception in older animals). In older adults, the parallel fibers look immature but normal, while the dendrites of the Purkinje cells have abnormally smooth contours and spines are lacking on their characteristic branchlets (Sidman, 1974; Sotelo and Changeux, 1974; Hirano and Dembitzer, 1975). Electrophysiological studies confirm that a major deficit exists in staggerer at the level of the Purkinje cells (Crepel et al., 1973; Crepel and Mariani, 1975). The parallel fibers indeed conduct action potentials, although slightly more slowly (0.258 ± 0.016 meters per sec) than in normal mice (0.361 ± 0.018 meters per sec), and have an absolute refractory period which is somewhat longer (2.81 ± 0.13 msec) than normal (1.61 ± 0.08 msec). In contrast, the antidromic response elicited by electrical stimulation of the axon is altered in about 60% of the Purkinje cells, and typical spontaneous or evoked responses to climbing fibers are never recorded (despite the fact that the climbing fiber-Purkinje cell synapses exist and are functional in *sg/sg* mice). Primarily the cell membrane of the Purkinje cell seems to be affected by the *sg* mutation, and it was suggested that this deficit is responsible for the absence of typical parallel fiber-Purkinje cell synapses. The staggerer cerebellum should, therefore, be an excellent material in which to identify the chemical determinants involved in the establishment of this particular category of synapse.

Another interesting mutant is the homozygous weaver (*wv/wv*) mouse, in which granule cells are absent. In normal cerebellum the afferent mossy fibers contact the granule cell dendrites at the level of the glomerulus (Fig. 4). But what happens to these fibers in weaver cerebellum when the normal target is missing? Ultrastructural studies disclose that, in addition to many free spines on Purkinje cell dendrites, a large number of them are occupied by mossy fiber terminals (Sotelo, 1975). Similar 'heterologous' synapses have also been found in the agranular cerebellum from virus infected ferrets (Llinas et al., 1973) and X-irradiated rats (Altman and Anderson, 1972; Crepel et al., 1976). Interestingly, these synapses seem to be quite functional. In the normal cerebellum, stimulation of the mossy fibers evokes a single spike discharge in Purkinje cells via the mossy fiber-granule cell pathway, with a latency of 2.2–6.0 msec (in rat) at threshold intensity. These responses are missing in the agranular cerebellum, and are replaced in 62% of the Purkinje cells by an early response with a much shorter latency (0.9–1.7 msec in the rat). Such short latencies indicate that monosynaptic transmission is taking place between mossy fibers and Purkinje cell.

The same category of functional heterologous synapses has also been found in 'reeler' cerebellum. There, a significant number of the Purkinje cells do not migrate, and remain packed as a central mass adjacent to the deep nuclei. The dendrites of these deep Purkinje cells, as in the case of the weaver mouse, do not receive parallel fibers in significant number, and similarly make functional heterologous contacts with the mossy fibers (Mariani et al., 1977). Occasionally, in the same cerebella, anatomical contacts were also observed between the soma of the granule cells, or even their dendrites, and the spines of the Purkinje cells. In any case, these observations clearly indicate that functional synapses may form between non-complementary pairs of cells, and it has even been suggested that the bioelectrical activity of these contacts is responsible, at least in part, for the behavioral deficit (Llinas et al., 1973). The recognition step between cell surfaces, therefore, does not require a complementarity of structure as stringent as one would expect from a strict chemoaffinity hypothesis. A 'compatibility' between cell surfaces (e.g., Changeux and Danchin, 1976) rather than complementarity might be sufficient for a synapse to form. The acquisition of

48

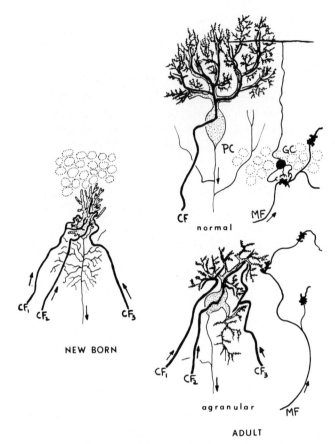

Fig. 4. The innervation of the Purkinje cell in normal and agranular cerebella from newborn and adult mouse or rat.

specificity has to be viewed as a progressive and sequential process, and other mechanisms in addition (or alternatively) to the recognition between cell surfaces have to be invoked in order to account for the sophisticated organization of neuronal connectivity in the adult.

In an attempt to obtain better definition of the possible role of the cell surface determinants responsible for such 'compatibility', biochemical investigations on the cerebellum from normal and mutant animals have been initiated. As already mentioned, the relative cellular homogeneity of the cerebellum renders this approach feasible. Moreover, the different categories of cells may be separated in significant amounts, according to cell size in dispersed cerebellar tissues. It is to be expected, simply from a consideration of the number of neurons present in the cerebellum, that the preparation of 'large cells' thus obtained should be enriched in Purkinje cells, and that granule neurons would be abundant in the 'small cell' fraction. When such cell separation is carried out under adequate conditions, the isolated cells may survive in vitro for days or even weeks, and develop characteristic neuritic processes (Monneron, personal communication).

In the weaver mutant mouse the cerebellum should show striking biochemical alterations, since it is deprived of the most abundant population of cerebellar neurons: the granule cell. Polyacrylamide gel electrophoresis under denaturing conditions (in sodium dodecylsulfate: SDS) of normal and weaver cerebellum indeed reveal marked biochemical differences (Mallet et al., 1976). The most striking difference concerns several protein bands with mobilities corresponding to those of purified histones. These bands appear markedly reduced in the agranular cerebellum, but are present in large amounts in the small cell preparation. This relative reduction in the histone bands was to be expected since there is a decrease in the total DNA content (6–7-fold) associated with the loss of granule cells. The high nucleus-to-cytoplasm ratio of the granule cells as compared to other neurons, and in particular the Purkinje cells, also explains the relative abundance of the histone bands in preparations of purified 'small cells', as well as their relative decrease in the extracts of agranular cerebella.

Anatomical and physiological evidence exists for an alteration of the Purkinje cells in staggerer cerebellum. In agreement with this conclusion, polyacrylamide gel electrophoresis in SDS of this mutant cerebellum shows that a protein with a very low mobility (apparent molecular weight of 400,000) is missing (Mallet et al., 1976). This P_{400} protein is present in purified suspensions of large neurons (mainly Purkinje cells) but not of small ones, and is missing in membrane fragments of adult *nervous* and *Purkinje cell degeneration* cerebellum where a majority of the Purkinje cells have died. It is therefore characteristic, if indeed not 'specific', for the Purkinje neuron. As expected, P_{400} is abundant in the agranular weaver cerebellum (although the observed enrichment in this mutant cerebellum may result simply from the absence of the granule cell component, rather than from an enhanced synthesis by the Purkinje cells caused by their deafferentation).

P_{400} is strongly 'membrane bound' (or 'particulate') and is present in large amounts in microsomal fractions prepared from crude cerebellum homogenates by the method of Whittaker (Whittaker and Barker, 1972). It can be purified from this fraction by successive extractions with Triton X-100, and cholate, followed by electrophoresis in SDS of the residual pellet. Amino acid analysis of the purified protein reveals that all the typical amino acids from globular proteins are present. On SDS gels, the P_{400} protein reacts with the periodic acid-Schiff reagent, and therefore possesses a glycosidic moiety. It is not yet known whether its low mobility on gels is due to (a) the high molecular weight of the chain, (b) to an incomplete unfolding of the molecule, or (c) to its carbohydrate component. In any case, P_{400} is highly susceptible to trypsin, and is split into smaller units in its presence.

The regional distribution of the P_{400} protein has been further investigated on preparations of isolated granular and molecular layers (Mikoshiba and Changeux, 1977). The molecular layer, granular layer and white matter can be separated by manual dissection from slices of beef cerebellum, in large enough quantities for carrying out standard biochemical studies (Fig. 5). The granular layer, containing a large number of cell somas with a particularly high nucleus-to-cytoplasm ratio, is indeed about 10 times richer in DNA (and histones) than the molecular layer and white matter. The relative RNA content is also larger in the molecular and granular layers than in the white matter, probably because of the abundance of myelin in the white matter (metabolically a rather inert structure). P_{400} is present almost exclusively in the isolated molecular layer, but also in the same layer separated from Purkinje cell somas. P_{400} is, therefore, also present in the dendritic arborization of the Purkinje cell, a finding consistent with the observation that this protein is missing in the cerebellum from the homozygous 'staggerer' mouse where Purkinje cells are present, but with abnormal dendritic arborizations.

In the course of these studies on isolated molecular and granular layers it was also found that, after homogenization, the isolated molecular layer takes up glutamic acid at a rate about 10 times faster per unit weight than the isolated granular layer (Table I). This result is consistent with the hypothesis that glutamic acid acts as the neurotransmitter of the parallel fiber-Purkinje cell synapse. Indeed, in the agranular cerebellum the content of

50

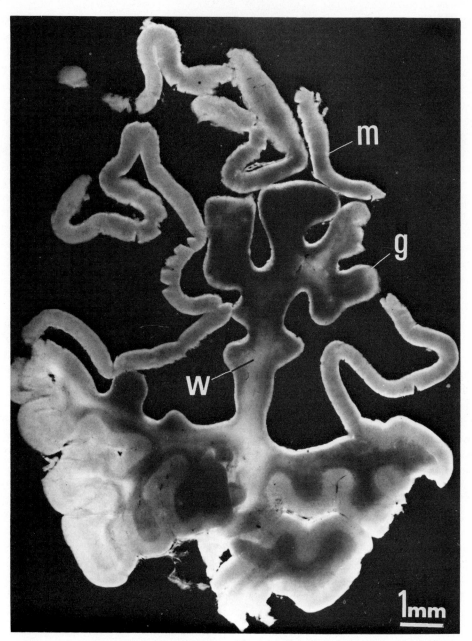

Fig. 5. Dissection of the molecular layer from a slice of bovine cerebellum without freezing. The slice was cut sagitally to the lobes with a razor blade and then dissected with fine forceps under a dissecting micro-scope. The clumps of granular layer were then cut off from white matter with small scissors. m, molecular layer; g, granular layer; w, white matter.

glutamic acid and the affinity uptake decrease (Mikoshiba et al., 1977). The parallel fibers are a major component of the molecular layer, and the homogenization procedure, however mild, destroys the granular cell bodies but preserves the parallel fibers. Moreover, the sub-cellular particles (Mikoshiba and Changeux, 1977; Mikoshiba et al., 1977) which take up

TABLE I

UPTAKE OF AMINO ACIDS BY ISOLATED MOLECULAR AND GRANULAR
LAYER

Amino acid incorporation into homogenates of molecular layer and granular layer
of bovine cerebellum.

	[^{3}H]Glutamate $(10^{-10}$ moles/mg protein/4 min)	[^{14}C]GABA
Molecular layer	23.12 ± 7.30 (3)	9.08 ± 2.87 (4)
Granular layer	2.55 ± 1.29 (3)	14.31 ± 2.33 (3)

glutamate can be separated by ultracentrifugation in Ficoll gradient from those which incorporate GABA. Fragmented parallel fibers can be further purified by using sucrose density gradient centrifugation, eliminating myelin. The same technique applied to the agranular weaver cerebellum fails to separate the same particles, again a result consistent with an eventual role of glutamic acid as the neurotransmitter of the parallel fibers. A continuation of these studies is expected to eventually result in the isolation of the pre- and post-synaptic partners of the parallel fiber-Purkinje spine synapse, thereby making possible the direct identification of their surface determinants.

Meanwhile an indirect, *immunological*, investigation on these surface determinants has been undertaken (Mallet and Changeux, unpublished observations). First of all, cell fractions enriched either in large cell bodies (mostly Purkinje cell perikarya), or in small ones (mostly granule cells), have been isolated from rat cerebellum and injected into rabbits. After several injections, the serum of the immunized rabbits give precipitation lines with crude extracts of cerebellar membrane fractions dissolved in non-denaturing detergent. The sera directed against the large cell fraction by the immunoperoxidase technique of Avrameas (1972) stain both isolated large and small cells. However, after adsorption on rat cerebellum, the sera react exclusively with the large cell bodies and give an unambiguous coloration of the Purkinje cell soma and dendrites on sections of normal rat (or mouse) cerebellum. Antibodies directed against Purkinje cells must therefore be present in these sera. This conclusion is further supported by the observations that the adsorbed sera do not stain any particular structure of the cerebellum from the 'nervous' mutant mouse, in which the Purkinje neurons are missing. Binding studies carried out with these particular sera (labeled with ^{125}I) confirm that antibodies directed against membrane-bound component(s) specific for the cerebellum have been raised in the rabbits.

In work done in collaboration with Alain Privat, these anti-'large-cell' sera have been tested on explants of newborn rat cerebella in tissue culture. Interestingly, after several days of culture these sera preferentially affect the Purkinje cells and rapidly cause their death. On the other hand, they do not show any noticeable effect on explants of rat cerebellum. The reasons for this selective death are not yet understood. Recently, antisera directed against P$_{400}$ protein have been raised in rabbit, and immunological investigation on this membrane (or particulate) protein undertaken (Mikoshiba et al., 1977). The anti-P$_{400}$ sera give a positive indirect peroxidase reaction with isolated large cell bodies (mostly Purkinje cell perikarya), but not with small cells. Preliminary observations indicate that the anti-P$_{400}$ serum affects the in vitro development of explants of newborn rat cerebellum. In these cultures, the spines on the dendrites of Purkinje cells, as well as the granule cell, may selectively disappear.

52

Chronic injections of these antisera in newborn mice seem to cause changes of behavior characteristic of a cerebellar syndrome. In any case, these still preliminary studies can be taken as illustrations of a method which may eventually lead to the identification of the cell surface components involved in the early steps of synapse formation.

THE SELECTIVE STABILIZATION OF DEVELOPING SYNAPSES AS A MECHANISM FOR THE SPECIFICATION OF NEURONAL NETWORKS

When it reaches its target cell, the growth cone of the developing nerve terminal adheres to its surface, but the mechanism of intercellular recognition alone is insufficient to explain the entire development of the synapse. Once formed, and even functional, a given synaptic contact need not be stable. Mechanisms of selective stablization are based on processes of cell surface recognition in the acquisition of the final specificity. The neuromuscular junction, despite its known 'rigidity' in the adult, is a simple system with which an analysis of this last category of mechanism becomes accessible to experimentation. The work of Bennett and Pettigrew (1974), and of others, has distinguished three principal steps in the formation of the adult neuromuscular junction (Figs. 6 and 7). First, the 'localization' of acetylcholine receptor and esterase is a strictly postsynaptic phenomenon. Under the growing nerve terminal, the density of acetylcholine receptor in the cytoplasmic membrane of the myotube and of acetylcholinesterase in the basement membrane increases, resulting in a well-defined and localized spot. Most often (in mammals), only one such spot forms per myotube, but in some instances (for example the avian latissimus dorsi (ALD)) several spots appear at regular intervals. Localization takes place as early as 12–13 days of incubation in chick embryo (the exact schedule varies from one given muscle to another) and 15 days of fetal life in the rat.

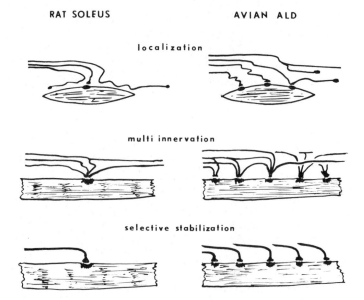

Fig. 6. Diagrammatic representation of three important steps in the development of the neuromuscular junction in skeletal muscles with focal and distributed innervation: (1) postsynaptic localization of the acetylcholine receptor; (2) transient polyneural innervation; (3) selective stabilization of a single nerve terminal per end-plate.

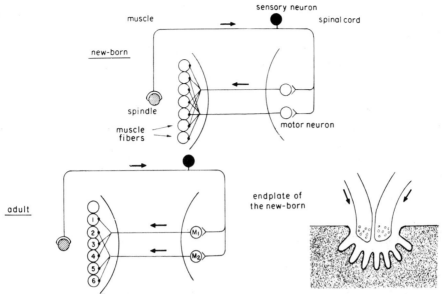

Fig. 7. The differentiation of motor units in a skeletal fast muscle by retrograde selective stabilization of nerve terminals. In the neonate one motor neuron innervates many more muscle fibers than in the adult, and each muscle fiber receives several nerve terminals. A few weeks after birth only one nerve terminal persists per muscle, the others having regressed (Changeux and Danchin, 1976).

Secondly, once localized the newly formed end-plate receives several nerve terminals converging from different neuronal somatas. The nerve terminals which contribute to this multi-innervation are usually functional; each muscle fiber is under the command of several neurons, which may also innervate other muscle fibers. A 'redundancy' of the innervation thus exists, but this redundancy is transient. Finally, the supernumerary nerve endings regress and a single axon terminal per muscle fiber persists in the adult. The stabilization of a single terminal per fiber seems to occur at random among the multiple nerve terminals and among the fibers of a given muscle. Yet all the muscle fibers become innervated and each motor neuron innervates approximately the same number of muscle fibers, giving rise to 'motor units' of regular size.

During this period of neuromuscular contact, the embryo moves actively. In the chick, for example, spontaneous movements begin as early as 3 days of incubation (Hamburger, 1970), are blocked by D-tubocurarine, and are of neurogenic origin (Ripley and Provine, 1972). The rat fetus also moves spontaneously as early as 15 days (Hamburger, 1970) in utero. Since a growth cone can liberate transmitter and give rise to typical end-plate potentials (Fischbach et al., 1976), it is obviously tempting to relate this precocious activity with the regulation of synapse formation. In any case, synapses are able to transmit nerve impulses, and do transmit them at very early stages of their development, long before the so-called 'anatomical' synapses are formed.

Postsynaptic localization of the acetylcholine receptor protein

The localization of acetylcholinesterase accompanies (or follows) that of the receptor protein, but less information is presently available than in the case of the receptor protein. Although the exact molecular mechanism of the localization of the acetylcholine receptor during development is still largely unknown, the following observations seem relevant to this question.

(a) The immobilization of the receptor protein in the adult synapse. In the adult neuro-muscular junction the density of acetylcholine receptor sites, as counted with radioactive snake α-toxins, is 100–1000 times greater than in extrasynaptic areas (e.g., Barnard et al., 1971). An average density of 8–9000 sites per μm^2 occurs in mouse junction, with greater densities at the top (30,000 ± 6,000 sites per μm^2) than at the bottom of the synaptic folds (Fertuck and Salpeter, 1974; Porter and Barnard, 1975). There are up to 50,000 ± 15,000 sites per μm^2 in *Electrophorus* electroplaque (Bourgeois et al., 1972). The subsynaptic mem-brane therefore consists of a closely packed assembly of receptor molecules. In the developing rat or chick myotube, the density of acetylcholine receptor sites lies in between that of the extra- and subsynaptic areas in the adult synapse (i.e. 1500–2000 sites per μm^2: (Fambrough, 1974). The actual translational mobility of the receptor protein in embryonic myotubes in vitro has been recently measured by labeling the acetylcholine receptor site with a fluorescent derivation of α-bungarotoxin, and then photobleaching with a laser beam (Axelrod et al., 1976). The mobility of the receptor protein in these extrasynaptic areas (outside the high density patches which appear spontaneously in vitro in the absence of nerve terminals) is that which is expected for an integral protein imbedded in a highly fluid lipidic environment (diffusion coefficient 5×10^{-11} cm^2/sec). By contrast, in the adult sub-synaptic membrane the receptor protein appears remarkably immobile. It is a well-known observation that, after denervation of skeletal muscle, the main anatomical features of the subsynaptic apparatus (Tello, 1917; Tower, 1939; Gutmann and Young, 1944) – the dense deposit of acetylcholinesterase revealed by the Koelle reaction (Birks et al., 1960) and the high sensitivity to iontophoretically applied acetylcholine (Axelson and Thesleff, 1959; Miledi, 1960) – persists for weeks. In *Electrophorus* electroplaque, the density of $[^3H]\alpha$-toxin sites measured by high resolution autoradiography in the remnants of the subsynaptic membrane decrease by less than 50% at 52 days after denervation, despite the fact that they are uncovered by the nerve terminal for that length of time (Bourgeois, 1974; Bourgeois et al., 1973). No significant tendency for lateral diffusion of the receptor protein exists in the adult neuromuscular junction under similar conditions (Lee et al., 1967; Frank et al., 1975). It therefore can be concluded that during the development of the synaptic contact the receptor protein becomes strongly immobilized in the area of the cytoplasmic membrane which underlies the nerve terminal.

(b) The turnover of the acetylcholine receptor in developing myotubes. In a study com-pleted in collaboration with the group of F. Gros, the metabolic stability of the receptor protein during development was explored in vitro on primary cultures of fetal calf muscle. Upon fusion of the myoblasts into myotubes, the total number of α-toxin sites increases markedly (Merlie et al., 1975). In order to determine whether this increase corresponds to a neosynthesis of receptor molecules, or whether to the unmasking of an hypothetical pre-cursor, primary cultures of myoblasts were labeled in vitro with $[^{35}S]$methionine; the receptor protein was extracted with Triton X-100, and then purified on a snake α-toxin affinity column. The purified product was characterized by centrifugation on sucrose gradients (using anti-receptor antibodies) (Merlie et al., 1975), or by electrophoresis in SDS (in one or two dimensions) (Merlie et al., 1976, 1978). The results were unambiguous: a neosynthesis of receptor molecules accounts for the increase of α-toxin sites which takes place upon fusion of the myoblasts. A similar conclusion was reached independently by measuring density shifts after incorporation of amino acids labeled with heavy isotopes (Devreotes and Fambrough, 1976).

Following the same methodology, but after pulse labeling (for 4 hr) with $[^{35}S]$methionine, the metabolic stability of the receptor protein could be determined (Merlie et al., 1976,

1978). First, it was confirmed that the intrinsic decay of the receptor–$[^{125}I]\alpha$-bungaro-toxin complex follows closely that of the pulse-labeled molecule. In other words, binding of the α-toxin does not significantly modify the half-life of the receptor molecule. Both methods give a half-life of 16—18 hr. The receptor protein in the sarcolemma of developing myotube, as in extrasynaptic areas of adult muscles following denervation (Chang and Huang, 1975; Berg and Hall, 1975), is metabolically a highly labile molecule. This behavior contrasts with that of the subsynaptic receptor from the adult neuromuscular junction. There, the values for the half-life obtained for the α-toxin—receptor complex are about 6—7 days, and fall in the range of those expected for the dissociation of α-bungarotoxin from the receptor site even in the absence of any receptor turnover. The stability of the subsynaptic receptor molecule in the adult synapse thus appears to be considerably higher than that of the extrasynaptic embryonic receptor. A major biochemical event which takes place during the maturation of the neuromuscular synapse, therefore, is the transformation of the receptor protein from a labile and mobile 'embryonic' form into a stable and immobile one.

(c) Structural differences between extra- and subsynaptic receptor molecules. The striking differences in metabolism noticed between extra- and subsynaptic receptor could result either from a basic dissimilarity in primary structure (the two proteins would be coded by distinct structural genes), or from differences in their local 'environment' (for instance, as a result of interactions between receptor molecules within the subsynaptic membrane, of anchoring to the basal membrane on the outside surface, or to the cytoskeleton on the inside membrane, etc). Pharmacological differences have been reported in vivo between the subsynaptic and the extrasynaptic receptors (Beranek and Vyskocil, 1967). In addition, noise measurements reveal that the opening time of the cholinergic ionophore increases after denervation (Katz and Miledi, 1972). Yet, they may not reveal differences in the primary structure of the two classes of receptor molecules, e.g. differences in packing or local environ-ment of the receptor protein in the membrane. In agreement with this interpretation are the following observations. (1) The in vitro binding constants for agonists and antagonists of the membrane bound receptor do not change in chick embryo leg muscles from 8 days (extra-synaptic) before hatching until 70 days after hatching (subsynaptic) (Giacobini, unpublished observations); the receptor proteins isolated from extra- and subsynaptic regions of rat diaphragm have been reported to show identical binding properties in two laboratories (Alper et al., 1974; Colquhoun and Rang, 1976), although different in a third laboratory (Brockes and Hall, 1975). (2) The equivalence points by immunoprecipitation seem to be identical for the two receptors (Brockes and Hall, 1975). (3) The two molecules have the same hydrodynamic properties, and only isoelectric focusing unambiguously separates the two receptors, revealing a charge difference (Brockes and Hall, 1975).

Two isoelectric forms of the receptor protein with similar properties have also been discovered in the electric organ of *Electrophorus* (Teichberg and Changeux, 1976), which offers a much more convenient material for biochemical studies than does skeletal muscle. Interestingly, these two forms can be interconverted in vitro. After treatment of a crude extract in the presence of NaF at 37 °C, the alkaline species disappears, while the opposite happens in the absence of fluorure (NaCl) (Teichberg and Changeux, 1976). The intercon-version between the two forms may therefore result from some covalent modification. A possible candidate for such a modification is a phosphorylation-dephosphorylation of the receptor protein by a protein kinase-phosphoprotein phosphatase present in the crude extract. The known inhibition of the phosphatase by fluoride ions would explain the dif-ferential effect of NaCl and NaF (Teichberg and Changeux, 1977). Recently, it has been shown by immunoelectrophoresis with an antiserum directed against the receptor protein purified by affinity chromatography from *E. electricus* electric organ, that in the crude extracts, after incubation with $[^{32}P]$-γ-ATP, the band corresponding to the receptor immunoprecipitate is ^{32}P-labeled. SDS electrophoresis of the immunoprecipitate reveals that the 48,000 rather than the 40,000 dalton chain of the receptor protein is preferentially phosphorylated (Teichberg et al., 1977).

There is no doubt that the receptor protein from *Electrophorus* electric organ can be covalently modified, but several questions still remain open about the biological significance of this modification. First of all, the 48,000 dalton component of the receptor molecule, and not the 40,000 one, appears to be the substrate of the phosphorylation reaction. Recent work on *Torpedo* receptor indicates that only the 40,000 dalton component, labeled by Karlin affinity reagent $[^{3}H]$MPTA (Sobel et al., 1977), would belong to the receptor molecule in the strict sense. On the other hand, two-dimensional SDS gel analysis of radiolabeled receptor from calf myotubes show a micro-heterogeneity of the 40,000 component which might also reveal a covalent modification of this particular chain (Merlie et al., 1978); secondly, there is no direct evidence yet that a phosphorylation of the receptor protein is involved in its stabilization during localization; the shift in isoelectric point can be taken only as *indirect* evidence. Thirdly, if such a modification were indeed responsible for the stabilization of the receptor molecule, it could represent only one among a cascade of reactions (not necessarily covalent) which finally lead to the genesis of the subneural apparatus of the adult neuromuscular junction.

(d) Factors regulating the postsynaptic localization of the acetylcholine receptor protein.
As already mentioned, the fusion of myoblasts into myotubes is accompanied by a marked increase of receptor synthesis, which manifests itself as an increase of the total number of receptor molecules in a given muscle. It is interesting to note that at the time when synapses are forming, the total content of muscle receptor molecules begins to decline (Betz et al., 1977). This is particularly striking after the 12th day of incubation in the fast, focally innervated posterior latissimus dorsi, or in the breast muscle of chick embryro (in the slow ALD with distributed innervation the total content in receptor tends to level off without any significant decrease). Two possibilities may account for such a behavior. Either the rate of degradation of the receptor protein in the extrasynaptic areas increases (for instance as a function of electrical activity: Stent (1973) proposed that the inversion of potential caused by the propagation of the action potential was responsible for enhanced degradation of the extrasynaptic receptor) or, alternatively, the synthesis of acetylcholine receptor stops, with the receptor protein under the nerve terminals becoming stabilized, and the extrasynaptic molecules continuing to be degraded at the same rate as in the embryonic (non-innervated) myotube.

Examination of the degradation of the α-bungarotoxin-labeled receptor in ovo does not reveal any gross increase of the degradation rate, but rather a tendency to slow down (Betz, unpublished observations). The overall decrease of receptor content should therefore result from a shut-off of its synthesis. An interesting possibility would then be that it is the activity of the muscle fiber (electrical, mechanical, or both) which, directly or indirectly, causes this shut-off. In agreement with this suggestion are the findings that stimulation of denervated rat diaphragm causes a decrease of total receptor content, without any increase in its rate of degradation (Hogan et al., 1976). Similar results have also been found as a consequence of in vitro electrical stimulation of developing myotubes (Shainberg and Burstein, 1976). The chemical nature of the signal which accounts for the shut-off is not known. Possible candidates are Ca^{2+} ions (Rasmussen, 1970; Rose and Loewenstein, 1975), cyclic nucleotides

(Tomkins, 1975; Greengard, 1976), or both. Ca^{2+} would be a rather simple 'shut-off' factor, since it could enter through either the cholinergic ionophore (Takeuchi, 1963; Kasai and Changeux, 1971; Evans, 1974) or the tetrodotoxin-sensitive ionic channels when these are activated. Signals directly coupled with the mechanical contraction of the muscle may also play a role. In any case, a first target for the regulation of acetylcholine receptor metabolism in the postsynaptic cell is the protein synthesis machinery. It is interesting to note that the onset of activity has a 'negative' effect on this synthesis.

Another target for the regulation of receptor metabolism is, as already mentioned, the area of the cytoplasmic membrane which underlies the ingrowing nerve terminal. At this level, sooner or later, the receptor molecule becomes immobilized and resistant to proteolysis. Again, the factors which regulate this process have not yet been identified. To test the possibility that the neurotransmitter is indeed such a factor, high doses of snake α-toxin were chronically injected into the yolk sac of chick embryo (at the 3rd, 8th, 12th day of incubation). Under these conditions the spontaneous movements of the embryo stop but the embryo does not die, although a serious atrophy of the skeletal muscles takes place. Localization of acetylcholinesterase was followed by the Koelle technique, which revealed very few end-plates in the chronically paralyzed embryos (Giacobini et al., 1973; Gordon et al., 1974; Gordon and Vrbova, 1975). The chronic injection of a postsynaptic blocking agent interferes directly or indirectly with the localization of the esterase. An 'anterograde' factor is involved, perhaps even the neurotransmitter itself. However, this role in localization of the receptor protein has been challenged (Steinbach et al., 1973), despite the fact that it provides a simple explanation for the segregation of different receptor molecules in a complex situation, such as that of a neuronal soma receiving nerve terminals with different neurotransmitters. Other factors liberated by the nerve terminals, such as ATP (Whittaker, 1973) or some of its degradation products, enzymes or polypeptide hormones, might have to be considered as well. Liberated ATP would offer a convenient energy supply for reactions taking place on the external surface of the membrane. Alternative (or additonal) processes which do not require the emission of a diffusible signal can also be envisioned, such as a 'patching' (Edelman, 1976) of the receptor molecules in the postsynaptic membrane, either spontaneously or resulting from direct physical contact with the nerve terminal.

In summary, to account for the localization of the receptor protein, it has been postulated (Changeux and Danchin, 1976) that:

(1) the receptor may exist in two interconvertible forms (L, labile diffusible, and S, immobilized and resistant to degradation);

(2) the S state derives from the L state by way of a stabilization reaction (L → S) which is not reversible, the reaction taking place when an anterograde factor is liberated by the nerve terminal during activity;

(3) the synthesis of the labile form of the receptor protein stops in the postsynaptic cell when activity starts in the myotube. An internal 'shut-off' factor would act selectively on the protein synthesis machinery. Accordingly, the selective localization process would correspond to the management of a fixed and limited stock of L via lateral diffusion and stabilization reactions.

The proposed model gives rise to several predictions which suggest experimental tests for the validity of its critical assumptions.

(1) If localization corresponds to the management of a limited pool of receptor protein, changing the size of this pool by selectively blocking receptor synthesis before the arrival of the nerve terminals should interfere with localization, and/or reduce the number of end-plates formed in a muscle like ALD. The 'immunity' to innervation of the extrasynaptic

areas in an adult muscle fiber would then result simply from the absence of receptor mole-cules available in the extrasynaptic membrane for forming a new end-plate.

(2) The activity of the postsynaptic cell is supposed to regulate the synthesis of receptor through the shut-off factor, but also to control the management of the membrane pool of receptor through the stabilization reaction. Once the synthesis of receptor has stopped, changes in the program of activity of the developing nerve terminals by chronic stimulation (or blocking) may lead to the formation of supernumerary end-plates (or prevent localiza-tion) or, thanks to the internal coupling factor for instance, modify the distance between end-plates. In ALD this may indeed occur. In agreement with these views is the recent observation that spontaneous activity markedly differs in the slow ALD with multiple end-plates and the focally innervated fast ALD from chick embryo (16—18-day-old) (ALD fires continuously at a rate of 0.2—5 Hz, Vrbova, unpublished observations). Chronic blocking of synaptic transmission might also modify the pattern of end-plates and their relative distance in these muscles (Gordon et al., 1974).

Presynaptic stabilization of the nerve terminals

In the chick embryo (Hamburger, 1934, 1958; Hamburger and Levi-Montalcini, 1949) and in amphibians (Prestige, 1965, 1967a, b) early limb bud extirpation causes a massive depletion of both motor neurons and sensory ganglion cells, accompanied by a decrease of the enzyme choline acetyltransferase in the spinal cord. Removal of the peripheral target cells dramatically enhances the 'normally occurring cell death'. An interaction with the periphery is therefore required for the neuron to continue its development. Similarly, in the mouse cerebellar mutant 'staggerer', a massive regression of the parallel fibers and granule cells occurs at late stages of development (Sotelo and Changeux, 1974), and has been attri-buted to the failure of parallel fibers to establish normal synapses with the Purkinje cells (which show electrophysiological signs of abnormality (Crepel and Mariani, 1975) and lack a characteristic membrane protein (Mallet et al., 1976)).

In both instances, the stabilization of the nerve terminals is regulated in a 'retrograde' manner, by their interaction with the target cell. To test the possibility that the activity of the postsynaptic cell has any effect on this regulation, several cholinergic agents or toxins known to selectively block neuromuscular transmission were injected into developing chick embryos. These drugs stop the spontaneous movements of the embryo which may, never-theless, survive until hatching. Such treatment causes a marked atrophy of skeletal muscles, which show signs of delayed differentiation and of regression (Giacobini et al., 1973; Giacobini-Robecchi et al., 1975, 1976), and, as already mentioned, interfere with the localization of acetylcholinesterase. Interestingly, some of these pharmacological agents, despite their almost exclusively postsynaptic site of action, affect the motor innervation of the muscle. Chronic injection of high doses of *Naja nigricollis* α-toxin (e.g., Giacobini et al., 1973) or of Flaxedil (Bourgeois, unpublished observations) causes a decrease in the total content of presynaptic choline acetyltransferase within the muscle (and also in the sciatic nerve), and a dramatic reduction in the total number of myelinated and non-myelinated axons in the ventral roots of the spinal nerves (no significant change takes place in the dorsal roots). A selective loss of the motor nerve terminals and of the motor neurons also occurs.

How can an essentially postsynaptic block influence the motor nerve terminal? The possibility that the α-toxin interferes with the 'recognition' step at the early stages of synapse formation is made unlikely by the observation that primitive junctions (as well as the content of choline acetyltransferase) in embryos injected at the 4th day of incubation do not differ significantly from those of the non-injected control until the 12th day of incubation. Similarly, D-tubocurarine or α-bungarotoxin do not prevent synapse formation in vitro (Crain and Peterson, 1971; Cohen, 1972; Steinbach, 1974) or prevent re-innervation of adult rat diaphragm (Van Essen and Jansen, 1974). Therefore it is the stabilization of the preformed neuromuscular contacts which requires a functional interaction with the muscle. The activity of the muscle apparently exerts, either in a direct or (most likely) an indirect manner, a positive feedback on the stabilization of its innervation.

Recent evidence indicates that the late phase of maturation of the neuromuscular junction, the regression of its polyneuronal innervation, is also coupled with the actual 'functioning' of the neuromuscular junction. One of the tendons of the sartorius muscle in infant rats was sectioned and the evolution of the polyneural innervation followed by electrophysiological techniques; the amplitude of the 'compound' end-plate potential increases stepwise as a function of stimulus strength, revealing the presence of several 'functional' motor axons converging to the same motor end-plate (Redfern, 1970; Bennett and Pettigrew, 1974; Benoit and Changeux, 1975; Brown et al., 1976). Tenotomy significantly delays the decrease in the number of steps of the compound end-plate potential observed during the first postnatal weeks (Benoit and Changeux, 1975). Partial deafferentation of the same muscle has similar consequences (Brown et al., 1976). In these two instances, however, it is not known how the chronic firing of the motor neuron is modified, but in both cases the mechanical contraction of the muscle appears seriously disturbed.

A more direct test of the effect of nerve activity on the stabilization of the motor terminals was carried out during re-innervation of soleus muscle in adult rats (Benoit and Changeux, 1977). Indeed, in the course of re-innervation following the crush of the sciatic nerve, a transient multi-innervation of the muscle fibers takes place, although to a smaller extent than during development. Application of a cuff of local anesthetic (lidocaine) on the regenerating terminal immediately after crushing the nerve enhances the magnitude of the transient multi-innervation and delays its regression. The most likely interpretation of this effect is that the local anesthetic, by blocking the activity of the motor nerve, causes the regressive process to slow down. In other words, the elimination of redundant nerve terminals and the consequent selective stabilization of one motor axon per muscle fiber is an 'active' process, regulated by the electrical activity of the motor nerve and/or its postsynaptic target.

A similar situation may take place in the cerebellum, although in this system only electrophysiological evidence is as yet available. In the adult, the majority (more than 90%) of the Purkinje cells receive only one climbing fiber (Eccles et al., 1966). Unit recordings in 8–9-day-old rats show that, at this early stage, the response of the Purkinje cell to climbing fiber stimulation is 'complex' or 'compound' as in the case of the immature neuromuscular junction (Crepel et al., 1976; Crepel and Mariani, 1976): more than 50% of the Purkinje cells would be innervated by at least two distinct climbing fibers. A subsequent regressive phenomenon leads, as early as 15 days after birth, to the one-to-one relationship seen in the adult. Several experimental situations exist where the major input of the Purkinje cells, the granule cells and their parallel fibers, is suppressed by X-irradiation of the newborn, or as a consequence of the mutations 'weaver' and 'reeler' (in which case only the Purkinje cells of the central mass are deafferented (Mariani et al., 1977)). In all these agranular cerebella the multiple innervation by climbing fibers persists into adulthood.

Despite the fact that little information is available on the *late* stabilization of the synapse, one may propose a rather simple model which could account for the selective stabilization of one motor axon per muscle fiber: (1) all the motor nerve terminals converging on a given end-plate receive the same average number of impulses, but in a randomly non-synchronous manner; (2) at the peak of the multi-innervation stage, all terminals share almost equivalent areas of the stabilized subsynaptic membrane surface, and/or dispose of a limited stock of a postsynaptic 'retrograde factor', x; (3) at this 'critical' stage, the arrival of impulses cause an increase of surface occupancy and/or of utilization of x; and (4) when the surface occupied by the nerve terminal (and/or the amount of x utilized) becomes lower than a critical value, this nerve terminal regresses.

This set of minimal assumptions can explain both the stabilization of a single nerve terminal and the constant size of the motor units. Accordingly, the size of the motor unit would be determined by the ratio of the number of muscle fibers to that of motor neurons, which prediction can be tested. An increase of surface occupancy by nerve terminals as a consequence of activity has been described, but the biochemical mechanisms by which a nerve terminal becomes stabilized once a critical surface of the postsynaptic membrane is occupied remains obscure. The postulated retrograde factor has not been identified chemically; in the case of the neuromuscular junction, the concentration of calcium or of nerve growth factor in the cleft are possible candidates. An interesting possibility would be that the retrograde effect consists in the covalent modification of presynaptic fibrillar or tubular proteins engaged in the maintenance of the shape of the nerve terminal by, for instance, regulating its internal 'cytoplasmic flow'. In this view, a 'shut-off' of the axoplasmic flow in a nerve terminal due to the lack of a retrograde factor would cause the regression of this nerve terminal.

CONCLUSIONS AND SUMMARY

From a biochemical point of view, the selective stabilization hypothesis appears to be quite plausible. Four different signalling mechanisms have been postulated to govern the evolution of a developing synapse: (a) *for the postsynaptic localization of the receptor protein*, one or more anterograde factor liberated by the nerve terminals (possibly the transmitter itself) which governs the localization and stabilization reactions of the receptor, an internal shut-off signal which informs the protein biosynthesis machinery (transcription and/or translation) of the activity of the postsynaptic cell (an internal coupling factor which permits exchange of information between synapses) and (b) *for the selective presynaptic stabilization of the nerve terminals*, a retrograde factor emitted by the postsynaptic cell. Additional mechanisms and regulatory signals may need to be postulated in the future to account for the complete stabilization and maturation of the synapse, which is certainly a complex process lasting for days or even weeks.

The basic assumption of the theory (Changeux et al., 1973; Changeux and Danchin, 1976), i.e. that an increase of 'specificity' accompanies the active stabilization of particular synapses (and the regression of others) at a 'critical period' of development, remains to be tested with neuronal networks (cerebellum, visual cortex) which are more complex than is the motor innervation of the striated muscle.

In a more general manner, these speculations place emphasis on critical features of developing neuronal networks which are directly accessible to experimentation: (1) their early activity (spontaneous or evoked) preceding synapse maturation; (2) the existence and limits of a transient redundancy (in the case of motor innervation the limits of the fluctuation are the boundaries of the muscle (Landmesser and Morris, 1975)); and (3) an eventual modification of this redundancy by chronic changes of the early activity.

Even if the limits of the redundancy are narrow, they may be sufficient to provide an opportunity for a significant saving of genes during the differentiation of neuronal networks, and also to provide a plausible biochemical mechanism for 'learning' without the necessity of postulating the synthesis of new molecular species.

REFERENCES

Alper, R., Lowy, J. and Schmidt, J. (1974) Binding properties of acetylcholine receptors extracted from normal and from denervated rat diaphragm, *FEBS Lett.*, 48: 130–134.

Altman, J. and Anderson, W. (1972) Experimental reorganisation of the cerebellum cortex. I. Morphological effects of elimination of all microneurons with prolonged X-irradiation started at birth, *J. comp. Neurol.*, 146: 355–406.

Avrameas, S. (1972) Enzyme-markers: their linkage with proteins and use in immuno-histochemistry, *Histochem. J.*, 4: 321–330.

Axelrod, D., Ravdin, P., Koppel, D.E., Schlessinger, J., Webb, W.W., Elson, E.L. and Podleski, T.R. (1976) Lateral motion of fluorescently labeled acetylcholine receptors in membranes of developing muscle fibers, *Proc. nat. Acad. Sci. (Wash.)*, 73: 4594–4598.

Axelson, J. and Thesleff, S. (1959) A study of supersensitivity in denervated mammalian skeletal muscle, *J. Physiol. (Lond.)*, 147: 178–193.

Barnard, E., Wieckowski, J. and Chiu, T.H. (1971) Cholinergic receptor molecules and cholinesterase molecules at mouse skeletal muscle junctions, *Nature (Lond.)*, 234: 297–309.

Bennett, M. and Pettigrew, A. (1974) The formation of synapses in striated muscle during development, *J. Physiol. (Lond.)*, 241: 515–545.

Benoit, P. and Changeux, J.P. (1975) Consequences of tenotomy on the evolution of multi-innervation in developing rat soleus muscle, *Brain Res.*, 99: 354–358.

Benoit, P. and Changeux, J.P. (1977) Effect of nerve activity on the evolution of multi-innervation at the regenerating neuromuscular junction of the rat, *Brain Res.*, in press.

Beranek, R. and Vyskocil, F. (1967) The action of tubocurarine and atropine on the normal and denervated rat diaphragm, *J. Physiol. (Lond.)*, 188: 53–66.

Berg, D. and Hall, Z.W. (1975) Loss of α-bungarotoxin from junctional and extrajunctional acetylcholine receptors in rat diaphragm muscle in vivo and in organ culture, *J. Physiol. (Lond.)*, 252: 771–789.

Betz, H., Bourgeois, J.P. and Changeux, J.P. (1977) Evidence for degradation of the acetylcholine (nicotinic) receptor in skeletal muscle during the development of the chick embryo, *FEBS Lett.*, 77: 219–224.

Birks, R., Katz, B. and Miledi, R. (1960) Physiological and structural changes at the amphibian myoneural junction in the course of nerve degeneration, *J. Physiol. (Lond.)*, 150: 145–168.

Bourgeois, J.P. (1974) *Localization du Site Récepteur de l'Acétylcholine sur l'Electroplaque Normale et Dénervée du Gymnote.* Doctoral dissertation, University of Paris.

Bourgeois, J.P., Popot, J.L., Ryter, A. and Changeux, J.P. (1973) Consequences of denervation on the distribution of the cholinergic (nicotinic) receptor sites from *Electrophorus electricus* revealed by high resolution autoradiography, *Brain Res.*, 62: 557–563.

Bourgeois, J.P., Ryter, A., Menez, A., Fromageot, P., Boquet, P. and Changeux, J.P. (1972) Localization of the cholinergic receptor protein in eel electroplax by high resolution autoradiography, *FEBS Lett.*, 25: 127–133.

Brockes, J. and Hall, Z.W. (1975) Acetylcholine receptors in normal and denervated rat diaphragm muscles. II. Comparison of junctional and extrajunctional receptors, *Biochemistry*, 14: 2100–2106.

Brown, M.C., Jansen, J.K. and Van Essen, D. (1976) Polyneuronal innervation of skeletal muscle in newborn rats and its elimination during maturation, *J. Physiol. (Lond.)*, 261: 387–422.

Cajal, S. Ramón y (1911) *Histologie du Système Nerveux de l'Homme et des Vertébrés*, Maloine, Paris.

Chang, C. and Huang, M. (1975) Turnover of junctional and extrajunctional acetylcholine receptors of the rat diaphragm, *Nature (Lond.)*, 253: 643–644.

Changeux, J.P., Courrège, P. and Danchin, A. (1973) A theory of the epigenesis of neuronal networks by selective stabilization of synapses, *Proc. nat. Acad. Sci. (Wash.)*, 70: 2974–2978.

Changeux, J.P. and Danchin, A. (1976) The selective stabilization of developing synapses as a mechanism for the specification of neuronal networks, *Nature (Lond.)*, 264: 705–712.

62

Cohen, M.W. (1972) The development of neuromuscular connections in the presence of D-tubocurarine, *Brain Res.*, 41: 457–463.

Colquhoun, D. and Rang, H.P., (1976) Effects of inhibitors on the binding of iodinated α-bungarotoxin to acetylcholine receptors in rat muscle, *Molec. Pharmacol.*, 12: 519–535.

Crain, S.M. and Peterson, E.R. (1971) Development of paired explants of fetal spinal cord and adult skeletal muscle during chronic exposure to curare and hemicholinium, *In Vitro*, 6: 373.

Crepel, F., Delhaye-Bouchaud, N. and Legrand, J. (1976) Electrophysiological analysis of the circuitry and of the corticonuclear relationships in the agranular cerebellum of irradiated rats, *Arch. ital. Biol.*, 114: 49–74.

Crepel, F. and Mariani, J. (1975) Anatomical, physiological and biochemical studies of the cerebellum from mutant mice. I. Electrophysiological analysis of cerebellar cortical neurons in the Staggerer mouse, *Brain Res.*, 98: 135–147.

Crepel, F. and Mariani, J. (1976) Multiple innervation of Purkinje cells by climbing fibres in the cerebellum of the Weaver mutant mouse, *J. Neurobiol.*, 7: 579–582.

Crepel, F., Mariani, J. and Delhaye-Bouchaud, N. (1976) Evidence for a multiple innervation of Purkinje cells by climbing fibres in the immature rat cerebellum, *J. Neurobiol.*, 7: 567–578.

Crepel, F., Mariani, J., Korn, H. et Changeux, J.P. (1973) Electrophysiologie du cortex cerebelleux chez la souris mutante 'Staggerer', *C.R. Acad. Sci.*, 277 D: 2761–2763.

Devreotes, P. and Fambrough, D.M. (1976) Synthesis of acetylcholine receptors by cultured chick myotubes and denervated mouse extensor digitorum longus muscles, *Proc. nat. Acad. Sci. (Wash.)*, 73: 161–164.

Eccles, J., Ito, M. and Szentagothai, J. (1967) *The Cerebellum as a Neuronal Machine*, Springer, Berlin.

Eccles, J.C., Llinas, R. and Sasaki, K. (1966) The excitatory synaptic action of climbing fibres on the Purkinje cells of the cerebellum, *J. Physiol. (Lond.)*, 182: 268–296.

Edelman, G.M. (1976) Surface modulation in cell recognition and cell growth, *Science*, 192: 218–225.

Evans, R.H. (1974) The entry of labelled calcium into the innervated region of the mouse diaphragm muscle, *J. Physiol. (Lond.)*, 240: 517–533.

Fambrough, D.E. (1974) Cellular and developmental biology of acetylcholine receptors in skeletal muscle. In E. de Robertis and J. Schacht (Eds.), *Neurochemistry of Cholinergic Receptors*, Raven Press, New York, pp. 85–113.

Fambrough, D. and Hartzell, H.C. (1972) Acetylcholine receptors: number and distribution at neuromuscular junctions in rat diaphragm, *Science*, 176: 189–191.

Fertuck, K. and Salpeter, M. (1974) Localization of acetylcholine receptor by ^{125}I-labelled α-bungarotoxin binding at mouse motor end-plate, *Proc. nat. Acad. Sci. (Wash.)*, 71: 1376–1378.

Fischbach, G., Berg, D., Cohen, S. and Frank, E. (1976) Enrichment of nerve-muscle synapses in spinal cord-muscle cultures and identification of relative peaks of ACh sensitivity at sites of transmitter release, *Cold Spr. Harb. Symp. quant. Biol.*, 40: 347–357.

Frank, E., Gautvik, K. and Sommershild, H. (1975) Cholinergic receptors at denervated mammalian end-plates, *Acta physiol. scand.*, 95: 66–76.

Gaze, R. (1970) *The Formation of Nerve Connections*, Academic Press, London.

Giacobini, G., Filogamo, G., Weber, M., Boquet, P. and Changeux, J.P. (1973) Effects of a snake α-neurotoxin on the development of innervated motor muscles in chick embryo, *Proc. nat. Acad. Sci. (Wash.)*, 70: 1708–1712.

Giacobini-Robecchi, M.G., Giacobini, G., Filogamo, G. and Changeux, J.P. (1975) Effects of the type A toxin from *C. botulinum* on the development of skeletal muscles and of their innervation in chick embryo, *Brain Res.*, 83: 107–121.

Giacobini-Robecchi, M.G., Giacobini, G., Filogamo, G. et Changeux, J.P., (1976) Effets comparés de l'injection chronique de toxine α de *Naja nigricollis* et de toxine botulinique A sur le développement des racines dorsales et ventrales de la moelle épinière d'embryons de poulet, *C.R. Acad. Sci. (Paris)*, 283: 271–274.

Gordon, T., Perry, R., Tuffery, A. and Vrbova, G. (1974) Possible mechanisms determining synapse formation in developing skeletal muscles of the chick, *Cell Tiss. Res.*, 155: 13–25.

Gordon, T. and Vrbova, G. (1975) Changes in chemosensitivity of developing chick muscle fibres in relation to end-plate formation, *Pflüger's Arch. ges Physiol.*, 360: 349–364.

Greengard, P. (1976) Possible role for cyclic nucleotides and phosphorylated membrane proteins in postsynaptic actions of neuro-transmitters, *Nature (Lond.)*, 260: 101–108.

Gutmann, E. and Young, J.Z. (1944) The reinnervation of muscles after various periods of atrophy, *J. Anat. (Lond.)*, 78: 15–43.

Hamburger, V. (1934) The effects of wing bud extirpation on the development of the central nervous system in chick embryos, *J. exp. Zool.*, 68: 449–494.

Hamburger, V. (1958) Regression versus peripheral control of differentiation in motor hypoplasia, *Amer. J. Anat.*, 102: 365–410.

Hamburger, V. (1970) In F.O. Schmidt (Ed.), *Neurosciences Second Study Program*, Rockefeller Univ. Press, New York, pp. 141–151.

Hamburger, V. and Levi-Montalcini, R. (1949) Proliferation, differentiation and degeneration in the spinal ganglia of the chick embryo under normal and experimental conditions, *J. exp. Zool.*, 111: 457–502.

Hartzell, C. and Fambrough, D. (1973) Acetylcholine receptor production and incorporation into membranes of developing muscle fibers, *Develop. Biol.*, 30: 153–165.

Hirano, A. and Dembitzer, H. (1975) The fine structure of Staggerer cerebellum, *J. Neuropathol. exp. Neurol.*, 34: 1–11.

Hogan, P., Marshall, J.P. and Hall, Z.W. (1976) Muscle activity decreases rate of degradation of α-bungarotoxin bound to extrajunctional acetylcholine receptors, *Nature (Lond.)*, 261: 328–330.

Jacobson, M. (1969) Development of specific neuronal connections, *Science*, 163: 543–547.

Kasai, M. and Changeux, J.P. (1971) In vitro excitation of purified membrane fragments by cholinergic agonists. II. The permeability change caused by cholinergic agonists, *J. Membr. Biol.*, 6: 24–57.

Katz, B. and Miledi, R. (1972) The statistical nature of the acetylcholine potential and its molecular components, *J. Physiol. (Lond.)*, 224: 665–699.

Landmesser, L. and Morris, D. (1975) The development of functional innervation in the hind limb of the chick embryo, *J. Physiol. (Lond.)*, 249: 301–326.

Landis, S. (1971) Cerebellar cortical development in the Staggerer mutant mouse, *J. Cell Biol.*, 51: 159a.

Lee, C.Y., Tseng, L. and Chiu, T. (1967) Influence of denervation on localization of neurotoxins from elapid venoms in rat diaphragm, *Nature (Lond.)*, 215: 1177–1178.

Levinthal, F., Macagno, E. and Levinthal, C. (1975) Anatomy and development of identified cells in isogenic organisms, *Cold Spr. Harb. Symp. quant. Biol.*, 40: 321–331.

Llinas, R., Hillman, D. and Precht, W. (1973) Neuronal circuit reorganization in mammalian agranular cerebellar cortex, *J. Neurobiol.*, 4: 69–94.

Mallet, J., Huchet, M., Pougeois, R. and Changeux, J.P. (1976) Anatomical, physiological and biochemical studies on the cerebellum from mutant mice. III. Protein differences associated with the Weaver, Staggerer and nervous mutations, *Brain Res.*, 103: 291–312.

Mariani, J., Crepel, F., Mikoshiba, K., Changeux, J.P. and Sotelo, C. (1977) Anatomical, physiological and biochemical studies of the cerebellum from Reeler mutant mouse, *Phil. Trans. B*, 281: 1–28.

Merlie, J., Changeux, J.P. and Gros, F. (1976) Acetylcholine receptor degradation measured by pulse chase labeling, *Nature (Lond.)*, 264: 74–76.

Merlie, J., Changeux, J.P. and Gros, F., (1978) Skeletal muscle acetylcholine receptor: purification, characterization and turnover in muscle cell cultures, *J. biol. Chem.*, in press.

Merlie, J., Sobel, A., Changeux, J.P. and Gros, F. (1975) Synthesis of acetylcholine receptor during differentiation of cultured embryonic muscle cells, *Proc. nat. Acad. Sci. (Wash.)*, 72: 4028–4032.

Mikoshiba, K. and Changeux, J.P. (1978) Morphological and biochemical studies on isolated molecular and granular layers from bovine cerebellum, *Brain Res.*, 142: 487–504.

Mikoshiba, K., Huchet, M. and Changeux, J.P. (1977a) Biochemical studies on P400 protein: a cerebellar protein. In *Proc. Int. Meet. Neurochem. Soc., Copenhagen* (abstract).

Mikoshiba, K., Teichberg, V.I. and Changeux, J.P. (1977b) Biochemical studies on the cerebellum of neurological mutants of mice: role for glutamic acid and cholinergic system. In *Proc. Int. Meet. Neurochem. Soc., Copenhagen* (abstract).

Miledi, R. (1960) The acetylcholine sensitivity of frog muscle fibres after complete or partial denervation, *J. Physiol. (Lond.)*, 151: 1–23.

Porter, C. and Barnard, E. (1975) The density of cholinergic receptors at the endplate postsynaptic membrane: ultra-structural studies in two mammalian species, *J. Membr. Biol.*, 20: 31–49.

Prestige, M.C. (1965) Cell turnover in the spinal ganglia of *Xenopus laevis* tadpoles, *J. Embryol. exp. Morphol.*, 13: 63–72.

Prestige, M.C. (1967a) The control of cell number in the lumbar spinal ganglia during the development of *Xenopus laevis* tadpoles, *J. Embryol. exp. Morphol.*, 17: 453–471.

Prestige, M.C. (1967b) The control of cell number in the lumbar ventral horns during the development of *Xenopus laevis* tadpoles, *J. Embryol. exp. Morphol.*, 18: 359–387.

64

Prestige, M. and Willshaw, D. (1975) On a role for competition in the formation of patterned neural connexions, *Proc. roy. Soc. B*, 190: 77–98.

Rakic, P. (1976) Synaptic specificity in the cerebellar cortex: study of anomalous circuits induced by single gene mutations in mice, *Cold Spr. Harb. Symp. quant. Biol.*, 40: 333–346.

Rasmussen, H. (1970) Cell communication, calcium ion and cyclic adenosine monophosphate, *Science*, 170: 404–412.

Redfern, P. (1970) Neuromuscular transmission in newborn rats, *J. Physiol. (Lond.)*, 209: 701–709.

Ripley, K.L. and Provine, R.R. (1972) Neural correlates of embryonic motility in the chick, *Brain Res.*, 45: 127–134.

Rose, B. and Loewenstein, W. (1975) Calcium ion distribution in cytoplasm visualized by aequorin: distribution in the cytosol is restricted due to energized sequestring, *Science*, 190: 1204–1206.

Sax, D.S., Hirano, A. and Shoper, R.J. (1968) Staggerer, a neurological murine mutant. An electron microscopic study of the cerebellar cortex in the adult, *Neurology (Minneap.)*, 18: 1093–1100.

Shainberg, A. and Burstein, M. (1976) Decrease of acetylcholine receptor synthesis in muscle cultures by electrical stimulation, *Nature (Lond.)*, 264: 368–369.

Sidman, R. (1974) In A. Moscona (Ed.) *The Cell Surface in Development*, Wiley, New York, pp. 221–253.

Sobel, A., Weber, M. and Changeux, J.P. (1977) Large scale purification of the acetylcholine receptor protein in its membrane-bound and detergent-extracted forms from *Torpedo marmorata* electric organ, *Europ. J. Biochem.*, 80: 215–224.

Sotelo, C. (1975) Anatomical, physiological and biochemical studies of the cerebellum from mutant mice. II. Morphological study of cerebellar cortical neurons and circuits in the Weaver mouse, *Brain Res.*, 94: 19–44.

Sotelo, C. and Changeux, J.P. (1974) Trans-synaptic degeneration 'en cascade' in the cerebellar cortex of Staggerer mutant mice, *Brain Res.*, 67: 519–526.

Sperry, R. (1963) Chemoaffinity in the orderly growth of nerve fiber patterns and connections, *Proc. nat. Acad. Sci. (Wash.)*, 50: 703–710.

Steinbach, J.H. (1974) Role of muscle activity in nerve-muscle interaction in vitro, *Nature (Lond.)*, 248: 70–71.

Steinbach, J.H., Harris, A.J., Patrick, J., Schubert, D. and Heinemann, S. (1973) Nerve-muscle interaction in vitro, *J. gen. Physiol.*, 62: 255–270.

Stent, G. (1973) A physiological mechanism for Hebb's postulate of learning, *Proc. nat. Acad Sci. (Wash.)*, 70: 997–1001.

Takeuchi, N. (1963) Effects of calcium on the conductance change of the end-plate membrane during the action of transmitter, *J. Physiol. (Lond.)*, 167: 141–155.

Teichberg, V. and Changeux, J.P. (1976) Presence of two forms with different isoelectric points of the acetylcholine receptor in the electric organ of *Electrophorus electricus* and their catalytic interconversion in vitro, *FEBS Lett.*, 67: 264–268.

Teichberg, V. and Changeux, J.P. (1977) Evidence for protein phosphorylation and dephosphorylation in membrane fragments isolated from the electric organ of *Electrophorus electricus*, *FEBS Lett.*, 74: 71–76.

Teichberg, V., Sobel, A. and Changeux, J.P. (1977) In vitro phosphorylation of acetylcholine receptor, *Nature (Lond.)*, 267: 540–542.

Tello, F. (1917) Genesis de las terminaciones nerviosas motrices y sensitivas. *Trab. lab. Invest. Biol. Univ. Madrid*, 15: 101.

Tomkins, G. (1975) The metabolic code, *Science*, 189: 760–763.

Tower, S. (1939) The reaction of muscle to denervation, *Physiol. Rev.*, 19: 1–48.

Van Essen, D. and Jansen, J.K. (1974) Reinnervation of the rat diaphragm during perfusion with α-bungarotoxin, *Acta physiol. scand.*, 91: 571–573.

Whittaker, V.P. (1973) The biochemistry of synaptic transmission, *Naturwissenschaften*, 60: 281–289.

Whittaker, V.P. and Barker, L.A. (1972) In R. Fried (Ed.), *Methods of Neurochemistry, Vol. 2*, Dekker, New York, pp. 1–28.

Wiesel, T. and Hubel, D. (1974) Ordered arrangement of orientation columns in monkeys lacking visual experience, *J. comp. Neurol.*, 158: 307–318.

DISCUSSION

SOTELO: How effective is the nerve cuff in the chronic anesthetic experiments: is it really blocking all impulse activity? In the cerebellar cortex lacking in parallel fibers, multiple innervation of the Purkinje cells by climbing fibers persists for the life of the animal.

CHANGEUX: Both in the cuff and in the tenotomy experiments, unfortunately, activity was blocked for only a limited period of time. As a consequence of the anesthetic cuff placed on the sciatic nerve, the leg is paralyzed for at least one week. In the case of tenotomy with newborn rats, a reinsertion of the tendon takes place after a week or two. This is the reason why, in the adult, the one-to-one relationship between motor nerve and muscle fiber becomes reestablished. The situation is more favorable in cerebellar mutants, because the mutation gives a completely irreversible lesion. On the other hand, it becomes difficult to decide if the nerve activity regulates only *synapse* development or the lack of parallel fibers per se.

JANSEN: In the case of the neuromuscular junction, there is indirect evidence that activity in the motor units cannot be the decisive factor. After normal development of the soleus muscle you end up with the original group of motor units, all approximately of equal size. If activity had been important, one might expect to have some motor units in the end that were very much larger than the others. Recently, moreover, we have also looked at the effect of prolonged reversible nerve blocks on the maturation of the pattern of innervation in newborn animals. With impulse activity blocked we find that, initially, the elimination of polyneuronal innervation proceeds normally. Then there is a second phase when the motor axons start to sprout, and we believe that this second stage is due to the inactivity of the muscle fibers.

CORNER: What do you think might be the 'purpose' during development of having a larger target area innervated, to begin with, than is necessary? I can understand the significance of having a given spot *multiply innervated*, but what about the converse side of the picture?

CHANGEUX: I think it is an easy way of getting every muscle innervated without precisely specifying which nerve terminal ends in which muscle fiber. A larger number than needed of synaptic contacts are established in a redundant manner, and the superfluous ones are eliminated, so that ultimately each muscle fiber is left with only one nerve terminal. This is an excellent way of getting the complete innervation of all the fibers from a given muscle to have a regular pattern of innervation and also a fixed size of motor units.

CORNER: I understand that, but it seems to me that this would be achieved simply by a large redundancy of motor neurons. Might not this question of the extensive initial field of a given efferent fiber in fact be a *different* phenomenon from the convergence of multiple innervation onto a single cell?

CHANGEUX: I think it is the same thing. To have multiply innervated muscle fibers means that each motor neuron has a larger field of innervation than if the muscle fibers were mono-innervated. Concerning the role of activity in this scheme: I think it might be an indirect one, in the sense that there could be factors which are liberated by the muscle cells only when they have reached a certain level of maturity. These factors are presumably present in limited amounts in the postsynaptic cell, and may be used to stabilize the nerve terminal by a retrograde action — but this is still quite speculative.

CORNER: To change the subject a bit, if it really were the case that in animals kept in continuous illumination (see Parnavelas, this volume) there occurs an increase in the background level of cortical excitation, and in addition a transient increase in structural connectivity, then I think we have a very interesting methodological problem relating to the hypothesis that you are proposing concerning the role of nerve function in development. This would predict changes in the *opposite* direction: neurophysiological function is not there in order to facilitate synaptogenesis, but rather to 'stabilize' certain synapses at the expense of others. We then have in the one view (Parnavelas) a mechanism where increased function will stimulate the growth of synapses, and we have another proposed mechanism (Changeux) where increased function will cause a *loss* of synapses, and in a very specific fashion. But what if *both* of these processes are operating simultaneously? I think that could make it very difficult to experimentally test these two alternatives.

CHANGEUX: I don't believe so. The experimental test is obvious: count the total number of connections formed throughout development. One can easily distinguish between an absolute increase in the number of connections, and a protection against a subsequent loss of connections. In light-reared animals, for instance, more spines might be counted than in a dark-reared animal. But perhaps at a certain stage of development, before the effect of light, many more synapses are formed than will be surviving in the end, with more synapses persisting in the light-reared animals than in the dark-reared ones.

SECTION II

CENTRAL AND SENSORY SYNAPTOGENESIS

In Vitro Approaches
to Positional Specification
in the Retinal-Tectal System

JACK LILIEN and JANNE BALSAMO

Department of Zoology, University of Wisconsin, Madison, Wisc. (U.S.A.)

INTRODUCTION

Functional integration within the nervous system demands that the component cells associate with each other in a highly regular and precise fashion. Such precision and regularity are exemplified in the vertebrate visual system, which has become a paradigm for studies on neuronal organization. Access to both cell bodies and axonal projections have allowed for precise anatomical and electrophysiological mapping of the spatial relations between cell bodies within the retina, and of axonal terminals within the tectum. Furthermore, the ability to manipulate both the retina and tectum has enabled investigators to accumulate a large body of information on the development of retinal-tectal connections. Such studies in a variety of organisms indicate that the pattern of functional connections of individual retinal axons in the tectum reflects the pattern of distribution of their respective cell bodies in the retina (reviewed by Gaze, 1970).

Topographic specificity appears to develop independently in the retina and tectum. Jacobson (1968) has shown in *Xenopus* embryos, following rotation of the eye at various developmental stages, that there are critical points in the differentiation of the retina when it acquires its unique position-dependent properties. In the chick embryo De Long and Coulombre (1965) and, more recently, Crossland et al. (1974), have analyzed the pattern of innervation of the tectum after ablation of segments from the optic cup at different stages. Ablation prior to 3 days of development resulted in a normal map, whereas beyond this time ablation resulted in uninnervated areas of the tectum. Thus, the topographic specificity of the retina seems to be determined as early as the third day of embryonic development, long before the actual connections in the tectum are made. In addition, the projection map that can be derived from such deletion experiments is roughly the same as that reported for *Xenopus* (De Long and Coulombre, 1965; Crossland et al., 1974). Retinal axons project onto the tectum in a roughly inverted position relative to the position of the cell bodies within the retina. Thus, dorsal retina projects to ventral tectum, ventral retina to dorsal tectum, nasal retina to posterior tectum, and temporal retina to anterior tectum. It should be stressed, however, that this description is an oversimplification: retinal axons from any one quadrant also project onto the adjacent tectal quadrants.

These studies firmly establish that retinal axons are destined to occupy a unique position within the tectum. However, they are unable to distinguish whether retinal axons sort themselves by assuming a relationship which determines their tectal orientation, or whether retinal elements are uniquely matched with their tectal counterparts. These alternatives can be clearly distinguished by mapping of projections to the tectum following translocation or duplication of tectal elements (goldfish: Yoon, 1974; *Xenopus*: Levine and Jacobson, 1974; Jacobson and Levine, 1975). The first alternative would predict that the pattern of retinal axons would remain constant, while the second would predict that retinal axons would 'seek' their unique position of the tectum. The results of such experiments are clear: retinal axons pair with their normal tectal elements regardless of position.

These in vivo experimental manipulations point firmly to a system of cellular recognition between retinal and tectal elements. What is the biochemical or molecular basis for such a system? To answer this question new experimental approaches are needed. It is the purpose of this paper to review several recent studies which have attempted to define the positional specificity of retinal-tectal connections using in vitro assays and thus set the stage for biochemical analyses.

IN VITRO ANALYSES OF RETINAL-TECTAL INTERACTIONS

The first in vitro analysis of retinal-tectal interactions was directed at ascertaining whether positional specification of retinal axons for a particular tectal region was reflected in the adhesive preferences of individual cells. To accomplish this, Barbera et al. (1973) utilized an assay which was originally developed for quantitative evaluation of adhesive specificity among embryonic cells (Roth and Weston 1967; Roth 1968). Isotopically labeled single cells were prepared from either the dorsal or the ventral halves of the retina by trypsinization, and then incubated with whole dorsal and ventral tectal halves. After 30 min of stationary culture, the tectal halves were washed and the radioactivity associated with each individual half was assumed to reflect the number of adherent single cells. Their results showed an adhesive selectivity which, within the regions tested, mimicked the retinotectal projections found in vivo. Dorsal retina cells display such selectivity immediately following trypsinization, and maintain it for at least 9 hr. However, cells prepared from ventral retinae adhere preferentially to ventral tectum soon after dissociation by trypsin. This selectivity is reversed when the cells are kept in nutrient medium for at least 5 hr prior to the assay. The authors suggest that the molecules responsible for recognition in the dorsal and ventral halves of the retina have different sensitivities to the trypsin treatment.

By incubating labeled cells and tectal halves in a reciprocating shaker, Barbera (1975) succeeded in decreasing the variability of the assay, and was able to test the adhesion of retina cells as young as 2.5–3 days of development. Already at this early stage, the specificity of binding of dorsal retina cells to ventral tectum is apparent. However, as with the older retina cells, cells prepared from the ventral halves of all ages of retina tested adhere preferentially to the *ventral* tectal half immediately following trypsinization. When the ventral retina cells are allowed to recover from trypsinization for 5–6 hr, there is a significant change in specificity only after day 6 of development. The expression of those molecules conferring specificity thus seems to progress from the dorsal to the ventral end of the retina.

More recently Marchase et al. (1977) have investigated the effects of glycosidases on adhesion of dorsal and ventral retina cells to dorsal and ventral tectal halves. It was found that treatment of only dorsal retina or dorsal tectum with β-N-acetylhexosaminidase reduced the regionally specific adhesion. Furthermore, GM_2 ganglioside (which terminates in N-acetylgalactosamine), when incorporated into dipalmitoyl lecithin vesicles, causes these vesicles to adhere preferentially to ventral tectum. The enzyme GM_1 synthetase, which adds the terminal galactosyl residue to GM_2, converting it to GM_1, appears to show greatest activity in homogenates of ventral retina, and decreasing towards the dorsal region. Thus, the authors suggest that complementarity between enzyme and acceptor (GM_2) may be involved in specification of axonal position within the tectum.

A direct interaction between retina and tectal cell surfaces has also been demonstrated by the work of Gottlieb et al. (1974). These authors prepared plasma membrane from optic tectum and neural retina of chick embryos. These membranes specifically inhibit the aggregation of homotypic cells, but retinal cell membranes in addition inhibit *tectal* cell adhesions. No inhibition of retina cell adhesion by tectal membranes was observed, however. Inhibition of adhesions by homologous membranes is age specific; membranes isolated from 7-, 8- and 9-day retina are most active in inhibiting adhesions among cells of the same age. This temporal specificity is also reflected in the inhibition of tectal cell adhesion: 8- and 9-day retina membranes are most effective on 8- and 9-day tectal cells, respectively. These data imply that both the retina and the tectum undergo a cell surface alteration between, 7, 8 and 9 days of development. Although the physiological significance of these temporal changes is as yet unclear, they do indicate that temporal changes in adhesive characteristics may occur in a coordinated fashion within both the retina and the tectum.

Temporal changes aside, retinal cell membranes (and by extrapolation, retina *cells*) are able to recognize specific components on the tectal cell surface, in accord with the results of Barbera et al. (1973) and Barbera (1975). The inability of optic lobe membranes to inhibit retina cell aggregation suggests that the recognition process occurs between two different complementary entities. As suggested by Merrell and Glaser (1973), these entities could be, respectively, a 'passive recognition site', which would remain intact in the isolated retina cell membranes, and an 'active' component, which is supplied by the live optic lobe cells.

Such an interpretation is also suggested by work done in our laboratory (Balsamo et al., 1976). Our previous work has established that embryonic chick neural retina and cerebral lobes release, into serum-free organ culture medium, glycoprotein ligands which bind selectively to homologous cells (Balsamo and Lilien, 1974a). The specificity inherent in binding is encoded in the saccharide moieties of the ligands (Balsamo and Lilien, 1975). The glycoprotein ligand is one of two extracellular components which participate in the formation of homotypic adhesive bonds. The second component is also tissue specific, and appears to interact with ligands on opposing cells to establish the adhesive bond (Balsamo and Lilien, 1974b; Lilien and Rutz, 1977; Lilien et al., 1977a; 1977b). The technology developed in these studies on the nature of homotypic adhesions was extended to examine the interaction of neural retina and optic tectum. Serum-free organ culture media labeled with [^{3}H]-glucosamine were prepared from 10-day neural retina, 10-day optic lobes and 10-day cerebral lobes. Binding of radioactive macromolecules in each of the culture supernatants to monolayers prepared from each cell type gave the following results: neural retina and cerebral lobe yield largely homotypic binding components, while components in optic lobe organ culture media bind both to optic lobe and neural retina monolayers.

These results further demonstrate the existence of regionally specific complementary molecules, whose pattern of distribution reflects the 'in vivo' pattern of innervation of the tectum by retinal axons. Organ culture-conditioned media were prepared from dorsal and ventral optic lobe halves, and from anterior and posterior halves. Retinal cells were prepared from dorsal, ventral, nasal and temporal quadrants. While culture supernatants prepared from all regions of the tectum were able to bind to cells prepared from all retina quadrants, the physiologically 'matching' combinations were favored: binding was greatest when optic lobe organ culture media from each of the four halves were matched with cells from that portion of the tectum which they ordinarily innervate.

Temporal differences in the production of retinal binding factors by optic lobes were also observed. There is a relative increase in the amount of nasal and ventral retina binding factor by optic lobes between 8 and 12 days of embryonic age. This is consistent with the normal pattern of innervation, which proceeds from the anterior-ventral to the posterior-dorsal pole of the lobes (Goldberg, 1974).

Another technique for investigating retinal-tectal interactions was made available by the findings of McDonough and Lilien (1975). These authors have reported that the induced capping of lectin receptors on trypsin-dispersed embryonic cells can be specifically inhibited by components which accumulate in organ culture medium. Thus, supernatants obtained from neural-retina and cerebral-lobe organ cultures inhibit capping of concanavalin A receptors on trypsin dissociated cells of only the homologous type. However, culture supernatants from optic lobes inhibit the capping of lectin receptors both on optic lobe cells and on retina cells. Furthermore, this inhibition is regionally specific, the effect being greatest for the following combinations: anterior optic lobe-temporal retina; posterior optic lobe-nasal retina; dorsal optic lobe-ventral retina and ventral optic lobe-dorsal retina.

These data on the inhibition of lectin-induced capping imply that many, if not all, of the cells of the retina are able to interact with optic lobe ligands. Within each quadrant, 70% of the cells are able to form lectin-induced caps; of this 70%, approximately 80% inhibition is seen in the presence of optic lobe ligands. Thus, a minimum of 55% of the population appears to have specific receptors for optic lobe ligands, many more than would be predicted if only the *ganglion* (i.e. optic nerve) cells were specified. This conclusion has also been reached by Barbera (1975) and Barbera et al. (1973). They showed that many more retina cells adhere to tectal halves than could be accounted for solely by ganglion cells. In addition, the finding that dorsal and ventral pigmented retina cells also show adhesive preferences to optic lobe halves argues for positional specification of the entire optic cup during early development.

Both the selective binding and the inhibition of capping exhibited by *neural-retina* organ culture conditioned media depend upon the presence of the same ligand terminal sugar, N-acetylgalactosamine. Similarly, both activities in *cerebral-lobe* organ culture conditioned media depend upon a terminal mannosamine-like residue (McDonough and Lilien, 1975). In addition, for neural retina the two activities appear to reside in a single molecular species (Lilien et al., 1977a). By analogy, therefore, the binding and inhibition of capping by optic lobe culture supernatants on retina cells may also reflect the activity of single molecular species, interacting through an oligosaccharide moiety.

INTERPRETATIONS AND DISCUSSION

The most compelling theoretical framework from which the topographic specificity of retinal axons for the tectum has been considered is that of Sperry (1963). Sperry suggests that the orderly projection of retinal axons onto the tectum is due to at least two complementary gradients of 'cytochemical affinities' between retinal axons and tectal surface, the two gradients being oriented perpendicular to each other. A majority of the existent data are consistent with such a hypothesis (see Jacobson, 1974).

This hypothesis makes two critical predictions: (1) the existence of positionally specific affinities between retinal axons and the tectal surface, and (2) the orientation of these affinities along a gradient. With respect to these predictions, data accumulated in three different laboratories suggest a definite correlation between selective adhesion and positional specification of retinal axons. While there is no direct evidence for the second prediction, the data have been interpreted in such a fashion. Barbera (1975) has suggested two gradients of complementary molecules running in opposite directions along the dorso-ventral axis of the retina. Two gradients, composed of identical molecules, would exist in the same orientation within the tectum (Fig. 1A). One prediction of this model is that dorsal retina cells should have a greater affinity for ventral retina cells than for each other, and vice versa. In a recent publication, Gottlieb et al. (1976) have demonstrated the existence of such a gradient by dividing the retina into six strips, along the dorso-ventral axis, and measuring the adhesion of radioactively labeled single cells to monolayers prepared from the most dorsal and most ventral regions. Attempts to show a similar gradient along the anterior-posterior axis were unfruitful.

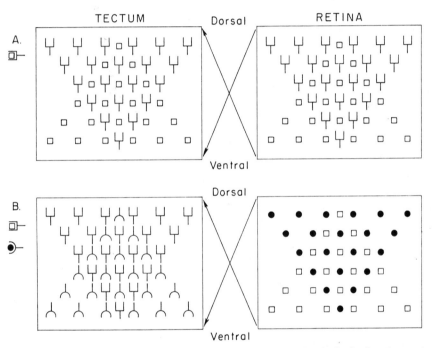

Fig. 1. Two possible models depicting gradients of complementary molecules in the dorsal-ventral axis of the retina and the optic tectum. (Similar gradients would exist in the anterior-posterior axis.) A: identical molecules forming the gradients in both retina and tectum: ५ is complementary to □ (redrawn after Barbera, 1975). B. molecules forming both of the retinal gradients are complementary to molecules forming the two tectal gradients: ५ is complementary to □; ⅄ is complementary to ●. Axonal position is determined by the greatest number of complementary interactions.

While such results agree with the model, it is difficult to accommodate the existence of gradients of identical molecules in both retina and tectum with the polar interactions observed by Gottlieb et al. (1974) and by Balsamo et al. (1976). The production by each optic lobe half of a component(s) which shows selective binding to, and inhibition of, capping among cells of the matching retinal quadrant, suggests that at least four qualitatively different components are synthesized by the tectum which are able to recognize distinct receptors on retina cells. These results can also be interpreted in terms of gradients of complementary molecules. Optic lobe binding components would exist as two opposite sets of gradients in the dorso-ventral axis, and two opposite sets along anterior-posterior axis, while the complementary molecules in the retina would exist as similar gradients of cell surface associated components (Fig. 1B).

Our findings that positionally specific tectal ligands are released into organ culture medium suggest that these components are soluble, whereas the presumed retinal receptors exist as insoluble surface components. Barbera (1975) has presented micrographs showing that pigmented retina cells (which also show positional adhesive specificity in the dorsal-ventral axis) are adherent to a non-cellular surface layer of the tectum even when the tecta are not innervated. This is consistent with data showing that retinal axons become organized on the tectal surface prior to penetration and synapse formation (goldfish: Attardi and Sperry, 1963; chick: Crossland et al., 1975). Taken together, these data imply that tectal ligands are also released from the cell surface in situ, and become incorporated into the non-cellular surface matrix of the tectum.

The results discussed above do not attempt to explain what forces direct the outgrowing retina axons to their proper target on the tectum, or how stable cellular patterns are maintained once the proper orientation is achieved. In this regard, McDonough and Lilien (1975) have suggested that inhibition of cell surface receptor capping by tissue-specific ligands reflects their ability to inhibit cell motility (for a discussion of the relation between capping and cell movement, see De Petris and Raff, 1973; also Lilien et al., 1977a). Thus, as the outgrowing axons reach their proper positions on the tectum (where interactions between retinal and tectal components are optimal), further movement over the tectum would be inhibited, and the axonal positions become stabilized.

ACKNOWLEDGEMENT

These studies were conducted in the laboratory of the senior author and were supported by a grant from NSF.

REFERENCES

Attardi, D.G. and Sperry, R.W. (1963) Preferential selection of central pathways by regenerating optic-fibers, *Exp. Neurol.*, 7: 46–64.

Balsamo, J. and Lilien, J. (1974a) Embryonic cell aggregation: kinetics and specificity of binding of enhancing factors, *Proc. nat. Acad. Sci. (Wash.)*, 71: 727–731.

Balsamo, J. and Lilien, J. (1974b) Functional identification of three components which mediate tissue-type specific embryonic adhesion, *Nature (Lond.)*, 251: 522–524.

Balsamo, J. and Lilien, J. (1975) The binding of tissue-specific adhesive molecules to the cell surface: a molecular basis for specificity, *Biochemistry*, 14: 167–171.

Balsamo, J., McDonough, J. and Lilien, J. (1976) Retinal-tectal connection in the embryonic chick: evidence for regionally specific cell surface components which mimic the pattern of innervation, *Develop. Biol.*, 49: 338–346.

Barbera, A.J. (1975) Adhesive recognition between developing retinal cells and the optic tecta of the chick embryo, *Develop. Biol.*, 46: 167–191.

Barbera, A.J., Marchase, R.B. and Roth, S. (1973) Adhesive recognition and retino-tectal specificity, *Proc. nat. Acad. Sci. (Wash.)*, 70: 2482–2486.

Crossland, W.J., Cowan, W.M., Rogers, L.A. and Kelly, J. (1974) The specification of the retino-tectal projection in the chick, *J. comp. Neurol.*, 155: 127–164.

De Long, G.R. and Coulombre, A.J. (1965) Development of the retino-topic projection in the chick embyro, *Exp. Neurol.*, 13: 350–363.

De Petris, S. and Raff, M.C. (1973) Fluidity of the plasma membrane and its implications for cell movement. In *Locomotion of Tissue Cells, Ciba Foundation Symposium 14*, Elsevier, Amsterdam, pp. 27–40.

Gaze, R.M. (1970) *The Formation of Nerve Connections*, Academic Press, New York.

Goldberg, S. (1974) Studies on the mechanics of development of the visual pathways in the chick embryo, *Develop. Biol.*, 36: 24–43.

Gottlieb, D.I., Merrell, R. and Glaser, L. (1974) Temporal changes in embryonal cell surface recognition, *Proc. nat. Acad. Sci. (Wash.)*, 71: 1800–1802.

Gottlieb, D.I., Rock, K. and Glaser, L. (1976) A gradient of adhesive specificity in developing avian retina, *Proc. nat. Acad. Sci. (Wash.)*, 73: 410–414.

Hunt, R.K. and Jacobson, M. (1974) Neuronal Specificity Revisited. In *Current Topics in Developmental Biology, Vol. 8*, Academic Press, New York, pp. 203–259.

Jacobson, M. (1968) Development of neuronal specificity in retinal ganglion cells of *Xenopus, Develop. Biol.*, 17: 202–218.

Jacobson, M. and Levine, R.L. (1975a) Plasticity in the adult frog brain: Filling the visual scotoma after excision or translocation of parts of the optic tectum, *Brain Res.*, 88: 339–345.

Jacobson, M. and Levine, R.L. (1975b) Stability of implanted duplicate tectal positional markers serving as targets for optic-axons in adult frogs, *Brain Res.*, 92: 468–471.

Levine, R. and Jacobson, M. (1974) Development of optic-nerve fibers is determined by positional markers in the frog's brain, *Exp. Neurol.*, 43: 527–538.

Lilien, J., Balsamo, J., McDonough, J., Hermolin, J., Cook, J. and Rutz, R. (1977a) Adhesive specificity sensory embryonic cells. In *Surfaces of Normal and Malignant Cells*, R. Hynes (Ed.), Wiley, London, in press.

Lilien, J., Hermolin, J. and Lipke, P. (1977b) Molecular interactions in specific cell adhesion. In *Specificity of Embryological Interactions*, D. Garrod (Ed.), Chapman-Hall, London, in press.

Lilien, J. and Rutz, R. (1977) A multicomponent model for specific cell adhesion. In *Cell and Tissue Interactions*, J. Lark and M. Bayer, (Eds.), Raven Press, New York, in press.

Marchase, R.B., Pierce, S. and Roth, S. (1977) Complementarity between the ganglioside GM_2 and the enzyme GM_1 synthetase as a possible mechanism in the chick retino-tectal projection. In *Cell Surface Carbohydrates and Biological Recognition*, 6th Annual ICN-UCLA Symposium.

McDonough, J. and Lilien, J. (1975) Inhibition of mobility of cell surface receptors by factors which mediate specific cell-cell interactions, *Nature (Lond.)*, 256: 416–417.

Merrell, R. and Galser, L. (1973) Specific recognition of plasma membranes by embryonic cells, *Proc. nat. Acad. Sci. (Wash.)*, 70: 2794–2798.

Roth, S. (1968) Studies on intercellular adhesive selectivity, *Develop. Biol.*, 18: 602–612.

Roth, S. and Weston, J. (1967) The measurement of intercellular adhesion, *Proc. nat. Acad. Sci. (Wash.)*, 58: 974–980.

Sperry, R.W. (1963) Chemoaffinity in the orderly growth of nerve fiber patterns and connections, *Proc. nat. Acad. Sci. (Wash.)*, 50: 703–710.

Yoon, M. (1973) Retention of the original topographic polarity by the 180° rotated tectal reimplant in young goldfish, *J. Physiol. (Lond.)*, 233: 575–588.

DISCUSSION

STIRLING: Is there just a simple gradient of these ligands over the tecta, or do you imagine that some of them are different in different places?

LILIEN: The data on binding and on inhibition of capping suggest that there are *four* qualitatively different interactions which mimick the projection of retinal axons onto the tectum. That is, dorsal, ventral, anterior and posterior optic lobe halves appear to produce ligands which interact specifically with ventral, dorsal, posterior and anterior retina, respectively. One cannot account for these differences in terms of *quantitative* differentials.

CHANGEUX: Comparing the effect of capping and the effect of binding, when you get capping you look at a discrete property of the cell: it either caps or it does not cap, is this not so? And when you get binding, you look at an *average* property of the whole situation.

LILIEN: One of the conclusions which I neglected to emphasize, but which we can infer from the capping assays, is that *all* the cells of the retina (not just the ganglion cells, which ultimately make the connections) appear to have the same unique positional specification. This conclusion is also supported by the studies of Barbera et al. (1973) showing that the pigmented retina shows the same dorsal-ventral adhesive specificity for optic lobe halves as does the neural retina. I therefore think we are looking at a gradient of specification which encompasses all the cells of the retina.

CHANGEUX: But you have, let's say, 20% of the cells which do not cap, which means that there is a heterogeneity of the cells. Do you find the same heterogeneity in binding properties?

LILIEN: We have not done any experiments which would definitely answer your question, but there is indeed heterogeneity in terms of capping. Approximately 70–75% of the cells will form caps, and of those we get about 80% inhibition. So there is clearly heterogeneity in *both* of these aspects.

LYNCH: You mentioned that some of your experiments were conducted on embryos at different ages. I wonder if your data show these molecular binding phenomena appearing at consecutive times in the life cycle of the cell, i.e. are the observed differences due to temporal differences in the production of ligands? For example, perhaps cerebral lobe cells make the same ligands as do optic lobe cells, but at a different time in development.

LILIEN: In answer to that, all I can say is that we have not done an extensive enough series of ages to permit rejection of such an alternative. For the ages which we *have* done, which are only those between 7 and 14 days of development, we don't find any qualitative changes in specificity.

STIRLING: How do you imagine the retinal cells become labeled in the eye during the development? The optic lobe is growing just at the back, while the retina grows circumferentially. There is a problem about how you decide to have you labels arranged in terms of cells being added to populations.

LILIEN: I really cannot add anything that has not been said in previous speculative discussions. Nothing we have done addresses the question of how (or when) the specification occurs.

HODDE: When you speak about ligands, do you think that there are any heavy metals involved in the binding?

LILIEN: We have shown that divalent cations, in any case, are not necessary for the binding of these protein ligands.

CHANGEUX: You said that you had two proteins, only one of which may be responsible for the binding? So, if you have purified one such protein, do you have any data as yet regarding the effects of an antibody against it?

LILIEN: You are a little ahead of us! We have only just begun to prepare antibodies against the neuro-retinal component.

REFERENCE

Barbera, A.J., Marchase, R.B. and Roth, S. (1973) Adhesive recognition and retinotectal specificity, *Proc. nat. Acad. Sci. (Wash.)*, 70: 2482–2486.

Synapse Selectivity in Somatic Afferent Systems

ROBERT E. BAKER

Netherlands Institute for Brain Research, IJdijk-28, Amsterdam-0 (The Netherlands)

Nerves,
  big nerves,
    tiny nerves,
      many nerves!–
galloped madly
   'til soon
     their legs gave way.

Vladimir Mayakovsky (*The Cloud in Trousers*)

INTRODUCTION

All animals monitor external and internal environmental changes and react with appropriate behavioral patterns to both pleasant and noxious stimuli. In all animals above the Porifera specialized sensory neurons perform these monitoring duties. Among vertebrates these neurons are usually monopolar, with the axon splitting shortly after leaving the perikaryon, and sending branches over extensive distances: centrally, into the CNS, and peripherally to various sensory end-organs. Inasmuch as sensory neurons serve as a bridge between the environment and motor responses, there is an inherent interest in understanding how this bridge comes about; in particular, whether or not sensory neurons behave developmentally as do centrally derived neurons (motor neurons and retinal ganglion cells) in selecting appropriate termination sites. Although we now know a great deal about the anatomy, physiology and timing of development for many types of sensory neurons, we still remain ignorant of the mechanisms which allow them to select their peripheral and central connections.

Although many studies have been reported on the formation of various interneuronal connections, few have been concerned with the formation of connections between *initial* nerve cell neurites and their end-organs. Most investigations rely on selective association between neurons and end-organs following early manipulation and re-innervation, or from examination of connections formed in tissue culture. One must assume, therefore, that both of these latter techniques sufficiently mirror the developmental processes to make them acceptable models upon which to formulate general connection hypotheses. However, some initial innervation studies have recently been conducted on organisms which afford access to very early stages of development, i.e. invertebrates, fish, amphibians and birds. These will be reviewed in the following section.

INITIAL EMBRYONIC NERVE CONNECTIONS

Experiments are now on record concerning the initial outgrowth and connection of sensory neurons in the antennae and limbs of locusts (Bates, 1976), the receptor cells of the retina in *Daphnia* (Lopresti et al., 1975), the retinotectal connections in *Xenopus* (Gaze et al., 1972), and neuromuscular (hindlimb) connections in frog (Lamb, 1974, 1976) and in chick (Landmesser and Morris, 1975).

Among the invertebrates examined, innervation is initiated by a few pioneering axons (the 'lead' axon in *Daphnia* retina, and two pioneering axons in the locust antenna and limb), with the subsequent addition of neurites using these earliest formed axons as a guidance system into the CNS. Such pioneering nerve cell neurites sometimes locate their preferred synaptic partners easily, due to the anatomical configurations of their environment which lead them directly to their end points (e.g. connections between the antennal fibers and the deuterocerebrum of the locust), whereas other fibers encounter numerous anatomical obstacles on the way to their preferred partners (i.e. various alternative muscle or sensory tissues which must be by-passed before a definitive connection is made with a given end-organ, as in the limbs of the locust).

In all of the developing limb systems examined, however, there clearly appears to be great pernickety on the part of the pioneering sensory neurites in locating and establishing contact with appropriate muscles or ganglia. If incorrect connections are formed in any of these developing systems, they appear to be short-lived. Temporary connections may be the rule in the developing tadpole retinotectal system, where a caudally directed shift in tectal cell association by ingrowing retinal fibers occurs during later stages of larval development, as additional ganglion cell axons arrive and acquire termination sites.

TRANSPLANTATION OF END-ORGANS

A frequently used method of examining neuronal target selectivity is the manipulation of end-organs or nerve trunks at selected stages of development, with observations of subsequent behavioral display and interneuronal connectivity patterns following regeneration. Re-innervation of many peripheral sensory end-organs, together with a return of normal behavior, physiology or central projection patterns in the regenerated system, have been observed in numerous disparate sensory systems (for cat Pacinian corpuscle: Burgess and Horch, 1973; Burgess et al., 1974; for sensory and neuromuscular systems of the crayfish limb: Bittner and Johnson, 1974; for frog Merkel cells: Nafstad and Baker, 1973; for heteromorph antennules of the lobster: Maynard, 1965; Maynard and Cohen, 1965; for leech interganglionic connectives, Jansen et al., 1974; Miyazaki et al., 1976; Baylor and Nicholls, 1971; for *Drosophila* antennapedia: Stocker et al., 1976; for cricket cercal cells: Edwards and Sahota, 1968; Edwards and Palka, 1971, 1973; McLean and Edwards, 1976; for axolotl limb cutaneous innervation, Johnston et al., 1975; Diamond, 1976; Stirling, 1973; Cooper and Diamond, 1977; Cooper et al., 1977).

Displacement of a sensory end-organ to a different body location results in its innervation by *new* sets of local sensory neurons, and often leads to abnormal behavioral responses in the host. Transplantation of trigeminal and vagal ganglia in salamander (Székely, 1959), cross-union of various sensory nerve trunks in urodeles and anurans (Sperry and Miner, 1949), and the addition of supernumerary sensory end-organs to the periphery all affect the host by producing behavioral changes which are maladaptive, and also impervious to experience. By the early stages of larval development frog skin structures are irreversibly specified, and will develop their characteristic morphological features even at atypical locations following transplantation and metamorphosis (e.g. Cole, 1922; Helf, 1931; Herrick, 1932; Rand and Pierce, 1932; Miner, 1956; Nafstad and Baker, 1973). Supernumerary limbs also retain characteristic skin pigmentation patterns of the limb, regardless of the site to which they are translocated.

Supernumerary limbs become sensitive to a variety of cutaneous stimuli, giving an appropriate and accurately aimed movement by the host's *normal* ipsilateral limb. Supernumerary limbs transplanted to the back of chick and frog embryros are innervated by dorsal nerve trunks in both types of animals (Miner, 1956; Székely and Szentagothai, 1962; Hollyday and Mendell, 1975), and become sensitive to cutaneous stimuli. As in salamanders, wings or limbs transplanted to thoracic levels on the back of frogs or chicks become ankylotic and atrophic, but provide the animal with cutaneous information responsible for 'correct' localization by the host of the point of stimulation (as monitored by the movements evoked in the normal limb). Such specific motor reactions consist of simple limb movements directed away from the disturbing mechanical stimuli or, as in the chick, may involve more complex behavioral patterns such as lame walking and preening in the normal limb when a continuous painful stimulus is applied to the transplant. The quality of information given to the host by a transplanted limb is not an absolute. Thus, hindlimbs transplanted to the brachial regions in both the chick and the frog exhibit wing or forelimb movements patterns in the host. Conversely, wings transplanted to the lumbar region in chicks will frequently exhibit leg-like movements.

One of the most striking findings to emerge from supernumerary limb transplantation studies has been that cutaneous neurons at thoracic levels are able to mediate well-directed reflex movements in a normal host limb, although they normally never provide innervation to limb skin. These behavioral findings have recently been extended electrophysiologically in *Xenopus*, where it has been shown that the sensory neurons providing sensory innervation to the supernumerary limb do not simultaneously provide innervation to the normal limb as well (Hollyday and Mendell, 1975). The most obvious conclusion which can be drawn from these experiments is that such reflexes might be mediated by synaptic associations between thoracic ganglion cells and hindlimb motoneurons within the spinal cord.

More than two decades ago Miner (1956) reported findings which correlated stereotypic wiping responses with grafted patches of rotated skin in the frog *Rana pipiens*. She noted that if a 180° rotation of trunk skin on one side of the frog's body were carried out at early stages of larval development (Fig. 1), the belly skin transplanted to the frog's dorsum differentiated as white skin, and gave rise to wiping reflexes directed towards its ventrum. Similarly, back skin differentiated as darkly pigmented skin (although located on the animal's ventrum) and caused the frog to direct its reflex responses towards the dorsum. Miner interpreted her results as evidence that the skin possessed a 'local sign', and that this local sign was somehow imparted to the innervating cutaneous neurons, which then selected their central associations so as to match the type of skin being innervated in the periphery. There did not appear to be any possibility that a selective return of the original nerve supplies had occurred, inasmuch as cutting the graft away from surrounding normal skin, and even dividing it at the middle, failed to eliminate the misdirected limb movements.

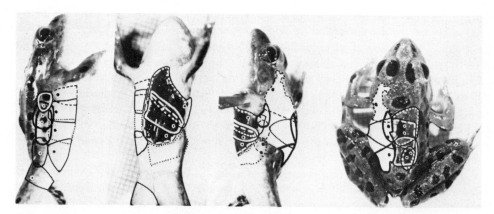

Fig. 1. Selected views of 180° skin-grafted *Rana pipiens* frog, showing cutaneous receptive fields (CRFs) for various body surfaces. Small circles within each CRF represents point at which the cutaneous nerve trunk appeared to enter the skin.

These various transplantation experiments form the basis of an unresolved problem. Cutaneous reinnervation of transplanted embryonic or larval skin structures can lead to abnormal behavioral displays in amphibians and birds. This can only be so either if (1) the original neurons of the transposed skin structures somehow manage to find their way back to the original end-organs (i.e. selective re-innervation), or (2) local neurons provide innervation to the grafted tissue, but are somehow informed of the change in peripheral end-organs and readjust their central connections accordingly (i.e. cutaneous 'modulation').

The only sensory systems which appear to lend in vivo support to the latter mechanism are the already mentioned regeneration studies in amphibians and birds. Attempts to demonstrate central synaptic readjustments following cross-uniting sensory and motor nerve trunks in newborn and adult mammals have failed to support this hypothesis (Sperry, 1941, 1943; Eccles et al., 1962; Mendell and Scott, 1975). It is not impossible, however, that switching of central connections would have occurred if such cross-unions were performed at stages of fetal development which paralleled the much earlier stages of development used in the lower vertebrate studies.

THE ANURAN CUTANEOUS SENSORY SYSTEM

One of the sensory systems employed to examine which of the two alternative mechanisms presented above might be responsible for behavioral changes, resulting from peripherally manipulated end-organs, has been that of epidermal relocations in anurans. The normal and experimental development of the amphibian dorsal root ganglia (DRG) and dorsal roots have been reported by numerous authors (e.g. Hardesty, 1899, 1900, 1905; Prestige, 1965; Hughes, 1959, 1961; Hughes and Tschumi, 1958; Baker et al., 1976; Baker and Richter, 1977). In *Xenopus*, two out of every three ganglion cells produced during larval stages degenerate before the end of metamorphosis. (This developmental scheme appears to prevail in the DRG of most vertebrates, even mammals: Hughes, 1973.) Similar losses also appear among fibers in the ventral roots and among motoneurons of the ventral horn in anurans (Hughes, 1959; Hughes and Tschumi, 1958; Prestige, 1976; Prestige and Wilson, 1972), even though the motoneurons of the frog (and perhaps chick ciliary ganglion cells as well; see Landmesser and Pilar, 1974a, b) had already made contact with peripheral musculature. It has been suggested, therefore, that contact alone is insufficient to ensure survival of any given neuron, but rather the number and type of connections made are the crucial factors.

The anatomy and development of the cutaneous sensory system has enjoyed considerable scrutiny in amphibians, inasmuch as it is accessible to experimentation at all stages of development. Morphological tracing of metamorphosing and adult frog dorsal root afferents has been performed using a variety of histological techniques (Brown, 1946; Liu and Chamber, 1957; Hughes et al., 1969; Fox, 1973; Székely, 1976) and also autoradiography (Joseph and Whitlock, 1966, 1968). In postmetamorphic *Rana pipiens* the number of dorsal root fibers increases as the animal increases in body size (Hardesty, 1899, 1900, 1905). Counts of brachial dorsal root fibers in pre-metamorphic tadpoles have recently been made and show a dramatic decline in the number of myelinated and unmyelinated fibers shortly before the completion of metamorphosis (Baker et al., 1976). Thus, the sensory system parallels the frog neuromuscular system (and chick ciliary ganglion) insofar as there is a dropping out of neurites from dorsal roots during given stages of development (Prestige, 1976; Prestige and Wilson, 1972; Landmesser and Pilar, 1974a, b). In a more recent study it has further been shown that dorsal root fiber counts in the frog *Discoglossus pictus* double between one and two weeks after metamorphosis (Baker and Richter, 1977).

Skin rotation experiments

A variety of skin grafts have been made on several anuran species, including back-to-belly rotations, head-to-tail rotations, left-right transpositions, patch graft interchanges, strip graft rotations, total trunk skin rotations, and even frogs with only one type of skin encircling its trunk. In all cases where misdirected reflexes develop in these skin-grafted animals, they do so in a more or less predictable manner. Small areas of the grafted skin, at the junction of two reflexogenous zones, give rise to misdirected responses either from the start of wiping reflex activity (i.e. during metamorphosis) or shortly thereafter (Fig. 2; also Jacobson and Baker, 1969; Baker et al., 1977). *Mixed* reflexes (i.e. normal as well as misdirected) occur from most areas of the grafted skin for a number of days following the completion of metamorphosis. After this transitional period, the misdirected behavioral responses usually become predominant over most of the grafted skin areas.

If one looks at the topography of cutaneous receptive fields (CRFs) in skin-grafted frogs, several interesting observations are immediately evident: most CRFs located near the graft border regions fail to cross the border to provide simultaneous innervation for both back skin and belly skin (see Fig. 1; also Jacobson and Baker, 1969; Baker and Jacobson, 1970; Sklar and Hunt, 1973). It is not a question of scar tissues forming an impenetrable barrier at such CRF boundary crossings, since overlap readily occurs at the borders in dorsal or ventral head-to-tail and left-right rotations, where the skin which is separated by the border scars is all of the same type (i.e. back skin or belly skin) (Jacobson and Baker, 1969; Scott and Sperry, 1975). Despite the exclusion-inclusion of CRFs, receptive fields for the major nerve trunks continue to occupy their usual places in the skin, both in late-stage tadpoles and in adult frogs (Jacobson and Baker, 1969). This latter observation would appear to support Miner's original contention that no peripheral searching by the cut afferent nerve fibers has occurred (see Fig. 3), the skin grafts thus being innervated exclusively by local cutaneous nerve sources.

Small patches of back skin which are excised and immediately reimplanted to the back of midlarval tadpoles become rapidly reinnervated (Nafstad and Baker: unpublished

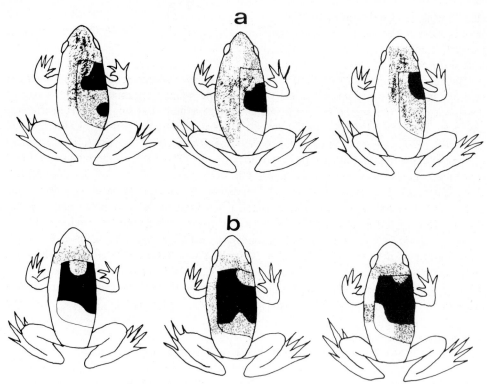

Fig. 2. Development of misdirected reflex responses in skin-grafted *D. pictus*. a: wiping reflexes in the first postmetamorphic week. Black areas show points on graft from which misdirected reflexes were elicited. Stippled areas gave rise to only normal reflexes, while from clear areas no reflex responses at all were elicited. b: wiping reflexes in the same animal on three successive days in the third postmetamorphic week. Color scheme as above. (From Baker et al., 1977.)

observations). Degenerative changes occur in the Merkel cells and the free nerve endings within 3 min after denervation, but intact intraepithelial nerve endings and normal appearing Merkel cells are observed as early as 20 min after return of the skin graft to the wound. Behavioral responsiveness to grafted skin in adult frogs occurs as early as 24 hr after the return of the graft (Scott and Sperry, 1975). Such observations seem to rule out any significant searching capabilities by severed cutaneous nerve cells in tadpoles at the time the various skin-grafting experiments mentioned above were performed. However, since nothing is known about long-term CRF morphology in these animals, one cannot definitely rule out the possibility of selective regrowth of given classes of neurites to their original sensory end-organs, given sufficient time. The fact that there is CRF exclusion-inclusion at graft borders suggests that distinct differences exist between back and belly skin. The neurons giving rise to one or the other behavioral reflex response might well be doing so, therefore, on the basis of some sort of selective recognition of skin type by individual sensory neurons.

Baker and Jacobson (1969, 1970) and Sklar and Hunt (1973) made all of their frog CRF recordings from peripheral nerve trunks near the point of entrance into the skin. These recordings showed that the nerves innervated the skin in the normal positions in both tadpoles and adults of *Rana pipiens*, leading the authors to conclude that restoration of the original sensory nerve connections could not be responsible for the development of misdirected responses in skin-grafted animals. Such peripheral recordings might appear

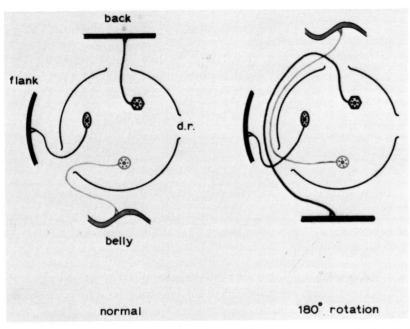

Fig. 3. Hypothetical schema of selective regrowth of cut peripheral cutaneous nerves back to their original skin types following a skin rotation on the trunk.

convincing at first glance, and yet could be masking selective return of nerve fibers via quite different pathways. Return of the original nerve fibers was in fact found following cross-union of motor nerve trunks in the leg of salamanders (Grimm, 1971). Stimulating the motor nerve trunks distal to the point of cross-union had suggested that the inappropriately matched nerve bundles were mediating the correct walking movements which had been observed in intact animals. Stimulation *proximal* to the point of nerve cross-union, however, evoked activity in the nerve trunk leading to the *appropriate* muscle, and effectively caused it to contract. Fibers from the original nerve trunk must therefore have managed to reconnect with the muscle via an unknown route.

EXPERIMENTAL STUDIES IN INVERTEBRATES

That a selective return of CRFs to near normal size and distribution might occur over extended periods of time has in fact been shown to occur in the leech. In leech, CRFs can be readily identified as belonging to ganglion sensory neurons of known modality, i.e. touch, pain or pressure (Nicholls and Baylor, 1968; Yau, 1977a). These CRFs normally have the same size, shape and position in all animals, reflecting the position of the cell body itself within the ganglion. In these animals, the cell body lies within a CNS ganglion, sending several long axons to the periphery where sensory connections are made (Yau, 1977b). The pattern of reinnervation of the skin following a peripheral nerve crush or cut is such that the original CRFs are correctly re-established (Fig. 4; also Baylor and Nicholls, 1971; van Essen and Jansen, 1976, 1977). Such re-establishment of CRFs to approximately their normal position and modality has also been noted in mammals, provided that sensory nerve trunks are merely crushed and not severed (e.g. Head and Rivers, 1905; Rivers and

84

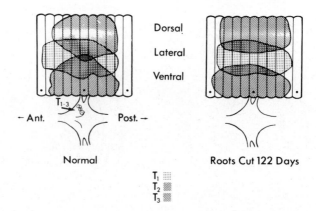

Fig. 4. Schema CRF in leech. Normal receptive fields (left) showing distribution of dorsal, lateral and ventral aspects of the body surface. Correct distribution of peripheral CRFs occur following a section of ganglionic nerve trunk 122 days previously (right). (From van Essen and Jansen, 1976.)

Head, 1908; Sharpey-Schafer, 1929, 1930; Weddell et al., 1941; Orgel et al., 1972). The return of appropriate cutaneous innervation, therefore, seems to be primarily dependent upon intact nerve channels remaining available to the regenerating afferent nerve fibers, rather than to their ability to find a particular area in the periphery.

If a sensory nerve trunk is severed, and a portion of the trunk is excised so that there is no direct abutment between the cut ends, the return of re-innervation is greatly diminished even in the leech, where only small CRFs located adjacent to the cut proximal stumps of the nerve are found (Fig. 5). Even here, however, the correct dorsal, lateral and ventral spacing of the CRFs is usually maintained (van Essen and Jansen, 1977). Moreover, regenerating neurons which do successfully locate the distal stump, and make functional connections, slowly extend their CRFs to occupy significantly larger areas of skin than in the original innervation; once again, this occurs in correct dorsoventral array. Although in the leech severed sensory neurons appear to preferentially re-innervate their original peripheral *territories* (i.e. dorsal, lateral and ventral areas of the body surface), it is not known whether they in fact re-innervate precisely the original termination *sites*.

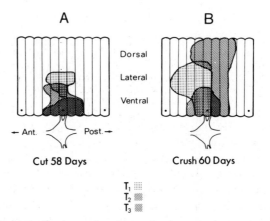

Fig. 5. Schema CRF in leech. Cutting and evulsion of peripheral nerve trunk 58 days previously (left) results in small CRFs located close to proximal cut end of the trunk. Such restruction does not occur if nerve trunk is merely crushed (right). (From van Essen and Jansen, 1976.)

Invertebrate axons frequently remain viable even when separated from their cell bodies. This is particularly true of the sensory neurons studied in the leech (Kuffler and Muller, 1974; Miyazaki et al., 1976; van Essen and Jansen, 1977). The old axons of the cut nerves continue to respond to stimulation of the pre-existing CRFs, while a new axonal sprout may provide superinnervation to the same areas of the integument. Superinnervation has also been noted in leeches possessing naturally occurring supernumerary sensory neurons: identical pathways and overlapping CRFs in the periphery. Thus, there appears to be a regrowth of cut axons to their original peripheral locations, provided the already established peripheral nerve trunks are available for guidance. Leech (and crustacean) nerves also can fuse with their cut distal ends, and thereby re-establish the correct innervation. Such fusions have been noted in various motoneurons of the crayfish (e.g. Hoy et al., 1967) and in the S-cell interneuron of the leech (Frank et al., 1975; Carbenetto and Muller, 1977). In order to do so, nerve fusions presumably rely upon some specific recognition factor operating at the level of the individual cell.

Superinnervation patterns, similar to that seen in the leech, can be chemically induced in salamander skin by treatment of one nerve trunk with colchicine, which results in collateral sprouting by adjacent nerve fibers. In this instance, both the treated fiber endings and the newly induced collateral endings are mechanically sensitive, and respond to touch by generating action potentials (Cooper et al., 1977).

CRITICAL TEST OF THE PERIPHERAL SEARCHING HYPOTHESIS

Recent work by Bloom and Tompkins (1976) on 180° skin-grafted *Rana pipiens* has shown that, if sensory nerve trunk recordings are made close to the DRG, a dorsally directed shift in the compound *ventral* CRFs is observed. Ventral CRFs apparently do not normally extend beyond the plica in this species of frog, but in 180°-grafted *R. pipiens*, with belly skin grafts now located on the dorsum, the ventral CRFs were found to have expanded dorsally to innervate modest portions of the belly skin on the back (portions from which some misdirected reflexes had been obtained). These data led the authors to believe that a selective return of appropriate nerve types to their original end-organs must have occurred, and was probably responsible for the development of misdirected wiping responses in these animals.

Our own studies have been conducted on the frog *Discoglossus pictus*, a species which also produces (when skin is grafted in a manner similar to that reported for *R. pipiens*) misdirected reflex behavior in post-metamorphic frogs (Fig. 6). Our recordings of the ventral and dorsal CRFs for such animals showed that the ventral CRFs indeed frequently crossed onto the dorsum to innervate grafted belly skin, while dorsal CRFs were never seen to cross the plica to provide innervation to flank or belly skin. Also in *normal D. pictus*, however, ventral CRFs frequently crossed the dorsal ridge to innervate varying areas of the dorsum (Fig. 7A), yet these animals never gave any misdirected reflexes upon stimulation of the normal back. When maps of the ventral CRFs in optimally skin-grafted frogs (i.e. grafts covering the entire dorsal and ventral surfaces of the animal) are compared with the behavioral maps given by the same animal over an extended period of time, it was noticed that even in cases where the ventral CRFs extended up to the midline of the back, misdirected reflexes might fail to be elicited outside of a small, laterally located area of the skin (Fig. 7B). Conversely, there were cases in which the ventral CRFs failed to include all of the grafted belly skin from which misdirected wiping responses could be elicited (Fig. 7C). Since

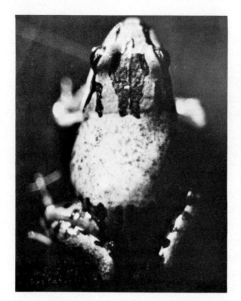
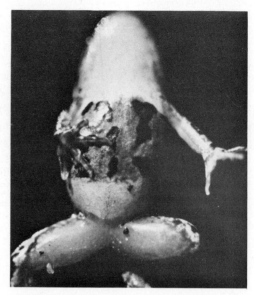

Fig. 6. Skin-grafted frogs (*Lymnodynastes peronii*). Left: with belly skin grafted on the back. Right: with back skin grafted on the belly.

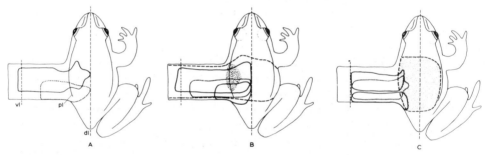

Fig. 7. CRFs and behavior in control and skin-grafted *D. pictus* frogs. A: ventral CRFs in control frog; CRFs for ventral nerve trunks VI and VII extend over lateral ridge to mid-dorsum, yet only normal behavioral wipes were noted. B: ventral CRFs for ganglia V, VI and VII extend over the lateral ridge to the dorsal midline in this 180° bilaterally grafted frog. Despite maximal CRF extension, only a small lateral area on the graft gave rise to misdirected reflex responses (stipple). C: ventral CRFs for ganglia V, VI and VII barely extend over the lateral ridge in this single belly skin-grafted frog. Misdirected forelimb wiping reflexes (stipple), however, were elicited from dorsal graft areas lying well outside of the ventral CRFs. (From Baker et al., 1977.)

such areas often lay well outside the dorsalmost extent of the ventral CRFs, expansion of ventral nerve trunk CRFs cannot very well be the factor which is primarily responsible for the development of misdirected reflexes. Rather, the *dorsal* nerve trunks must be carrying most of the nerve fibers which mediate misdirected (i.e. ventrally directed) wiping reflexes upon stimulation of the back.

To test this deduction, four animals with large belly skin grafts on the dorsum, each giving rise to misdirected wiping reflexes aimed at the ventrum, were subjected to crushing of all the thoracic dorso-medial nerve trunks on one side of the body (Baker et al., 1977). In all four animals, the misdirected wiping responses disappeared from the entire ipsilateral area alongside the midline incision, and covering most of the grafted skin. The remainder of the graft produced behavioral maps similar to those obtained in earlier test sessions. These data demonstrate that misdirected reflexes must be elicited chiefly by nerve fibers reaching the back skin via the dorsal nerve trunks, and at best only in part from ventral CRF extensions.

Since enlargement of regenerated CRFs occurs both in the leech (van Essen and Jansen, 1976) and in the frog (Baker et al., 1977), I suggest that the dorsal extensions observed by Bloom and Tompkins (1976) in their *Rana pipiens* were a non-selective reaction to the skin-grafting operation itself, and cannot be more than marginally responsible for such reflexes. Several recently concluded experiments have provided further evidence which supports this conclusion. First of all, ventral CRFs spread equally well in single-skin animals which failed to give misdirected reflexes from skin grafts located on the ventrum. Secondly, the ventrolateral (VL) nerve trunk is the peripheral nerve trunk most affected by graft rotations, always providing the dorsalmost portion of ventral CRFs (i.e. that portion of the compound ventral CRF most likely to be associated with graft areas giving rise to misdirected reflexes). Yet in several single-skin and 180° graft-rotated animals, the VL's CRF extended all the way to the *ventral* midline without evoking any misdirected reflexes. Lastly, CRFs of the dorsal nerve trunk were never observed to extend ventrally even in frogs which *did* give misdirected reflexes from ventrally located back skin grafts, as would be expected if fibers within these trunks were responsible for misdirected wiping responses.

The confirmation that misdirected belly responses are indeed mediated by fibers within the dorsal nerve trunks raised the following question. Do the fibers coursing in the dorsal trunks belong to belly or to back skin neurons within the DRG? If they belong to belly neurons, then the responses elicited by mechanical stimulation of the rotated belly skin are appropriate to the cell types providing innervation, but their location in the dorsal nerve trunk is anomalous. If they are back neurons, on the other hand, their location in dorsal nerve trunks is correct but the wiping responses are now reversed. Further, by what mechanism are misdirected hindlimb wiping responses evoked from back skin grafts located on the ventrum? The question still to be answered, then, is could a selective growth of belly and back skin neurites to the rotated skin grafts occur via mechanisms other than that of peripheral searching?

CRITICAL TEST OF THE 'MULTIPLE BRANCHING' HYPOTHESIS

A second possibility for explaining the behavior of skin-grafted frogs on the basis of selective afferent innervation of the skin, one which does not require any assumptions about directed outgrowth of nerve fibers, would be for each ganglion cell to initially send multiple collaterals to the periphery, with persistence of only those which happpen to properly match the sensory receptor encountered (Fig. 8). In this model, animals with a single type of skin on both belly and back (and showing misdirected wiping reflexes, of course) would be expected to have many units either possessing more than one CRF or having abnormally large receptive fields. Branched CRFs have been occasionally observed in normal adult frogs, and could represent vestigial remnants of a once more extensive embryonic condition (Adrian et al., 1931; Verveen, 1963).

The above prediction turned out not to be the case in a series of all-belly skin preparations which we examined electrophysiologically (Corner et al., 1977; also Mendell and Hollyday, 1976, for single-unit recordings from supernumerary legs in *Xenopus*). Only one out of more than 250 neurons studied in 6 frogs showed anything remotely approaching the predicted

88

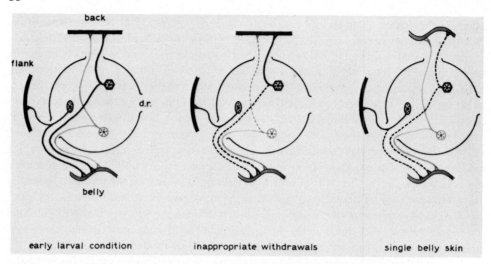

early larval condition   inappropriate withdrawals   single belly skin

Fig. 8. Hypothetical schema of multiple branching in spinal ganglion sensory neurons. Left: normal larval condition. Middle: withdrawal of one branch which had erroneously connected with an incompatible skin type. Right: the experimental situation with a single belly skin-grafted animal; both branches of the belly skin neuron remain viable, while back skin neurons, lacking an appropriate periphery, die.

receptive field pattern (Fig. 9). Neither of the two split-field CRFs which were found provided simultaneous innervation to *both* normal belly skin and grafted belly skin on the animals dorsum, but rather innervated normal belly and flank skin areas. Thus, sensory ganglion cells rarely possess split receptive fields, and even when they do the location of the two fields is not able to explain misdirected wiping responses arising from the atypically located skin-graft. The multiple-collateral hypothesis, therefore, must be rejected as being insufficient to account for the development of misdirected reflex responses in skin-grafted anurans.

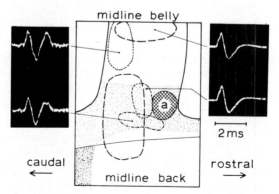

Fig. 9. CRFs of three unusual cutaneous neurons. Two possess split receptive fields, on both belly and flank skin, while the third extends from normal belly skin on the ventrum to the grafted belly skin graft on the dorsum. The recorded action potentials from the separated fields are shown for the two belly/flank cells (left: triphasic extracellular spike, 1.5 mV peak-to-peak; right, 7 mV positive spike, quasi-intracellular, with large afterpotential). Excised forelimb stub indicated by 'a'. (From Corner et al., 1977.)

CRITICAL TEST OF THE 'DEGENERATION-REGENERATION' MECHANISM

The final selective growth mechanism to be considered is for the nerves involved in the grafting experiments to undergo a selective degeneration-regeneration sequence (Fig. 10). After axon section and initial regrowth, through a short-lived association with rotated skin, the neurons would come to 'know' that their connections are with an inappropriate sort of skin. These atypical connections would then be broken, with the neurite degenerating back to the cell body, and sending out a new neurite in the direction of its orginal end-organs (now located at an atypical site on the animal's body). In this way, belly neurons of the DRG would send their neurites to the dorsum via nerve branches which originally carried only back skin neurons, and vice versa. The CRF maps obtained by recording from the peripheral branches would be indistinguishable from maps reported for control nerve trunks, and are therefore incapable of deciding between the two major hypotheses. While the degeneration-regeneration hypothesis perhaps presupposes unrealistic demands on a neuron's growing capabilities, it is an alternative which nevertheless needs to be examined experimentally before drawing any firm conclusions.

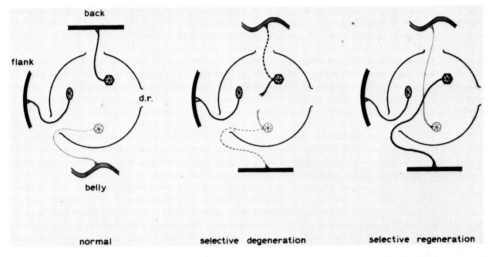

Fig. 10. Hypothetical schema of selective degeneration-regeneration of peripheral cutaneous nerve cells associated with skin grafts in the frog. Left: normal condition. Middle: nerve fibers come into contact with foreign skin types, break connections, and degenerate back to cell bodies in the ganglion. Right: new fibers regenerate out existing nerve trunks towards original skin types, regardless of where that skin might be located on the body.

In order to test the possibility of selective return of innervation to grafted skin in *D. pictus*, we have been recording the topographical locations of cell types in the thoracic DRG of this species of frog (Baker, Corner and Veltman, in preparation). In adult *Rana esculenta* and *D. pictus* the overall topography, despite considerable individual variations, shows that the ventral surface of thoracic DRG projects predominantly to the animal's belly (Fig. 11). This differential projection pattern is strongest in the caudal half of the ganglia, where almost twice as many neurons were found projecting to belly as to back skin. The pattern is reversed for the dorsal surface, where the majority of the cutaneous units project to back skin.

90

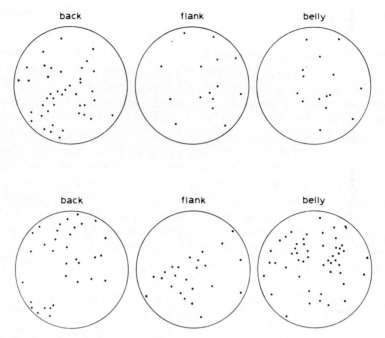

Fig. 11. Composite of cutaneous nerve cell topography in the thoracic ganglia of *Rana esculenta* (from about 30 animals). Top: dorsal aspect of ganglia V–VII showing distribution of back, flank and belly neurons. Bottom: ventral aspect of ganglion VI showing distribution of back, flank and belly skin neurons.

The hypothesis of selective degeneration-regeneration of previously determined classes of nerve fibers (in this instance, belly and back cutaneous afferents) means, in effect, that misdirected reflexes are caused by the back and/or the belly neurons managing to find the appropriately matching skin despite its abnormal location on the body. As such, a switch in peripheral terminations ought to be readily demonstrable: regions within the spinal ganglia which normally project heavily to the frog's ventrum should now project largely to the (belly) skin grafted onto the dorsum, whereas predominantly back skin regions of the DRG should acquire a heavy projection to the ventrum. This would be the case, furthermore, regardless of the route taken by the fibers to reach the proper skin type (see Figs. 3, 8 and 10).

The topographical location of cutaneous mechanoceptive neurons was studied, therefore, in thoracic spinal ganglia of *D. pictus* frogs in which large portions of back and belly skin had been interchanged prior to metamorphosis. Four of the nine animals studied gave excellent misdirected reflex responses *both* from belly skin on the dorsum and from back skin on the ventrum. (The other five animals were not able to be tested satisfactorily on the ventral side, but gave misdirected reflexes from the dorsum – the ganglion topography was the same as in the first four animals, however; four additional skin-rotated frogs were not used for the ganglion mapping experiments because the back skin grafts on the frog's ventrum evoked only *normal* forelimb responses). We found that the distribution of back and belly skin neurons within the DRG in this group of nine operated frogs was indistinguishable from that observed in control frogs (Table I). The data thus indicate that no switch in CRF projection patterns from the DRG is likely to have occurred in 180° skin-rotated *D. pictus*.

The degeneration-regeneration mechanism too does not seem, therefore, to be the correct explanation for the development of misdirected responses in these animals. Although

TABLE I

PROPORTIONS OF CUTANEOUS SENSORY UNITS IN THORACIC DORSAL ROOT GANGLIA OF CONTROL AND 180° GRAFT-ROTATED *D. PICTUS* FROGS

n, number of units recorded per ganglion. Numbers in parentheses after graft description represent number of animals per group. v, ventral side; d, dorsal side of the ganglia. Be, belly; Ba, back neurons.

Ganglion	Controls (10)					180° Rotation graft (9)				
	V	VI	VII	Total		V	VI	VII	Total	
n	62	97	71	230	73	88	111	56	255	29
Belly	0.35	0.43	0.38	0.40	0.27	0.33	0.32	0.39	0.34	0.34
Flank	0.31	0.31	0.31	0.31	0.37	0.40	0.43	0.30	0.39	0.21
Back	0.34	0.26	0.31	0.30	0.36	0.27	0.24	0.30	0.27	0.45
Be/Ba	1.05	1.68	1.23	1.34	0.77	1.21	1.33	1.29	1.28	0.77
	(Ventral)			(v)	(d)	(ventral)			(v)	(d)

none of the experiments offer any support for selectivity in the establishment of cutaneous innervation patterns in skin-grafted frogs, the topography of functional cell types within the ganglion nevertheless indicates that axonal outgrowth from the ganglion is not a random process. Since all or most neurons first send their axons into the interior of the ganglion, where they divide to form central and peripheral branches (Fig. 12), the

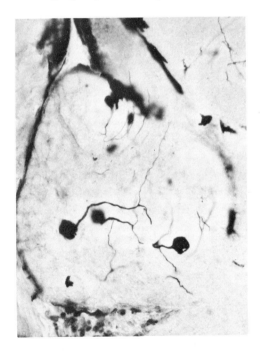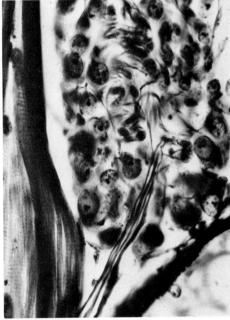

Fig. 12. Spinal ganglion histology in early larval *D. pictus*, showing three sensory neurons (left) with their axons projecting towards the center of the ganglion, where they bifurcate into a larger branch projecting to the periphery, and a smaller branch projecting into the spinal cord: Golgi-Cox preparation. Right: Bodian silver-stained preparation showing the relatively peripheral location of nerve cell bodies, with the afferent fibers coursing into the center of the ganglion.

differential location of belly and back skin cells implies that each class of nerve fibers must have grown out preferentially along one of several possible routes. This surmise is confirmed when the topography of neurons projecting to the *flank* is also taken into consideration. Thus, despite the fact that flank nerve fibers travel for a long distance together with belly fibers in the ventral nerve trunk, the ratio of flank to belly units differs significantly between the medial and lateral halves of the thoracic spinal ganglia, both in *D. pictus* and *R. esculenta* (see Fig. 11).

SINGLE-SKIN GANGLION TOPOGRAPHY

If one looks at the topography of the neurons in the DRG of single-skin animals, a striking deviation from the topography seen in control animals is observed: the ventral surfaces of thoracic DRG in single belly skin animals project predominantly to the dorsum instead of to the ventrum (Table II). Since no such change in innervation pattern had been found in the 180°-rotated skin preparations, however, a role in the occurrence of reversed tactile reflexes seems highly questionable. This doubt becomes a virtual certainty when the findings in frogs with only back skin grafts are examined. These preparations gave only *normal* wiping responses from all graft areas, but nevertheless underwent a clearcut change in the pattern of innervation of the body surface, a change which was precisely opposite to that seen in the all-belly skin frogs (Table II). Thus, the dorsal surfaces of the ganglia projected primarily to the ventrum instead of to the dorsum in this group of animals, and there was a greatly reduced proportion of dorsally projecting units found on the ventral surfaces as well.

A possible explanation for these effects in single skin frogs is that, rather than certain ganglion cells *shifting* their peripheral connections (as in selective regrowth mechanisms, as discussed above), there has been an actual *loss* of certain classes of nerve fibers. In belly skin preparations these would be the belly units, and in back skin frogs the back units. The common factor in both cases is that skin from a sibling tadpole (i.e. homografting rather than autografting) had been grafted at those places where nerve connections seem to have disappeared. An immunological response to the foreign skin is known to occur in tadpoles of other

TABLE II

PROPORTIONS OF CUTANEOUS SENSORY UNITS IN THORACIC DORSAL ROOT GANGLIA OF SINGLE SKIN-GRAFTED *D. PICTUS* FROGS

n, number of units recorded per ganglion. Numbers in parentheses after graft description represent number of animals per group.

Ganglion n	Single skin, belly (7)					Single skin, back (6)				
	V *49*	*VI* *75*	*VII* *58*	*V* *22*	*VI* *30*	*V* *44*	*VI* *63*	*V* *32*	*VI* *45*	*VII* *25*
Belly	0.27	0.25	0.31	0.32	0.27	0.39	0.40	0.28	0.42	0.40
Flank	0.24	0.40	0.47	0.27	0.37	0.45	0.51	0.41	0.53	0.48
Back	0.49	0.35	0.22	0.41	0.37	0.16	0.10	0.31	0.04	0.12
Be/Ba	0.54	0.73	1.38	0.78	0.73	2.43	4.17	0.90	9.50	3.33
		(ventral)		(dorsal)		(ventral)		(dorsal)		

anurans, and can be severe enough even to cause rejection of the graft (e.g. Hadley, 1929; Borbjerg, 1966; Hildemann and Hass, 1959). If the integrity of their peripheral innervation is crucial to the survival of cutaneous neurons, then perhaps the loss of the sensory end-organ at a critical stage of development results in the death of those neurons associated with the degenerating end-organ. Such losses might then be partially, or even wholly, compensated for by later maturing cells ('spare' neurons), presumably located deeper within the ganglion.

The possibility that neuronal survival depends upon intact peripheral innervation offers a plausible alternative mechanism for consideration as the means by which selective reflex connections become established. On the sensory side, each skin type might be presented during ontogeny with a mixed population of nerve fibers (arising from prespecified 'back' and 'belly' neurons), with only the neurites which properly match the skin type encountered becoming stabilized in the course of maturation. In this model of selective growth, skin transplanted early enough to an abnormal site would receive its definitive nerve supply from cells which, under normal circumstances, would have disappeared or become inactivated with further development. I hasten to point out, however, that directed outgrowth of sensory axons (as suggested by the normal ganglionic topography: see Fig. 11 and Table I) should not be thought of in absolute terms inasmuch as fibers sometimes reach the dorsum via a ventral instead of a dorsal nerve trunk.

CONCLUSIONS

During development, sensory neurons send out neurites connecting the periphery with the CNS and, in those cases where the initial outgrowth of a sensory neurite has been directly observed, they selectively innervate peripheral and/or central structures. These connections may be formed with varying degrees of 'searching'. Minimal searching occurs in those neurites which are channelled directly towards their preferred partners via simple anatomical routing. Maximal searching occurs when neurites grow into organs or areas where many possible sites for occupancy are available. Such neurites may bypass targets of similar type, i.e. other muscles, skin, etc., and selectively connect with a given end-organ only after a tortuous route has been negotiated. In this latter instance, some system of multiple cues must operate in directing these neurites to their preferred synaptic partners.

Tissue culture and regeneration studies on invertebrate and vertebrate sensory systems confirm the observations presented above: when given an opportunity for doing so, neurons will selectively reconnect with particular end-organs. Whether regenerating neurites, in selecting their appropriate end-organs, respond to the same cues which were experienced by the first outgrowing neurites, is unknown. It is also not known whether the selectivity of re-innervation by any regenerating neurite is specific for a given site, or simply for a given area and/or modality.

Many sensory neurons, unlike centrally derived nerve cells, originate from neural crest cells. In most instances, therefore, two long processes are required to link up the periphery with a central network. It is not known to what extent, if any, the periphery might act in directing the final selection of central connections. Since the outgrowth of sensory neurites (whether initially, during regeneration, or in tissue culture) does not appear to be a random process, and since tortuous routes may be taken by such neurites in locating their appropriate end-organs, great reservations must be held in assigning to the periphery any role in directing central synaptic connections.

On the other hand, many studies on supernumerary limb transplants in frogs and chicks, and on rotated skin grafts in frogs, have suggested that the peripheral end-organ could be playing a significant role in determining central reflex connections in these animals. Wherever non-random outgrowth and selective innervation have been observed in sensory neurons, it has always been in *either* the peripheral or the central branch but never in both simultaneously. Thus, we simply do not know how one branch might behave when the other is experimentally interfered with. Two basic alternatives are thus open to us regarding the question of the basis for selectivity in cutaneous afferent innervation patterns. Either (1) the sensory neurons preferentially select their pathways and their end-organs, thereby (re)establishing the correct correspondence between peripheral and central connections (*selective innervation*), or (2) sensory neurons traverse any peripheral pathway and innervate whatever end-organ is found at the end of it, but then select the central synaptic sites appropriate for that end-organ (*sensory 'modulation'*).

None of the selective innervation mechanisms discussed in this review proved to be compatible with our newest experimental findings. Innervation of translocated skin grafts via expansion of the cutaneous receptive fields, for instance, was found to be untenable because large areas of grafted skin could lie outside the expanded fields and still give rise to misdirected wiping responses. Multiple branching of neurites from single neurons, so as to innervate different body areas, does not occur with a high enough frequency to be taken seriously as a mechanism underlying the misdirected response phenomenon. Selective degeneration-regeneration of cutaneous afferents is highly unlikely, finally, because no differences were observed between normal and experimental topographical maps for belly and back neurons within the sensory ganglia after the skin was rotated through 180°.

We are now faced with the challenge of designing an experimental strategy which would allow us to detect possible ganglion cell losses, associated with replacement by 'spare' neurons, following the innervation of an inappropriate skin type. The major difficulty here is that most of the predictions which can be deduced from the *'spare' neuron* hypothesis are consistent with the *cutaneous specification* hypothesis as well. A crucial experiment to distinguish between these two mechanisms still remains to be formulated.

ACKNOWLEDGEMENTS

The most recent experiments, carried out over the last few years at the Netherlands Institute for Brain Research, were done in collaboration with Drs. Michael Corner and Wim Veltman, ably assisted by Ton Richter and Jos van de Nes. The Hubrecht Embryological Laboratory in Utrecht was always a most generous and enthusiastic supplier of *Discoglossus pictus* tadpoles (the backbone of our experimental program) for which the author owes Mrs. Verhoeff-Fremery, Chris Gorlec and Prof. Pieter Nieuwkoop a large debt of gratitude.

REFERENCES

Adrian, E.D., Cattell, M. and Hoagland, H. (1931) Sensory discharges in single cutaneous nerve fibres, *J. Physiol. (Lond.)*, 72: 377–391.

Baker, R.E., Corner, M.A. and Veltman, W.A.M. (1977) Cutaneous receptive field enlargement following skin-grafting at larval stages in the frog, *Discoglossus pictus, Brain Res. Bull.*, 2: 475–477.

Baker, R.E., and Jacobson, M. (1970) Development of reflexes from skin grafts in *Rana pipiens*: influence of size and position of grafts, *Develop. Biol.*, 22: 476–494.

Baker, R.E. and Richter, A.Ph.J. (1977) Development of dorsal root III afferent in postmetamorphic juveniles of the frog, *Discoglossus pictus, Neuroscience*, 2: 271–273.

Baker, R.E., Richter, A.Ph.J. and Piller, N. (1976) A light and electron microscopic examination of dorsal root afferent development in three species of anurans, *Neuroscience*, 1: 367–370.

Baker, R.E., Veltman, W.A.M. and Corner, M.A. (1977) Effect of cutaneous stimulation on the development of misdirected wiping reflexes in skin-grafted *D. pictus, Develop. Psychobiol.*, 10: 299–304.

Bate, C.M. (1976) Pioneer neurones in an insect embryo, *Nature (Lond.)*, 260: 54–56.

Baylor, D.A. and Nicholls, J.G. (1971) Patterns of regeneration between individual nerve cells in the central nervous system of the leech, *Nature (Lond.)*, 232: 268–269.

Bittner, G.D. and Johnson, A.L. (1974) Degeneration and regeneration in crustacean peripheral nerves, *J. comp. Physiol.*, 89: 1–21.

Bloom, E.M. and Tompkins, R. (1976) Selective reinnervation in skin rotation grafts in *Rana pipiens, J. exp. Zool.*, 195: 237–246.

Borbjerg, A.M. (1966) Rejection of skin homografts in larvae of *Rana pipiens, J. exp. Zool.*, 161: 69–80.

Brown, M.E. (1946) The histology of the tadpole tail during metamorphosis, with special reference to the nervous system, *Amer. J. Anat.*, 78: 79–113.

Burgess, P.R. and Horch, K.W. (1973) Specific regeneration of cutaneous fibers in the cat, *J. Neurophysiol.*, 36: 101–114.

Burgess, P.R., English, K.B., Horch, K.W. and Stensaas, L.J. (1974) Patterning in the regeneration of type I cutaneous receptors, *J. Physiol. (Lond.)*, 236: 57–82.

Carbonetto, S. and Muller, K.J. (1977) A regenerating neurone in the leech can form an electrical synapse on its severed axon segment, *Nature (Lond.)*, 267: 450–452.

Cole, W.H. (1922) The transplantation of skin in frog tadpoles, with special reference to the adjustment of grafts over eyes, and to the local specificity of integument, *J. exp. Zool.*, 35: 353–420.

Cooper, E. and Diamond, J. (1977) A quantitative study of the mechanosensory innervation of the salamander limb, *J. Physiol. (Lond.)*, 264: 695–723.

Cooper, E., Diamond, J. and Turner, C. (1977) The effects of nerve section and of colchicine treatment on the density of mechanosensory nerve endings in salamander skin, *J. Physiol. (Lond.)*, 264: 725–749.

Corner, M.A., Baker, R.E. and Veltman, W.A.M. (1977) Receptive fields of cutaneous mechanoreceptive neurons in the frog, *Discoglossus pictus*, following skin transplantation at larval stages, *Brain Res. Bull.*, 2: 393–395.

Diamond, J. (1976) Sprouting: regeneration and competition in salamander skin innervation, *Neurosci, Res. Prog. Bull.*, 14: 337–346.

Eccles, J.C., Eccles, R.M., Shealy, C.N. and Willis, W.D. (1962) Experiments utilizing monosynaptic excitatory action on motoneurons for testing hypotheses relating to specificity of neuronal connections, *J. Neurophysiol.*, 25: 559–580.

Edwards, J. and Sahota, T.S. (1968) Regeneration of a sensory system: the formation of central connections by normal and transplanted cerci of the house cricket *Acheta domesticus, J. exp. Zool.*, 166: 387–396.

Edwards, J.S. and Palka, J. (1971) Neural regeneration: delayed formation of central contacts by insect sensory cells, *Science*, 172: 591–594.

Edwards, J.S. and Palka, J. (1973) Neural specificity as a game of cricket: some rules for sensory regeneration in *Acheta domesticus*. In *Developmental Neurobiology of Arthropods*, J. Young (Ed.), Cambridge Univ. Press, pp. 131–146.

Essen, D. van and Jansen, J.K.S. (1976) Repair of specific neuronal pathways in the leech, *Cold Spr. Harb. Symp. quant. Biol.*, 40: 495–502.

Essen, D.C. van and Jansen, J.K.S. (1977) The specificity of re-innervation by identified sensory and motor neurones in the leech, *J. comp. Neurol.*, 171: 433–454.

Fox, H. (1973) Degeneration of the nerve cord in the tail of *Rana temporaria* during metamorphic climax: study by electron microscopy, *J. Embryol. exp. Morph.*, 30: 377–396.

Frank, E., Jansen, J.K.S. and Rinvik, E. (1975) A multisomatic axon in the central nervous system of the leech, *J. comp. Neurol.*, 159: 1–14.

Gaze, R.M., Chung, S.H. and Keating, M.J. (1972) Development of the retinotectal projection in *Xenopus, Nature (Lond.)*, 236: 133–135.

Grimm, L.M. (1971) An evaluation of myotypic respecification in axolotls, *J. exp. Zool.*, 178: 479–496.

Hadley, C.E. (1929) The compatibility of the skin of *Rana pipiens* and *Rana clamitans* as tested by transplantations, *J. exp. Zool.*, 54: 127–155.

Hardesty, I. (1899) The number and arrangement of the fibers forming the spinal nerves of the frog (*Rana virescens*), *J. comp. Neurol.*, 9: 64–112.

Hardesty, I. (1900) Further observations on the conditions determining the number and arrangement of the fibers forming the spinal nerves of the frog (*Rana virescens*), *J. comp. Neurol.*, 10: 323–354.

Hardesty, I. (1905) On the number and relations of the ganglion cells and medullated nerve fibers in the spinal nerves of frogs of different ages, *J. comp. Neurol.*, 19: 17–56.

Head, H. and Rivers, W.H.R. (1905) The afferent nervous system from a new aspect, *Brain*, 28: 99–115.

Helf, O.M. (1931) Studies on amphibian metamorphosis. IX. Integumentary specificity and dermal plicae formation in the anuran, *Rana pipiens*, *Biol. Bull*, 60: 11–22.

Herrick, E.H. (1932) Mechanism of movement of epidermis, especially its melanophores, in wound healing, and behaviour of skin grafts in frog tadpoles, *Biol. Bull.*, 63: 271–286.

Hildemann, W.H. and Haas, R. (1959) Homotransplantation immunity and tolerance in the bullfrog, *J. Immunol.*, 83: 478–485.

Hollyday, M. and Mendell, L. (1975) Area specific reflexes from normal and supernumerary hindlimbs of *Xenopus laevis*, *J. comp. Neurol.*, 162: 205–220.

Hoy, R.R., Bittner, G.D. and Kennedy, D. (1967) Regeneration in crustacean motoneurons: evidence for axonal fusion, *Science*, 156: 251–252.

Hughes, A. (1959) Studies in embryonic and larval development in amphibia. I. The embryology of *Eleutherodactylus ricordii*, with special reference to the spinal cord, *J. Embyrol. exp. Morph.*, 7: 22–38.

Hughes, A. (1961) Cell degeneration in the larval ventral horn of *Xenopus laevis* (Daudin), *J. Embryol. exp. Morph.*, 9: 269–284.

Hughes, A. (1973) The development of dorsal root ganglia and ventral horns in the opossum. A quantitative study, *J. Embryol. exp. Morph.*, 30: 359–376.

Hughes, A. and Tschumi, P.A. (1958) The factors controlling the development of the dorsal root ganglia and ventral horn in *Xenopus laevis* (Daudin), *J. Anat. (Lond.)*, 92: 498–527.

Hughes, A., Egar, M. and Turner, T. (1969) Degeneration of nerve fibres within the embryonic spinal cord, *Nature (Lond.)*, 221: 579–581.

Jacobson, M. and Baker, R.E. (1969) Development of neuronal connections with skin grafts in frogs: behavioural and electrophysiological studies, *J. comp. Neurol.*, 137: 121–142.

Jansen, J.K.S., Muller, K.J. and Nicholls, J.G. (1974) Persistent modification of synaptic interactions between sensory and motor nerve cells following discrete lesions in the central nervous system of the leech, *J. Physiol. (Lond.)*, 242: 289–305.

Johnston, B.T., Schrameck, J.E. and Mark, R.F. (1975) Re-innervation of axolotl limbs. II. Sensory nerves, *Proc. roy. Soc. B*, 190: 59–75.

Joseph, B.S. and Whitlock, D.G. (1966) Central connections of caudal dorsal root ganglion in the toad (*Bufo marinus*), *Anat. Rec.*, 154: 364.

Joseph, B.S. and Whitlock, D.G. (1968) Central projections of selected spinal dorsal roots in anuran amphibians, *Anat. Rec.*, 160: 280–288.

Kuffler, D.P. and Muller, K.J. (1974) The properties and connections of supernumerary sensory and motor nerve cells in the central nervous system of an abnormal leech, *J. Neurobiol.*, 5: 331–348.

Landmesser, L. and Pilar, G. (1974a) Synapse formation during embryogenesis on ganglion cells lacking a periphery, *J. Physiol. (Lond.)*, 241: 715–736.

Landmesser, L. and Pilar, G. (1974b) Synaptic transmission and cell death during normal ganglionic development, *J. Physiol. (Lond.)*, 241: 737–749.

Landmesser, L. and Morris, D.G. (1975) The development of functional innervation in the hindlimb of the chick embryo, *J. Physiol. (Lond.)*, 249: 301–326.

Lamb, A.H. (1974) The timing of the earliest motor innervation to the hindlimb bud in the *Xenopus* tadpole, *Brain Res.*, 67: 527–530.

Lamb, A.H. (1976) The projection patterns of the ventral horn to the hind limb during development, *Develop. Biol.*, 54: 82–99.

Liu, C.N. and Chambers, W.W. (1957) Experimental study of anatomical organization of frog's spinal cord, *Anat. Rec.*, 127: 326.

Lopresti, V., Macagno, E.R. and Levinthal, C. (1973) Structure and development of neuronal connections in isogenic organisms: cellular interactions in the development of the optic lamina of *Daphnia*, *Proc. nat. Acad. Sci. (Wash.)*, 70: 433–437.

MacLean, M. and Edwards, J.S. (1976) Target discrimination in regenerating insect sensory nerve, *J. Embyrol. exp. Morph.*, 36: 19–39.

Maynard, D.M. (1965) The occurrence and functional characteristics of heteromorph antennules in an experimental population of spiny lobsters, *Panularus argus, J. exp. Biol.*, 43: 79–106.

Maynard, D.M. and Cohen, M.J. (1965) The function of a heteromorph antennule in a spiny lobster, *Panularus argus, J. exp. Biol.*, 43: 55–78.

Mendell, L.M. and Scott, J.G. (1975) The effect of peripheral nerve cross-union on connections of single Ia fibers to motoneurons, *Exp. Brain Res.*, 22: 221–234.

Mendell, L.M. and Hollyday, M. (1976) Spinal reflexes with altered periphery. In *Frog Neurobiology*, R. Llinas and W. Precht (Eds.), Springer, Heidleberg, pp. 793–810.

Miner, N. (1956) Integumental specification of sensory fibers in the development of cutaneous local sign, *J. comp. Neurol.*, 105: 161–170.

Miyazaki, S., Nicholls, J.G. and Wallace, B.G. (1976) Modification and regeneration of synaptic connections in cultured leech ganglia, *Cold Spr. Harb. Symp. quant. Biol.*, 40: 483–493.

Nafstad, P.H.J. and Baker, R.E. (1973) Comparative ultrastructural study of normal and grafted skin in the frog, *Rana pipiens*, with special reference to neuroepithelial connections, *Z. Zellforsch.*, 139: 451–462.

Nicholls, J.G. and Baylor, D.A. (1968) Specific modalities and receptive fields of sensory neurons in CNS of the leech, *J. Neurophysiol.*, 31: 740–756.

Orgel, M., Aguayo, A. and Williams, H.B. (1972) Sensory nerve regeneration: an experimental study of skin grafts in the rabbit, *J. Anat. (Lond.)*, 111: 121–135.

Prestige, M.C. (1965) Cell turnover in the spinal ganglia of *Xenopus laevis* tadpoles, *J. Embryol. exp. Morph.*, 13: 63–72.

Prestige, M.C. (1967) The control of cell number in the lumbar ventral horns during the development of *Xenopus laevis* tadpoles, *J. Embryol. exp. Morph.*, 18: 359–387.

Prestige, M.C. (1976) Evidence that at least some of the motor nerve cells that die during development have first made peripheral connections, *J. comp. Neurol.*, 170: 123–134.

Prestige, M.C. and Wilson, M.A. (1972) Loss of axons from ventral roots during development, *Brain Res.*, 41: 467–470.

Rand, H.W. and Pierce, M.E. (1932) Skin grafting in frog tadpoles: local specificity of skin and behavior of epidermis, *J. exp. Zool.*, 62: 125–172.

Rivers, W.H.R. and Head, H. (1908) A human experiment in nerve division, *Brain*, 31: 323–450.

Scott, M.Y. and Sperry, R.W. (1975) Tests for left-right chemospecificity in frog cutaneous nerves, *Brain Behav. Evol.*, 11: 60–72.

Sharpey-Schafer, E. (1929) The effects of denervation of a cutaneous area, *Quart. J. exp. Physiol.*, 19: 85–107.

Sharpey-Schafer, E. (1930) The permanent results of denervation of a cutaneous area, *Quart. J. exp. Physiol.*, 20: 95–99.

Sklar, J. and Hunt, R.K. (1973) The acquisition of specificity in cutaneous sensory neurons: a reconsideration of the integumental specification hypothesis, *Proc. nat. Acad. Sci. (Wash.)*, 70: 3684–3688.

Sperry, R.W. (1941) The effect of crossing nerves to antagonistic muscles in the hind limb of the rat, *J. comp. Neurol.*, 75: 1–19.

Sperry, R.W. (1943) Functional results of crossing sensory nerves in the rat, *J. comp. Neurol.*, 78: 59–90.

Sperry, R.W. and Miner, N. (1949) Formation within sensory nucleus V of synaptic association mediating cutaneous localizations, *J. comp. Neurol.*, 90: 403–423.

Stirling, V. (1973) The effect of increasing the innervation field sizes of nerves on their reflex response time in salamanders, *J. Physiol. (Lond.)*, 229: 657–679.

Stocker, R.F., Edwards, J.S., Palka, J. and Schubiger, G. (1976) Projection of sensory neurons from a homeotic mutant appendage, attennapedia, in *Drosophila melanogaster, Develop. Biol.*, 52: 210–220.

Székely, G. (1959) Functional specificity of cranial sensory neuroblasts in urodela, *Acta biol. Acad. Sci. hung.*, 10: 107–116.

Székely, G. (1976) The morphology of motoneurons and dorsal root fibers in the frog's spinal cord, *Brain Res.*, 103: 275–290.

Székely, G. and Szentagothai, J. (1962) Reflex and behaviour patterns elicited from implanted supernumerary limbs in the chick, *J. Embryol. exp. Morph.*, 10: 140–151.

Verveen, A.A. (1963) Fields of touch receptors in frog skin, *Exp. Neurol.*, 8: 482–492.

Weddell, G., Guttmann, L. and Gotmann, E. (1941) The local extension of nerve fibres into denervated areas of skin, *J. Neurol. Psychiat.*, 4: 206–225.

Yau, K.W. (1977a) Physiological properties and receptive fields of mechanosensory neurones in the head ganglion of the leech: comparison with homologous cells in segmental ganglia, *J. Physiol. (Lond.)*, 263: 489–512.

Yau, K.W. (1977b) Receptive fields, geometry and conduction block of sensory neurones in the central nervous system of the leech, *J. Physiol. (Lond.)*, 263: 513–538.

DISCUSSION

CHANGEUX: In your experiments, have you mapped the sensory ganglia in the very early stages? Also, is there any dependence of the results of the skin-rotation experiments as a function of the time?

BAKER: We have not examined what ganglionic changes may be occurring in the metamorphic or immediate post-metamorphic periods. Receptive fields were mapped only in frogs of at least 6 months post-metamorphic age. If you skin-graft late in larval development, at near-metamorphic stages or later, you will no longer get any misdirected reflex responses. One then finds only normal reflex responses, regardless of what kind of grafting is done.

CHANGEUX: Are there nerves present in the skin at the time you are doing the graft?

BAKER: There are nerve fibers already present when the skin grafting operation is made (you can see them actually being torn away as the skin is pulled from the body), and more nerve fibers are added throughout the larval stages. But there also appears to be a rather sudden ingrowth of dorsal root fibers immediately after metamorphosis.

STIRLING: You mentioned that there is a relationship between the appearance of the reflex, as a wiping reflex, and an increase in the number of fibers in the nerve trunk. Could it be that certain neurons degenerate, and in fact what you get at metamorphosis is a new sensory nervous system with a new pattern of connections?

BAKER: The idea of cell replacement is certainly an attractive possibility, but one which would be extremely difficult to prove in the frog systems we now use. As you know, naturally occurring ganglia and spinal cord degenerations are taking place throughout the period of reflex development. It would be difficult to differentiate between this naturally occurring degeneration and possible graft-induced degeneration. Similarly, all of the possible mechanisms presented above for inducing misdirected reflexes in stable nerve systems, would still have to be checked out for neurons which were in the process of replacing dying nerve cells. In other words, do the cutaneous fibers grow out selectively to given skin types in the periphery and similarly make selective central connections based on genetic instructions, or do they grow out willy-nilly, and then make central connections according to the information which they receive there?

Transplantation Techniques
for the Study of Regeneration
in the Central Nervous System

ULF STENEVI and ANDERS BJÖRKLUND

Departments of Ophthalmology and Histology, University of Lund, Lund (Sweden)

INTRODUCTION

The intention of this paper is to briefly describe three transplantation techniques designed for the study of regenerative growth of central and, to some extent, also peripheral neurons. The literature on regeneration in the central nervous system (CNS) has been extensively reviewed by several authors (see Windle, 1956; Clemente, 1964; Moore et al. 1973; Stenevi et al., 1973), and will not be recapitulated here. In short, one can state that interest in CNS regeneration is again increasing, mostly due to the development of new experimental techniques as well as new, sensitive, and selective histochemical and biochemical analytical techniques. Certainly, many contradictory results in the past can now be understood against the background of inadequate techniques. This was already recognized in 1956 by Windle when he stated: "Past failure to recognize fully the possibility of central regeneration may have been due, partly, to casual experimentation with inadequate or even inept techniques, unskilled surgical procedures resulting in massive tissue damage, improper selection of histological methods to reveal regeneration and to wrong timing of experiments. However, there can be no doubt that it was mainly lack of knowledge regarding the means of creating or maintaining a milieu favourable to forward growth of sprouting axons in brain and cord lesions that prevented earlier recognition of the possibilities".

One difficulty inherent in the study of CNS regeneration is the problem of selectivity, i.e. the ability to distinguish newly formed nerve fibers from pre-existing fibers within the CNS tissue. This difficulty is greatly reduced by using the techniques of tissue grafting into the brain and observing the growth of neurites into or out from the transplant. Many investigators have used this classical approach through the years, and have transplanted several types of tissues to many intracerebral locations in different experimental animals. Common to all the experiments involving mammals was their low reproducibility, quite in contrast to the neuronal tissue transplantation or reimplantation experiments performed on lower vertebrates. Thus, most of our current knowledge stems from these latter experiments, and not until recently have adequate techniques been available for mammals (for details and references see Svendgaard et al., 1975 and Stenevi et al., 1976).

Using the transplantation techniques described below, the growth capacity and growth characteristics of different neuron types have been studied. Other features of growing and developing neurons can be studied with the elegant technique of tissue culture (see Crain, 1976, for details). In such an in vitro system interaction between neurons and/or target cells can be followed, intra- and extracellular recordings from the neurons can be made, and the effects of drugs can be conveniently observed. Also, the classical method of transplanting various tissues to the anterior eye chamber have been employed for the study of neuronal development and growth (see Olson and Malmfors, 1970; Olson and Seiger, 1972). In this in vivo 'growth chamber', transplants of sympathetic ganglia or pieces of embryonic brain tissue survive, grow and develop; Olson and co-workers have demonstrated the potential of this culturing technique for the study of development and growth of peripheral and central neurons (for references see Olson and Seiger, 1972 and Seiger and Olson, 1977).

Our own studies were at first concentrated on the regenerative capacity of monoamine-containing neurons in the CNS. For this purpose we have used three different approaches: (1) transplantation of non-nervous tissue to the CNS; (2) transplantation of non-nervous tissue to the retina; (3) transplantation of central or peripheral neurons to the CNS. Each technique will be described and for detailed results references will be given. The recipient animals have always been adult female rats and, in order to avoid interference from regenerating peripheral sympathetic fibers, bilateral cervical sympathectomy has been performed prior to or at the same time as the transplantation.

TRANSPLANTATION OF NON-NERVOUS TISSUE TO THE BRAIN

Sprouting and regenerative growth from axotomized central monoamine neurons following an electrolytic or mechanical lesion was first described in 1971 by Katzman et al. The time course of the sprouting process was subsequently studied for central noradrenaline (NA), dopamine (DA), and indoleamine (IA) neurons (Björklund et al., 1971). To prove once and for all that the nerve fibers newly appearing under the microscope were in fact newly *formed*, the following transplantation technique was introduced and later modified (Björklund and Stenevi, 1971; Stenevi et al., 1974). The rationale was the following: when a peripheral transplant lacking intrinsic neurons is placed inside the brain or spinal cord, then if nerve fibers later appear in the transplant, they must have grown into the transplant and (provided interference by sprouting fibers of peripheral origin is ruled out) they can only be of central origin.

The transplant to be used should either be naturally thin or be trimmed down. Transplants with dimensions of up to 1—2 mm wide and 5—6 mm long have been found to be feasible. The transplant is dissected out with sterile or aseptic instruments and stored in sterile saline at room temperature. The head of the anesthetized rat is fixed conveniently in a stereotactic apparatus, shaved, washed, and the skin opened. The bone overlying the transplantation site is removed and, again with sterile instruments, the dura is opened. If bleeding occurs this is stopped with gel-foam. The transplant is now transferred to the top of the brain with one end covering the opening in the dura. The placement in the brain is performed with a thin glass rod about 1 mm wide and 0.2 mm thick (Fig. 1). The glass rod catches the transplant at that end overlying the opening in the dura. By free hand the rod and the transplant are carefully lowered into the desired position in the brain whereafter the rod is removed in the same fashion. The transplant is thus left in close apposition to the transected axons whose regenerative capacity is to be studied (see Fig. 1). In most of our studies the rat iris has been used as a transplant, but other tissues can be used as well (Björklund and Stenevi, 1971; Björklund et al., 1975, 1976).

The iris has certain advantages that make it particularly useful as a transplant. It is thin and is of the right size, its normal peripheral innervation is well known (Ehinger and Falck, 1966), it survives well, is rapidly vascularized from the surrounding brain vessels and it lacks intrinsic

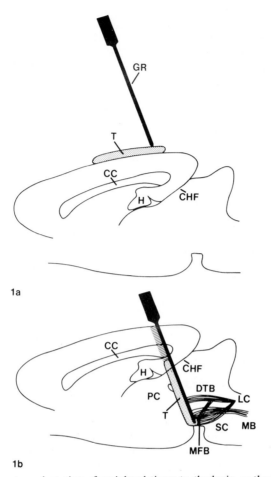

Fig. 1. Diagrams showing transplantation of peripheral tissue to the brain. a: the transplant (T) is placed on top of the brain and the glass rod (GR) catches the posterior portion of the transplant. b: the rod and the transplant have been lowered into position and in the next step the rod is carefully removed, leaving the transplant within the brain tissue. CC, corpus callosum; CHF, choroidal fissure; DTB, dorsal tegmental CA bundle; GR, glass rod; H, hippocampus; LC, locus coeruleus; MB, medullary CA bundle; MFB, medial forebrain bundle; PC, posterior commissure; SC, nucleus subcoeruleus; T, transplant.

neurons (Svendgaard et al., 1975). Finally, it can be transplanted autologously without serious consequences to the experimental animal and, at the end of the experimental period, it can easily be dissected out for further processing (see below).

The placement of the transplant is of course entirely dependent upon what neuronal system or systems are to be investigated (Stenevi et al., 1974; Svendgaard et al., 1975, 1976; Emson et al., 1977). The iris, or an equivalent peripheral tissue, probably can survive in most positions within the brain or spinal cord. Most favorable are those sites where the transplant is in direct contact with pial vessels, since those are the most efficient source of revascularization. Provided that bleedings and infections are avoided, the transplants survive well, and with our techniques no obvious signs of rejection of either autologous or homo- logous grafts can be observed. In a limited number of experiments with *heterologous* grafts of neuronal tissue the survival rate has been poor (cf. Zalewski, 1971 and Zalewski and Singer, 1976). By altering the transplantation site it is possible to have central NA, DA, and IA neurons grow into the iris at the same time, but it is also possible to separate the different

104

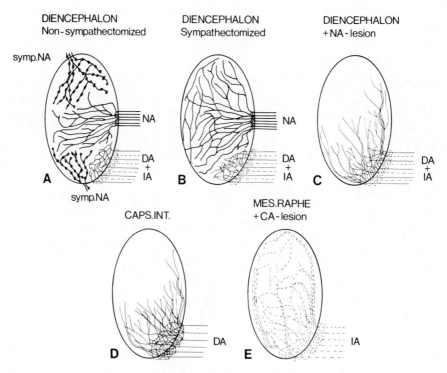

Fig. 2. Diagrams representing schematically the principal features of the ingrowth and extent of sprouting of the different types of monoaminergic neurons: sympathetic NA; central NA; DA; and IA, in irides transplanted under the various experimental conditions. A: non-sympathectomized host animal. Sympathetic and central NA fibers compete with each other in the reinnervation of the transplant, whereas the DA and IA sprouts remain restricted to the region close to their site of ingrowth. B: sympathectomized host animal. Central NA fibers expand over the entire iris, whereas the DA and IA sprouts remain restricted as in A. C: sympathectomized host animal with a lesion of the ascending NA fibers. DA sprouts expand over large parts of the transplant, whereas IA sprouts still remain restricted. D: transplant to the nigro-striatal DA pathway in a sympathectomized host animal. DA sprouts behave principally as in C. E: transplant implanted caudal to the mesencephalic DA cell groups in a sympathectomized host animal with a lesion of the ascending CA fibers. In the absence of growing CA fibers, IA sprouts expand over the entire graft. (From Svendgaard et al. 1975.)

neuronal systems and let each neuron type grow in separately (Fig. 2). In this way the specific growth characteristics of central monoamine neurons, as well as of central cholinergic and GABA neurons have been described (Björklund and Stenevi, 1971; Svendgaard et al., 1975, 1976; Emson et al., 1976, 1977).

At the end of the experimental period the iris is dissected out, freed from surrounding brain tissue, and carefully stretched on a microscope slide (Figs. 3 and 4); with the transplant as a whole mount it can now be readily analyzed using the histochemical technique of choice. Whole mount preparations offer an improved possibility for observations of the distribution and patterning of regenerating fibers in the graft, as compared with the in situ situation, where the grafts must be serially sectioned. For the preparation of the whole mounts, the brain or the eye (see below) is rapidly removed and the iris transplant extirpated under a stereomicroscope (6–16 X). Still under the operating microscope (25–40 X), the grafts are unfolded on a microscope slide with a pair of fine watch-maker forceps. This procedure is facilitated by allowing the first unfolded part to dry enough to attach itself to

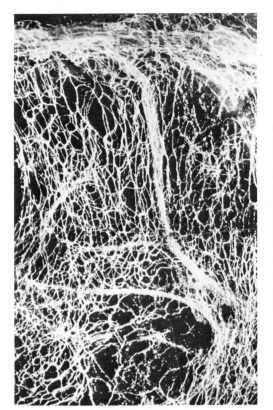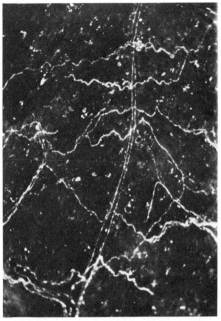

Fig. 3. Left: photomicrograph from an iris transplanted to the caudal diencephalon shown in Fig. 1. One month survival. Central NA neurons from the locus coeruleus form a mature ground plexus. × 135. Right: photomicrograph from an iris transplanted to the retina, one month survival. Retinal DA neurons have grown into the transplant but no mature ground plexus is formed. × 135. In both animals the superior cervical ganglia were removed prior to transplantation.

the slide. The unfolding is carried out with the aim of reproducing the original shape of the iris and to stretch it uniformly. Iris transplants with a survival age of 9–21 days are the easiest to unfold. In younger grafts, edema may cause difficulties, while in older grafts adhesions and infiltrating brain tissue make the unfolding and stretching more difficult. In electron microscopic studies it is better to perfuse the brain before the transplant is removed (Ljungdahl and Stenevi, unpublished information).

In addition to morphological studies, the transplant and the nerve fibers 'trapped' inside it can be assayed for transmitter content and transmitter-related enzymes. In a recent study, the time-course and extent of sprouting were measured at different time intervals using: tyrosine hydroxylase, aromatic amino acid decarboxylase, choline acetyltransferase, acetylcholinesterase, and glutamic acid decarboxylase as markers for, respectively, catecholamine, cholinergic and GABA-producing fibers (Emson et al., 1977). The transplants have also been found suitable for electrophysiological experiments in vitro. With this technique it has been shown that regenerating central NA and cholinergic fibers can establish functional connections with smooth muscle cells within the transplant (Björklund et al., 1975).

It is important to note that, unless the superior cervical ganglia are removed bilaterally, peripheral sympathetic fibers will grow into the transplants and become a potential cause of

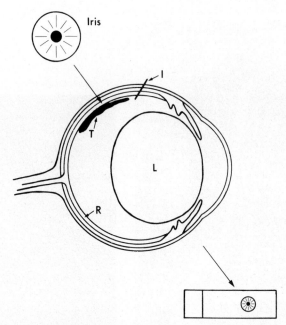

Fig. 4. Schematic drawing of transplants of peripheral tissue to the retina. The iris is dissected and, through the incision (I), placed in contact with the retina (R). For analyses the iris is removed from the eye and stretched on a microscope slide as a whole-mount preparation (see text). I, incision; L, lens; R, retina; T, transplant.

error in this type of investigation. In certain locations in the brain parasympathetic cholinergic axons may also reach the transplant (Svendgaard et al., 1976). To check for such unwanted phenomena, it is essential to include the appropriate miscroscopical controls.

TRANSPLANTATION OF PERIPHERAL TISSUE TO THE RETINA

The retina is part of the CNS. Very little is known about regenerative growth in the adult retina, as opposed to other parts of the visual system (Cunningham, 1972; Goodman et al., 1973; Goodman and Horel, 1966; Hichey, 1975; Lund and Lund, 1971; Stenevi et al., 1973). Degenerative states in the retina are a well-known clinical observation, and 'destructive' treatment in the form of photocoagulation is frequently used against several forms of retinal disease. Most retinal transmitters are still unknown, however, including that of the ganglion cells. DA has been identified in retinal amacrine cells and several amino acids have been proposed as retinal transmitters (see Bouting, 1976, for references). Transplants to the retina can therefore be used with the double purpose of studying retinal regeneration and of identifying the transmitter substance of the regenerating neurons (Stenevi and Björklund, 1978).

The transplant is prepared as described previously. With the rat under general anesthesia, a suture is placed in the upper eyelid in order to expose the anterior portion of the eye. With sterile instruments the conjunctiva is freed from the limbus, and the sclera is exposed to well beyond the ciliary body. One of the rectus muscles is conveniently used to fix the eyeball while operating. The sclera is opened posterior to the ciliary body and, with the same type of thin glass rod described above, the transplant is gently pushed into the eye in contact with the retina (Fig. 4). The cut in the sclera is made under a muscle so that there is no need for sutures. In fact, if the opening in the conjunctiva is made small enough there is no need for any sutures at all. The rat eye has a relatively large lens which might be damaged during the transplantation, resulting in cataract formation. If the lens is damaged, or if an inflammatory reaction occurs within the eye, it should be discarded.

At the end of the experimental period the iris is easily dissected out and further processed as described above. The regenerative growth of retinal DA neurons is shown in Fig. 3, right (Stenevi and Björklund, unpub.). It is important to note that unless the superior cervical ganglia are removed bilaterally, peripheral sympathetic fibers can grow into the transplants, and are thus a potential source of error in this type of investigation.

TRANSPLANTATION OF PERIPHERAL OR CENTRAL NEURONS TO THE BRAIN

Transplantation of neurons to the CNS of mammals has been tried many times through the years but with little success (for references see Stenevi et al., 1976). The survival rate of the transplanted neurons has been low and the reproducibility poor. Adult brain tissue does not seem to survive transplantation at all. Sensory ganglia, on the other hand, partially survive transplantation (Le Gros Clark, 1942; Ranson, 1914; Tidd, 1932), and CNS tissue from young or fetal animals can also be used. Survival of young or fetal CNS tissue transplanted to the brain of very young rats have been observed (Das and Altman, 1971; Lund and Hauschka, 1976). The most extensive study of the survival of transplanted CNS tissue to date is that of Seiger and Olson (1977) using pieces of brain stem grafted into the anterior eye chamber. This study should be consulted for further details on survival of transplants taken from donors of different ages.

The incentive for the development of the following transplantation technique was in order to study axonal growth and regeneration within the adult CNS from transplanted peripheral or central neurons. The transplants used so far have been pieces of adult superior cervical ganglia, pieces of fetal brain stem tissue containing different monoamine-containing cell groups or pieces of fetal cerebellum, cerebral cortex, hippocampus or septum (Kromer et al., 1978). The most critical factor for obtaining good survival of the neural grafts is their rapid and efficient revascularization. This is ensured provided that they are transplanted to a milieu rich in blood vessels, such as the choroidal fissure overlying the thalamus and the tectum (as illustrated in Fig. 5). Nygren et al. (1977) have recently shown that embryonic brain stem tissues survive grafting to the spinal cord. Also in this case, it is

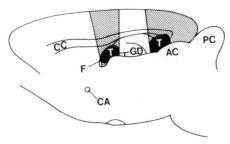

Fig. 5. Schematic representation of the position of the transplants placed onto the pia in the choroidal fissure in the rostral and caudal sites. The hatched area is removed by suction and the bleeding stopped before the transplantation. For details, see text. AC, anterior colliculus; CA, anterior commissure; CC, corpus callosum; F, fornix; GD, dentate gyrus; PC, posterior colliculus; T, transplant. (Redrawn from Stenevi et al., 1976.)

likely that revascularization from pial vessels is the prime factor promoting survival of the graft.

In the transplantation site shown in Fig. 5, the occipital cortex and adjacent parts of subiculum and presubiculum are removed by suction under visual control. The vascular bed of the choroidal fissure is exposed and the lesion reaches the most posterior part of the dentate gyrus. The transplant is then placed on the choroidal fissure in contact with the dentate gyrus and is covered by a piece of gel foam to fill the resection cavity. In the more rostrally situated transplantation site (Fig. 5), the cortex and the hippocampal fimbria overlying the anterior thalamus are removed by suction in order to expose the blood vessels of the choroidal fissure. The transplant is placed onto the vessels in contact with the anterior part of the transected hippocampus.

The transplants survive well in either position, and the regenerating axons will grow into the hippocampal formation either caudally or rostrally (Stenevi et al., 1976; Björklund et al., 1976; Björklund and Stenevi, 1977a, b). Stenevi et al. (1976) have estimated that only about 10–20% of the immature NA neurons of the embryonic locus coeruleus region survive the grafting, whereas the figure is still lower for adult sympathetic ganglionic neurons (about 1–3%). Still, several hundreds of nerve cells survive, which is sufficient for extensive fiber outgrowth.

There are three major inputs to the hippocampus: the perforant path from the entorhinal cortex, the septo-hippocampal pathway, and the commissural fibers from the contralateral hippocampus. Each of these pathways can readily be lesioned before, during or after the time of transplantation. The effect of these different denervating lesions on the regenerative growth of different transplants is under study. When studying the growth of monoamine neurons, the normal NA and/or IA innervation of the hippocampus is removed prior to any transplantation (Stenevi et al., 1976). Different neuron types pattern themselves differently in their new environment inside the adult hippocampus. Whereas the innervation pattern of transplanted NA neurons mimics the normal NA innervation of the hippocampus, the regenerating DA and IA neurons distribute themselves entirely differently (for details see Björklund et al., 1976 and Björklund and Stenevi, 1977a). Central cholinergic neurons, too, have been shown to regenerate into the hippocampus when transplanted as described above (Björklund and Stenevi, 1977b).

Also with this type of transplantation technique, it is important that the superior cervical ganglia are removed bilaterally. In fact, the transplantation lesion or an electrolytic lesion can by itself trigger growth of peripheral sympathetic fibers into the hippocampus, thus being a potential source of erroneous conclusions (Stenevi and Björklund, 1978).

CONCLUSIONS AND SUMMARY

Regenerative growth of different CNS neurons can conveniently be studied with peripheral transplants to the CNS; the whole mount preparations of the transplants makes the morphological analyses both rapid and convenient, while modern micromethods make it possible to analyse the transplant both for transmitter content and for transmitter synthesizing enzymes. In the study of Emson et al. (1977) as many as four different enzymes (choline acetyltransferase, acetylcholinesterase, aromatic amino acid decarboxylase and glutamic acid decarboxylase) could be assayed simultaneously in one and the same iris transplant. The high reproducibility and survival rate of the neuronal transplants to CNS makes it possible, for the first time, to study regenerative growth from such transplants in the adult brain. It also makes it possible to study factors regulating axonal regeneration in the CNS. We have earlier stressed the importance of an aseptic technique in these types of operative procedures, not because this concept is in any way new but because it is of vital importance for the survival of the transplants. Bleeding should be avoided in all of the operations described since hematomas are deleterious for the graft. If bleeding occurs it should, therefore, be stopped completely before the transplantation is carried out. It should again be pointed out that, in all three procedures described above, regenerative growth from peripheral autonomic fibers is a potential source of error. Thus, all experimental animals should have their superior cervical ganglia removed bilaterally before surgery. In addition, acetylcholinesterase histochemistry should be employed whenever needed, to rule out interference by parasympathetic fibers.

Although these techniques were all designed for the study of CNS regeneration, it is obvious that the method of grafting neurons into the CNS can be used for many other purposes as well. This technique can be used as a simple in vivo 'culture technique'. It offers possibilities for developmental studies of isolated CNS pieces or combination of different regions. Two or more simultaneous transplants survive quite well, and the innervation patterns from one transplant to another are currently under study.

ACKNOWLEDGEMENT

This study was supported by grants from the Magnus Bergvall Foundation and the Swedish Medical Research Council (No. 04X-3874).

REFERENCES

Björklund, A., Johansson, B., Stenevi, U. and Svendgaard, N.A. (1975) Re-establishment of functional connections by regenerating central adrenergic and cholinergic axons, *Nature, (Lond.)*, 253: 446–447.

Björklund, A., Katzman, R., Stenevi, U. and West, K.A. (1971) Development and growth of axonal sprouts from noradrenaline and 5-hydroxytryptamine neurons in the rat spinal cord, *Brain Res.*, 31: 21–33.

Björklund, A. and Stenevi, U. (1971) Growth of central catecholamine neurons into smooth muscle grafts in the rat mesencephalon, *Brain Res.*, 31: 1–20.

Björklund, A. and Stenevi, U. (1977a) Experimental reinnervation of the rat hippocampus by grafted sympathetic ganglia, *Brain Res.*, in press.

Björklund, A. and Stenevi, U. (1977b) Reformation of the severed septohippocampal cholinergic pathway by transplanted septal neurons, *Cell. Tiss. Res.*, 185:289–302.

Björklund, A., Stenevi, U. and Svendgaard, N.A. (1976) Growth of transplanted monoaminergic neurons into the adult hippocampus along the perforant path, *Nature (Lond.)*, 262: 787–790.

Bonting, S.L. (1976) *Transmitters in the Visual Process*, Pergamon Press, London.

Clemente, C.D. (1964) Regeneration in the vertebrate central nervous system, *Int. Rev. Neurobiol.*, 6: 257–301.

Crain, S. (1976) *Neurophysiologic Studies in Tissue Culture*, Raven Press, New York.

Cunningham, T.J. (1972) Sprouting of the optic projections after cortical lesions, *Anat. Rec.*, 172: 298.

Das, G.D. and Altman, J. (1971) Transplanted precursors of nerve cells: their fate in the cerebellum of young rats, *Science*, 173: 637–638.

Ehinger, B. and Falck, B. (1966) Concomitant adrenergic and parasympathetic fibres in the rat iris, *Acta physiol. scand.*, 67: 201–207.

Emson, P.C., Björklund, A. and Stenevi, U. (1976) Possible regeneration of γ-aminobutyric acid containing fibres into irides transplanted into the central nervous system, *Nature (Lond.)*, 259: 567–570.

Emson, P.C., Björklund, A. and Stenevi, U. (1977) Evaluation of the regenerative capacity of central

110

dopaminergic, noradrenergic and cholinergic neurons using iris implants as targets, *Brain Res.*, in press.

Goodman, D.C., Bodasararian, R.S. and Horel, J.A. (1973) Axonal sprouting of ipsilateral optic tract following opposite eye removal, *Brain Behav. Evol.*, 8: 27–50.

Goodman, D.C. and Horel, J.A. (1966) Sprouting of optic tract projections in the brain stem of the rat, *J. comp. Neurol.*, 127: 71–88.

Hichey, T.L. (1975) Translaminar growth of axons in the kitten dorsal lateral geniculate nucleus following removal of one eye, *J. comp. Neurol.*, 161: 359–382.

Katzman, R., Björklund, A., Owman, Ch., Stenevi, U. and West, K.A. (1971) Evidence for regenerative axon sprouting of central catecholamine neurons in the rat mesencephalon following electrolytic lesions, *Brain Res.*, 25: 579–596.

Kromer, L., Björklund, A. and Stenevi, U. (1978) Intracephalic implants – a technique for studying neuronal interactions. *Ann. Meet. Amer. Ass. Anatomists*, abstract.

Le Gros Clark, W.E. (1942) The problem of neuronal regeneration in the central nervous system. I. The influence of spinal ganglia and nerve fragments grafted in the brain, *J. Anat. (Lond.)*, 77: 20–48.

Lund, R.D. and Lund, J.S. (1971) Synaptic adjustment after deafferentation of the superior colliculus of the rat, *Science*, 171: 804–807.

Lund, R.D. and Hauschka, S.D. (1976) Transplanted neural tissue develops connections with host rat brain, *Science*, 193: 582–584.

Moore, R.Y., Björklund, A. and Stenevi, U. (1973) Growth and plasticity of adrenergic neurons. In *Neurosciences Third Study Program*, F.O. Schmitt (Ed.), MIT Press, Cambridge, Mass., pp. 961–977.

Nygren, L.-G., Olson, L. and Seiger, A. (1977) Monoaminergic reinnervation of the transected spinal cord by homologous fetal brain grafts, *Brain Res.*, 129: 227–235.

Olson, L. and Malmfors, T. (1970) Growth characteristics of adrenergic nerves in the adult rat. Fluorescence histochemical and ³H-noradrenaline uptake studies using tissue transplantation to the anterior chamber of the eye, *Acta physiol. scand.*, Suppl. 348: 1–112.

Olson, L. and Seiger, A. (1972) Brain tissue transplanted to the anterior chamber of the eye. 1. Fluorescence histochemistry of immature catecholamine and 5-hydroxytryptamine neurons reinnervating the rat iris, *Z. Zellforsch.*, 135: 175–194.

Ranson, S.W. (1914) Transplantation of the spinal ganglion, with observation on the significance of the complex types of spinal ganglion cells, *J. comp. Neurol.*, 24: 547–558.

Seiger, A. and Olson, L. (1977) Quantitation of fiber growth in transplanted central monoaminergic neurons, *Cell Tiss. Res.*, 179: 285–316.

Stenevi, U., Bjerre, B., Björklund, A. and Mobley, W. (1974) Effects of localized intracerebral injections of nerve growth factor on the regenerative growth of lesioned central noradrenergic neurons, *Brain Res.*, 69: 217–234.

Stenevi, U. and Björklund, A. (1978) Growth of vascular sympathetic axons into the hippocampus after lesions of the septo-hippocampal pathway: a pitfall in brain lesion studies, *Neurosci. Lett.*

Stenevi, U., Björklund, A. and Moore, R.Y. (1972) Growth of intact central adrenergic axons in the denervated lateral geniculate body, *Exp. Neurol.*, 35: 290–299.

Stenevi, U., Björklund, A. and Moore, R.Y. (1973) Morphological plasticity of central adrenergic neurons. *Brain Behav. Evol.*, 8: 110–134.

Stenevi, U., Björklund, A. and Svendgaard, N.A. (1976) Transplantation of central and peripheral monoamine neurons to the adult rat brain: techniques and conditions for survival, *Brain Res.*, 114: 1–20.

Svendgaard, N.A., Björklund, A. and Stenevi, U. (1975) Regenerative properties of central monoamine neurons, *Ergebn. Anat. Entwickl.-Gesch.*, 51: 1–77.

Svendgaard, N.A., Björklund, A. and Stenevi, U. (1976) Regeneration of central cholinergic neurons in the adult rat brain, *Brain Res.*, 102: 1–22.

Tidd, C.W. (1932) The transplantation of spinal ganglia in the white rat. A study of the morphological changes in the surviving cells, *J. comp. Neurol.*, 55: 531–543.

Windle, W.F. (1956) Regeneration of axons in the vertebrate central nervous system, *Physiol. Rev.*, 36: 427–440.

Zalewski, A.A. (1971) The effect of Ag-B locus compatibility and incompatibility on neuron survival in the transplanted sensory ganglia in rats, *Exp. Neurol.*, 33: 576–583.

Zalewski, A.A. and Silvers, W.K. (1976) The fate and functional capacity of neonatal neurons in allografts of ganglia in normal and immunologically tolerant rats, *Exp. Neurol.*, 52: 507–514.

DISCUSSION

WILKIN: What type of connections do the nerve transplants make? For example, you showed fibers going to the cerebellum. Do those monoaminergic fibers form connections on Purkinje cells, or do they grow straight past them?

STENEVI: What I showed was serotonin fibers growing into a piece of transplanted cerebellum. With serotonin there is a specific problem, and that is that so far there is no really good histochemical technique for visualizing the terminals. To visualize the terminals one has nowadays to use techniques that result in visualizing not only serotonin but also noradrenaline. So, no one has a technique that is sensitive enough and histochemically specific for the serotonin endings. On the electron microscopic level it might be different, but I do not have any information about that.

ZIMMER: When you make a lesion in the fimbria on one side you in fact cause denervation in both hippocampi. But only on the side where you get the lesion do you have a proliferation of the fibers normally found on blood vessels. That means that it is probably not denervation which causes the proliferation and the extensions of fibers from the vascular bed, but that rather the lesion causes new vessels to form.

STENEVI: That could be, but we think that when we make these lesions we damage some of the nerves to the blood vessels. These peripheral sympathetic nerves start to grow, and they find their way very easily in the cut end of the fimbria; they then continue to grow in that direction. Denervation also seems to play a part, since an electrolytic lesion of the septum can also induce this type of growth.

ZIMMER: Have you seen them grow along the fimbria in the *other* direction?

STENEVI: No, they always grow into the hippocampus; we have not seen such growth into the septum. It would be just as plausible that they would sense that there is denervation going both ways, and that there are open channels going back both ways. But if you place a transplant towards the septum and leave it a millimeter or two from the fimbria, it will not grow into the septum but will return and grow into the hippocampus.

SOTELO: In the early work of your laboratory there was a very nice correlation between the type of peripheral transplant you put into the brain and the amount of reinnervation that you would get, also in the iris, and there was a constant relationship between receptors and the amount of innervation. However, the story became much more complicated with the GABA-neurons, because the iris has no GABA-receptors, or at least very few. The question then is if this is a biochemical artifact: how was the transplant taken from the brain, and how much contamination was there?

STENEVI: One piece of evidence that it is not an artifact is that the amount of GAD in the transplanted iris goes up. Of course it is also possible that this is located in glia cells, but if you remove the transplant and take it to another transplantation site, like the anterior eye chamber, the amount of GAD will drop dramatically — just as one would expect for the degenerating GABA-terminals. Glia cells would certainly survive such a transplantation. And there is another piece of evidence that shows that GABA-neurons really grow in: if you look at it in the electron microscope you will see that there is GABA uptake in certain cells, but there is also uptake in nerve terminals. However, as you noted at the tail end of the graph, the GAD again declines drastically. As I indicated, maybe it is so that the only thing that really grows very well into (and remains in) the transplant are the cholinergic and the noradrenaline fibers, which *should be* there to start with. I did not show the slide that shows that dopamine fibers grow very inefficiently. The only thing that seems to inhibit the ingrowth of central noradrenaline fibers is the presence of other noradrenaline fibers. But that does not hold true for the dopamine and the serotonin fibers. So far, every type of transmitter that we look at is growing into the transplant. It might be, therefore, that when you lesion the axons they will grow into the transplant, whether it is an iris or a muscle, but after a while only the appropriate ones will remain. That could be the reason why the GABA disappears if it is left in the brain, because there is certainly no degeneration to speak of in the transplant.

STIRLING: You just mentioned muscles. Have you actually put muscle tissue into the brain?

STENEVI: We have tried different types of muscle. One is ordinary skeletal muscle, and that does not survive very well. We used portal veins for looking at the formation of synapses within the transplant, and the muscles *in* the portal vein survive very well (because the spontaneous contractions of the normal portal vein keep going when you take out the transplants, even after a couple of months). By means of stimulation it can be shown that the type of activation of the synapses is unchanged when the innervation is coming from the brain instead of the normal innervation. However, we have not looked at the morphology; we only checked that there really were fibers in there, both cholinergic and noradrenergic ones.

STIRLING: The transplants were done between adults, were they not?

STENEVI: All recipients are adults, and the portal vein and peripheral transplants are all taken from either the same animal or from littermates. Also, the superior cervical ganglion is taken from the same animal because you have to remove those ganglia anyway. So we used these ganglia as a transplant.

UYLINGS: Are there limits to the size of tissue which you transplant into the brain? Do you get into trouble if, for instance, the transplant is too thick?

STENEVI: We thought at the beginning that you needed very small pieces in order to have them survive. That is not true: you even can use pieces that are several millimeters in diameter. A substantial amount of tissue can survive, for example, four to six adult ganglia.

DE GROOT: Did you observe any growth of the transplant itself within the brain compartment, or did it merely survive there?

STENEVI: The transplants will grow in some instances, as has been very nicely demonstrated by Olson and his coworkers (Berger and Olson, 1977), while using a similar technique in order to transplant both peripheral and central neurons to the anterior eye chamber. And this seems to be dependent on how old the fetus is when you do the transplantation. They have made measurements, and it is very easy to see from their curves when you should take your transplants if you want it to stay the same size, and when if you want it to grow. We ourselves have not done measurements, but we have made the same observations: the transplant sometimes stays the same size and sometimes it grows.

CHANGEUX: This is a continuation of the same question. If you take newborn cerebellum, for instance, and you put in into an adult brain, what is the sequence of development for the cerebellum?

STENEVI: We have never worked with cerebellum except for one slide that I showed you, which was only to establish that it is possible to have an artificial situation where you can look at the reinnervation from one transplant to another. This might be an experiment well worth doing, but we don't have the facilities that you and Dr. Sotelo have. You could have pieces of cerebellum from normal mice and from mutants, and then study the development of each tissue alone or together. But this is a quite new approach to me: we don't work with that type of problem!

LYNCH: In your iris transplants into the fimbria you found a rise in GABA. The only GABA in the hippocampus is thought to be contained in *inter*neurons. Is the GABA that is growing in indeed coming from interneurons within the hippocampus?

STENEVI: Well, if we had a GABA-specific histochemical technique I could probably answer that, but we do not yet have such a technique.

REFERENCE

Berger and Olson (1977) *Cell Tiss. Res.,* 179: 285–316.

Neuroplasticity in the Hippocampal Formation

GARY LYNCH, CHRISTINE GALL and THOMAS V. DUNWIDDIE

Department of Psychobiology, University of California, Irvine, Calif. 92717 (U.S.A.)

INTRODUCTION

Information becomes available to an animal throughout its life, and some of this is selected and faithfully stored. How can an organ such as the brain which, despite constant allusions to circuits and cables, is composed of organelles and membranes which are constantly being broken down and rebuilt, make permanent analogues of experiences which might last only a few seconds? This problem has long fascinated neuroscientists and psychologists but, despite prolonged and often very clever experiments into the biology of learning, a satisfactory explanation has yet to be advanced (see, for example, Bennett and Rosenzweig, 1975). In part because of this and in part because of continuing technological gains, new strategies for the study of behavioral (and physiological) adaptability have begun to evolve.

Much of this work is found in an area which is often referred to as 'neuroplasticity'. In this, the emphasis is placed first on the identification of cellular processes which possess the capability for persistent change or adjustment; the hope is that once such processes are found and characterized, then tests of their involvement in behavioral phenomena such as learning will be possible. Put simply, the emphasis in this approach is from the cellular level to the behavioral, rather than vice versa. The present chapter will review a limited segment of this rapidly expanding field: specifically, evidence will be discussed which indicates that the neural circuitries of the rat hippocampal formation possess remarkable capacities for both functional and structural changes. Before beginning, it is necessary that we briefly consider certain of the anatomical and physiological features of the hippocampus, and emphasize some of the unique advantages possessed by this structure for studies of plasticity.

THE HIPPOCAMPUS AS A MODEL SYSTEM FOR THE STUDY OF NEUROPLASTICITY

The mammalian hippocampal formation has come under intense investigation from several subfields of neurobiology in recent years, and our understanding of its structure and operating characteristics has increased accordingly. However, in the following sections only those aspects which bear on studies of neuroplasticity will be considered in any detail. As can be seen in Fig. 1, the hippocampus is composed of two major groups of neurons: the pyramidal and granule cells, whose somata are organized into two densely packed, spatially isolated cell layers. The dendritic tree of pyramidal cells emerges and ramifies from both the apical

114

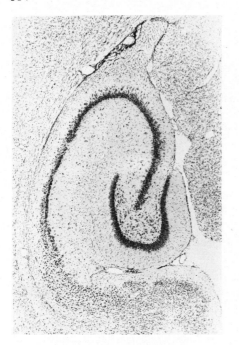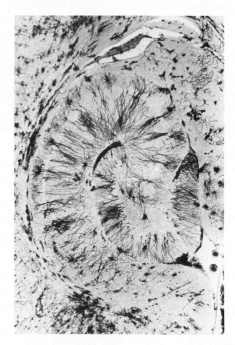

Fig. 1. Photomicrographs of horizontal sections of the rat hippocampal formation, as seen in cresyl violet (left) and Golgi-Cox (right) impregnated material.

and the basal poles of the cell body, whereas granule cells have only an apical dendritic tree. The organization of the afferents to these dendrites maintains the theme of simplicity seen in the cytoarchitecture of the hippocampus.

Two massive fiber systems invade the hippocampal formation: the perforant path, which originates in the ipsilateral entorhinal cortex, and the commissural projections from the contralateral hippocampal pyramidal cells (much smaller projections from the brain stem, septum, and contralateral entorhinal cortex are also present, but these will not be discussed). The entorhinal axons generate terminal fields which occupy the outer portions of the apical dendrites of the granule and pyramidal cells, while the commissural afferents densely inner-vate the proximal segments of these same dendrites. (The commissural fibers also terminate on the basal dendrites of the pyramidal cells). The two afferents thus form complementary laminations on the dendrites of the target cells, abutting against but not overlapping each other (Blackstad, 1956; Gottlieb and Cowan, 1973; Hjorth-Simonsen and Jeune, 1972; Mosko et al., 1973). Neurophysiological studies have shown that the two inputs are excita-tory (Anderson, 1975; Anderson et al., 1966; Deadwyler et al., 1975, in preparation); their transmitters are not known, although recent work suggests that glutamate and aspartate are likely candidates (Nadler et al., 1976).

There are three major projection systems within the hippocampus that need to be con-sidered. The granule cells of the dentate gyrus emit axons which terminate upon the apical and basal dendritic shafts of the pyramidal cell, at the point where these emerge from the somata. This projection, the mossy fibers, extends only about one-half of the distance around the arch of pyramidal cells. This portion of the pyramidal cell layer is known as the regio inferior (Cajal, 1911). The pyramidal cells themselves generate the two remaining internal fiber systems; one of these projects back to the granule cells (the 'associational'

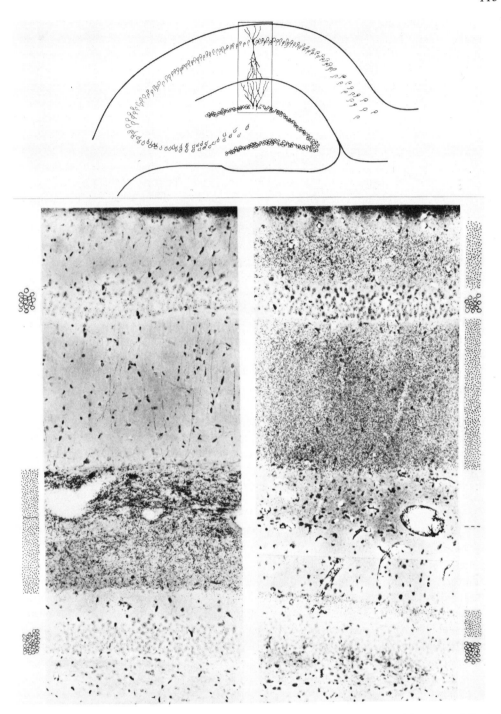

Fig. 2. Photomicrographs of terminal degeneration within a zone of the hippocampal formation, following the removal of that structure's major extrinsic afferents: the hippocampal-commissural (right) and ipsilateral entorhinal (left) afferent systems. Each micrograph extends from below the dorsal granule cell layer to the superficial edge of the hippocampus, including the dendritic fields of both the granule and pyramidal cells (indicated on the accompanying line drawing). The position of the cell layers and degeneration fields are highlighted by circles and stippling adjacent to each micrograph. (Fink-Heimer stain.)

system: Dunwiddie and Lynch, in preparation; Gottlieb and Cowan, 1973; Zimmer, 1974), while the other travels forward to the pyramidal cells which did not receive mossy fiber inputs (the 'regio superior': Cajal, 1911). These fibers are known as the Schaffer collaterals. The pyramidal cells of the regio inferior are also the source of the commissural fibers which travel to the contralateral hippocampus. Like the *external* inputs to the hippocampus, the intrinsic projections systems are rigidly laminated. Specifically, the associational and Schaffer projection terminate precisely in the regions of the commissural fibers, and do not mingle with the entorhinal fibers and terminals (Lynch and Cotman, 1975). Finally, all three of the intrinsic projections are almost certainly excitatory (Anderson, 1975; Schwartzkroin and Wester, 1975; West et al., 1975). The hippocampus also contains interneuron systems and other intrinsic connections, but these are not germane to the topic of this review.

From this necessarily brief sketch, it can be understood why the hippocampus is becoming increasingly popular as a model system for the study of cellular phenomena such as plasticity. First, there are the factors of simplicity and homogeneity. There are only two major classes of neurons within the hippocampus, and even these two are spatially segregated. This makes it possible to establish which cells and circuits are involved in both anatomical and physiological studies, as well as greatly simplifying the task of relocating these elements from experiment to experiment. More important, these features make it possible to interpret events in groups of cells in terms of the behavior of individual neurons. A second advantage of the hippocampus lies in the lamination of its afferent inputs and cellular elements. This allows an experimenter to selectively manipulate the inputs to particular dendritic regions and to observe the interactions of afferents which are spatially separated but which terminate on the same neuron.

It should also be noted that 'slices' of adult hippocampus can be maintained for hours in vitro (e.g. Algar and Taylor, 1976; Deadwyler et al., 1975; Schwartzkroin and Wester, 1975; Yamamoto, 1972). These slices show many of the physiological characteristics seen in the hippocampus under in vivo circumstances. Because of the stereotyped nature of hippocampal anatomy, it is possible to prepare individual slices which contain all of the circuitries described above. As will be seen, the use of these slices opens the way to experiments on plasticity which would be impossible to conduct with intact preparations.

PHYSIOLOGICAL PLASTICITY IN THE HIPPOCAMPUS

Long-term potentiation

Neuroscientists have long searched for physiological analogues of memory, and one of the favored areas of investigation has been the study of effects of prolonged usage on synaptic transmission. In a casual sense this is reasonable: it is plausible that learning might involve altered usage patterns in particular brain circuitries and if so, experiments on the effects of usage upon the subsequent 'strength' of connections could prove most informative. However, experiments using several different preparations and designs have shown that even extreme stimulation conditions produce increases in circuit strength which begin to decay very quickly, and return to control levels over a period of minutes or hours (Beswick and Conway, 1965; Lloyd, 1949). Thus, while the obtained effects might well be related to some short term aspects of learning, the experiments failed to identify physiological processes which possessed the extreme duration of memory. A new and dramatic dimension to this type of investigation was provided by the experiments of Bliss and Lømo (1973), in which they used repetitive stimulation of the primary afferent input to the hippocampus, the

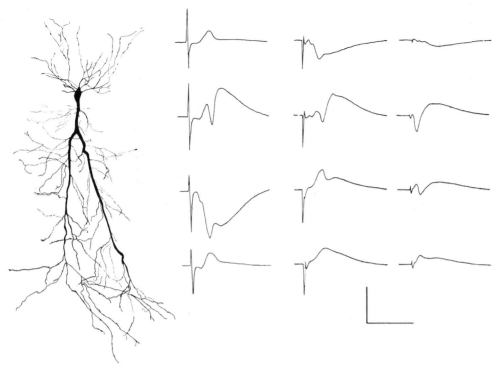

Fig. 3. A comparison of the potentials recorded from various depths in the CA1 region of the hippocampus with a camera lucida drawing of a typical pyramidal cell found in this region (drawn from a Golgi-Cox stained section). The columns of potentials were evoked by stimulation of stratum radiatum near the CA3 region (left column); stratum oriens (middle column); and antidromic stimulation of the CA1 pyramids (right column). The vertical location of the records corresponds to the depth (on the camera lucida figure) from which they were recorded. These may be compared with corresponding records before and after potentiation, as seen in Fig. 4. Calibration marks indicate 5 mV and 10 msec; upwards deflections represent positive polarity.

perforant path. They found that relatively brief stimulation trains produced pronounced increases in the postsynaptic response of the target cells to subsequent single pulse stimulation of this pathway. Furthermore, these changes developed quite rapidly, and often persisted without decrement for hours. Later experiments, using 'chronic' animals, indicated that the potentiation in fact lasted for days or even months (Bliss and Gardner-Medwin, 1973; Douglas and Goddard, 1975); this effect has been aptly labeled 'long-term potentiation' (LTP), and has now been found in several hippocampal pathways (Alger and Taylor, 1976; Deadwyler et al., 1975; Schwartzkroin and Wester, 1975).

Long-term potentiation possesses two key features which make it an intriguing analogue of memory: it occurs rapidly, and in some cases it persists indefinitely. Beyond this, the stimulation parameters required to produce it, while extreme, are not so very unlike events sometimes encountered in the 'real-world', i.e. in the behaving animal. LTP lasting without decrement for hours — usually the duration of the experimenter's patience — can be produced by trains of 100 Hz stimulation lasting for less than a second. Experiments in which recordings were taken from the dentate gyrus of a rat, in the process of learning various behaviors, showed that many granule cells do discharge at high frequencies for nearly a second (Deadwyler et al., 1976).

118

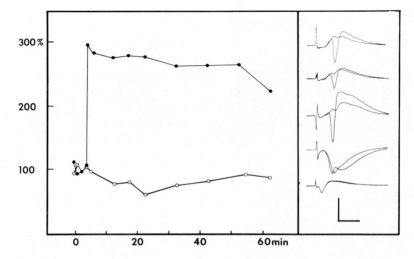

Fig. 4. The left-hand figure illustrates the duration of the long-term potentiation observed in the in vitro hippocampal slice preparation. A 1-sec train of 100 pulses was delivered to the stratum radiatum (primarily Schaffer and commissural) pathway at 5 min, which resulted in potentiation of that response, while control stimulation (in the stratum oriens) caused no potentiation. The slight depression of the heterosynaptic response following potentiation was commonly observed in this preparation. All points represent population-spike amplitude, as a percentage of the control responses obtained during the prestimulus period. On the right hand side are displayed superimposed averaged waveforms, taken before and 5 min following a 100 per sec train of 1-sec duration, delivered to stratum radiatum near the subicular and CA1-CA3 borders (top two traces), and to stratum oriens (middle trace) as recorded from the cell layer. The large negative spike seen in each of the records following potentiation (referred to as the population spike) reflects synchronous firing of the pyramidal neurons, and shows the greatest relative degree of change following potentiation; increasing in amplitude and decreasing in latency. This component was largely absent from the recordings made prior to stimulation. The second trace from the bottom was recorded from the dendritic region being activated by a stratum radiatum volley, and is considered to be the reflection of synaptic currents (EPSPs) generated in the vicinity of the recording electrode. As can be seen, this response undergoes potentiation as well, although of lesser relative magnitude than the population spike, while the antidromic response seen in the cell layer (lowest trace) is unaffected by tetanic stimulation. Calibration marks represent 5 mV and 5 msec.

The locus of potentiation

Any attempt to understand the substrates of potentiation must first deal with the problem of which element in the circuit is changing; is it the axon, its terminal, the synapse itself, the postsynaptic sites, or perhaps the entire target neuron? The answer to this is not yet at hand, but several of the alternatives just mentioned have been shown to be rather unlikely. Repetitive stimulation of hippocampal afferents does not change the antidromic volley produced by these axons (Schwartzkroin and Wester, 1975), nor does it appear to influence the magnitude of the presynaptic volley recorded at the target site (Anderson et al., 1977). Therefore, it is unlikely that LTP is due to any alterations in the axons of the afferent system under study. Similarly, generalized changes in the postsynaptic target cells can be excluded. This has been shown in experiments (using the in vitro slice preparation) in which the response of the target neurons to their unstimulated afferents has been studied and found to be actually depressed following repetitive stimulation of one input (Dunwiddie and Lynch, 1977; Lynch et al., 1977; see Fig. 4). Possibly related to this is the observation that the responsivity of the dendrites of the target cells to iontophoretically applied glutamic acid is reduced following the induction of LTP (Lynch et al., 1976). Even projections to the same dendritic regions as the 'potentiated' afferents are depressed. This effect, hetero-synaptic depression (or 'HSD'), can last for more than 15 min and represents a surprising type of plasticity in its own right. For the purposes of the present discussion, however, it is enough to note that the potentiation is limited to that afferent which has been repetitively activated, and thus cannot represent a generalized change in the target neuron.

This leaves either the terminals, the synapses or the spines as the locus of the potentiation. It will be extremely difficult, and perhaps impossible using purely physiological approaches, to identify which of these is the critical element. However, a likely answer may yet emerge from pharmacological and biochemical studies of the mechanisms responsible for potentiation.

Mechanisms responsible for LTP

The analysis of the mechanisms responsible for long-term plasticity might reasonably be cased in terms of (a) what triggers it, (b) what are the cellular processes which produce it, and (c) what is its final form? Studies directed at these questions have only just begun, and at present only a few tantalizing clues have been obtained. Taking the first issue, the 'triggers for potentiation', we might start with an analysis of the stimulation train which causes LTP. In the slice preparation LTP can be elicited by stimulation parameters which range from 5 to more than 100 Hz, and it appears that the higher frequencies are the most effective (Dunwiddie and Lynch, 1978). This is useful information, because these parameters of stimulation produce very different postsynaptic response patterns during the train. The field responses produced by low frequency trains 'follow' the stimulation trains (a response is obtained for each pulse); these wax and wane during the trains but gradually increase in size. High frequency stimulation produces a very different pattern — specifically, field responses are obtained only to the first few pulses, and then essentially no responses are found. It seems, therefore, that LTP is being produced under conditions in which trans-mission has failed, suggesting that some factor (other than repetitive synaptic transmission) associated with stimulation is the factor responsible for the LTP.

One reasonable candidate of this type is *calcium*, synaptic transmission involves an influx of calcium, and it has been suggested that repetitive stimulation results in an accumulation of this cation in nerve terminals (Weinrich, 1971). Furthermore, there is evidence that this accumulation (or 'charging') is responsible for some of the short-term forms of plasticity seen in the peripheral nervous system (Rosenthal, 1969; Wilson and Skirboll, 1974). If increases in intraterminal calcium initiate LTP, then it should be possible to interfere with the induction of the potentiation effect by lowering the extracellular calcium concentration to such a point that release and transmission will still accompany high frequency stimulation, but at which accumulation of calcium will be less likely to occur. Studies of this sort have shown that LTP is indeed extremely difficult to obtain in low-calcium medium, despite the occurrence of robust synaptic transmission during the stimulation period (Dunwiddie and Lynch, in press). It was also noted in these studies that *short*-lived forms of plasticity, such as paired-pulse and frequency facilitation, work extremely well in the lowered calcium concentrations. These experiments provide indirect support for the hypothesis that long-term potentiation is triggered by calcium 'charging', probably of the nerve terminals. This in turn implies that LTP is caused by some process which has a requirement for intraterminal calcium levels well above that required for normal release and transmission.

There are at least three types of mechanism by which calcium might act. First, LTP might be the consequence of a supranormal amount of activation of the postsynaptic cell, elicited during the stimulation train. This seems unlikely, however, because the optimal parameters for inducing LTP do not correspond to those which produce the maximum set of post-synaptic responses to the stimulation train. Furthermore, it appears that the postsynaptic potentials generated during repetitive stimulation are as great in low calcium as they are in normal medium, suggesting again that repetitive transmission (in the sense of repeated EPSPs) is not a key event in generating potentiation. Second, LTP might result from some unusual aspect of the normal release process which only occurs during *repetitive* stimulation, such as transmitter or vesicle depletion, postsynaptic depolarization block, and similar phenomena. Some mechanism of this sort could trigger a second, more enduring, reaction which is responsible for potentiation. It is certainly plausible, and perhaps even likely, that extreme events of this type are brought about by high levels of calcium accumulated in the terminals by repetitive stimulation; lowering the calcium might hinder these events, and hence block LTP.

As a third possibility, long-term potentiation could result from unique processes not directly related to release: e.g. by mechanisms which can only be initiated by calcium concentrations higher than those reached during normal transmission but which are achieved with repetitive stimulation. An increasing body of evidence shows that calcium can act as a 'second messenger' in the cytosol, in much the same way as cAMP does (Rasmussen and Goodman, 1977). There are a number of proteins which are altered by calcium (often via phosphorylation brought about by calcium-sensitive protein kinases) to produce specific cellular reactions, and many proteins of this type are found in the brain (Bennett and Rosenzweig, 1975; Kretsinger, 1976). It has been hypothesized that various processes of this type have different requirements for calcium and that some specificity of action is achieved by requiring successively higher calcium concentrations to trigger different kinds of processes. In the context of the present discussion, the process which produces LTP could be a biochemical reaction which has a higher threshold than transmitter release, this threshold being reached only during high frequency stimulation.

Further understanding of the initial events leading to LTP can only come from additional experimentation. Particularly valuable would be studies in which synaptic transmission was blocked by other means than reduction of calcium. Depending upon the outcome of such studies, it should be possible to further define the minimum conditions required for the production of LTP, and to assess the balance in favor of one or the other of the hypotheses described above. (If, for example, blockade of postsynaptic responses did not prevent the occurrence of potentiation this would clearly point to a presynaptic locus of the initial events in the induction of LTP; the opposite result would suggest some exotic postsynaptic effects.)

It is likely, though by no means certain, that biochemical changes are interposed between the transient events surrounding repetitive stimulation and the permanent adjustments which constitute LTP. There are several candidates for a process of this sort, and correlating the occurrence of any of them with potentiation might provide a clue as to the nature of LTP. One possibility which deserves attention is a change in protein synthesis; for example, the target cell might increase the synthesis of particular classes of polypeptides, and these could somehow influence subsequent transmission. Over the years many efforts have been made to demonstrate that protein synthesis is essential for the formation of long-term memory and, while many investigators seem to feel that this has been satisfactorily established (Barondes, 1970), the issue remains controversial. In any event, recent experiments have shown that protein synthesis is not required for the initiation or maintenance of long-term potentiation (Deadwyler et al., 1977). Following incubation of slices in cycloheximide (or other inhibitors) for 10–15 min, protein synthesis was shown to be almost completely blocked; despite this, robust LTP was generated by high frequency stimulation. However, it was found that 30–40 min of protein inhibition markedly reduced the probability of obtaining LTP. This latter result is open to two interpretations. First, the longer inhibition could have produced any of several side effects known to be associated with these drugs, and have impeded the potentiation process in a non-specific fashion. Second, it might be the case that some short-lived protein is required for the induction of LTP. In any event, the 15 min incubation experiments establish that the synthesis of new proteins per se is not a prerequisite for LTP.

Protein phosphorylation is another attractive candidate for a biochemical intermediate in the production of long-lasting changes in synaptic operation. Many proteins change their operational status according to the extent to which they are phosphorylated, and this process can occur in seconds and persist for minutes, or even longer. This provides a mechanism by which brief events can have enduring consequences. Furthermore, most (but not all) protein phosphorylation is accomplished via the action of protein kinases, some of which demonstrate calcium sensitivity (Brostrum et al., 1972). The time course, persistence, and possible role of calcium in these types of biochemical processes make it reasonable to examine the possibility that phosphorylation is involved in LTP.

We have done several types of experiments to test this possibility (Browning et al., in preparation). Repetitive stimulation which produces potentiation has been found to cause changes in the amount of phosphate incorporated into a specific synaptosomal protein, with a molecular weight of about 40,000 daltons, during a subsequent 'broken cell' assay. In these experiments, synaptosomes were prepared from 'potentiated' hippocampal slices and then exposed to radioactive ATP; proteins were then separated on polyacrylamide gels and the amount of phosphate per band of protein measured by autoradiography. These results show that stimulation influences the phosphorylation status of protein(s) of a particular weight, a result that might reflect activation of the phosphorylation machinery during repetitive synaptic activation. If in future experiments it appears that the phosphoprotein change correlates with the occurrence of LTP, then the possibility that this change is an intermediate in the production of LTP would have to be seriously considered. Protein synthesis and phosphorylation do not begin to exhaust the possible biochemical intermediaries which could be links in the chain of events leading to LTP: pharmacological and biochemical experiments using the slice preparation should allow tests to be made of other mechanisms as well.

The extreme persistence of LTP invites the speculation that it might represent an anatomical type of change, but it is also possible that 'regenerative' types of biochemical events are responsible. Neuroanatomical studies have suggested the presence of numerous positive feedback 'loops' within the hippocampus (Zimmer, 1971) and recent neurophysiological work from this laboratory has verified that such circuits are functionally operative (Deadwyler et al., 1975). Potentiation of a particular synaptic locus might alter patterns of discharge throughout an entire neuronal circuit, in such a way as to increase activity across the originally potentiated synapse. Thus positive feedback could provide a mechanism by which a transient biochemical process could be maintained indefinitely.

The alternative to the regeneration hypothesis is that long-term potentiation represents a quasi-permanent change in the synaptic complex (terminal, synapse, spine, and surrounding glia). Ultrastructural adjustments of this type are certainly within the capabilities of hippocampal circuitries. Studies from this laboratory have shown that afferents in the adult hippocampus are capable of generating entirely new synaptic connections if their neighbors are surgically eliminated and that, once started, the formation of new connections can occur quite rapidly. Since mature terminals retain a vigorous growth capacity, it is possible that

122

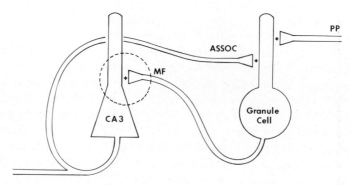

Fig. 5. A schematic illustration of one type of positive feedback loop which has been demonstrated in the hippocampus, and which could serve to sustain potentiation. Granule cells are driven by the perforant path (PP) input, and in turn stimulate CA3 cells via mossy fiber (MF) connections. These in turn provide excitatory synaptic input via the associational (ASSOC) fibers, which terminate in the inner zone of the dentate molecular layer. Potentiation of the mossy fiber synapse (broken circle) would result in greater activity of CA3 cells following a subsequent perforant path volley; this increased activity would exert positive feedback on the granule cells, and result in elevated frequencies of transmission across the mossy fiber synapse. This increased level of activity in this circuit would act to prolong the potentiated character of the granule cell-CA3 connection.

this can be used to augment the strength of a particular collection of afferents. It should also be noted that experiments in the peripheral nervous system have shown that the morphology of nerve is changed by repetitive stimulation (Pysch and Wiley, 1972).

The only test for possible anatomical changes attendant to LTP has been that of Van Harreveld and Fifkova (1975). They used an ingenious freeze substitution technique to provide extremely rapid (within seconds) fixation of the dentate gyrus after high frequency stimulation of the entorhinal cortex. They found evidence that the spines in the outer molecular layer — the target zone of the entorhinal axons — were swollen in comparison to spines in the inner molecular layer, and suggested that these changes may alter the electrotonic coupling between the spine and the rest of the neuron. However, without supporting electrophysiological evidence it could not be determined whether or not LTP occurred in this situation, or even if the swollen spines were synaptically activated by the stimulation trains. Since potentiation is not always seen following stimulation of the perforant path (Bliss and Gardner-Medwin, 1973; Bliss and Lømo, 1973), electrophysiological recordings will be required before spine changes can be regarded as a substrate for potentiation.

NEUROANATOMICAL PLASTICITY IN HIPPOCAMPAL CIRCUITRIES

The sprouting effect

The preceding section reviewed studies showing that hippocampal circuitry is capable of semi-permanent functional change. In the following section, we will consider the evidence that these connections also possess the capacity for a different type of plasticity: changes in the density and distribution of their synaptic domains. The ability of the fiber connections to grow and change is a question of real importance to theories of behavioral plasticity. If, for example, axons are able to increase or decrease the number of their synaptic contacts, then the relative permanence of phenomena such as memory becomes, if not yet understandable, at least less mysterious.

In order to study possible anatomical growth in the circuitries of the adult hippocampus, it is necessary to provide a situation in which such growth might be detected. This can be accomplished by surgically removing one collection of afferents and measuring the response of residual inputs to the presence of newly denervated dendritic space (Goodman and Horel, 1966; Raisman, 1969). Experiments of this kind have shown that the remaining afferents undergo growth responses ('sprouting') and re-innervate the vacated territory (Lee et al., 1977; Lund and Lund, 1971; Matthews et al., 1976; Raisman, 1969; Raisman and Field, 1973). Several forms of growth have been identified. For example, unilateral removal of the hippocampus results in a 25% loss in the terminal and synaptic population of the inner molecular layer of the remaining, contralateral, dentate gyrus. However, when the same region is examined with the electron miscroscope some 6 weeks later, it is found that the deafferented zone possesses an essentially normal population of terminals and synaptic connections (McWilliams and Lynch, 1978). An even more dramatic example of this effect is shown in Fig. 6; here the entorhinal cortex has been removed, with a resulting loss of as much as 90% of the terminals of the middle molecular layer. However, beginning at 5 to 6 days after the lesion the terminal and synaptic population begins to be replaced, so that 5 days after sprouting has begun nearly 20% of the normal synaptic bouton density is recovered (Lee et al., 1977). Light microscopic studies have provided strong evidence that these 'replacements' come from branches, emitted from the intact axons found in the lower part of the dendritic tree (Lynch et al., 1973, 1976, 1977). It is interesting to note that the sprouting response has been measured in this circumstance in both adult and juvenile rats, and that growth is much more vigorous in the younger animals (Lynch et al., 1973). These experiments — and there are several others (Matthews et al., 1976; Nakamura et al., 1974; Tsukahara and Fujito, 1976) — show that the adult brain retains the ability to increase the number and distribution of synaptic contacts formed by specific afferents.

Furthermore, there is evidence that the new circuitries formed in this fashion are functional. It was shown above that the commissural projections to the inner molecular layer invade the middle molecular layer 5—6 days after that region has lost its primary input following

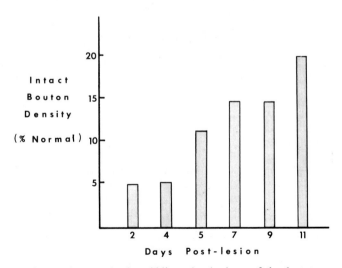

Fig. 6. The density of intact boutons in the middle molecular layer of the dentate gyrus, expressed as a per cent of the normal intact bouton density, and shown as a function of survival time following entorhinal lesion (in days).

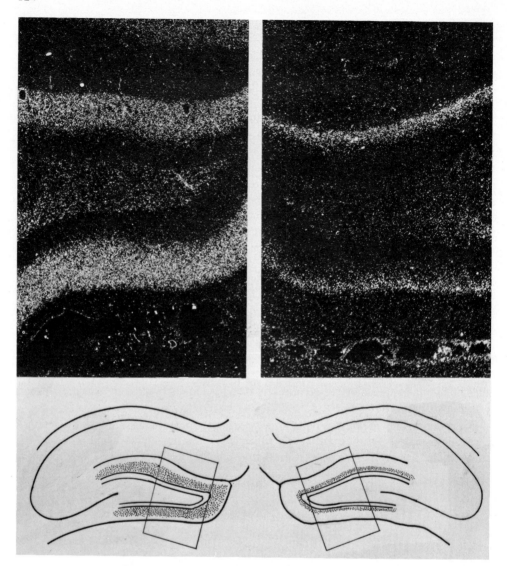

Fig. 7. Dark field photomicrographs of autoradiographic material from two animals in which the commissural terminal field in the dentate gyrus was labeled by transport of [³H]leucine. The adjacent line drawings illustrate the field from which each micrograph was taken. The commissural fibers normally terminate within the proximal fourth of the dentate molecular layer, as pictured on the right. The left dentate in this case was deafferented at 14 days post-natal, by removal of the ipsilateral entorhinal cortex, resulting in the expansion of the commissural terminal field into the more distal (deafferented) molecular layer.

lesions of the entorhinal cortex. Between 9 and 10 days after the lesion, the distribution of field potentials generated in the dentate gyrus by electrical stimulation of the commissural afferents to the inner molecular layer begins to extend itself out of the dendritic trees (West et al., 1975). This suggests that the new synapses formed by this projection in the middle molecular layer are beginning to function. Still more direct evidence that 'sprouted' synaptic systems are operational has come from studies on another system, the afferents of the red nucleus. Electron microscopic studies have shown that the number of axo-somatic contacts generated by cortical projections to the red nucleus increases after cerebellar inputs to the cell body are surgically eliminated (Tsukahara and Fujito, 1976). Furthermore, intracellular recording from these cells revealed that the rise time of the EPSPs generated by stimulation of the cortex increases after the lesion, a result that would be predicted if the newly formed contacts were operational.

Afferents in the hippocampus and elsewhere are capable of rather dramatic growth, and there is reason to believe that this growth produces permanent functional change. Is it possible that this growth plays a role in the normal operation of the brain? A first step in answering this would be to establish that 'sprouting' in some form occurs in circumstances other than surgically produced deafferentation. In an extremely interesting paper, Sotelo and Palay (1971) reported evidence that degenerating endings and terminal growth profiles are found in the brains of 'normal' rats, and suggested that sprouting may be a continuous process. If so, then the possibility is strengthened that examples of physiological (such as LTP) and behavioral change might be due to the directed usage of growth capacities of brain circuits. The next section will consider this question in more detail.

RELATING NEURAL PLASTICITY TO BEHAVIORAL PHENOMENA

In the preceding sections we have seen that circuits in the hippocampus can be made to increase their functional strength rapidly and for indefinite periods of time. Furthermore, evidence has been reviewed which indicates that these fiber systems can grow new synapses and terminals, and that it is likely that these are functional. But can these physiological and anatomical phenomena be linked to events which actually occur in the behaving animal? At least two very formidable problems make investigation of this question most difficult. The first of these is that of detecting a particular form of cellular plasticity in a behaving animal. Perhaps the best hope for this lies in finding biochemical mechanisms which are responsible for – or at least correlate with – LTP, sprouting, etc. If mechanisms of these types were to be identified, and if it were technically possible to measure them after sacrificing an animal, then it might be possible to establish the occurrence of these phenomena during learning.

The second problem is one of where and when to look for putative substrates of plasticity. There is no reason to assume that every system in the hippocampus will undergo cellular change during learning or, for that matter, that the effects might not be formed and then erased. Clearly what is needed is an analysis of the behavior of the circuits of the hippo-campus as the rat acquires and uses specific memories. Several experiments (cf. Segal et al., 1972) of this type have been conducted, using firing rates of neurons recorded from various areas of the hippocampus, but it is difficult to relate results of this type to changes in the behavior of specific circuits. However, a more recent study has provided an analysis of the operation of the perforant path-granule cell circuit during learning (Deadwyler et al., 1978a, b). In these experiments, recording microelectrodes were lowered into the termination zone of the entorhinal projections to the dentate (i.e. the middle molecular layer), using the physiological responses evoked by stimulation of the commissural and entorhinal afferents of this region as guides. The rat was then required to learn that a tone was the cue for it to perform a response to obtain a water reward. Initially, the middle molecular layer did not respond to the tone but, as the animal acquired the learning, a very marked negative evoked potential gradually appeared in this layer. However, when the microelectrode was lowered into the granule cell layer, it was found that the neurons did not reliably respond to the signal. If, however, a second tone — which was 'negative', in that the animal was not rewarded for a response — was added to the paradigm, then *both* cues evoked field responses in the entorhinal zone, and consistently 'drove' the granule cells. Eventually, as the rat learned to respond only to the correct signal, the cell discharge patterns to the two cues changed dramatically; a long burst of cell firing was elicited by the positive cue, but only a short burst followed the incorrect tone. Reversing the significance of the tones reversed the firing patterns that they evoked.

These results illustrate the complex changes that hippocampal circuitries undergo during learning. It appears that the perforant path-dentate gyrus connection begins to operate during acquisition of the learning, but this is not an adequate condition to control the behavior of the granule cells. When the rat is faced with discriminating between a previously learned cue and a new (but similar) stimulus, then the granule cells fire and, presumably, the remainder of the hippocampus is brought into play. Finally, some mechanism works upon this cell firing in such a way that it reacts differentially to correct and incorrect tones.

None of the above phenomena necessarily involves neural plasticity of synaptic connections of the dentate gyrus: the entire process could be regulated by agencies *outside* the hippocampus (for example, changes could be going on in projections leading to the hippocampus). Alternatively, and more optimistically, the types of functional and anatomical plasticity described in earlier sections can readily account for the behaviorally induced changes in the operation of hippocampal circuits seen during the learning task just described. Furthermore, many of the effects recorded in the dentate gyrus are fairly close to conditions which might be expected to produce physiological changes of the type seen in neuroplasticity experiments (e.g. prolonged firing of the granule cells could induce LTP). Hopefully, as our understanding of both behavioral physiology and cellular plasticity becomes more refined, better opportunities for relating these fields will become available.

ACKNOWLEDGEMENTS

Supported by Research Grants MH 19793 from NIMH and BM 76–17370 from NSF; G.L. is a recipient of a Research Career Development Award from NIH (NS-00043).

REFERENCES

Alger, B.E. and Teyler, T.J. (1976) Long-term and short-term plasticity in the CA1, CA3, and dentate regions of the rat hippocampal slice, *Brain Res.*, 110: 463–480.

Anderson, P. (1975) Organization of hippocampal neurons and their connections. In *The Hippocampus, Vol. 1.*, R.L. Isaacson and K.H. Pribram, (Eds.), Plenum Press, New York, pp. 155–176.

Anderson, P., Holmquist, B. and Voorhoeve, P.E. (1966) Excitatory synapses on hippocampal apical dendrites activated by entorhinal stimulation, *Acta physiol. scand.*, 66: 461–471.

Anderson, P., Sundberg, S.H., Sveen, O. and Wigstrom, H. (1977) Specific long-lasting potentiation of synaptic transmission in hippocampal slices, *Nature (Lond.)*, 266: 736–737.

Barondes, S.H. (1970) Cerebral protein synthesis inhibitors block long-term memory, *Int. Rev. Neurobiol.*, 12: 177–205.

Bennett, E. and Rosenzweig, M. (1975) In *Neural Mechanisms of Learning and Memory*, MIT Press, Cambridge, Mass., pp. 544–546.

Beswick, F.B. and Conroy, R.T.W.L. (1965) Optimal conditioning of heteronymous monosynaptic reflexes, *J. Physiol. (Lond.)*, 180: 134–146.

Blackstad, T.W. (1956) Commissural connections of the hippocampal region in the rat, with special reference to their mode of termination, *J. comp. Neurol.*, 105: 417–537.

Bliss, T.V.P. and Gardner-Medwin, A.T. (1973) Long-lasting potentiation of synaptic transmission in the dentate area of the unanaesthetized rabbit following stimulation of the perforant path, *J. Physiol. (Lond.)*, 232: 357–374.

Bliss, T.V.P., and Lømo, T. (1973) Long-lasting potentiation of synaptic transmission in the dentate area of the anaesthetized rabbit following stimulation of the perforant path, *J. Physiol. (Lond.)*, 232: 331–356.

Brostrum, C., Huang, Y.C., Breckenridge, B.M. and Wolff, D.J. (1975) Identification of a calcium-binding protein as a calcium-dependent regulator of brain adenylate cyclase, *Proc. nat. Acad. Sci. (Wash.)*, 72: 177–205.

Brostrum, C.O., Hunksler, F.L. and Krebs, E.G. (1972) The regulation of skeletal muscle phosphorylase, *J. biol. Chem*, 246: 1961–1967.

Cajal, S. Ramón y (1911) *Histologie du Système Nerveux de l'Homme et des Vertébrés*, Intituto Ramón y Cajal, Madrid.

Deadwyler, S.A., Dudek, F.E., Cotman, C.W. and Lynch, G. (1975) Intracellular responses of rat dentate granule cells in vitro: post-tetanic potentiation to perforant path stimulation, *Brain Res.*, 88: 80–85.

Deadwyler, S.A., West, J.R., Cotman, C.W. and Lynch, G.S. (1975) A neurophysiological analysis of the commissural projections to the dentate gyrus of the rat, *J. Neurophysiol.*, 38: 167–184.

Deadwyler, S.A., West, J.R., Cotman, C.W. and Lynch, G.S. (1975) Physiological studies of the reciprocal connections between the hippocampus and the entorhinal cortex, *Exp. Neurol.*, 49: 35–57.

Deadwyler, S.A., West, M. and Lynch, G. (1978a) Activation of the hippocampal circuitry during conditioning. I. Discharge of the perforant path, *Brain Res.*, in press.

Deadwyler, S.A., West, M. and Lynch, G.S. (1978b) Activation of hippocampal circuitry during conditioning. II. Discharge of the granule cells, in preparation.

Douglas, R.M. and Goddard, G.V. (1975) Long-term potentiation of the perforant path-granule cell synapse in the rat hippocampus, *Brain Res.*, 86: 205–215.

Dunwiddie, T.V. and Lynch, G.S. (1978) Long-term potentiation and depression of synaptic responses in the hippocampus: localization and frequency dependency, *J. Physiol. (Lond.)*, 276: 353–364.

Fifkova, E. and Van Harreveld, A. (1977) Long-lasting morphological changes in dendritic spines of dentate granule cells following stimulation of the entorhinal area, *J. Neurocytol.*, 6: 211–230.

Goodman, D.C. and Horel, J.A. (1966) Sprouting of optic tract projections in the brain stem of the rat, *J. comp. Neurol.*, 127: 71–88.

Gottlieb, D.E. and Cowan, W.M. (1973) Autoradiographic studies of the commissural and ipsilateral associational connections of the hippocampus and dentate gyrus of the rat. I. The commissural connections, *J. comp. Neurol.*, 149: 393–422.

Hjorth-Simonsen, A. and Jeune, B. (1972) Projection of the lateral part of the entorhinal area to the hippocampus and fascia dentata, *J. comp. Neurol.*, 146: 215–232.

Kretsinger, R. (1976) Calcium-binding proteins, *Ann. Rev. Biochem.*, 45: 240–266.

Lee, K., Stanford, E.J., Cotman, C.W. and Lynch, G.S. (1977) Ultrastructural evidence for bouton proliferation in the partially deafferented dentate gyrus of the rat, *Exp. Brain Res.*, 129: 475–485.

Lloyd, D.P. (1949) Post-tetanic potentiation of response in monosynaptic reflex pathways of the spinal cord, *J. gen. Physiol.*, 33: 147–170.

Lund, R.D. and Lund, J.S. (1971) Synaptic adjustment after deafferentation of the superior colliculus of the rat, *Science*, 171: 804–807.

Lynch, G., Stanfield, B. and Cotman, C.W. (1973) Developmental differences in post-lesion axonal growth in the hippocampus, *Brain Res.*, 59: 155–168.

Lynch, G., Gall, C., Rose, G. and Cotman, C.W. (1976) Changes in the distribution of the dentate gyrus associational system following unilateral or bilateral entorhinal lesions in the adult rat, *Brain Res.*, 110: 57–71.

Lynch, G., Gall, C. and Cotman, C.W. (1977) Temporal parameters of axon 'sprouting' in the brain of the adult rat, *Exp. Neurol.*, 54: 179–183.

Lynch, G., Gribkoff, V. and Deadwyler, S.A. (1976) Long-term potentiation is accompanied by a reduction in dendritic responsiveness to glutamic acid, *Nature (Lond.)*, 263: 151–153.

Lynch, G., Dunwiddie, T.V. and Gribkoff, V. (1977) Heterosynaptic depression: a postsynaptic correlate of long-term potentiation, *Nature (Lond.)*, 266: 737–739.

Lynch, G. and Cotman, C.W. (1975) The hippocampus as a model for studying anatomical plasticity in the adult brain. In *The Hippocampus, Vol. I*, R. Isaacson and K. Pribram (Eds.), Plenum Press, New York, pp. 123–155.

128

Matthews, D.A., Cotman, C.W. and Lynch, G. (1976) An electron microscopic study of lesion-induced synaptogenesis in the dentate gyrus of the adult rat. II. Reappearance of morphologically normal synaptic contacts, *Brain Res.,* 115: 23–41.

McWilliams, J.R. and Lynch, G. (1978) Ultrastructural analysis of preterminal sprouting after modest deafferentation, *J. comp. Neurol.,* in press.

Mosko, S., Lynch, G. and Cotman, C.W. (1973) The distribution of the septal projections to the hippo-campus of the rat, *J. comp. Neurol.,* 152: 163–174.

Nadler, J.V., Vaca, K.W., White, W.F., Lynch, G.S. and Cotman, C.W. (1976) Aspartate and glutamate as possible transmitters of excitatory hippocampal afferents, *Nature (Lond.),* 260: 537–539.

Nakamura, Y., Mizuno, N., Kunishi, A. and Saka, M. (1974) Synaptic reorganization of the red nucleus after chronic deafferentation from cerebello-rubral fibers: an electron microscope study in the cat, *Brain Res.,* 82: 298–301.

Olds, J.E. (1975) Unit recordings during Pavlovian conditioning. In *Brain Mechanisms in Mental Retardation,* Buchwald and Brazier (Eds.), Academic Press, New York, pp. 343–371.

Pysch, J.J. and Wiley, R.G. (1972) Morphologic alterations of synapses in electrically stimulated superior cervical ganglia of the cat, *Science,* 176: 191–193.

Raisman, G. (1969) Neuronal plasticity in the septal nuclei of the adult rat, *Brain Res.,* 14: 25–48.

Raisman, G. and Field, P.A. (1973) A quantitative investigation of the development of collateral rein-nervation after partial deafferentation of the septal nuclei, *Brain Res.,* 50: 241–264.

Rassmussen, H. and Goodman, D. (1977) Relationship between calcium and cyclic nucleotides in cell activation, *Physiol. Rev.,* 57: 421–501.

Rosenthal, J. (1969) Post-tetanic potentiation at the neuromuscular junction of the frog, *J. Physiol. (Lond.),* 203: 121–133.

Schwartzkroin, P.A. and Wester, K. (1975) Long-lasting facilitation of a synaptic potential following tetanization in the in vitro hippocampal slice, *Brain Res.,* 89: 107–119.

Segal, M.E., Disterhoft, J. and Olds, J. (1972) Hippocampal unit activity during classical aversive and appetitive conditioning, *Science,* 175: 791–794.

Sotelo, C. and Palay, S.L. (1971) Altered axons and axon terminals in the lateral vestibular nucleus of the rat: possible example of axonal remodelling, *Lab. Invest.,* 25: 653–673.

Steward, O., Cotman, C.W. and Lynch, G. (1973) Growth of a new fiber projection in the brain of adult rats: reinnervation of the dentate gyrus by the contralateral entorhinal cortex following ipsilateral entorhinal lesions, *Exp. Brain Res.,* 18: 396–414.

Tsukahara, N. and Fujito, Y. (1976) Physiological evidence of formation of new synapses from cerebrum in the red nucleus neurons following cross-union of forelimb nerves, *Brain Res.,* 106: 184–188.

Van Harreveld, A. and Fifkova, E. (1975) Swelling of dendritic spines in the fascia dentata after stimula-tion of the perforant path fibers as a mechanism of post-tetanic potentiation, *Exp. Neurol.,* 49: 736–749.

Weinrich, D. (1971) Ionic mechanism of post-tetanic potentiation at the neuromuscular junction of the frog, *J. Physiol. (Lond.),* 212: 431–446.

West, J.R., Deadwyler, S.A., Cotman, C.W. and Lynch, G. (1975) Time-dependent changes in commissural field potentials in the dentate gyrus following lesions of the entorhinal cortex in adult rats, *Brain Res.,* 97: 215–233.

Wilson, D. and Skirboll, L. (1974) Basis for post-tetanic potentiation at the mammalian neuromuscular junction, *Amer. J. Physiol.,* 227: 92–95.

Yamamoto, C. (1972) Activation of hippocampal neurons by mossy fiber stimulation in thin brain section in vitro, *Exp. Brain Res.,* 14: 423–435.

Zimmer, J. (1974) Proximity as a factor in the regulation of aberrant axonal growth in postnatally deaf-ferented fascia dentata, *Brain Res.,* 72: 137–142.

Zimmer, J. (1971) Ipsilateral afferents to the commissural zone of the fascia dentata, demonstrated in decommissurated rats by silver impregnation, *J. comp. Neurol.,* 142: 393–416.

DISCUSSION

SOTELO: From the many mechanisms that have been advanced for postsynaptic potentiation one, of course, has been concerned with calcium and the increasing concentration of this cation. But a second one, already speculated upon, is that postsynaptic spines might increase in size, possibly at the spine neck. I believe Fifková and Van Harreveld have some anatomical evidence on this.

LYNCH: The trouble with the experiments to which you refer is that the anatomical studies were not accompanied by physiological recording. Consequently, it is not certain that the regions sampled for electron microscopy actually contained 'potentiated' synapses. Beyond this those experiments were conducted with acute animals and the spine swelling was found in the great majority of the cases. However, in animal experiments potentiation is often difficult to achieve. The kind of stimulation conditions used by Van Harrevald and Fifková commonly produces seizures and their effects might be correlated with these rather than potentiation. The results are intriguing but I am not satisfied that they are related to potentiation.

CORNER: You have given some very good direct evidence that short high-frequency bursts could really appear to have a long-lasting potentiation effect. But have you tried to find how extensive the bursts need be before you get any such potentiation?

LYNCH: Yes. I am talking of long-term potentiation in the slice, which is a non-decrementing response that goes on for an hour or two. That is, until the experimenter runs out of patience. When you find potentiation that is not decremented for 5 or 10 minutes then it lasts for very long periods. This is the preparation from which I have collected data relevant to your question. In the slice, we have been able to produce the effect with 20 pulses; I would suspect that 20 or 30 pulses is down near the lower limit.

STIRLING: When you are looking at these granule cells firing off, do you think they fire throughout the hippocampus? If you try to do a visual test in your animal would you expect the same thing? And would you expect it in all parts of the hippocampus, or are you just looking at one part, basically?

LYNCH: Visual input by itself does not appear to drive the cells. I think a visual input *would* drive the cells if it was used as the kind of operant cue as the tone was. Regarding the second question: we have only recorded at one septal-temporal segment of the hippocampus in all of these experiments. And so, whether it is happening along the whole structure or not, I don't know. In some sense I would be disappointed if it were.

BLOM: Is the frequency of the granule cells that you observed at about the same range as what you see with at the visual stimulation? And do you see this effect happening only in a very special type of behavioral experiment, for example what in the human we would call motivation or something similar? Then, it would not appear to matter what the modality of the input is, whether visual, auditory or whatever.

LYNCH: I don't think it is purely a question of motivational level. The animals go through a period before they have learned the task in which they are deprived, etc., and the test tones will not drive the granule cells. The tones only begin to drive the cells as the animal learns it (the tone) has significance to him.

McEWEN: Is this task one which the animal will learn if the hippocampus is removed?

LYNCH: No. From the literature I suspect that rats will learn the one tone test missing the hippocampus. But it is doubtful that they could adequately learn the task when we add a second tone.

JANSEN: In the experiments where you saw sprouting, do you have any information on the functioning of these sprouts? And secondly: what happens to them once the innervation returns?

LYNCH: In this situation the innervation does not return. With regard to functioning of the sprouts we have stimulated these 'sprouted' afferents and observed we find that the responses can be recorded much farther out the dendritic tree. In the adult animal at about 9 days after the lesion one can see the post-synaptic responses to the stimulation of the sprouting afferents beginning to ascend the dendrite. There are other examples from people who have attempted to show that the new connections are functional, in which they recorded intracellularly and had new synapses appearing closer to the cell body, and found the expected changes in the characteristics of the intracellular potentials. But the issue, I would say, is still not settled. It is difficult to imagine experiments that would be absolutely satisfactory, since the deafferentation procedure needed to elicit sprouting causes considerable changes in the target cell. So it may be changing the physiological properties of the postsynaptic cell, and that may be responsible for some of the physiological changes recorded after stimulation of the sprouted afferent. But what you *do* see is in accordance with what you would expect to find if the sprout were functional.

ZIMMER: You have this situation where you have a perforant path input which does not fire the granule cells, but by changing the stimuli you induce them to fire. Which other pathway, would you think, could be involved in releasing the activity?

LYNCH: I suspect that the afferents to the hippocampus coming from the septum and possibly the monoaminergic ones from the brain stem may be responsible; we have hypothesized that these are terminating in large part in a population of interneurons. And many of these interneurons are known to generate axons which go on to the granule cells and ramify there extensively. So my guess is (and it is nothing more than speculation) that the septal cholinergic and brain stem monoaminergic inputs regulate the excitability of the granule cells via interneurons.

ADRIEN: I would be very interested to see what happens if instead of non-discriminantly stimulating your brain slices you would use spike trains resembling those seen in the intact animal and see if the potentiation is generated in the slice.

LYNCH: There is an experiment by Douglas and Goddard (*Brain Research*, 1975) in which they used spike trains which resembled the discharge pattern of pyramidal cells, and I believe they reported excellent potentiation.

JANSEN: In your stimulation experiments what you get with electrical stimulation is activity in the whole bundle of afferent axons. And that is obviously a much different situation from anything that you would normally expect to see in vivo. So it is tempting to guess that you will have changes immediately in the surrounds of the terminals on account of the synchronous activity and these changes may be involved in potentiation.

LYNCH: Your point is well taken. We are assuming that what we see is a multiplication of what goes on at the single cell level. That may not be the case. It may be that the synchronous stimulation is required to create a change in the milieu which produces potentiation. In some of these hippocampal systems it may be possible to electrically stimulate single cells and record from single cell targets and experiments of this sort may be required to answer your question.

SECTION III

GENETIC PROGRAMMING
OF NERVOUS DEVELOPMENT

Environmental and Genetic Determinants of Connectivity in the Central Nervous System — An Approach Through Dendritic Field Analysis

MARTIN BERRY, PHILIP BRADLEY and SALVADOR BORGES

Anatomy Department, Medical School, University of Birmingham, Birmingham BL5 2TJ (Great Britain)

INTRODUCTION

The mechanisms which underlie the establishment of neural connections in the mammalian central nervous system are largely unknown, although several propositions have been advanced which could form the basis of experimental studies. For example, Altman (1967) and Jacobson (1974) put forward the idea that two classes of neuron exist: (a) *macroneurons,* which are tightly constrained genetically, and (b) highly plastic *microneurons,* whose growth is largely determined by environmental factors. Macroneurons are generally formed first during ontogeny and establish major axon tracts between neural centers, whereas microneurons are formed later in development and have short axons which make local connections. The maturation of many microneurons coincides with the acquisition of an adaptive behavioral repertoire, and thus the plasticity of these cells could be important in the development of such neural activities as learning and memory.

Morest (1969) studied the development of dendritic networks in a variety of regions of the mammalian brain and concluded that dendritic growth was associated with the formation of contacts between axons and membrane specializations of the developing dendritic tree called *filopodia.* The significance of Morest's observation was not fully realized until Skoff and Hamburger (1974) and Vaughn et al. (1974) discovered synaptic profiles on dendritic filopodia, enabling the latter workers to formulate their filopodial synaptogenic hypothesis of dendritic growth. This simple theory proposed that dendritic trees develop their ramifications under the influence of axonal synaptic contacts on dendritic filopodia. However, it has been shown that such contacts are probably not exclusively synaptic but can also be established merely by selective adhesiveness between axonal and dendritic membrane (Merrell et al., 1975, 1976; Hinds and Hinds, 1976a, b; Merrell and Glaser, 1973).

Since dendritic parameters such as size of tree, patterns of branching, and synaptology are surely among the prime determinants of the information processing capabilities of a neuron, it follows that a study of the mechanisms underlying dendritic growth ought to help in elucidating the natural history of neural connectivity. We have investigated the relative contribution of nurture and nature in the formation of dendritic trees in both cerebellar and cerebral cortex by (1) studying the effects of changes induced by altering afferent connections, and (2) investigating growth in the murine mutants 'weaver' and 'staggerer'. We present here a summary of the main results and conclusions of these studies, and outline a general hypothesis of connectivity to explain our findings.

GROWTH OF DENDRITES OF PURKINJE CELLS IN THE NORMAL CEREBELLUM

Purkinje cell trees are ideally suited to dendritic growth studies. They are arranged in a fan-like fashion, with a very small depth to their field, so that minimal projection artefact is obtained during analysis (Berry et al., 1972). Afferent connections are well understood and consist, in the main, of two spatially and morphologically distinct fiber systems: *climbing fibers,* probably originating exclusively from the inferior olive and engaging the 'smooth' surfaces of the proximal branches, and *parallel fibers*, stemming from granule cells, which contact spines on the more distal branches (Palay and Chan-Palay, 1974). These two projection systems can be ablated differentially, and the effects of such treatments on the developing dendritic tree have provided good evidence that the growth of spiny branches is induced through the axo-spinous contacts of parallel fibers (Altman and Anderson, 1972; Berry and Bradley, 1976c, Bradley and Berry, 1978a, b) and that climbing fibers probably exert only a minor influence on the formation of the tree (Sotelo et al., 1975; Bradley and Berry, 1976a, b; Sotelo and Arsenio-Nunes, 1976; Kawaguchi et al., 1975), although this latter conclusion is by no means universally accepted (Hámori, 1973; Kornguth and Scott, 1972; Eccles, 1977). Once the Purkinje cell has received the inductive stimulus from parallel fibers, the development of the dendritic tree may proceed at a constant rate, and branching patterns become determined by adhesive interactions between the growth cone filopodia and the axonal arborizations.

Support for this dendritic filopodial attachment theory has come from the results of quantitative analyses of growing Purkinje cell networks (Bradley and Berry, 1976a; Berry and Bradley, 1976b). In particular, the theory predicts that: (i) the branching patterns of dendritic trees are established by growth at the terminals and, if the density of axons is uniform about the tree, the branching will be at random; (ii) dendrites become directed into areas in which the density of growing axons is maximal; (iii) segment lengths are inversely related to the density of axons; (iv) the number of segments – and also (v) the relative frequencies of dichotomy, trichotomy, etc. – are directly correlated with the density of growing axons in the neuropil about the developing tree (Bradley and Berry, 1976a; Berry et al., 1975; Berry and Bradley, 1976a; Berry, 1976a).

All these predictions have so far been borne out by quantitative analysis of Purkinje cell dendritic trees in normal rats (Berry and Bradley, 1976b; Hollingworth and Berry, 1975) and mice (Bradley and Berry, 1978a), in 'weaver' and 'staggerer' mutant mice (Bradley and Berry, 1978a), and in experimental studies on partially (Bradley and Berry, 1976a, 1978b; McConnell and Berry, 1978b) or almost completely (Berry and Bradley, 1976c) agranular rat cerebellar cortex. The results of these analyses suggest that genes program the formation of postsynaptic sites on the surface of dendrites, but that other parameters of the dendritic field are regulated to a considerable degree by environmental factors.

GROWTH OF DENDRITIC TREES OF PURKINJE CELLS IN MUTANT MICE

Homozygous 'weaver' mutant mouse

In the 'weaver' condition very few parallel fibers are formed (Hirano and Dembitzer, 1974), since most granule cells degenerate within the external granular layer before they can migrate (Rakic and Sidman, 1973a, b). The dendritic tree of the 'weaver' is often improperly oriented and elaborates only 12% of the normal number of segments, but segment lengths are the same as equivalent proximal segments in the normal tree (Bradley and Berry,

1978a). The number of trichotomous nodes and the topology of the branching patterns are also identical with the normal proximal parts of the tree (Fig. 1).

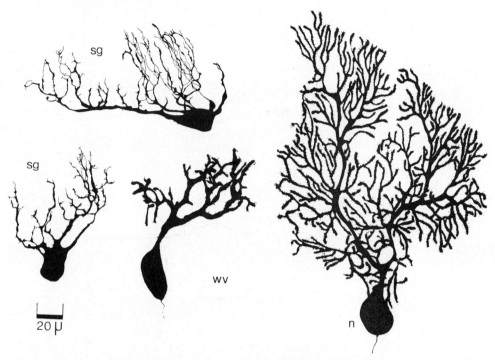

Fig. 1. Representative drawings of Golgi-Cox impregnated Purkinje cells from 20-day-old normal (n) 'weaver' (wv) and 'staggerer' (sg) mice. The small tree size of the two mutants is obvious, and results from a failure in formation of segments rather than a reduction in segment lengths. See text and Fig. 2B. (The two examples of 'staggerer' cells show the range of variation seen in this mutant.)

These results indicate that, although the dendritic trees of Purkinje cells in the 'weaver' mutant can be disorientated, they otherwise develop normally for a certain period, but that their growth is curtailed at an early stage in development. Quantitative comparison between the development of normal and 'weaver' trees unequivocally identifies the time of arrest at about the 7th day post partum (pp), when parallel fibers begin to be laid down in the molecular layer of the normal mouse (Fig. 2). Since only a very few granule cells are formed in this mutant strain (Hirano and Dembitzer, 1974), the most obvious conclusion to be drawn is that direct synaptic contact by a critical number of parallel fibers with the primordial tree on the 7th day is a prerequisite to further growth (i.e. parallel fiber synaptic contacts induce a *secondary* phase of growth).

Before the stage of presumed parallel fiber induction, normal growth occurs in the proximal dendritic segments of the 'weaver' Purkinje cell (Fig. 2). Such growth may be either autonomous (Calvet et al., 1976; Gona, 1975), or directly induced by climbing (Berry and Bradley, 1976b) or by monoaminergic fibers (Rakic, 1974), which are both known to arborize about the Purkinje cell somata at this early time. Experimental evidence indicates that monoaminergic fibers are involved in the initiation and maintenance of early growth (Bloom, 1974), and they could thus control the resorption of perisomatic processes, the organization of apical polarity, and the elaboration of proximal segments in the Purkinje

136

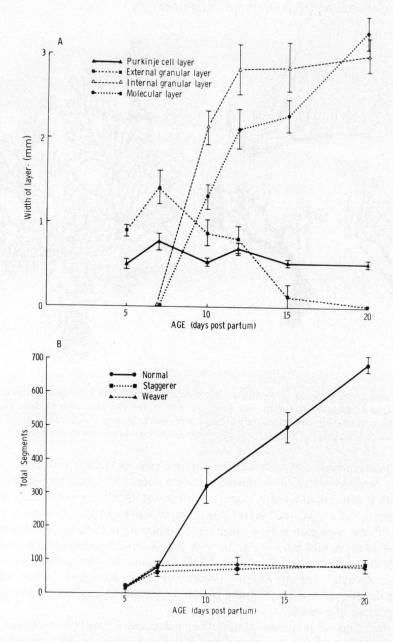

Fig. 2. A: graph summarizing the development of the normal mouse cerebellum, by analysis of the thickness of the composite layers. Note that the migration of granule cells begins by about the 7th day post partum, and that this is accompanied by an increase in the thickness of the molecular layer as parallel fibers are deposited and the Purkinje cell dendritic tree expands. Migration is completed by about the 15th day post partum as the external granule layer disappears and the internal granule layer stabilizes to a constant thickness. B: graph of total number of segments in normal, 'weaver' and 'staggerer' trees at different ages. No more segments are added to 'weaver' or 'staggerer' trees after 7 days of age, the time when parallel fiber deposition in the normal cerebellum begins to initiate the exponential phase of dendritic growth.

cell dendritic tree. However, some features of early growth might be influenced by still other afferent fibers or by neuron-glia interactions. For example, resorption of perisomatic processes and the development of apical polarity could be organized by basket cell axons (Altman, 1976), and orientation towards the pial surface achieved by contact guidance with the radial processes of Bergmann glia. The latter proposition is supported by the observation that when Bergmann glia are reduced in number by degranulating procedures, or if they are hypoplastic (as in the 'weaver' mouse), the normal orientation is lost in many Purkinje cells (Altman and Anderson, 1972; Berry and Bradley, 1976b; Hirano et al., 1972; Rakic and Sidman, 1973a, b; Woodward et al., 1975).

Homozygous 'staggerer' mutant mouse

It has been suggested that in the 'staggerer' mouse the primary genetic defect results in a failure of spine development on Purkinje cell dendrites (Sidman, 1972). Granule cells secondarily degenerate in the internal granular layer since their axons fail to make synaptic contacts with the Purkinje cell tree (Sotelo and Changeux, 1974). Another explanation is that the effect of the mutation is pleiotropic involving both Purkinje cells and granule cells (Yoon, 1974). The dendritic tree of the Purkinje cell in the 'staggerer' mutant is multipolar, nonspiny and has fewer segments than in normal mice. The tree, however, is normally orientated and planar, with a normal topology and frequency of trichotomy (Fig. 1) (Bradley and Berry, 1978a). Comparison of the development of 'staggerer' and normal Purkinje cell trees shows that the mutant tree stops growing at about the 7th day post partum, like that of the 'weaver', and presumably for the same reason: failure of parallel fibers to elicit their inductive effect. A few junctions do form between 'staggerer' Purkinje cell dendrites and parallel fibers (Landis and Sidman, 1978; Landis and Rees, 1976; Sotelo, 1973, 1975a), but these never develop into mature axo-spinous synapses. Induction of a secondary phase of growth therefore appears to be contingent on the elaboration of mature axo-spinous contacts.

The density of climbing fibers within the 'staggerer' cerebellum is much lower than in the normal cerebellum, making it unlikely that all Purkinje cells are innervated by them (Sotelo, 1975b). Indeed, electrophysiological investigations (Crepel et al., 1973) have obtained climbing fiber responses in only 40% of tested Purkinje cells. Although Hámori (1973) has suggested that spine development on the Purkinje cell dendritic tree is conditional on heterotopic induction* by climbing fibers, the uniform loss of spines in 'staggerer' mice, plus recent experimental evidence of spine redistribution rather than loss after either neonatal or adult climbing fiber ablation (Bradley and Berry, 1976a, b; Sotelo and Arsenio-Nunes, 1976; Kawaguchi et al., 1975) refute this view. Alternatively, Kim (1975) has suggested that only a very small number of parallel fiber contacts is needed to induce spine formation, since a few granule cells do survive in 'weaver' mice, and also after most other degranulation procedures. However, within the present state of knowledge, it seems equally reasonable to suppose that the postsynaptic apparatus of dendritic spines is formed without any kind of presynaptic induction. Thus, the frequency of dendritic spines per unit area of dendritic shaft membrane could be genetically determined and, for a given species, be constant over the entire surface of the tree. Whether the ratio of excitatory and inhibitory

---

* Heterotopic induction: "specific afferents would induce the host cells to develop and maintain postsynaptic receptors for axon terminals at other sites" (Hámori, 1973).

138

synapses is also predetermined over the membrane is uncertain. Climbing fibers have the property of effecting spine resorption as they invade the tree during growth (Berry and Bradley, 1976b; Larramendi, 1969; Larramendi and Victor, 1966, 1967), and spines are not resorbed during the development of the tree if climbing fibers are absent (Bradley and Berry, 1976a; Sotelo and Arsenio-Nunes, 1976; Kawaguchi et al., 1975). Moreover, spines reappear on the 'smooth' proximal branches after climbing fiber deafferentation of the mature Purkinje cell dendritic tree (Sotelo et al., 1975; Bradley and Berry, 1976b).

Dendritic growth in partially agranular cortex

Prolonged low level irradiation during the neonatal period (Altman and Anderson, 1972) or the administration soon after birth of methylazoxymethanol acetate (MAM) (Hirano et al.,

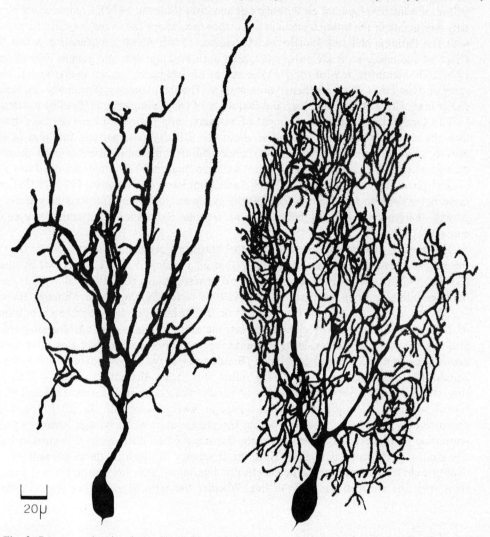

20μ

Fig. 3. Representative drawings of two 30-day-old rat Purkinje cells from a normal animal (right) and from a rat irradiated with 200 rads daily for the first 10 days of life (left). Note the long segment lengths in the treated cell and the normal path lengths.

1972; Woodward et al., 1975), destroys most granule cells. In the presence of a reduced number of parallel fibers, Purkinje cell trees have a few, very long spiny segments with a low frequency of trichotomy, although the mean distance from dendrite tips to the cell body is normal (Fig. 3; Berry and Bradley, 1976c; Bradley and Berry, 1978b). This result was largely predictable from the dendritic filopodial attachment hypothesis. The normal path lengths suggest that induction by parallel fibers, through axo-spinous synapses on dendritic shaft membrane, has occurred in the partially agranular cortex. This would mean firstly, that the formation of only a small number of such synapses is needed to mediate induction, and secondly, that the rate of subsequent growth is constant. The frequencies of different topologies of dendrites in partially agranular cortex deviate somewhat from the normal random terminal distribution, and this is probably correlated with a non-random interaction between growth cones and their tissue substrate in the neuropil of MAM-treated and irradiated animals. The frequency of spines per unit area of Purkinje cell dendritic membrane is normal (approximately 1.5 spines/unit area of membrane) in irradiated and MAM-treated animals, despite the demonstration by other workers that in partially agranular cerebellar cortex many of the spines are not engaged by synapses (Kim, 1975; Altman and Anderson, 1972; Hirano et al., 1972; Privat, 1975; Privat and Drian, 1976).

It is clear that if Purkinje cells can be classed as macroneurons, then the idea that they are rigidly constrained by genetic programming must be incorrect. The number of dendritic segments elaborated, their length and the topology of the tree, are environmentally controlled (specifically by interactions with parallel fibers) and, as mentioned above, genetic influences may be confined to the designation of the density of postsynaptic spine sites over the dendritic membrane, and to the nature of the receptor membrane for adhesion and synaptogenesis. (The Purkinje cell peripheral dendritic membrane surfaces appear to have an almost exclusive affinity for parallel fibers (Sotelo, 1973, 1975b; Llinas et al., 1973).)

At the time of attachment between Purkinje cell dendritic filopodia and parallel fibers, the parent granule cells probably have not yet become engaged by mossy fibers, since such granule cells are still in transit along their migratory path to the internal granule layer, and because mossy fiber contacts in the glomeruli of the internal granule layer mature relatively late (Altman, 1972). Thus, Purkinje cell dendritic filopodial/parallel fiber interactions would not be influenced by volleys of afferent unit activity, but be entirely determined by the number and spatial distribution of potentially contactable axons (the latter being directly related to the number of granule cells produced). The ratio of granule cells to Purkinje cells increases during phylogenesis and brain evolution. For example, the ratio in man is 2991:1, in the rat 897:1, and in the mouse 778:1 (Lange, 1975), and this parameter is directly correlated with the number of segments elaborated by the Purkinje cell tree in each species (Bradley and Berry, 1978a; Hollingworth and Berry, 1975; Nieuwenhuys, 1972).

DEVELOPMENT OF NEOCORTICAL NEURONS

Macroneurons

The observations of Van der Loos (1965) on 'improperly' orientated neocortical pyramidal cells indicated that dendritic growth of these macroneurons may be little affected by the environment, although deafferentation in neonates (Valverde, 1968; Berry and Hollingworth, 1973; Globus and Scheibel, 1967a, b; Coleman and Riesen, 1968; Jones and Thomas, 1962) and rearing in enriched environments (Holloway, 1966; Volkmar and Greenough, 1972; Greenough and Volkmar, 1973; Greenough et al., 1973; Uylings et al., this volume) does produce quantitatively detectable changes. Although these results might suggest that the dendritic fields of neocortical macroneurons are largely under genetic control, the geometry of their trees may in fact be refined by local tissue factors, randomly distributed in space, so that dendrites form the same patterns regardless of their orientation within the cortex. Analysis of branching patterns supports this view, since it has been demonstrated that basal dendritic fields grow by random terminal branching (Hollingworth and Berry, 1975), implying a random distribution of adhesive sites for dendritic filopodial attachment about the somata. Furthermore, the basal dendrites bifurcate without preference for any particular direction (Uylings and Smit, 1975). The apical dendrites of neocortical pyramids form first when newly migrated neurons are within the molecular layer. As later arriving migrating cells ascend into the molecular layer, expansion of the cortex is achieved by accretion of cells onto the pial surface of the cortical plate (Berry and Rogers, 1965). This causes a relative displacement of the tips of established apical dendrites outwards away from their somata. The shafts of apical dendrites are formed pari passu with displacement (Berry, 1974), and their orientation is determined largely by the initial orientation of somata immediately after migration has ceased (Berry and Eayrs, 1966). The collateral branches of apical dendrites do, however, grow by random terminal branching (Hollingworth and Berry, 1975).

The spines which develop on pyramidal cell dendrites are remarkably sensitive to environmental changes during ontogeny (Globus and Scheibel, 1966, 1967a, b; Fifkova, 1970a, b; Ruiz-Marcos and Valverde, 1969; Valverde, 1967, 1968, 1971; Valverde and Estéban, 1968; Valverde and Ruiz Marcos, 1969) and in the adult (Valverde, 1971; Rutledge et al., 1974). Two populations of spines may exist: those that develop under *genetic* control, i.e. are largely insensitive to changes in afferent input, and those that are highly 'plastic' in response to stimulation (Valverde, 1971). This latter group may be induced either (a) *directly* by specific afferents (Globus and Scheibel, 1967b; Schapiro and Vukovich, 1970; Jones and Powell, 1970), (b) *indirectly* by internuncial axons (Valverde and Ruiz-Marcos, 1969), or (c) *heterotopically* (Hámori, 1973). Another explanation is that *all* spines are genetically determined, but that intact afferents invade vacated synaptic regions after deafferentation, causing resorption of spines, much as do the climbing fibers on Purkinje cell dendrites during development (Berry and Bradley 1976b; Larramendi, 1969; Larramendi and Victor, 1966, 1967).

Microneurons

Stellate cells in the neocortex are classified as microneurons, and there now seems to be good evidence that their dendritic trees establish connections largely under the influence of environmental conditions (Altman, 1967; Jacobson, 1974). For example, stellate cell dendritic trees in layer IV of the mouse visual cortex become directed into the supragranular and infragranular laminae after enucleation at birth (Valverde, 1968) and, in the dark-reared rat, preferential reorientation of stellate cell dendrites occurs towards the pial surface (Borges and Berry, 1976, 1978) (Fig. 4). This latter abnormality could be caused by filopodia on the terminal dendritic growth cones, i.e. in the superficial part of the stellate cell tree, which adhere to a greater number of growing axons than is possible for filopodia in the lower part of the tree. This would mean that dark-reared rats have fewer axons in layer IV of their visual cortices than do normally reared animals, and that the adhesiveness between growing axons and stellate cell dendritic filopodia may be non-specific.

It has been argued that dendritic branching patterns are organized by adhesive interaction between axons and dendrites independent of synaptic activity. Thus, if the frequency of firing in retinal ganglion cells modifies protein synthesis in LGN cells which, in turn, dictates the degree of intracortical branching of geniculostriate axon terminals, a means by which the visual environment could affect neural connections in the striate cortex would be established. There is good evidence for a direct correlation between RNA synthesis and neural activity (Watson, 1976), but at present there is little idea of where new proteins are being incorporated. In the visual system, however, the normal traffic of patterned visual input through the visual radiations appears to be a prerequisite for normal development (Berry, 1976b). Thus, geniculostriate axons fail to arborize normally within the visual cortex after visual deafferentation (Singer et al., 1977; Thorpe and Blakemore, 1975) whereas, in the normal

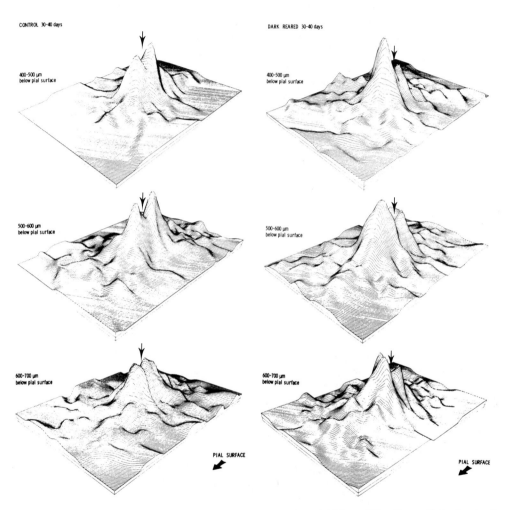

CONTROL 30-40 days   DARK REARED 30-40 days

400-500 μm below pial surface

500-600 μm below pial surface

600-700 μm below pial surface

PIAL SURFACE

Fig. 4. Average dendritic density distribution about the somata of 18 layer IV stellate cells in the visual cortex of the rat, normally reared to 30–40 days post partum (control 30–40 days), and animals reared in darkness to 30–40 days (dark-reared 30–40 days). In each case the somata (arrowed) are centered on a 250 μm × 350 μm sampling area. The computed surface of the grid has a standard orientation with respect to the pial surface, and represents the dendritic density calculated from the averaged grid values. Stellate cell dendrites in dark-reared animals are distributed such that a significantly higher dendritic density (as measured by t-tests) is present in the dorsal half of the averaged dendritic field. Conversely, in the ventral half of the field, there is a significant reduction in dendritic density in the dark-reared animals.

animal a surge in the production of neural processes in the visual cortex, as judged by tubulin production, occurs immediately after eye-opening (Cronly-Dillon and Perry, 1976). All of which suggests, of course, that the level of incoming axonal activity is an important factor in the regulation of terminal branching.

IMPLICATIONS FOR A THEORY OF CONNECTIVITY

The following generalizations may be useful as a basis for planning future work. In *macroneurons,* which are formed relatively early in ontogeny, (i) *primary induction* occurs to initiate differentiation and organize early growth; this might be mediated by catecholamine (CA) fibers. (ii) Growth of dendrites proceeds for a limited period after induction, under the trophic influence of CA fibers and other afferent input, but a *secondary induction* is required if growth is to continue. (iii) Secondary induction is mediated through specific fiber systems by synaptic engagement, e.g. parallel fiber axo-spinous synapses on Purkinje cell dendrites. (iv) After secondary induction, growth proceeds at a constant rate in all terminals for a constant duration. Segment lengths become designated by the frequency of branch formation, which results from adhesive interactions between dendritic filopodia and specific axon groups. The number of segments generated by a given tree, and the frequency of different orders of magnitude of branching, are directly related to the frequency of adhesions formed. The growth of dendrites is directed into areas of neuropil where the density of axons with matching affinities is highest. (v) Dendritic shaft synaptogenesis is genetically controlled, and postsynaptic sites elaborated at a constant frequency per unit surface area of membrane. The number of postsynaptic sites normally elaborated is, however, generally consistent with the number of presynaptic elements present, because of the constraints of both secondary induction and the specificity of dendritic filopodial-axon adhesiveness. Postsynaptic activity per se might not influence dendritic branching patterns since in most macroneurons growth is well underway before functional connections are formed. However, the formation of functional connections could have a trophic influence on growth (Smith and Kreutzberg, 1976).

In the case of *microneurons,* which on the whole are formed later in ontogeny, the environment influences dendritic branching by controlling the relative densities of different functional groups of projection fibers in the developing neuropil. This might be brought about if the frequency of unit activity, conducted through a neural chain, controls protein synthetic processes which support the growth of terminal axon arborizations. Primary and secondary induction of dendritic growth, dendritic filopodial axon adhesiveness and synaptogenesis are weakly specified in microneurons, although selective synaptic stabilization might ultimately be achieved (Changeux and Danchin, 1976; Changeux and Mikoshiba, this volume).

This hypothesis for the establishment of neural connections proposes that cell autonomous gene expression is confined to the development of synaptic membranes and the glycocalyx, whilst the size of the dendritic tree (number and length of segments), orientation and topology are controlled by the number and species of growing axons ramifying within dendritic fields. The 'environment' may, in turn, control the relative numbers of different species of axon growing about the dendritic tree and, in this way, modulate its growth (along with the subsequent qualitative and quantitative characteristics of synaptic connectivity). Such a scheme meets the requirements for 'gene-saving' mechanisms in the specification of neural networks (Changeux and Danchin, 1976; Wolpert and Lewis, 1975) and strikes a compromise between preformist and empiricist views.

REFERENCES

Altman, J. (1967) Postnatal growth and differentiation of the mammalian brain with implications for a morphological theory of memory. In *The Neurosciences, A Study Programme*, G.C. Quarton, T. Melnechuk and F.O. Schmitt (Eds.), Rockefeller University Press, New York, pp. 723–743.

Altman, J. (1972) Postnatal development of cerebellar cortex of the rat. III. Maturation of the components of the granular layer, *J. comp. Neurol.*, 145: 465–514.

Altman, J. and Anderson, W.J. (1972) Experimental reorganisation of the cerebellar cortex. I. Morphological effects of elimination of the microneurons with prolonged X-irradiation started at birth, *J. comp. Neurol.*, 143: 355–406.

Altman, J. (1976) Experimental reorganisation of the cerebellar cortex. V. Effects of early X-irradiation schedules that allow or prevent the acquisition of basket cells, *J. comp. Neurol.*, 165: 31–48.

Berry, M. (1974) Development of the cerebral neocortex of the rat. In *Studies on the Development of Behavior and the Nervous System, Vol. 2*, G. Gottlieb (Ed.), Academic Press, New York, pp. 7–67.

Berry, M. (1976a) Topological analysis of dendritic trees. In *Proceedings of the Fourth International Congress for Stereology*, E.E. Underwood (Ed.), National Bureau of Standards Special Publications 431, Washington D.C., pp. 49–54.

Berry, M. (1976b) Plasticity in the visual system and visually guided behaviour. In *Advances in Psychobiology, Vol. III*, A.H. Riesen and R.F. Thompson (Eds.), John Wiley, New York, pp. 125–192.

Berry, M. and Bradley, P. (1976a) The application of network analysis to the study of branching patterns of large dendritic fields, *Brain Res.*, 109: 111–132.

Berry, M. and Bradley, P. (1976b) The growth of the dendritic trees of Purkinje cells in the cerebellum of the rat, *Brain Res.*, 112: 1–35.

Berry, M. and Bradley, P. (1976c) The growth of the dendritic trees of Purkinje cells in irradiated agranular cerebellar cortex, *Brain Res.*, 116: 361–387.

Berry, M. and Eayrs, J.T. (1966) The effects of X-irradiation on the development of the cerebral cortex, *J. Anat. (Lond.)*, 100: 707–722.

Berry, M. and Hollingworth, T. (1973) Development of isolated cortex, *Experientia (Basel)*, 29: 204–207.

Berry, M., Hollingworth, T., Anderson, E.M. and Flinn, R.M. (1975) Application of network analysis to the study of the branching patterns of dendritic fields. In *Physiology and Pathology of Dendrites, Advances in Neurology, Vol. 12*, G.W. Kreutzberg (Ed.), Raven Press, New York, pp. 217–245.

Berry, M., Hollingworth, T., Flinn, R.M. and Anderson, E.M. (1972) Dendritic field analysis – A reappraisal. *T.-I.-T. J. Life Sci.*, 2: 129–140.

Berry, M. and Rogers, A.W. (1965) The migration of neuroblasts in the developing cerebral cortex, *J. Anat. (Lond.)*, 99: 691–709.

Bloom, F.E. (1974) The role of cyclic nucleotides in central synaptic function, *Rev. Physiol. Biochem. Pharmacol.*, 74: 1–103.

Borges, S. and Berry, M. (1976) Preferential orientation of stellate cell dendrites in the visual cortex of the dark-reared rat, *Brain Res.*, 112: 141–147.

Borges, S. and Berry, M. (1978) Recovery of the cerebral cortex from the effects of dark rearing after exposure to light, *J. comp. Neurol.*, in press.

Bradley, P. and Berry, M. (1976a) The effects of reduced climbing and parallel fibre input on Purkinje cell dendritic growth, *Brain Res.*, 109: 133–151.

Bradley, P. and Berry, M. (1976b) Quantitative effects of climbing fibre deafferentation on the adult Purkinje cell dendritic tree, *Brain Res.*, 112: 133–140.

Bradley, P. and Berry, M. (1978a) Development of Purkinje cells in the murine mutants 'weaver' and 'staggerer', *Brain Res.*, 142: 135–141.

Bradley, P. and Berry, M. (1978b) Effects of methylazoxymethanol acetate on the development of the cerebellum of the rat, *Brain Res.*, 143: 499–511.

Bradley, P. and Berry, M. (1978c) The effects of thiophen on the dendritic tree of the Purkinje cell of the adult rat, *Brain Res.*, in press.

Calvet, M., Lepault, A. and Calvet, J. (1976) A Procion yellow study of cultured Purkinje cells, *Brain Res.*, 111: 399–406.

Changeux, J.P. and Danchin, A. (1976) Selective stabilisation of developing synapses as a mechanism for the specification of neural networks, *Nature. (Lond.)*, 264: 705–712.

Coleman, P.D. and Riesen, A.H. (1968) Environmental effects on cortical dendritic fields. I. Rearing in the dark, *J. Anat. (Lond.)*, 102: 363–374.

Crepel, F., Mariani, J., Korn, H. and Changeux, J.P. (1973) Electrophysiologie du cortex cerebellar chez la souris mutant "staggerer" *C.R. Acad. Sci. (Paris)*, 277: 2761–2763.

Cronly-Dillon, J.R. and Perry, G.W. (1976) Tubulin synthesis in developing rat visual cortex, *Nature (Lond.)*, 261: 581–583.

Eccles, J.C. (1977) An instruction-selection theory of learning in the cerebellar cortex, *Brain Res.*, 127: 327–352.

Fifkova, E. (1970a) The effects of monocular deprivation on the synaptic contacts of the visual cortex, *J. Neurobiol.*, 1: 285–294.

Fifkova, E. (1970b) The effects of unilateral deprivation of visual centres in rats, *J. comp. Neurol.*, 140: 431–438.

Globus, A. and Scheibel, A.B. (1966) Loss of dendritic spines as an index of presynaptic terminal patterns. An experimental application of the Golgi method, *Nature (Lond.)*, 212: 463–465.

Globus, A. and Scheibel, A.B. (1967a) Synaptic loci in cortical neurons of the rabbit; the specific afferent radiation, *Exp. Neurol.*, 18: 116–131.

Globus, A. and Scheibel, A.B. (1967b) The effect of visual deprivation on cortical neurons. A Golgi study, *Exp. Neurol.*, 19: 331–345.

Gona, A.G. (1975) Golgi studies of cerebellar maturation of frog tadpoles, *Brain Res.*, 95: 132–136.

Greenough, W.T., and Volkmar, F. (1973) Pattern of dendritic branching in occipital cortex of rats reared in complex environments, *Exp. Neurol.*, 40: 491–504.

Greenough, W.T., Volkmar, F. and Juraska, J.M. (1973) Effects of rearing complexity on dendritic branching in frontolateral and temporal cortex of the rat, *Exp. Neurol.*, 41: 371–378.

Hámori, J. (1973) The inductive role of presynaptic axons in the development of post-synaptic spines, *Brain Res.*, 62: 337–344.

Hinds, J.W. and Hinds, P.L. (1976a) Synapse formation in the mouse olfactory bulb. I. Quantitative studies, *J. comp. Neurol.*, 169: 15–40.

Hinds, J.W. and Hinds, P.L. (1976b) Synapse formation in the mouse olfactory bulb. II. Morphogenesis, *J. comp. Neurol.*, 169: 41–62.

Hirano, A. and Dembitzer, H.M. (1974) Observations on the development of the 'weaver' mouse cerebellum, *J. Neuropath. exp. Neurol.*, 33: 354–364.

Hirano, A., Dembitzer, H.M. and Jones, M. (1972) An electron microscopic study of cycasin-induced cerebellar alteration, *J. Neuropath. exp. Neurol.*, 13: 113–125.

Hollingworth, T. and Berry, M. (1975) Network analysis of dendritic fields of pyramidal cells in the neocortex and Purkinje cells in the cerebellum of the rat, *Phil. Trans. B*, 270: 227–262.

Holloway, J.R., Jr. (1966) Dendritic branching: some preliminary results of training and complexity in rat visual cortex, *Brain Res.*, 2: 393–396.

Jacobson, M. (1974) A plentitude of neurons. In *Studies on the Development of Behavior and the Nervous System, Aspects of Neurogenesis, Vol. 2*, G. Gottlieb (Ed.), Academic Press, New York, pp. 151–166.

Jones, H.W. and Thomas, D.B. (1962) Changes in the dendritic organisation of neurons in the cerebral cortex following deafferentation, *J. Anat. (Lond.)*, 96: 375–381.

Jones, E.G. and Powell, T.P.S. (1970) An electron microscopic study of terminal degeneration in the neocortex of the cat, *Phil. Trans. B*, 257: 29–43.

Kawaguchi, S., Yamamota, T., Mizuno N. and Iwahori, N. (1975) The role of climbing fibres in the development of Purkinje cell dendrites, *Neurosci. Lett.*, 1: 301–304.

Kim, S.V. (1975) Formation of unattached spines of Purkinje cell dendrites in organotypic cultures of mouse cerebellum, *Brain Res.*, 88: 52–58.

Kornguth, S.E. and Scott, G. (1972) The role of climbing fibres in the formation of Purkinje cell dendrites, *J. comp. Neurol.*, 146: 61–82.

Landis, D.M.D. and Reese, T.S. (1976) Structure of the Purkinje cell membrane in 'staggerer' and 'weaver' mutant mice, *J. comp. Neurol.*, 171: 247–260.

Landis, D.M.D. and Sidman, R.L. (1978) Electron microscopic analysis of postnatal histogenesis in the cerebellar cortex of 'staggerer' mutant mice, *J. comp. Neurol.*, in press.

Lange, W. (1975) Cell number and cell density in the cerebellar cortex of man and some other mammals, *Cell Tiss. Res.*, 157: 115–124.

Larramendi, L.M.H. (1969) Analysis of synaptogenesis in the cerebellum of the mouse. In *Neurobiology of Cerebellar Evolution and Development*, R. Llinas (Ed.), American Medical Association, Chicago, pp. 803–843.

Larramendi, L.M.H. and Victor, T. (1966) Soma-dendritic gradient of spine resorption in the Purkinje cell of the cerebellum of the mouse during post-natal development. An electron microscopic study, *Anat. Rec.*, 154: 373.

Larramendi, L.M.H. and Victor, T. (1967) Synapses in the Purkinje cell spines in the mouse: an electron microscopic study, *Brain Res.*, 5: 15–30.

Llinas, R., Hillman, D.E. and Precht, W. (1973) Neuronal circuit reorganisation in mammalian agranular cortex, *J. Neurobiol.*, 4: 69–74.

McConnell, P. and Berry, M. (1978a) The effects of undernutrition on Purkinje cell dendritic growth in the rat, *J. comp. Neurol.*, 177: 159–172.

McConnell, P. and Berry, M. (1978b) The effects of refeeding on Purkinje cell dendritic growth in the neonatally starved rat, *J. comp. Neurol.*, 178: 759–772.

Merrell, R. and Glaser, L. (1973) Specific recognition of plasma membranes by embryonic cells, *Proc. nat. Acad. Sci. (Wash.)*, 70: 2794–2797.

Merrell, R., Gottlieb, D.I. and Glaser, L. (1975) Embryonal cell surface recognition. Extraction of an active plasma membrane component, *J. biol. Chem.*, 250: 5655–5659.

Merrell, R., Gottlieb, D.I. and Glaser, L. (1976) Membranes as a tool for the study of cell surface recognition. In *Neural Recognition*, S.H. Barondes (Ed.), Chapman and Hall, London, pp. 249–273.

Morest, D.K. (1969) The growth of dendrites in the mammalian brain, *Z. Anat. Entwickl.-Gesch.*, 128: 290–317.

Nieuwenhuys, R. (1972) Comparative anatomy of the cerebellum. In *The Cerebellum, Progr. Brain Res.*, *Vol. 25*, P.C.A. Fox and R.S. Snider (Eds.), Elsevier, Amsterdam, pp. 1–93.

Palay, S.L. and Chan-Palay, V. (1974) *Cerebellar cortex: Cytology and Organisation*, Springer, New York.

Privat, A. (1975) Dendritic growth in vitro. In *Physiology and Pathology of Dendrites, Advances in Neuropathology, Vol. 12*, G.W. Kreutzberg (Ed.), Raven Press, New York, pp. 201–216.

Privat, A. and Drian, M.J. (1976) Postnatal maturation of rat Purkinje cells culturated in the absence of two afferent systems: an ultrastructural study, *J. comp. Neurol.*, 166: 201–244.

Rakic, P. (1974) Intrinsic and extrinsic factors influencing the shape of neurons and their assembly into neuronal circuits. In *Frontiers in Neurology and Neuroscience Research*, P. Seeman and G.M. Brown (Eds.), University of Toronto Press, pp. 112–132.

Rakic, P. and Sidman R.L. (1973a) 'Weaver' mutant mouse cerebellum defective neuronal migration secondary to specific abnormality of Bergmann glia, *Proc. nat. Acad. Sci. (Wash.)*, 70: 240–244.

Rakic, P. and Sidman, R.L. (1973b) Sequence of development abnormalities leading to granule cell deficit in cerebellar cortex of 'weaver' mutant mice, *J. comp. Neurol.*, 152: 103–132.

Ruiz-Marcos, A. and Valverde, F. (1969) The temporal evolution of the distribution of dendritic spines in the visual cortex of normal and dark raised mice, *Exp. Brain Res.*, 8: 284–294.

Rutledge, L.T., Wright, C. and Duncan, J. (1974) Morphological changes in pyramidal cells of mammalian neocortex associated with increased use, *Exp. Neurol.*, 44: 209–228.

Schapiro, S. and Vukovich, R.R. (1970) Early experience effects upon cortical dendrites: a proposed model for development, *Science*, 167: 292–294.

Sidman, R.L. (1972) Cell interactions in developing mammalian central nervous system. In *Cell Interactions*, L.G. Silvestri (Ed.), North-Holland Publ., Amsterdam, pp. 1–13.

Singer, W., Holländer, H. and Vanegas, H. (1977) Decreased geniculate neurons following deafferentation, *Brain Res.*, 120: 133–137.

Skoff, R.P. and Hamburger, V. (1974) Fine structure of dendritic and axonal growth cones in embryonic chick spinal cord, *J. comp. Neurol.*, 53: 107–148.

Smith, B.H. and Kreutzberg, G.W. (Eds.) (1976) *Neurosciences Research Program Bulletin, Vol. 14 (No. 13), Neuron-Target Cell Interaction*, pp. 225–259.

Sotelo, C. (1973) Permanence and fate of paramembranous synaptic specialization in 'mutant' and experimental animals, *Brain Res.*, 62: 345–351.

Sotelo, C. (1975a) Dendritic abnormalities of Purkinje cells in the cerebellum of neurological mutant mice ('weaver' and 'staggerer'). In *Physiology and Pathology of Dendrites, Advances in Neurology, Vol. 12*, G.W. Kreutzberg, (Ed.), Raven Press, New York, pp. 335–351.

Sotelo, C. (1975b) Anatomical, physiological and biochemical studies on the cerebellum from mutant mice. II. Morphological study of cerebellar cortical neurons and circuits in the 'weaver' mouse, *Brain Res.*, 94: 19–44.

Sotelo, C. and Arsenio-Nunes, M.L. (1976) Development of Purkinje cells in the absence of climbing fibres, *Brain Res.,* 111: 389–395.

Sotelo, C. and Changeux, J.P. (1974) Trans-synaptic degeneration 'en cascade' in the cerebellar cortex of 'staggerer' mutant mice, *Brain Res.,* 67: 519–526.

Sotelo, C., Hillman, D.E., Zamora, A.K. and Llinas, R. (1975) Climbing fibre deafferentation its action on Purkinje cell dendritic spines, *Brain Res.,* 98: 574–581.

Thorpe, P.A. and Blakemore, C. (1975) Evidence for a loss of afferent axons in the visual cortex of monocularly deprived cats, *Neurosci. Lett.,* 1: 271–276.

Uylings, H.B.M., Kuypers, K. and Veltman, W.A.M. (1978) Environmental influences on neocortex in later life, this volume.

Uylings, H.B.M. and Smit, G.J. (1975) Three-dimensional branching structure of pyramidal cell dendrites, *Brain Res.,* 87: 55–60.

Valverde, F. (1967) Apical dendritic spines of the visual cortex and light deprivation in the mouse, *Exp. Brain Res.,* 3: 337–352.

Valverde, F. (1968) Structural changes in the area striata of the mouse after enucleation, *Exp. Brain Res.,* 5: 274–292.

Valverde, F. (1971) Rate of and extent of recovery from dark-rearing in visual cortex of the mouse, *Brain Res.,* 33: 1–11.

Valverde, F. and Estéban, M.E. (1968) Peristriate cortex of mouse: location and effects of enucleation on the number of dendritic spines, *Brain Res.,* 9: 145–148.

Valverde, F. and Ruiz-Marcos, A. (1969) Dendritic spines in the visual cortex of the mouse: introduction to a mathematical model, *Exp. Brain Res.,* 8: 269–283.

Van der Loos, H. (1965) The 'improperly' orientated pyramidal cell in the cerebral cortex and its possible bearing on the problems of neuronal growth and cell orientation, *Bull. Johns. Hopk. Hosp.,* 117: 228–250.

Vaughn, J.E., Henrikson, C.K. and Grieshaber, J.A. (1974) A quantitative study of synapses in motor neuron dendrite growth cones in developing mouse spinal cord, *J. Cell Biol.,* 60: 664–672.

Volkmar, F.N. and Greenough, W.T. (1972) Rearing complexity affects branching of dendrites in the visual cortex of the rat, *Science,* 176: 1445–1447.

Watson, J. (1976) *Cell Biology of Brain,* Chapman and Hall, London, pp. 155–164.

Wolpert, L. and Lewis, J.H. (1975) Towards a theory of development, *Fed. Proc.,* 34: 14–20.

Woodward, D.J., Bickett, D. and Chanda, R. (1975) Purkinje cell dendritic alteration after transient developmental injury of the external germinal layer, *Brain Res.,* 97: 195–214.

Yoon, C.H. (1976) Pleiotropic effects of the 'staggerer' gene, *Brain Res.,* 109: 206–215.

DISCUSSION

CHANGEUX: I have a question about the comparison between Staggerer and Weaver mutants, in which you mentioned that the growth of the tree is blocked in the cerebellum. How do you explain the fact that in the Weaver there are spines and in the Staggerer not?

BERRY: The hypothesis put forward is that the secondary phase of Purkinje cell growth, i.e. beyond the 7th day, which one sees in the normal animal, requires induction by parallel fibers. In the case of the Weaver this induction is not able to occur, because the parallel fibers are not present (since the granule cells don't migrate, and degenerate in the external granular layer). In the Staggerer, parallel fiber induction is also unable to occur, but in this case because no spines have formed on the dendritic tree, even though the granule cells migrate normally and establish an internal granular layer. Thus, the common denominator between the Staggerer and Weaver is a failure of contact of parallel fibers with the dendritic tree, and accordingly induction fails and dendritic growth is arrested.

PARNAVELAS: I would like to know how you selected the cells on which you made the measurements. As you know, there are various types of non-pyramidal cells in layer IV, some of which (type a) have dendrites which are randomly oriented, whereas others (type b) have two groups of dendrites which radiate, one towards the pial surface and one towards the white matter. If you selected relatively more of the latter type of cells, that would bias the result, it seems to me.

UYLINGS: Along the same lines, do you have some numbers about the proportion between the different types of non-pyramidal cells present in the dark rearing material as compared with normal material? And a second question I would like to ask: in these dark-rearing experiments, did you find with the density procedure a reduction in the number of segments, or rather a reorientation of the whole dendritic tree?

BERRY: We selected the cells in Golgi-Cox specimens just as we came across them, thus presumably completely at random. We did not make any kind of distinction between them. However, the dendritic pattern of most cells used was that of type-7 of Jones, also called 'star cells' by Cajal and, more recently, 'spurious stellates' by Lund and Valverde. A very few of the cells included in the analysis were type-5 of Jones, with smooth peri-somatically distributed dendrites. The number of segments, as measured by the number of terminals, was normal in each case, and so was the number of primary dendrites emanating from the soma. The number of branches in the upper half of the dark-reared field was always greater than in the lower half. In the normals, in contrast, the number of branches in both halves is the same. These results demonstrate that growth is inhibited in the lower field and enhanced in the upper field of dark-reared animals. With respect to the first question, the cells used for analysis were mainly types-7 and -5, using the classification of Jones. The difference between these two sorts of cells is that type-7 has spiny dendrites, whereas type-5 has smooth dendrites. Both cells have similarly oriented dendritic fields.

STIRLING: When you are talking about filopodial extension, do you believe that the synapses have to make contact with the growing dendrites in order for them to continue growing, or do you think that there may be attraction at a distance? I have been looking at the Reeler mouse, and the dendrites in the dentate granule cells are situated right in the middle of the hippocampal hilus, and there you have extremely long dendrites. Unlike the granule cells in normal mice, they send their dendrites straight out, with hardly any branching, as if they were 'searching' for the perforant path.

BERRY: The hypothesis states that actual contact must be established. I suspect that normally in the growing central nervous system – if this filopodial-axonal contact idea is correct – interaction between axons and dendritic filopodia occurs with a high frequency, such that it controls further growth. Now, if you don't have any axons around as, for example, when you take a cell out of the central nervous system and place it in a culture situation, the dendrites still branch, but they do so with a very much lower frequency than in vivo and they have very long segments. The low frequency of branching of the dendrites in the tissue culture situation may thus be similar to the situation that you are looking at in the intact hippocampus where, in the absence of compatible axons, branching results from non-specific adhesive interaction of dendritic growth cones with their physical substrate. Thus, segments are long and branching is infrequent.

WILKIN: Is it possible to change the behavioral pattern of the mutant Purkinje cells, for example by putting them side by side with normal tissue in culture, or by doing transplantation experiments?

BERRY: Well, of course, such types of experiments provide a fascinating opportunity for making an attempt to resolve the 'nature/nurture' conflict with respect to a given tissue. In the mutant mouse chimera, for example, there exists a mosaic of the genetically defective and the normal tissue: environmental and genetic factors are all operating to produce the overt defect in the CNS displayed by the mutant. By looking at the interface between the two sorts of tissue in the same animal, the chimera technique offers a means of dissecting genetic and environmental factors. For example, a cerebellar chimera of Weaver and normal would be made up of a mosaic of groups of Weaver and normal Purkinje cells, interdigitating with one another. In such chimeras we would predict that if the primary genetic defect leads to the degeneration of granule cells, the disorientation and stunted growth of the typical Weaver Purkinje cell would be averted at the interface between mosaics of tissue, where Weaver Purkinje cells grow in a normal environment of parallel fibers.

Purkinje Cell Ontogeny:
Formation and Maintenance
of Spines

CONSTANTINO SOTELO

*Laboratoire de Neuromorphologie (U-106 INSERM), Centre Médico-Chirurgical FOCH, 92.150 Suresnes
(France)*

INTRODUCTION

The tridimensional shape and the connectivity of neurons are the two fundamental features which underlie neural function. However, the way in which these parameters become established still remains a largely unanswered question. The Purkinje cells of the cerebellar cortex of small mammals, such as the mouse and the rat, offer a favorable material to at least partially solve these questions. Indeed, cerebellar circuitry and the normal processes of cell migration, differentiation and synaptogenesis (Ramón y Cajal, 1911) are better understood in the cerebellum than in any other central nervous region. In addition, in the mouse cerebellum there are several mutations affecting a specific kind of neuron or a single type of synapse (Sidman et al., 1965). Finally, in the cerebellum of small mammals most of the developmental processes take place during the first 3 postnatal weeks, thus allowing the experimental impairment of afferent fibers and/or interneurons derived from the external granular layer. Therefore, the study of the cerebellum in mutant mice and in rats devoid of climbing fibers, or of granule, stellate and basket cells, has proved to be very useful in elucidating some of the above mentioned problems. This has been the subject of our work during the last years (Sotelo, 1973, 1975a, b, 1977; Sotelo and Changeux, 1974a, b; Sotelo et al., 1975; Sotelo and Arsenio-Nunes, 1976; Mariani et al., 1977).

The present review will be concerned only with the morphological analysis of microenvironmental factors influencing the molding of the Purkinje cell dendritic tree. Particular emphasis will be given to the problem of the formation and maintenance of dendritic spines, since they are by far the most numerous receptor sites in these neurons.

PURKINJE CELL DEVELOPMENT IN NORMAL CELLULAR ENVIRONMENT

During normal development, Purkinje cell differentiation occurs in a concomitant manner with the development of its synaptic inputs. Climbing fibers reach Purkinje cells, establishing early axo-somatic synapses (Ramón y Cajal, 1911) which are already functional by day 3 post-natally (Crepel, 1971). This pericellular climbing plexus originates from 3–4 different climbing fibers (Crepel et al., 1976). The further development of the Purkinje cell dendritic tree parallels the growth of climbing fibers and the maturation of their synapses (Ramón y Cajal, 1911). By day 12–15, the climbing fiber varicosities make synapses on thorns emerging from the thick Purkinje cell dendritic branches (Larramendi and Victor,

1967). At this stage the immature multiple innervation is transformed into the definitive one-to-one relationship, which characterizes the climbing fiber-Purkinje cell synapses in adult animals (Crepel et al., 1976). During the 2nd and 3rd postnatal weeks, migration of the bulk of granule cells takes place, giving rise to the millions of parallel fibers found in the molecular layer (Ramón y Cajal, 1911). The development of parallel fibers (accounting for more than 95% of the synaptic input to Purkinje cells) is accompanied by the formation of thin terminal branches of the Purkinje cell dendritic arborization, the so-called *spiny branchlets*, and by the achievement of the *espalier* arrangement of these dendritic trees which give to the Purkinje cells their unique tridimensional shape (Ramón y Cajal, 1911). According to its synaptic investment, the dendritic arborization of a mature Purkinje cell can be divided into two different compartments: (i) a proximal one which consists of the thick (and almost smooth) dendritic branches and which is postsynaptic both to climbing fibers and to inhibitory terminals, and (ii) a distal compartment formed by the numerous spiny branchlets, and contacted exclusively by parallel fibers. The former grows earlier than the latter. Therefore, the study of the development of Purkinje cells under normal conditions gives us a complete schedule of the cellular interactions which occur during the molding of their dendritic arborizations. It does not, however, tell us about which part in this final dendritic arrangement is due to the intrinsic program of Purkinje cells, and which derives from the cellular interactions taking place during their development. As mentioned above, we expected that the study of Purkinje cell development in various abnormal cellular environments would help to solve this problem.

PURKINJE CELLS IN AGRANULAR CEREBELLA

The most appropriate natural situation to study the development of Purkinje cells in the absence of parallel fibers is offered by the homozygous 'weaver' (*wv*) mutant. In these mice, granule cells fail to migrate, and die in the external granular layer at the stage of postmitotic neuroblasts, before forming any parallel fibers (Rakic and Sidman, 1973a). Phenocopies of the 'weaver' mutation can be obtained by damaging the external granular layer in newborn animals, and we have used repeated postnatal doses of X-rays (Altman and Anderson, 1972) to destroy all neuronal elements derived from this germinative layer. Although important differences exist between the 'weaver' cerebellum and the agranular cerebellum obtained by X-rays (mainly due to the presence of stellate and basket cells in the 'weaver', and their absence in the irradiated cerebellum; Sotelo, 1977), the morphological characteristics of Purkinje cells are similar in both cases. These can be summarized as follows: the total length of the dendritic tree is severely reduced, the dendrites are randomly oriented, and the whole dendritic tree is often inversed (Fig. 1); in addition, although they do not develop spiny branchlets, the primary and secondary branches are rather thick and exhibit an irregular rough surface, which is obviously due to the presence of numerous spines (Fig. 2) (see refs. in Sotelo, 1975a and in Berry and Bradley, 1976).

In agreement with these general characteristics, the large dendritic trunks of the Purkinje cells are widespread from the white matter up to a subpial band, in which the general appearance of the molecular layer is preserved. The Purkinje cell perikarya have a smooth contour, although in some instances somatic immature-like spines can be present. The hillock and initial segment of the axon emerge from the cell body, and only in one case of Purkinje cell situated near the pial surface was the initial segment identified as arising from a dendritic profile. As previously described (Hirano and Dembitzer, 1973; Rakic and Sidman, 1973b;

Sotelo, 1973), the electron microscopic picture which characterizes the agranular cerebellum is the presence at all cortical levels of innumerable dendritic spines, similar to those normally arising from spiny branchlets but devoid of presynaptic elements. When observed at higher magnification, it can be demonstrated that lateral segments of the spinous unit-membrane bear fuzzy cytoplasmic material, identical to a normal postsynaptic differentiation, and that these segments appear to be coated with a granular extracellular material resembling the one commonly observed at normal synaptic clefts. In the large majority of cases, the post-synaptic and cleft differentiations are facing a normal looking unit-membrane belonging to a Bergmann fiber. With the application of the freeze-fracture technique to the study of the rodent cerebellum (Landis and Reese, 1974; Palay and Chan-Palay, 1974) it has been pos-sible to disclose a conspicuous specialization in the internal organization of the membranes of Purkinje spines. At the synaptic interface between parallel fibers and Purkinje spines, the postsynaptic membrane of the latter contains an aggregate of homogeneous particles asso-ciated with their E face. Therefore, this aggregate characterizes the receptor site of the spine membrane, and might be related to some of the specific proteins which could play an active role during synaptic transmission. Similar studies on 'weaver' cerebellum (Hanna et al., 1976; Landis and Reese, 1977) have demonstrated that the membranes of free Purkinje spines also contain these characteristic particle aggregates on their external halfs (E faces), making these spines morphologically identical to the innervated ones in normal cerebellum. Spines with a shorter stalk and a more rounded head, similar to those present in the primary and secondary dendritic branches of normal Purkinje cells, have also been observed in this cerebellum; as in normal animals, they make synaptic contacts with the climbing fibers.

PURKINJE CELLS IN THE 'REELER' CEREBELLUM

This autosomal recessive mutation not only causes extensive perturbations in the de-velopment of the cerebellar cortex (see refs. in Mariani et al., 1977) but also affects other cortical regions: the cerebral cortex and the hippocampal formation (Caviness and Sidman, 1972, 1973; Caviness, 1973, 1976). The main defect in all these cortical structures is a sys-tematic malposition of different neuronal classes. Thus, in the cerebellum, only a few Purkinje cells are located at their normal position in a discrete zone of the cerebellar cortex; along with a shallow but distinct molecular layer and an internal granular layer. On the con-trary, the large majority of Purkinje cells does not reach their normal position, and are dispersed throughout the granular layer, the white matter and the deep cerebellar nuclei. According to their location, various Purkinje cells grow their dendritic trees in different cellular environments (thus differing from the 'weaver' cerebellum, in which the whole Purkinje cell population becomes mature in the same cellular environment). The 'reeler' cerebellum therefore offers the best 'natural experiment' to analyze the factors which determine or modulate the shape of Purkinje cell dendritic trees.

In the 'reeler' cerebellum, as a consequence of the mispositioning, the Purkinje cells can be found in four different environments, and, interestingly, the shape of these cells differs in each position:

(1) Purkinje cells normally positioned in the superficial cortex

These exhibit identical morphological features to the Purkinje cells in control mice. However, due to the reduced thickness of the molecular layer, most of these Purkinje cell dendritic arborizations extend laterally (always in the sagittal plane) for longer distances

152

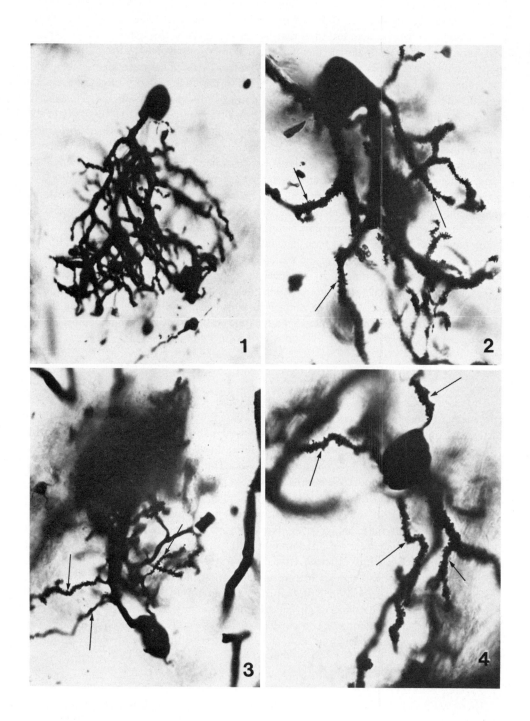

than in the normal mouse. In 1 μm thick plastic sections, the secondary dendrites can be seen running horizontally, parallel to the pial surface. In Golgi impregnated material, the dendritic arborizations of these Purkinje cells keep their typical *espalier* arrangement. From a qualitative point of view, secondary and tertiary thick dendritic trunks are present, as well as the spiny branchlets.

Electron microscopic studies confirm the scarcity of Purkinje cells in their normal positions. The narrow molecular layer contains numerous dendritic profiles of Purkinje cells. Some of the thick profiles give rise to spines which may be contacted by climbing varicosities and stellate axon terminals but also occasionally by parallel fibers. The large majority of spines originating from spiny branchlets make contact with parallel fibers; free spines are practically non-existent.

(2) Purkinje cells dispersed within the granular layer of the superficial cortex

Rows of Purkinje cell perikarya are observed in the inner part of the granular layer and in the white matter, exactly as if they were 'invading' the cortex from the white matter. As a result, the broad horizontal band of the granular layer is partitioned by vertical septa distributed at irregular intervals. Within this layer, Golgi impregnation discloses three main types of Purkinje cells, differing by the shape of their dendritic arborizations.

(i) The Purkinje cells 'en parapluie': their perikarya lie at different depths in this layer. A main dendritic branch emerges from the apical pole and ascends, without branching, in a vertical direction to the molecular layer (where it branches profusely). Clusters of stubby spines are present on the main vertical branch, while in the molecular layer the dendritic arborizations resemble those of normal Purkinje cells, and even spiny branchlets are well developed.

(ii) The 'multipolar' Purkinje cells: in addition to the presence of a main dendritic trunk, one to three thinner dendrites arise from the perikarya. Shortly after its emergence the main dendritic trunk ramifies profusely. The entire dendritic arborization of these multipolar Purkinje cells ends within the granular layer. Both the medium-sized and the thin branches of the dendritic arborizations are studded with spines.

(iii) The third class of dispersed Purkinje cells is a mixture of the two previous ones. The dendritic tree generally emerges from one apical trunk which, during its ascension within the granular layer, branches in a dichotomous manner, giving off medium-sized dendritic trunks (Fig. 3). Those branches which succeed in reaching the molecular layer ramify profusely, in a similar way as in the case of the first type of dispersed Purkinje cells.

Ultrastructural study of the granular layer discloses an abnormal arrangement of its neuropil, which is characteristic for the 'reeler' cerebellum. The ascending dendrites of the Purkinje cells, which occupy most of the volume of the vertical septa, are in the vicinity of

Figs. 1–4. Golgi-impregnated Purkinje cells (Golgi-Rio-Hortega technique).

Fig. 1. Purkinje cell in an irradiated cerebellum. The dendritic tree emerges from a unique stem but is completely inversed. Note the absence of spiny branchlets. × 420.

Fig. 2. Disoriented Purkinje cell in an irradiated rat cerebellum. All of the dendritic branches are studded with spines (arrows). × 800.

Fig. 3. 'Reeler' cerebellum: mixed type of Purkinje cell within the granular layer. Its main dendritic branches give rise to dendritic trunks (arrows) spreading within the granular layer. The terminal branches in the molecular layer are out of focus. × 500.

Fig. 4. 'Reeler' cerebellum. Multipolar Purkinje cell located at the central cerebellar mass. This cell has randomly oriented dendrites, which are studded with spines (arrows). × 800.

154

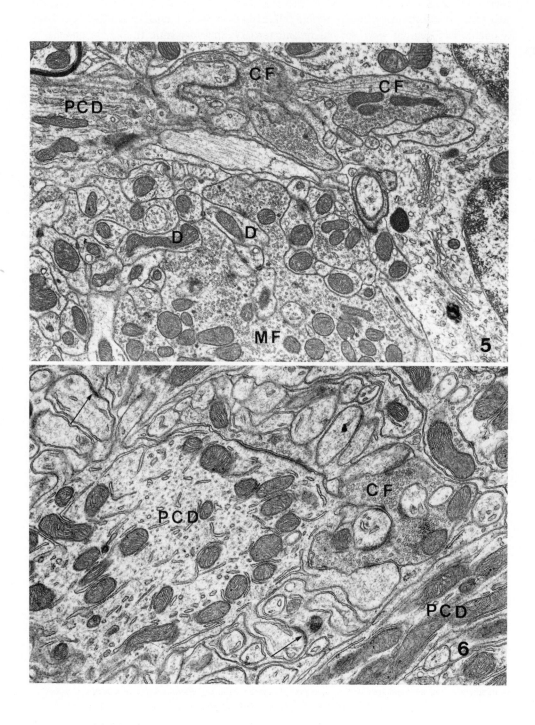

the cerebellar glomeruli (Fig. 5). The spines emerging from these ascending dendrites are mainly in contact with climbing fiber varicosities (Fig. 5).

(3) Purkinje cells intermingled with the white matter in the central mass

The majority of such Purkinje cells are concentrated in the central area. In Golgi impregnated material they exhibit a large variety of shapes (Rakic, 1976; Mariani et al., 1977), all of them resembling neurons described in agranular cerebella. Indeed, the central mass is devoid of granule cells, giving the Purkinje cells a cellular environment similar to that in 'weaver' and irradiated cerebella. Multipolar Purkinje cells (Fig. 4) represent extremes in a continuous series of shapes derived from the disoriented (but monopolar) dendritic tree commonly observed in agranular cerebella.

Similar to what was described above for the 'weaver' cerebellum, the neuropil of the central mass is mainly formed by profiles of randomly oriented Purkinje dendrites (Fig. 6). The presence of innumerable spines devoid of innervation is also characteristic of these dendrites (Fig. 6). Postsynaptic-like differentiations are observed on these free spines (Figs. 6 and 7), which closely resemble the spines which originate from the spiny branchlets in normal Purkinje cells. Some of these spines are innervated by axon terminals, mainly climbing varicosities (Figs. 6 and 7) (Mariani et al., 1977).

Another very important characteristic of Purkinje cell dendrites in this region is the presence of postsynaptic-like dense cytoplasmic material, undercoating membrane segments of variable length at the dendritic smooth surface. This postsynaptic web-like material displays a morphology similar to that which is characteristic of postsynaptic differentiations in Gray type-1 synapses (Fig. 8). Such dendritic segments can face glial elements, naked spines, or, more often, axon terminals of stellate cells. In general, these axon terminals develop neither presynaptic dense projections nor clustering of synaptic vesicles facing the dendritic postsynaptic differentiation. Similar differentiations were also observed in the 'weaver' cerebellum (Sotelo, 1975a).

(4) Purkinje cells penetrating the deep cerebellar nuclei

A clear-cut border exists between the central region containing the Purkinje cell perikarya and the region occupied by the cell bodies of the deep cerebellar nuclei. Such a distinction does not exist for the dendritic tree, however. Indeed, Purkinje cells in the vicinity of the cerebellar nuclei send all or part of the dendritic tree into the nuclear territory. The shapes of these Purkinje neurons resemble those encountered in the white matter. With the electron microscope, dendritic profiles clearly identified as belonging to Purkinje cells can be found side by side with dendritic profiles of cerebellar nuclear neurons (Fig. 9). The spines of these Purkinje dendrites may either be free of innervation or be postsynaptic to their own normal inputs (mainly climbing varicosities), or apposed to the axon terminals present in the cerebellar nuclei.

Figs. 5 and 6. Electron micrographs from adult 'reeler' cerebellum.

Fig. 5. Characteristic arrangement of the neuropil in the granular layer in 'reeler'. A cerebellar glomerulus, composed by a central mossy rosette (MF) synapsing on granule cell dendrites (D), is near to a Purkinje cell dendritic profile (PCD). The spines emerging from this dendrite are contacted by climbing varicosities (CF). × 19,000.

Fig. 6. Neuropil in the central cerebellar mass. Two Purkinje dendritic profiles of different diameters (PCD) occupy most of the surface of this micrograph. Numerous spines emerge from the larger dendrite; some of them are postsynaptic to a climbing varicosity (CF), while others exhibit a postsynaptic density (arrows) facing glial processes. × 27,000.

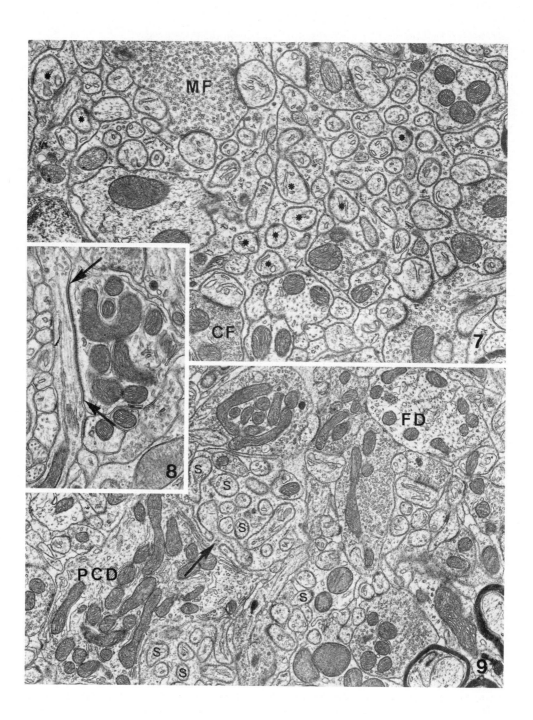

The results described above and obtained in the 'weaver', the irradiated and the 'reeler' cerebella clearly demonstrate that the presence of all normal inputs to the Purkinje cell is necessary for the achievement of the planar disposition and the normal branching pattern of their dendrites (see refs. in Mariani et al., 1977). Indeed, as already suggested by Ramón y Cajal (1929), the parallel fibers are the main organizing element for the 'espalier' disposition of the Purkinje cell dendrites, and they are essential for the induction of spiny branchlets. It seems clear, however, that there is an intrinsic mechanism which allows the Purkinje cell dendrites to grow autonomously in a random manner, explaining the existence of aberrant multipolar forms as illustrated in Fig. 4. Complementary information on the existence of such intrinsic mechanism can be obtained from in vitro studies of cerebellar explants, cultivated in presence of an antimitotic agent. In this situation, almost totally deafferented Purkinje cells are still able to grow randomly oriented dendritic arborizations (Calvet et al., 1976).

DEVELOPMENT OF PURKINJE CELL DENDRITIC SPINES

Despite the disorientation of their dendritic trees, Purkinje cells developing in an agranular milieu are studded with numerous dendritic spines. As described above, two main types of spines can be observed: (i) a large majority which is similar to the spines emerging from spiny branchlets in the normal cerebellum; and (ii) some spines with shorter stalks and more rounded heads, resembling those normally present in the proximal dendritic compartment. The former are almost completely devoid of innervation, whereas the latter are postsynaptic to climbing fibers. Since both types of spines can be present on the same dendritic segment, the characteristic normal compartmentalization of Purkinje cell dendrites does not occur in the agranular cerebellum.

In the absence of parallel fibers, therefore, Purkinje dendrites are capable of spine formation, and even of developing the two well defined categories of spines present in normal Purkinje cells. Two main questions arise from these results: (i) are Purkinje cells able of an autonomous formation of postsynaptic receptor sites?; and if so (ii) is the production of the two categories of spines controlled by the same intrinsic mechanism? A partial answer to the last question can be obtained by the study of the cerebellum in the 'staggerer' mutant mouse.

Figs. 7–9. Electron micrographs from adult 'reeler' cerebellum.

Fig. 7. Free Purkinje spines in the neuropil of the central mass. Many of them (asterisks) bear postsynaptic differentiations in absence of presynaptic elements. Only some of them are postsynaptic to climbing fibers (CF) or to mossy fibers (MF). × 25,000.

Fig. 8. Neuropil of the central cerebellar mass. The arrows point to the boundaries of a long postsynaptic differentiation undercoating the smooth surface of a Purkinje dendrite. A neuronal process is facing this postsynaptic density. Note the absence of presynaptic vesicular grid in the axonal profile. × 22,000.

Fig. 9. Neuropil of the fastigial nucleus. A Purkinje dendritic profile (PCD) is in the vicinity of a fastigial neuron dendrite (FD), confirming the overlapping of Purkinje dendrites on a deep cerebellar nucleus. A branching spine (arrow) emerges from the Purkinje dendrite; numerous free spines(s) are surrounded by glia. × 16,000.

158

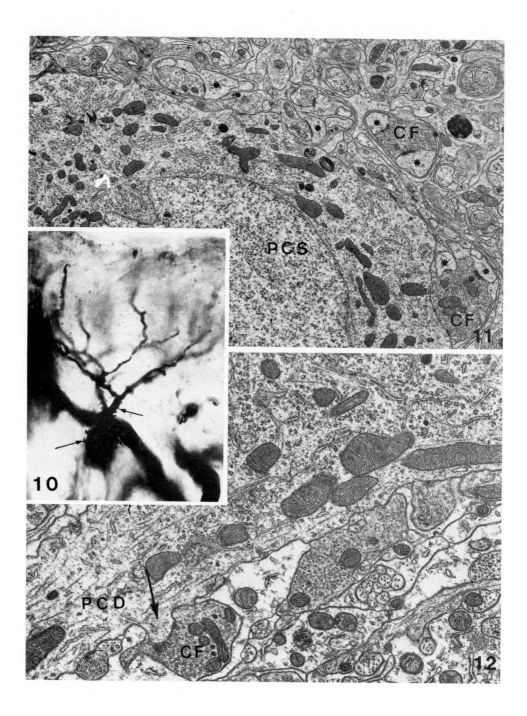

PURKINJE CELLS IN THE 'STAGGERER' CEREBELLUM

This recessive mutation mainly affects the Purkinje cells; the major phenotypical expression in 'staggerer' mice being the selective, and almost complete, absence of parallel fiber Purkinje cell synapses (Landis, 1971; Sidman, 1972; Sotelo and Changeux, 1974a; Hirano and Dembitzer, 1975; Sotelo, 1975a). In this mutant, and contrary to what was described above for the 'weaver', granule cells can accomplish migration (although in much smaller number than in control cerebellum), therefore forming normally oriented parallel fibers which give rise to a well defined molecular layer (Figs. 13 and 14). Since the Purkinje cells do not form branchlet spines on time, the parallel fibers are devoid of their postsynaptic targets, and undergo a degenerative process which ends with the cell death of the inner granule cells, resulting in an almost completely agranular cerebellum (Sidman, 1972). The homozygous 'staggerer' animals generally do not survive beyond the end of the first postnatal month; in our laboratory the oldest 'staggerer' mice obtained were 40–50 days old, but the large majority of the studied animals were younger than 30 days.

In Golgi impregnated cerebella from about 1-month-old 'staggerer' mice, the Purkinje cells display a wide spectrum of shapes, ranging from cells which give off one main dendritic trunk (Fig. 10) to true multipolar neurons, giving rise to up to 8 dendritic trunks (Sotelo, 1975b). The multipolar appearance of some of the Purkinje cells was considered as a remnant of their immature stage (in which the normal resorption of all somatic filopodia fails to occur) with some of these processes continuing to develop into real dendrites (Sotelo, 1975b). The 'staggerer' Purkinje cells have dendritic trees which are greatly reduced in size, and on which spiny branchlets are absent. The only spines present on these neurons emerge from the soma and from primary branches, exclusively on segments close to the cell body (Fig. 10).

The ultrastructural study confirms the immature appearance of the Purkinje cells. Their perikarya are not contacted by the normal basket cell terminals, but instead give rise to numerous perisomatic processes which make synaptic contacts with the climbing fibers (Fig. 11). Some of the primary dendritic segments are also provided with spines (as illustrated in Fig. 12) which are postsynaptic to climbing varicosities. The number of these stubby spines is much lower than on the main dendritic trunk of normal Purkinje cells. These results, concerning the somatic disposition of climbing fibers and their decreased density on dendritic spines, may partially explain the abnormal responses to climbing inputs observed by Crepel and Mariani (1975). The superficial two-thirds of the molecular layer are occupied mainly by clusters of closely packed parallel fibers, glial processes and some dendritic profiles (Figs. 13 and 14), dendritic spines being practically absent. The differences

---

Figs. 10–12. Adult 'staggerer' cerebellum.

Fig. 10. Golgi impregnated Purkinje cell in a 32-day-old 'staggerer' cerebellum. Note that the soma as well as the primary dendrites have a rough contour, due to the presence of spines (arrows). The dendritic branches spreading in the molecular layer, on the contrary, are smooth; spiny branchlets do not exist. × 600.

Fig. 11. Electron micrograph of a Purkinje cell soma (PCS) in a 28-day-old 'staggerer'. Climbing varicosities (CF) surround the cell body, and establish synaptic contacts with somatic spines (asterisks). The pericellular nest location of climbing fibers is an indication of the retardation in maturation of Purkinje cells in this type of cerebellum. × 10,000.

Fig. 12. Electron micrograph of the region of emergence of the primary dendritic stem of a Purkinje cell (PCD) in a 28-day-old 'staggerer'. Note the stubby spine (arrow) arising from this dendrite. The spine is postsynaptic to a climbing fiber varicosity (CF). × 18,000.

160

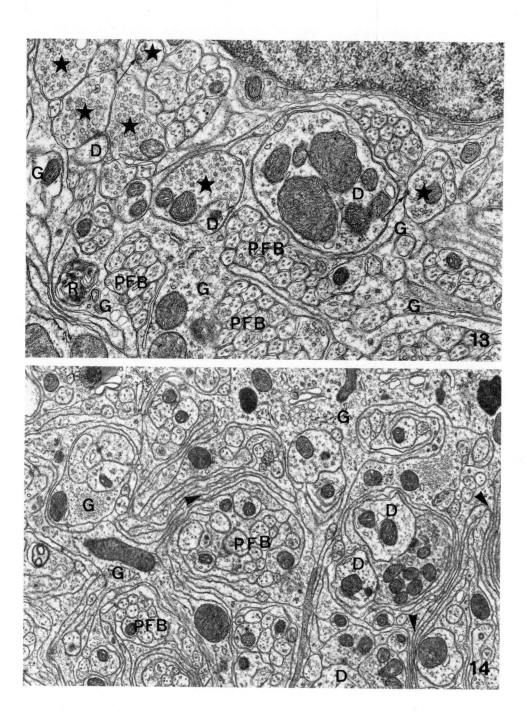

between the molecular layer in 1-month-old and in 45-day-old 'staggerer' cerebella are illustrated in Figs. 13 and 14. Bundles of parallel fibers are more abundant in the younger cerebellum, whereas gliosis is much more extensive in the older one. In both instances, however, most of the Purkinje dendrites are smooth, and granule cells are still present in the inner granular layer.

These results in 'staggerer' cerebellum indicate that the Purkinje cells are directly affected by the mutation. The alteration of their receptive surfaces primarily involves the spines, normally postsynaptic to parallel fibers, which last fail to develop. On the contrary, somatic spines are formed, as well as some of the stubby spines on primary dendrites, both of them being postsynaptic to climbing fibers. It can be concluded that only the formation of branchlet spines is impaired by the 'staggerer' mutation, and that the development of both categories of Purkinje spines must therefore be controlled by different intrinsic mechanisms.

CLIMBING FIBERS AND PURKINJE SPINES

Several hypotheses have been advanced to explain the presence of free Purkinje spines in 'weaver' and in irradiated cerebella. The most obvious explanation is that they are formed by an intrinsic mechanism, independent of interactions with parallel fibers. A different interpretation has been suggested by Hámori (1973), who postulates an indirect or heterotopic induction of Purkinje spines by the climbing fibers, which exhibit an abnormally high density in these agranular cerebella (see refs. in Sotelo, 1975a). According to Hámori, climbing fibers would be necessary during development for the *induction* of Purkinje spines, and throughout the whole life of the animal for the *maintenance* of these spines. If this assumption is correct, it would represent a morphological basis for the theory advanced by Marr (1969) for 'learning in the cerebellum'. Indeed, Marr predicted that 'the synapses from parallel fibers to Purkinje cells are facilitated by the conjunction of presynaptic and climbing fiber (or postsynaptic) activity'.

A series of experiments has recently been carried out in order to see if the presence of climbing fibers is necessary for the formation and maintenance of the spines attached to the spiny branchlets (Sotelo and Arsenio-Nunes, 1976; Sotelo et al., 1975). A review of these studies will be summarized below.

(1) Climbing fibers and Purkinje spines formation

According to recent electrophysiological studies (Crepel et al., 1976), climbing fibers establish their first functional synapses with Purkinje cells in the rat by day 3 postnatally,

Figs. 13 and 14. Electron micrographs from 'staggerer' cerebellum.

Fig. 13. Sagittal section through the molecular layer of a 28-day-old 'staggerer' cerebellum. The dendritic profiles (D) are smooth, and no spines are present in this neuropil. Numerous parallel fibers occupy the large majority of the surface of the micrograph. The non-synaptic segments of these fibers run in bundles (PFB), keeping their normal orientation. The bundles are separated by glial processes (G). Dark degenerative debris (R) probably belonging to parallel fibers are present in the glial processes. Presynaptic segments of parallel fibers (stars), containing synaptic vesicles, either establish contacts with small dendritic profiles or are found facing the glial processes (arrows). × 29,000.

Fig. 14. Molecular layer of a 45-day-old 'staggerer' cerebellum. As in the younger animal of Fig. 13, the dendrites (D) are smooth and spines are absent. The important differences between both mice are: (i) a decrease in the number of parallel fibers within the bundles (PFB), and (ii) an increase of the gliosis (G); the bundles are now segregated by various layers of enwrapping thin glial processes (arrow heads). × 21,000.

in such a way that the immature Purkinje cells receive a multiple innervation by climbing fibers. The adult one-to-one relationship is only attained by day 15. In order to avoid the possible inductive action of climbing fibers, the left inferior peduncle was destroyed within the first 48 hr after birth. Since the vast majority of olivo-cerebellar fibers (which give rise to the climbing fibers) reaches the cerebellum via the inferior peduncle, most of the Purkinje cells in the left cerebellar hemisphere following this type of lesion will develop in absence of climbing fibers.

Under such circumstances, the dendritic arborization of the deafferented Purkinje cells spreads out in the same vertical plane, and with the same tridimensional shape, as observed in Purkinje cells with intact inferior olivary input. In addition, there are primary, secondary and tertiary branches, as well as spiny branchlets, present on the dendritic tree. However, some important differences exist between climbing fiber-deafferented and normal Purkinje cells (Kawaguchi et al., 1975; Bradley and Berry, 1976a; Sotelo and Arsenio-Nunes, 1976): (i) the dendritic tree is reduced in length, although it is larger than for Purkinje cells in agranular cerebella; (ii) the amount of branching of the main dendritic segments is smaller than in normal cells; (iii) some of the distal dendritic segments run in a straight vertical direction, at right angles to the longitudinal axis of the folium; and (iv) instead of being almost smooth (as in normal cells, where only a few clusters of stubby spines are present), the thick dendritic trunks in some of the deafferented cells are studded with spines. The ultrastructural analysis discloses the presence of numerous long-necked spines emerging from the thick dendritic branches. These ectopic spines are mainly postsynaptic to parallel fibers (Sotelo and Arsenio-Nunes, 1976).

The above results clearly show that initial dendritic outgrowth, as well as the formation of spines, is independent of any inductive role by the climbing fibers. In conclusion, although climbing fibers are not necessary for the development of parallel fiber-Purkinje cell synapses, they seem necessary both for the complete growth of the dendritic arborization of the Purkinje cells, and for the compartmentalization of their dendritic trees.

(II) Climbing fibers and Purkinje spine maintenance

The most convincing argument put forward by Hámori (1973) to support his hypothesis of the 'indirect or heterotopic induction of Purkinje spines' was the fact that the majority of Purkinje spines disappear after chronic isolation of the adult cat cerebellar cortex. Since undercutting the cerebellar white matter produced (among other things) degeneration of the climbing fibers, Hámori concluded that the presence of this system of afferences must be necessary for maintenance of the spines. We have re-examined this problem using the *rat* cerebellum, and a different experimental approach. Chemical destruction of the inferior olives was performed with an intraperitoneal injection of 3-acetylpyridine (3-AP), which causes climbing fiber degeneration within 18–24 hr (Desclin, 1974; Sotelo et al., 1975;

Fig. 15. Light micrograph of a plastic section stained with toluidine blue. Sagittal section of the left hemisphere of a rat cerebellum, 7 days after electrolytic lesion of the white matter. The right lower corner of the micrograph is occupied by the evolutive lesion, which at this place has also destroyed part of the granular layer. Except for the axotomy produced close to the cell body by the lesion, Purkinje cells (arrows) keep their normal appearance. Abundant microglial cells, with a dark appearance, are spread throughout the molecular layer, where no cell death is visible. × 200.

Fig. 16. Golgi impregnated Purkinje cell from the cerebellum of a rat sacrificed two years after 3-AP administration. Within the superficial two-thirds of the molecular layer, all Purkinje cell dendrites are studded with spines. Spiny branchlets (big arrows) are maintained, and the large dendritic trunks bear many more abundant spines (small arrow) than in normal Purkinje cells. × 2500.

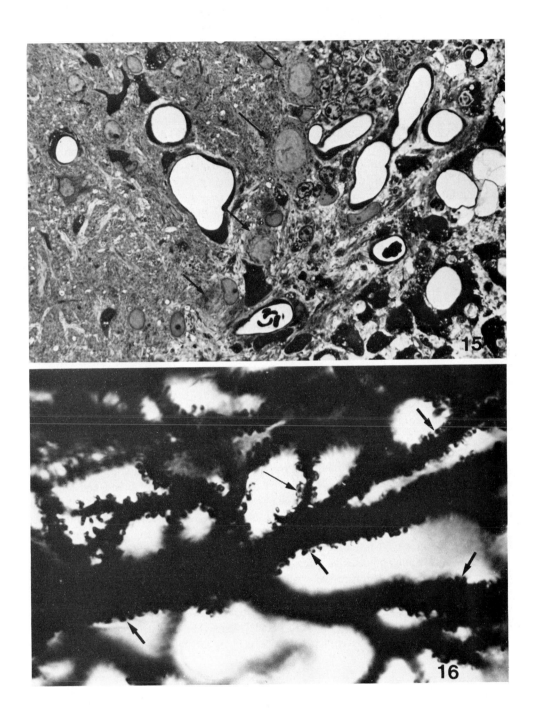

Llinas et al., 1975). The 3-AP was administrated according to the schedule proposed by Llinas et al. (1975), resulting in a highly specific and almost complete olivary lesion. Within a few days after 3-AP administration the cerebellar cortex had become totally devoid of climbing fibers, as could be established with either morphological (Desclin, 1974; Sotelo et al., 1975) or electrophysiological (Llinas et al., 1975) techniques.

In the chronic experiments reported by us (Sotelo et al., 1975), the survival times ranged between 7 days and 3 months after 3-AP injection. A surprising finding was not only the maintenance of spiny branchlets, but also an unexpected increase in the number of spines emerging from secondary and tertiary thick dendritic trunks. These results have since been corroborated in other laboratories; Bradley and Berry (1976b) described the Golgi-stained Purkinje cells in rats 60 days after 3-AP administration. They reported that: 'there was a larger number of spines more proximally situated on the main-stem dendrites than in control groups. The level of spine density in the spiny branchlets of the climbing fiber deafferented cells and normal was identical'. These results demonstrate a de novo formation of spines in adult Purkinje cells, occupying an ectopic position on the thick dendritic segments. They further indicate that climbing fibers are not necessary for the maintenance of Purkinje spines but that, on the contrary, their absence *induces* spine formation.

The nature of the chemical specificity of the 3-AP on the inferior olive of the rat is still unknown. Although several groups of investigators have demonstrated the selectivity of action of this drug (Denk et al., 1968; Desclin and Escubi, 1974; Llinas et al., 1975), it can be suggested that 'besides killing climbing fibers, the poison may act on their synaptic sites on the Purkinje cell dendrites to cause the observed increase in spines' (Eccles 1977). In order to test this hypothesis (Sotelo and Llinas, unpublished observations), a slightly different mechanical approach from the one used by Hámori (1973) was employed. Adult rats were anesthetized by i.p. injection of chloral hydrate (35 mg/100 g body weight), and fixed in a stereotaxic instrument. A dorsal craniectomy was made in order to expose the cerebellum, and a single stainless steel electrode, insulated except for the tip, was lowered in an oblique lateral direction through the vermis. The electrode tip was directed towards the left central white matter overlying the lateral nucleus, where an extensive electrolytic lesion was made. The rats were intracardially perfused with fixative 5 or 7 days after the operation; the left hemisphere was embedded in Araldite and prepared for electron microscopy; sections were made on the sagittal plane. Contrary to what has been reported by Brand and Mugnaini (1976) in the isolated vermal cerebellar folia of the cat, the large majority of Purkinje cells in the hemisphere folia had a normal appearance. Even those Purkinje cells which were close to the lesion (Fig. 15) did not degenerate. Ultrastructural study of the molecular layer, in folia directly overlying the extensive lesion, disclosed an almost total absence of climbing fibers. Abundant reactive microglia cells were dispersed throughout this layer, but almost no degenerating remnants were left behind. Concerning Purkinje dendrites, many of their thick profiles in the upper two-thirds of the molecular layer did not show a smooth contour; on the contrary, they give rise to numerous long-necked spines (Fig. 17). Most of these ectopic spines were postsynaptic to parallel fibers. The ultrastructural appearance of these Purkinje cells closely resembles that observed in cerebella of adult rats 7 days after 3-AP administration.

The electrolytic lesion of the white matter not only induces the degeneration of climbing and mossy fibers but also causes axotomy of the Purkinje cells. In this respect it reproduces the experiments of Hámori (1973) on the isolated cerebellar folia. The results obtained in the two series of experiments are contradictory, however. Hámori reported that 'after chronic isolation of the cerebellar cortex, the vast majority of Purkinje dendritic spines

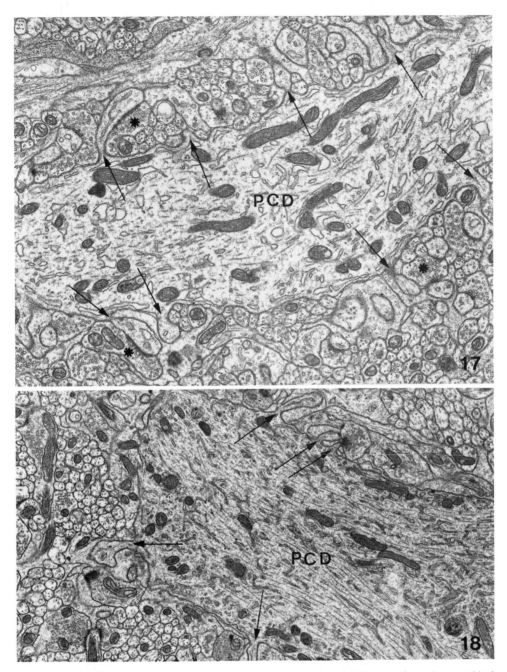

Fig. 17. Electron micrograph of a large Purkinje cell dendritic profile (PCD) taken from the same block as in Fig. 15. Numerous long-necked spines emerge from the dendrite (arrows). Some of them are post-synaptic to parallel fibers (asterisks) within the plane of the section. × 18,000.

Fig. 18. Electron micrograph of a large Purkinje cell dendritic profile (PCD) from a rat treated with 3-AP two years before sacrifice. Abundant spines emerge from this dendritic profile (arrows). × 12,000.

disappear in spite of the presence of many surviving granule cells and their parallel fibers'. In our experiments, however, not only do spiny branchlets survive but new spines are formed on the main-stem 'smooth' dendrites. This discrepancy can be partly explained in the light of the results of Brand and Mugnaini (1976). The last authors demonstrated that when cerebellar folia are undercut with a knife to produce cortical slabs, the Purkinje cells near the lesion undergo an electron-dense type of degeneration which is obvious 6 hr after the operation; 4–10 days after the lesion their dendritic trees become fragmented and phagocytozed. The undercutting produces a fulminant Purkinje cell death. It is therefore quite possible that in the cerebellar slabs studied by Hámori (1973), the disappearance of Purkinje spines two months after the undercutting was not due to climbing fiber deafferentation but rather to the fulminant death of Purkinje cells.

The experiments described above on the adult rat cerebellum lead to the conclusion that the spinogenesis observed after chemical lesion of the inferior olive must be due to climbing deafferentation, and not to an indirect effect of the 3-AP upon the Purkinje cell membrane. Therefore, confident of the validity of using the action of 3-AP to study Purkinje changes related only to climbing deafferentation, we have extended our work to survival times of over two years (almost the entire life of the rats) to see if climbing fibers are really necessary for the maintenance of Purkinje spines. The results obtained in these old rats were exactly the same as those observed in the much shorter survival time experiments. The Golgi picture shows the maintenance of spiny branchlets, as well as a large increase in the number of spines emerging from secondary and tertiary thick dendritic trunks (Fig. 16). The ultra-structural analysis confirms the reality of these ectopic spines (Fig. 18). We can therefore once again conclude that climbing fibers are not necessary at all for the maintenance of dendritic spines but, on the contrary, their absence induces the formation of spines.

ACKNOWLEDGEMENTS

This work was supported by grants from the INSERM, the CNRS and the DGRST.

REFERENCES

Altman, J. and Anderson, W.J. (1972) Experimental reorganization of the cerebellar cortex. I. Morphological effects of elimination of all microneurons with prolonged X-irradiation started at birth, *J. comp. Neurol.*, 146: 355–406.

Berry, M. and Bradley, P. (1976) The growth of the dendritic trees of Purkinje cells in irradiated agranular cerebellar cortex, *Brain Res.*, 116: 361–387.

Bradley, P. and Berry, M. (1976a) The effects of reduced climbing and parallel fibre input on Purkinje cell dendritic growth, *Brain Res.*, 109: 133–151.

Bradley, P. and Berry, M. (1976b) Quantitative effects of climbing fibre deafferentation on the adult Purkinje cell dendritic tree, *Brain Res.*, 112: 133–140.

Brand, S. and Mugnaini, E. (1976) Fulminant Purkinje cell death following axotomy and its use for analysis of the dendritic arborization, *Exp. Brain Res.*, 26: 105–119.

Calvet, M.C., Lepault, A.M. and Calvet, J. (1976) A Procion yellow study of cultured Purkinje cells, *Brain Res.*, 111: 399–406.

Caviness, V.S., Jr. (1973) Time of neuron origin in the hippocampus and dentate gyrus of normal and 'reeler' mutant mice; an autoradiographic analysis, *J. comp. Neurol.*, 151: 113–120.

Caviness, V.S., Jr. (1976) Patterns of cell and fiber distribution in the neocortex of the 'reeler' mutant mouse, *J. comp. Neurol.*, 170: 435–448.

Caviness, V.S., Jr. and Sidman, R.L. (1972) Olfactory structures of the forebrain in the 'reeler' mutant mouse, *J. comp. Neurol.*, 145: 85–104.

Caviness, V.S., Jr. and Sidman, R.L. (1973) Time of origin of corresponding cell classes in the cerebral cortex of normal and 'reeler' mutant mice: an autoradiographic analysis, *J. comp. Neurol.*, 148: 141–152.

Crepel, F. (1971) Maturation of climbing fiber responses in the rat, *Brain Res.*, 35: 272–276.

Crepel, F., Mariani, J. and Delhaye-Bouchaud, N. (1976) Evidence for a multiple innervation of Purkinje cells by climbing fibers in the immature rat cerebellum, *J. Neurobiol.*, 7: 567–578.

Denk, H., Haider, M., Koyac, W. und Studynka, G. (1968) Verhaltensänderung und Neuropathologie bei der 3-Acetylpyridinvergiftung der Ratte, *Acta neuropath. (Berl.)*, 10: 34–44.

Desclin, J.C. (1974) Histological evidence supporting the inferior olive as the major source of cerebellar climbing fibers in the rat, *Brain Res.*, 77: 365–384.

Desclin, J.C. and Escubi, J. (1974) Effects of 3-acetylpyridine on the central nervous system of the rat, as demonstrated by silver methods, *Brain Res.*, 77: 349–364.

Eccles, J.C. (1977) An instruction-selection theory of learning in the cerebellar cortex, *Brain Res.*, 127: 327–352.

Hámori, J. (1973) Developmental morphology of dendritic postsynaptic specialization. In *Recent Developments of Neurobiology in Hungary, Results in Neuroanatomy, Neuroendocrinology, Neurophysiology, Behavior and Neuropathology, Vol. IV*, Akadémiai Kiado, Budapest, pp. 9–32.

Hanna, R.B., Hirano, A. and Pappas, G.D. (1976) Membrane specializations of dendritic spines and glia in the 'weaver' mouse cerebellum: a freeze-fracture study, *J. Cell Biol.*, 68. 403–410.

Hirano, A. and Dembitzer, H.M. (1973) Cerebellar alterations in the 'weaver' mouse, *J. Cell Biol.*, 56: 478–486.

Hirano, A. and Dembitzer, H.M. (1975) The fine structure of 'staggerer' cerebellum, *J. Neuropath. exp. Neurol.*, 34: 1–11.

Kawaguchi, S., Yamamoto, T., Mizuno, N. and Iwahori, N. (1975) The role of climbing fibers in the development of Purkinje cell dendrites, *Neurosci. Lett.*, 1: 301–304.

Landis, D. (1971) Cerebellar cortical development in the 'staggerer' mutant mouse. In Abstracts of papers of *Eleventh Annual Meeting, American Society for Cell Biology*, p. 159.

Landis, D.M.D. and Reese, T.S. (1974) Differences in membrane structure between excitatory and inhibitory synapses in the cerebellar cortex, *J. comp. Neurol.*, 155: 93–126.

Landis, D.M.D. and Reese, T.S. (1977) Structure of the Purkinje cell membrane in 'staggerer' and 'weaver' mutant mice, *J. comp. Neurol.*, 171: 247–260.

Larramendi, L.M.H. and Victor, T. (1967) Synapses on the Purkinje cell spines in the mouse. An electron microscopic study, *Brain Res.*, 5: 15–30.

Llinas, R., Walton, K., Hillman, D.E. and Sotelo, C. (1975) Inferior olive: its role in motor learning, *Science*, 190: 1230–1231.

Mariani, J., Crepel, F., Mikoshiba, K., Changeux, J.P. and Sotelo, C. (1977) Anatomical, physiological and biochemical studies of the cerebellum from 'reeler' mutant mouse, *Phil. Trans. B*, 281: 1–28.

Marr, D.A. (1969) A theory of cerebellar cortex, *J. Physiol. (Lond.)*, 202: 437–470.

Palay, S.L. and Chan-Palay, V. (1974) *Cerebellar Cortex*, Springer Verlag, Berlin.

Rakic, P. (1976) Synaptic specificity in the cerebellar cortex: study of anomalous circuits induced by single gene mutations in mice, *Cold Spr. Harb. Symp. quant. Biol.*, 11: 333–346.

Rakic, P. and Sidman, R.L. (1973a) Sequence of developmental abnormalities leading to granule cell deficit in cerebellar cortex of 'weaver' mutant mice, *J. comp. Neurol*, 152: 103–132.

Rakic, P. and Sidman, R.L. (1973) Organization of cerebellar cortex secondary to deficit of granule cells in 'weaver' mutant mice, *J. comp. Neurol.*, 152: 133–162.

Ramón y Cajal, S. (1911) *Histologie du Système Nerveux de l'Homme et des Vertébrés*, Paris, Maloine.

Ramón y Cajal, S. (1929) Etude sur la neurogénèse de quelques vertébrés. In *Studies on Vertebrate Neurogenesis*, Thomas, Springfield, Ill., 1960.

Sidman, R.L. (1972) Cell interactions in developing mammalian central nervous system. In *Cell Interactions, Proc. 3rd LePetit Symp.*, North-Holland Publ., Amsterdam.

Sidman, R.L., Green, M.L. and Appel, S.H. (1965) *Catalog of the Neurological Mutants of the Mouse*, Harvard University Press, Cambridge, Mass.

Sotelo, C. (1973) Permanence and fate of paramembranous synaptic specializations in 'mutants' and experimental animals, *Brain Res.*, 62: 345–351.

Sotelo, C. (1975a) Anatomical, physiological and biochemical studies of the cerebellum from mutant mice. II. Morphological study of cerebellar cortical neurons and circuits in the 'weaver' mouse, *Brain Res.*, 94: 19–44.

Sotelo, C. (1975b) Dendritic abnormalities of Purkinje cells in the cerebellum of neurologic mutant mice (weaver and staggerer). In *Advances in Neurology, Vol. 12*, G.W. Kreutzberg (Ed.), Raven Press, New York.

Sotelo, C. (1977) Formation of presynaptic dendrites in the rat cerebellum following neonatal X-irradiation, *Neuroscience*, 2: 275–283.

Sotelo, C., Hillman, D.E., Zamora, A.J. and Llinas, R. (1975) Climbing fiber deafferentation: its action on Purkinje cell dendritic spines, *Brain Res.*, 98: 574–581.

Sotelo, C. and Changeux, J.P. (1974a) Transsynaptic degeneration 'en cascade' in the cerebellar cortex of 'staggerer' mutant mice, *Brain Res.*, 67: 519–526.

Sotelo, C. and Changeux, J.P. (1974b) Bergmann fibers and granular cell migration in the cerebellum of homozygous 'weaver' mutant mouse, *Brain Res.*, 77: 484–491.

Sotelo, C. and Arsenio-Nunes, M.L. (1976) Development of Purkinje cells in absence of climbing fibers, *Brain Res.*, 111: 389–395.

DISCUSSION

CHANGEUX: Concerning the morphology of the spines, you stated that there can be apparently perfect morphological equivalence, but certainly the neurotransmitters have to be different.

SOTELO: Few things are known with certainty about the kinds of neurotransmitter present in the various types of presynaptic axons involved in the cerebellar cortical circuitry. There is, however, some evidence that Purkinje cell axon collaterals, as well as stellate, basket and Golgi cell axons are all *GABA-ergic,* that parallel fibers are *glutaminergic,* and that some mossy fibers are *cholinergic* whereas others use *serotonin* as the neurotransmitter. No information is available for the bulk of the mossy fibers, nor for the climbing fibers. In the normal cerebellum the Purkinje cell spines can be postsynaptic to parallel fibers, climbing fibers, ascending collaterals of the basket axons, stellate axons, and recurrent collaterals of the Purkinje cell axons. With the exception of the morphological differences between the spines arising from thick dendritic trunks (and which are postsynaptic to climbing fibers) and those emerging from spiny branchlets, there are no obvious differences among all these types of spines. What I am saying, therefore, is that the morphology of the spine cannot be a tool to identify the nature of the presynaptic axon and, thus, of its neurotransmitter. In agranular cerebella, Purkinje spines which are morphologically similar to those normally arising from spiny branchlets can be postsynaptic to mossy fibers and/or Golgi cell dendrites — something which never occurs under normal conditions. Therefore, if the postsynaptic spine in these heterologous synapses has a receptor which is complementary to the transmitter being released by the new presynaptic element, this complementarity could be attained either by (a) inducing a change on the receptor, or (b) changing the nature of the neurotransmitter released by the presynaptic axon.

VRENSEN: You have studied genetic aberrants such as Staggerer and Weaver, and what do they really tell us about the organization of Purkinje cells? For you say that the climbing fibers are sometimes missing. Can it be that the same genetic influence which changes the climbing fibers also affects the granule cells, or the climbing fibers *and* the Purkinje cells at the same time? Perhaps it is not the 'moulding' effect of the climbing fibers which is missing, but *both* factors are missing: the Purkinje cell cannot develop normally, *and* the climbing fibers are not arriving. I don't see that there is necessarily a causal relationship.

SOTELO: In both of the mutants discussed, Weaver and Staggerer, climbing fibers are present in the cerebellum. However, it is true that we do not know with certainty what is the primary cellular target in either the Weaver or the Staggerer mutation. From a morphological point of view, the only thing we can say is that, in early stages of postnatal development, postmitotic granule cells die at the external granular layer in the Weaver, and that Purkinje cell dendrites fail to form spines in the Staggerer. For these and other reasons (Sotelo and Changeux, 1974a, b), we have considered that the Weaver locus primarily affects the granule cells, while the Staggerer locus affects the Purkinje cell receptor areas, with the aberrant shape of Purkinje cells in Weaver and the granule cell death in Staggerer being secondary or transsynaptic events. This interpretation is, of course, only a working hypothesis, and we don't at all feel that we have the final answer. Different working hypotheses have been advanced by other investigators. For instance, Rakic and Sidman (1973) consider that the primary cellular target in Weaver is the Bergmann glia, and Yoon (1976) interprets the hypoplasia of the Staggerer cerebellum as being due to a pleiotropic action of the mutation, which affects the external granular layer and the Purkinje cells independently. In this respect, I want to mention the recent results obtained by the group of Sidman (Trenker et al., 1976) using in vitro experiments with dissociated cells from the external granular layer of homozygous Weaver mice. When these cells are cultivated with the serum obtained from Weaver mice (serum which contains high concentrations of lipids and cholesterol), neuronal death proceeds at a high rate in the cultures. When the concentrations of these substances are reduced by lipid extraction, the viability of external granule cells in the culture increases, which indicates that the effect of the Weaver gene locus upon granular cell death is an indirect one.

VRENSEN: Could it be that receptor sites for the climbing fibers on the main shaft after destroying climbing fibers elevate so as to resemble spines?

SOTELO: In the granular cerebellum some of the numerous, autonomously formed, Purkinje spines can be innervated by heterologous presynaptic elements. The local cellular milieu must play an important role in this remodeling of cerebellar circuitry. In fact, in the two different agranular cerebella which we have studied, i.e. the Weaver genetic mutation, and the cerebellum experimentally obtained by X-irradiation, the local cellular milieu for Purkinje cells is quite different: only the granule cells are missing in the former, whereas also stellate and basket cells are missing in the latter. In Weaver, mossy fibers can establish *wrong* synaptic connections with the Purkinje spines, whereas in the irradiated cerebellum not only the mossy fibers are able to effect Purkinje spine innervations but also Golgi cells (the only inhibitory interneuron left in this cortex) can be involved in heterologous synapse formation, mainly through presynaptic dendrites. Thus, absolute specificity in synaptic formation is not preserved in these agranular cerebella. A different problem concerns the matching of the presynaptic neurotransmitter with the spine receptor. Morphological criteria are obviously not enough to disclose if the spine membrane contains a receptor for glutamate, or for GABA, or for any other neurotransmitter.

CORNER: How good is the evidence for there being only one process which is disturbed, a process which is specifically localized in one particular cell type in one particular cell region, rather than a *general* failure of migration, for instance? In a mutation where you find that there is a failure of migration of granule cells in the cerebellum, if you look at other sites in the brain, might you not find evidence of a disturbed migration of certain types of cells there too?

SOTELO: Of the 7 known neurological mutants with cerebellar disturbances, only two show altered migration patterns: (i) the Weaver, in which postmitotic granule cells fail to migrate, and then degenerate in the external granular layer, and (ii) the Reeler, in which there is a malpositioning of the Purkinje cells. Only the Reeler mutation also affects the cerebral cortex and the hippocampal formation, where there are indeed serious anomalies in the alignment and in the dendritic polarity of many pyramidal cells.

ZIMMER: When you remove the climbing fibers experimentally you see the terminals degenerate, and after a while you see spines along the dendrites. Do you ever see unoccupied synaptic sites, such as empty postsynaptic thinnings or spines devoid of presynaptic elements? That is, which is first: the spine or the parallel fiber?

SOTELO: Purkinje cells react to climbing fiber deafferentation by increasing the number of spines which originate from the proximal dendritic compartment. Indeed, 5–7 days after the lesion of the inferior olive, most of these newly formed ectopic spines can be already visualized with the Golgi impregnation. The electron microscopic analysis of these ectopic spines shows that when the spine bears a postsynaptic differentiation, it is facing a parallel fiber varicosity. In contrast, when the spine is *not* in direct relationship with a presynaptic axon within the plane of the section, it is devoid of postsynaptic differentiation – with very rare exceptions. Therefore, the formation of spines in adult Purkinje cells mimicks the morphological events described during development, where it is impossible to distinguish if the spine induces the formation of the presynaptic varicosity, or vice versa. However, by analogy to what happens in agranular cerebella, in which Purkinje cells can form spines in absence of parallel fibers (and also due to the presence of some rare spines free of innervation but bearing postsynaptic differentiations) it can be suggested that in climbing deafferentation the spine formation *precedes* the sprouting of parallel fibers.

Development of the Hippocampus and Fascia Dentata: Morphological and Histochemical Aspects

JENS ZIMMER

Institute of Anatomy B, University of Aarhus, DK 8000 Aarhus C (Denmark)

INTRODUCTION

Compared with most other areas of the cerebral cortex, the hippocampus and the fascia dentata display a relatively simple cytological organization, each having only one main cell layer (Fig. 1). Moreover, the terminations of the major afferent fiber systems are segregated along the dendrites of both the dentate granule cells and the hippocampal pyramidal cells in a strictly laminated fashion (Figs. 1 and 2). Due to this apparently simple – and highly characteristic – structure, the hippocampus and the fascia dentata have been widely used as models for studies on the cerebral cortex.

In the following sections, certain aspects of the development of the hippocampus and the fascia dentata in the rat will be reviewed. The emphasis will be placed on the developmental changes which take place during the *first postnatal month*. To illustrate the different developmental stages, including the laminar differentiation of the afferent fiber systems, results obtained with the Timm sulfide silver method will be used. This histochemical method provides an excellent means for monitoring and screening en bloc the development of the afferent systems to the hippocampal region. A full presentation of these results, obtained in collaboration with Dr. F.-M. Haug, will appear elsewhere (Zimmer and Haug, 1978). In addition to our own results, this review will incorporate results available from laboratories where the hippocampal development has been studied by other methods. At the end, a separate paragraph will be devoted to examples of *experimental approaches*, which involve the hippocampus and the fascia dentata, and which help to clarify which factors are important for the formation and laminar segregation of nervous connections. This last paragraph will include preliminary results obtained by *transplantation* of hippocampal and dentate tissue from neonatal rats into the CNS of littermates and adult rats.

THE TIMM SULFIDE SILVER METHOD

Since this histochemical method, originally introduced by Timm (1958) for detection of heavy metals, may not be familiar to most readers, the method and its application will be

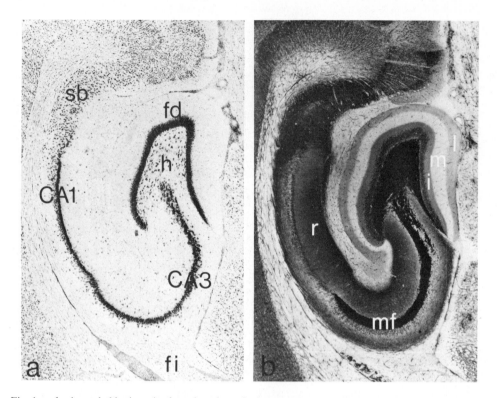

Fig. 1. a: horizontal thionin-stained section through the posterior part of the hippocampus and the fascia dentata, illustrating the main cell layers. b: adjacent Timm-stained section. The differentially stained laminae of the hippocampal and dentate neuropil correspond to the terminal areas of the major afferent systems. CA1, region superior of hippocampus; CA3, regio inferior of hippocampus; fd, fascia dentata; fi, fimbria; h, hilus of fascia dentata (CA4); i, commissural-ipsilateral zone; l, lateral perforant path zone; m, medial perforant path zone; mf, mossy fiber zone; r, str. radiatum of CA1; sb, subiculum. × 22.

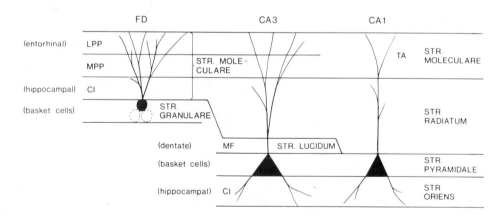

Fig. 2. Schematic drawing showing the different layers of the hippocampus and fascia dentata, and the distribution of the afferent systems within them. CI, commissural and ipsilateral associational systems; LPP, lateral perforant path; MF, mossy fiber system; MPP, medial perforant path; TA, temporo-ammonic tract.

dealt with specifically at this point. Since fuller descriptions of the method are already available (Timm, 1958; Haug, 1973; Danscher and Zimmer, 1978), only the main principles of the method will be presented here. For details about Timm staining in developing rats, the reader is referred to Zimmer and Haug (1978).

In brief, the Timm method is applied to brain tissue as follows. The animal is perfused with a sodium sulfide solution, which causes metallosulfides to form and precipitate in the tissues. Following removal, the brain is frozen and cut into 20—40 μm thick sections in a cryostat. The sections are thawed onto glass slides, allowed to dry, fixed in alcohol, and then subjected to physical development (Voigt, 1959) to visualize the metallosulfides, onto which metallic silver precipitates. The metals which can be demonstrated by the Timm method are heavy metals, and transitional and group IIb metals. These include biologically occurring metals such as zinc and copper, but also lead, mercury and cadmium, if present.

This method does not distinguish among these different metals by the way in which the tissues are stained. Observed differences in staining instead reflect different concentrations of the total amount of stainable metals present within the tissues. The fact that one metal may be present in an especially high concentration in certain structures, for example zinc in the hippocampal mossy fiber boutons (mf, Fig. 1b), is a separate matter. In brain structures, the Timm staining pattern in the hippocampus and fascia dentata is especially striking.

The evidence that the staining here is localized in nerve terminals is the following:
(a) strict correspondence between the Timm stained laminae in the neuropil and the terminal fields of known afferent systems (Fig. 1b) (Haug, 1974);
(b) detailed, bouton-like, appearance of the precipitate under the light microscope;
(c) localization of the precipitate within terminals, as revealed by electron microscopy (Haug, 1967, 1975; Ibata and Otsuka, 1968; Danscher and Zimmer, 1978);
(d) rapid loss (within 10 hr to 2 days) of staining from the terminal fields of lesioned Timm positive pathways (Haug et al., 1971; Haug, 1976);
(e) spread of Timm staining into denervated laminae, parallel to the collateral sprouting of Timm positive systems (Zimmer, 1973a, b, 1974a, b, 1976).

MORPHOGENESIS OF THE HIPPOCAMPUS AND FASCIA DENTATA

Results along this line have been obtained by several authors using Golgi and Nissl stained material from several species (Godina and Barassa, 1964; Brown, 1966; Humphrey, 1966; Stensaas, 1967, 1968). Especially informative, however, are the studies using autoradiographic methods after injections of tritiated thymidine, which is incorporated into the DNA of dividing cells. In this way, it has been possible to demonstrate when the different neurons form and where and how they migrate and settle within different layers of the hippocampus and fascia dentata (Angevine, 1965, 1975; Altman and Das, 1965; Hine and Das, 1974; Bayer and Altman, 1974; Schlessinger et al., 1975; Banker and Cowan, 1977).

In brief, these studies have shown that *all* pyramidal cells of the hippocampus are formed before birth, while as many as 85% of the dentate granule cells are formed postnatally during the first three weeks. A recent study has demonstrated a slight ongoing proliferation of granule cells even in adulthood (Kaplan and Hinds, 1977). Another conclusion to be drawn from these studies is that several *morphogenetic gradients* exist within the hippocampus and fascia dentata (Fig. 3). Within the hippocampus, the pyramidal cells of the CA2 field (a transitional field between CA3 and CA1) and the adjacent, lateral part of CA3 (CA3a) form ahead of the corresponding cells in both CA1 and the medial part of CA3, which lies adjacent

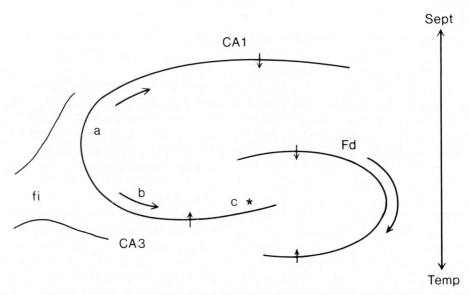

Fig. 3. Schematic drawing of the main cell layers of the hippocampus and fascia dentata as seen in a horizontal section. The developmental gradients mentioned in the text are indicated by arrows. Asterisk, part of CA3 (CA3c) displaying a reverse, outside-in sequence in BALB/cJ mice. abc, subfields of CA3; sept, direction towards the septum along the longitudinal axis of the hippocampus; temp, direction towards the temporal part of the hippocampus.

to the fascia dentata (CA3c). In general, the CA3 cells are formed before the cells in CA1. In all hippocampal fields, the first formed pyramidal cells settle in what becomes the deep part of the pyramidal cell layer, while the later formed cells migrate past these to occupy increasingly more superficial positions. This is referred to as the *inside-out sequence,* and is found in most other parts of the cerebral cortex.

Within the fascia dentata there are three morphogenetic gradients: from *temporal to septal,* from *lateral to medial,* and from *outside-to-inside.* Thus, more cells settle earlier in the temporal parts than in the septal parts (with a great overlap, however). The first formed cells at all septo-temporal levels align themselves laterally opposite CA1 and subiculum, and start forming the lateral blade of the granule cell layer. By subsequent addition of new cells, this layer expands medially until, by postnatal day 5, a medial blade (lying opposite the brain stem) also becomes recognizable. Within the granule cell layer, the first formed cells take up what becomes a superficial position; the later formed cells are then added on the deep side of these in an *outside-in* fashion, i.e. the reverse of the situation in the hippo-campal pyramidal cell layer.

The morphogenetic gradients outlined here should be kept in mind in the following when the cytological differentiation and the laminar differentiation of the afferent systems are considered.

CELLULAR DIFFERENTIATION OF HIPPOCAMPAL AND DENTATE NEURONS

The differentiation of the cellular processes of the hippocampal pyramidal cells and the dentate granule cells has been studied mainly by the Golgi method (Godina and Barassa, 1964; Stensaas, 1967, 1968; Purpura and Pappas, 1968; Minkwitz, 1976a–c; Minkwitz and

Holz, 1975), but a few electron microscopic studies are also available (Schwartz et al., 1968; Cotman et al., 1973; Crain et al., 1973; LaVail and Wolf, 1973; Bliss et al., 1974). The reader is referred to these studies, and to Stirling and Bliss (this volume), for a more detailed account. Here, only the general principles will be reviewed, plus a few observations of interest for the interpretation of the laminar differentiation of the Timm staining.

The hippocampal pyramidal cells follow the same pattern of differentiation as do the other cortical pyramidal cells. Thus, they generate and differentiate their apical dendrites in advance of the basal ones, and spines are first generated on the apical dendrites. With regard to spine formation, Minkwitz (1976a) noticed that the CA3 pyramidal cells (from his description, presumably in CA3a) appeared to be in advance of the pyramidal cells in CA1. The most intense spine formation takes place during the second and third postnatal weeks: the spine density in CA1, for instance, increases by 4-fold from day 5–10, and an additional 2.5-fold from day 10–20 (Minkwitz, 1976c). As regards the mutual width of the layers within which different parts of the pyramidal cell dendrites distribute themselves, the studies of Stensaas (1967, 1968) and of Minkwitz and Holz (1975) show that in CA1 the layer containing the apical end branches (str. moleculare) progressively narrows relative to the underlying layer (str. radiatum) which contains the apical stem dendrites (see Fig. 6 in Minkwitz and Holz, 1975). This implies *intralaminar* growth of the shaft of the apical dendrite, and argues against growth of dendrites exclusively at their tips.

The differentiation of the granule cells follows the general morphogenetic gradient of the structure from lateral to medial, but the differentiation of the dendrites is delayed relative to the settling of cell bodies within the granule cell layer. For an illustration of this, the reader should consult the work of Godina and Barassa (1964), based on the development of the sheep hippocampus and fascia dentata. In the rat, spines are observable on the granule cell dendrites in Golgi preparations by day 7, and are already much more common by day 10 (Stirling, personal communication). In an electron microscopic study, Cotman et al. (1973) found that dentate spines continue to develop after day 25.

LAMINAR DIFFERENTIATION OF NEUROPIL AND AFFERENT FIBER CONNECTIONS

Considering the development of fiber connections in animals born in an immature state, like the rat, there has been a tendency to expect these connections to develop rather late, i.e. during the third postnatal week, or later. It is somewhat contradictory then, that references have often been made to the Golgi studies of Cajal (1893, 1911) and of Lorente de Nó (1934) in order to confirm the existence of cell types and fiber pathways found in adult brains, since a great number of their illustrations and observations are based on 'immature' animals (8–12 days old: Fig. 4). Such references nevertheless are often justified, because the different cell types and fiber connections in fact do differentiate and develop quite early.

In the following sections the development of each of the major afferent pathways is presented, based upon the differentiation of Timm staining characteristics (Figs. 5–8), and upon information available from other studies, using either fiber tracing techniques or electron microscopy.

The mossy fiber system

The mossy fibers (MF) are axons of the dentate granule cells, projecting onto the modified pyramidal cells of the dentate hilus (CA4) and the CA3 pyramidal cells (Figs. 1b and 2) (Blackstad et al., 1970). The boutons are of giant size and stain very intensely by the Timm

176

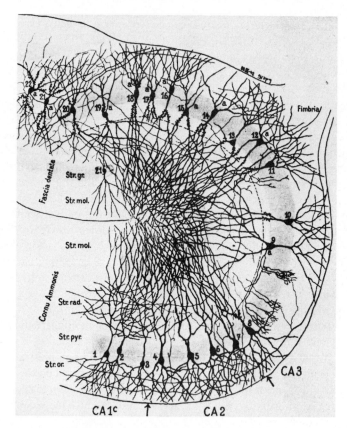

Fig. 4. Picture of cells in the fascia dentata and the hippocampus from a 12-day-old mouse, stained with the Golgi method (Fig. 9 of Lorente de Nó, 1934).

method (Fig. 1b) because of their content of, especially, zinc (Euler, 1967; Maske, 1965; Hu and Friede, 1968; Danscher et al., 1976).

At day 1, the presence of the MF system is suggested by an enhanced Timm staining both of the lateral part of the hilus and of a rather diffusely delimited zone just above the CA3 pyramidal cell layer (Fig. 5). By day 3, individually stained particles resembling small MF boutons are identifiable. The outline of the stained lamina (the MF zone) in CA3 has also sharpened by this age. Following a subsequent increase in the staining density, the size and number of the individual particles (boutons), and the width of the layer itself through day 5 to 12 (Figs. 6–8), the staining of the MF system appears to be mature by day 18. The infrapyramidal MF in CA3c, which arises from granule cells of the medial blade of the fascia dentata, is first seen by day 5, reflecting the latero-medial developmental gradient in the fascia dentata. Developmental gradients are also found within the suprapyramidal part of the MF layer in CA3. Thus, at days 3–9 there is a decrease in staining in the *proximo-distal* direction (from CA3b to CA3a). In the latter subfield, moreover, the staining tends to be concentrated along the *superficial* part of the layer.

The results obtained by the Timm method should be compared with those of Bliss et al. (1974), who studied the structural and functional development of the MF system both by electron microscopy and by electrophysiological means. These observations as well as more recent findings are specifically dealt with by Stirling and Bliss (this volume).

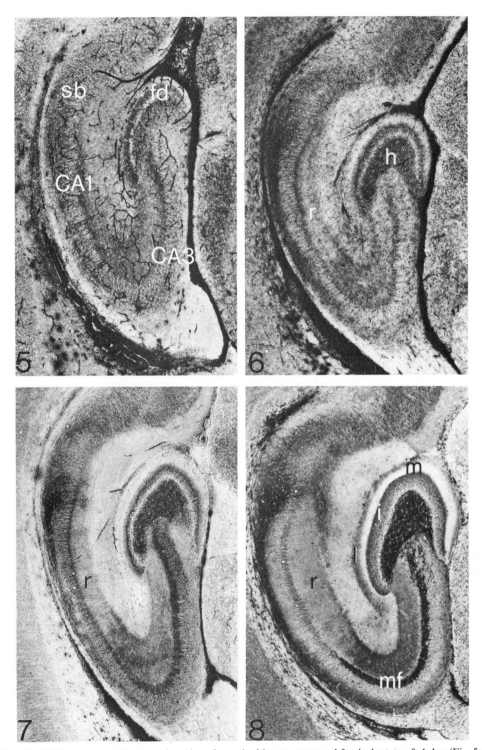

Figs. 5–8. Timm-stained, horizontal sections from the hippocampus and fascia dentata of: 1-day (Fig. 5; × 40), 5-day (Fig. 6; × 30), 7-day (Fig. 7; × 30), and 12-day (Fig. 8; × 28) old rats, illustrating the laminar differentiation of the neuropil. Abbreviations as in Fig. 1.

The perforant path

This pathway (Cajal, 1911) consists of two separate fiber connections, both of which project from the entorhinal area to the fascia dentata and to the CA3 field of the hippocampus (Hjorth-Simonsen and Jeune, 1972; Hjorth-Simonsen, 1972; Steward, 1976). The lateral perforant path (LPP) arises in the lateral part of the entorhinal area, and terminates in the outer part of the molecular layer of fascia dentata and CA3 (Fig. 2). It stains moderately with the Timm method (l, Fig. 1b). The medial perforant path (MPP) arises in the medial part of the entorhinal cortex, and terminates in the middle of the dentate molecular layer and the inner half of the str. moleculare in CA3 (Fig. 2). The MPP zone is characterized by the total absence of Timm staining (m, in Fig. 1b). At least 85% of the terminals in the PP zones of the dentate molecular layer belong to these systems (Matthews et al., 1976).

The earliest indications with Timm staining of the presence of LPP and MPP in the dentate molecular layer are seen in the lateral blade at day 5 (in the form of a slight accumulation of staining in the outer part, and a bleaching of the middle part: Fig. 6). The changes are thought to reflect the formation and differentiation of an increasing number (and volume) of moderately stained and of unstained LPP and MPP terminals. Perforant path afferents, however, appear to be present in the outer parts of the molecular layer at least a couple of days before this. Thus, fiber tracing studies by Fricke and Cowan (1977) and Loy et al. (1977) have demonstrated the presence of entorhinal afferents within the dentate by day 3 and 4, respectively. At these ages, the afferents occupy their appropriate laminar positions in relation both to each other (Fricke and Cowan, 1977) and to the commissural and ipsilateral hippocampo-dentate afferents in the inner zone (see below).

The commissural and ipsilateral associated systems to the fascia dentata

These systems arise from cells in the hilus of fascia dentata (CA4) and in the adjacent part of CA3 (CA3c): cells in these fields project bilaterally to the *inner* zone of the dentate molecular layer (Figs. 1b and 2) (Blackstad, 1956; Zimmer, 1971; Gottlieb and Cowan, 1972, 1973). The majority of the terminals in this zone belong to the ipsilateral association system (Gottlieb and Cowan, 1972; McWilliams et al., 1975), and this system is also responsible for most, if not all, of the Timm staining in the zone (Zimmer, 1974a; Zimmer and Laurberg, 1976). At day 1 this staining is already present laterally (Fig. 5), and then spreads medially as the medial blade of the granule cell layer progressively forms (Figs. 6–8). Parallel to this spread the zone gradually widens, and its superficial border towards the MPP zone sharpens. A quite mature Timm staining *pattern*, including all three zones of the dentate molecular layer, has formed in this way by day 9. Smaller adjustments of the abolute and relative widths of the laminae and their staining densities still go on, however.

In accordance with the Timm staining results, Fricke and Cowan (1977) and Loy et al. (1977) have shown the existence of ipsilateral afferents to the lateral blade of fascia dentata already by day 3 and 4. (For technical reasons, no results on younger animals have as yet been obtained.) Also the commissural afferents were found at that age (4 days) too, by Loy et al. (1977), whereas Fricke and Cowan (1977) were able to demonstrate these only from day 6. Later arrival and maturation of the commissural afferents is in accordance with the hypothesis of *temporal competition* for synaptic sites, presented by Gottlieb and Cowan (1972) to explain why there are more ipsilateral than commissural terminals in the lateral blade.

To conclude this section on the development of afferent pathways to fascia dentata, both the Timm staining and the fiber tracing studies demonstrate a latero-medial progression in development, in accordance with the *latero-medial morphogenetic gradient*. In Timm staining, moreover, there is a slight tendency for the temporal to mid-posterior levels to differentiate before the more septal ones. Such a *septo-temporal* gradient may correspond to the morphogenetic findings that granule cells at the temporal levels form slightly ahead of the more septal ones (Schlessinger et al., 1975). Within the molecular layer, both the fiber tracing and the Timm staining studies show that the three main afferent systems are segregated into histochemically characteristic laminae very early in postnatal development. By none of the methods, however, has it been possible to establish the time at which the first afferents arrive. For this reason, it is not possible to either prove or disprove the existence of an initial overlap in the spatial distribution of the afferent systems, like the one displayed by the visual systems at the earliest stages of development (Rakic, 1977).

Commissural and ipsilateral associational systems to the hippocampus

These systems arise from the pyramidal cells of CA3 and CA4 in the contralateral and ipsilateral hippocampus, and terminate in the str. radiatum and oriens of CA3 and CA1 (Fig. 2) (Blackstad, 1956; Hjorth-Simonsen, 1973; Gottlieb and Cowan, 1973). The ipsilateral projections are traditionally divided into a longitudinal association path, intrinsic to CA3, and the Schaffer collaterals from CA3–4 to CA1 (Lorente de Nó, 1934). The systems stain moderately to intense by the Timm method, and there are also septo-temporal, latero-medial and basal-apical differences in the staining densities of the fields (Fig. 1b, and Haug, 1974). These differences in the adult rat may to some degree reflect a sequential development of subsystems having different stainabilities, belonging to the total commissural-associational projection complex. Thus along the *septo-temporal* axis, the temporal parts of CA3 and CA1 attain their characteristic staining before the more septal parts. Along the transverse, *medio-lateral* axis, CA3a matures at all septo-temporal levels before CA1 and the rest of the CA3 complex, with CA3c being the latest. An earlier arrival of afferents to CA3a than to CA1 or CA3b, c has also been found by Loy et al. (1977). Within the str. radiatum in both CA3 and CA1, the apical parts stain earlier than do more basal parts of the layer, indicating the existence of an *apical to basal* developmental gradient along the apical dendrites of the pyramidal cells.

There are two very characteristic features of the Timm staining differentiation between CA3 and CA1. Firstly, there is a delayed (but then rapid) accumulation of staining in str. radiatum and oriens at the septal levels, taking place between day 8 and day 12. Secondly, during the same period, the str. radiatum of CA1 grows in width to such an extent that the situation from the first postnatal week (where the overlying str. moleculare is the wider of the two) becomes reversed. Both features are comparable with events observed in Golgi-stained material: the accumulation of staining in str. radiatum from 8–12 days occurs parallel to extensive dendritic branching and formation of spines within this layer (Minkwitz, 1976c), while the growth spurt in the str. radiatum of CA1 corresponds to an elongation of apical pyramidal cell dendrites, relative to the distal end branches (Minkwitz and Holz, 1975).

The temporo-ammonic tract

This pathway connects the entorhinal area with the str. moleculare of CA1 and the adjacent part of the subiculum both on the ipsilateral (ipsilateral temporo-ammonic (TA)-tract) and on the contralateral side (crossed TA-tract) (Blackstad, 1956; Steward, 1976). While the perforant path (PP) fibers to fascia dentata and CA3 originate mainly in entorhinal layer II, the TA fibers arise mainly in layer III (Steward and Scoville, 1976). Similar to the PP, there is a topographical organization of the TA fibers, with those of medial entorhinal origin terminating in CA1 closest to CA3, whereas the fibers of lateral entorhinal origin end more posteriorly towards the subiculum (Steward, 1976). The two terminal fields have a different appearance with Timm staining: the 'medial' is unstained, while the 'lateral' is moderately stained (Fig. 1b).

During postnatal development, the Timm staining of str. moleculare of CA1 is already distinct from that of the underlying str. radiatum at day 1 (Fig. 5). Whether the paleness of str. moleculare at that age is due to the presence of unstained or poorly stained TA afferents is not known, however. During the first week a significant bleaching of the part closest to CA3 takes place, while the part closest to the subiculum gradually attains the yellowish hue characteristic of the adult staining (Fig. 8).

As mentioned earlier, the growth rates of the commissural-ipsilateral terminal zone (str. radiatum) and of the TA zone (str. moleculare) in CA1 differ during the postnatal period. Thus, the mutual width of the two layers reverses from birth up to days 9–12, by which time the commissural-ipsilateral zone has become the wider of the two. In this way, the ratio between width of the commissural-ipsilateral and width of the entorhinal zones in CA1 changes, in the postnatal period, opposite to this ratio in the dentate molecular layer. Here, the total width of the *entorhinal* zones increases during development, relative to the inner commissural-ipsilateral zone (cf. Loy et al., 1977).

Functional maturation of the afferent pathways to the hippocampus and fascia dentata

The only available study on this question in the rat is the study on the electrophysiological and ultrastructural maturation of the mossy fiber system by Bliss et al. (1974). They recorded the first functional mossy fibers by day 5. In related experiments the same authors found functional Schaffer collaterals by day 2 and functional perforant path fibers by day 7 (Bliss, personal communication).

EXPERIMENTAL APPROACHES TO THE UNDERSTANDING OF THE LAMINAR SEGREGATION OF THE HIPPOCAMPAL AND DENTATE AFFERENT PATHWAYS

(i) Removal of afferents and collateral reinnervation

In this type of experiment one or more of the afferent systems are lesioned, either during the period of development or in adulthood, to see how this operation effects the interaction between the target neurons and the remaining fiber systems. Such experiments have mainly involved the fascia dentata and its afferent systems, and a remarkable degree of connective plasticity, in the sense of aberrant axonal growth and collateral reinnervation, has been found (e.g. Lynch et al., 1975; Zimmer, 1976). The general conclusion from these experiments, with regard to the present context, is that *no absolute specification* of the termination of the afferent systems onto distinct dendritic segments does exist within the fascia dentata. Afferents normally restricted in termination to one lamina along the dentate granule cell dendrites can therefore invade adjacent laminae following lesioning of the normal afferents to these laminae (Fig. 9).

(ii) Removal of target cells

Another type of experiment involves the removal not of the afferent fibers but of the target cells. Taking advantage of the postnatal formation of most of the dentate granule cells, their proliferation can be inhibited by early postnatal X-irradiation (Bayer and Altman, 1975). As many as 80–85% of the dentate granule cells fail to form and differentiate in such

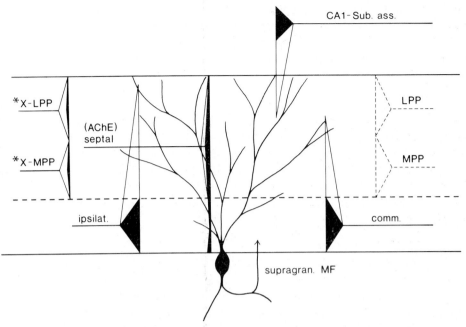

Fig. 9. Schematic illustration of the laminar reorganization of terminal fields in the dentate molecular layer which follows an early postnatal removal of the perforant pathways. The dentate molecular layer is between the solid lines; above the upper line (hippocampal fissure) is str. moleculare of CA1 and subiculum. Both commissural (comm.) and ipsilateral (ipsilat.) fibers extend into the denervated perforant path zones (above broken line), within which AChE-containing septal afferents proliferate. At the most septal levels, where sparse crossed perforant pathways (asterisks) are normally present, the afferent fibers proliferate and expand. More posteriorly and temporally, these systems are replaced by CA1-subiculum associated afferents (CA1-sub. ass.) which cross the hippocampal fissure. An extension of mossy fiber collaterals into the commissural-ipsilateral zone is also observed (supragran. MF).

preparations, hereby depriving the perforant path of a substantial proportion of its normal target cells. Under these conditions, however, the LPP and the MPP still terminate in a normal laminar fashion in the residual fascia dentata; they even do so in an aberrant termination formed by an induced elongation of the basal dendrites of CA3c pyramidical cells (Laurberg and Hjorth-Simonsen, 1977). In the latter area it is not the dentate granule cells (which never form in sufficient numbers to make up a medial blade) that determine the laminar pattern of the PP terminations. The basal dendrites of the CA3c pyramidal cells may possibly mimic the response which is normally mediated by the apical end branches of the same cells (with which the PP are normally connected). Even with this reservation, these experiments nevertheless demonstrate the important role of afferent fibers in triggering and modulating dendritic growth.

(iii) Transplantation of immature hippocampus and fascia dentata

Transplantation of nervous tissue from a given area of the brain into corresponding or different areas of other brains, opens the possibility of studying the effect of intrinsic and extrinsic factors — and of afferent systems — on the development and differentiation of the transplanted cell types (Das, 1975). Transplantation experiments using pieces of immature fascia dentata, including adjacent parts of the hippocampus, have been initiated for this purpose in collaboration with Dr. N. Sunde. Some of the results, where the Timm method has been used to monitor the changes in synaptology and afferent lamination, will be presented below. A description of the technique used for the transplantations is available from the author, and will be published separately (Zimmer and Sunde, in preparation).

Following transplantation of neonatal fascia dentata from 1-day-old rats into the cerebellum of littermates or adult rats the transplants are able to grow, differentiate, and survive for at least two months. They attain an apparently normal cytological organization, with a distinct granule cell layer, molecular layer and hilus (Fig. 10). Compared to the normal fascia dentata, however, both the granule cell layer and the molecular layer are reduced in width. The pattern of Timm staining is not normal (Fig. 11), since the laminae characteristic of the perforant pathways are absent. These are replaced by a darker staining of coarser granularity, which normally is related to the ipsilateral associational systems of the hippocampus and fascia dentata. In addition, an intense supragranular band of mossy fiber staining develops. These features are typical of dentate tissue which has been severely deafferented and isolated, but otherwise left in situ in its normal position within its 'own' brain.

No cytological barrier, in the form of an accumulation of pial or glial cell bodies, is recognizable at the interface between the transplant and the host tissue. Moreover, Timm stainable elements (i.e. terminals) arising from the transplant — the cerebellum does not normally display any Timm staining — are found to invade the adjacent cerebellar neuropil of the host (Fig. 12). With the limitations of the methods kept in mind, it nonetheless seems reasonable to conclude that, although there presumably are some interactions and exchanges of afferent connections (especially at the interface between the transplant and the host tissue; also see Fig. 13), the major intrinsic organization of the transplant is not affected by the surrounding cerebellar tissue. Thus, a dentate transplant in the cerebellum is not basically different from dentate tissue allowed to develop and differentiate in situ, but deprived of its normal major extrinsic afferents.

A more profound action of host afferent fibers on the synaptic organization of transplants occurs when dentate tissue is transplanted into the fimbria, which is the normal route for commissural afferents to the fascia dentata and the hippocampus. In that situation, the outer parts of the molecular layer still suffer from removal of the perforant pathways, and resemble a non-transplanted fascia dentata which has been deprived of entorhinal input. The inner zone of the dentate molecular layer of the transplant, however, develops into an almost normal looking commissural-ipsilateral zone (Fig. 14). The invasion of the transplant by fimbrial fibers (Fig. 15) accordingly prevents the formation of the anomalous supragranular mossy fiber staining. This situation is comparable to that found in *non*-transplant cases with heavy denervation of the commissural-ipsilateral zone, in which the presence of even a small residual amount of the original associational or commissural afferents is found to abolish, or restrict, the formation of the supragranular mossy fiber staining which is otherwise induced (Zimmer and Laurberg, 1976).

Figs. 10–13. Horizontal sections through the cerebellum of an adult rat, showing a graft of dentate and hippocampal tissue. The graft was obtained from a 1-day-old rat, and was transplanted into the host animal one month before it was sacrificed.

Fig. 10. Thionin-stained section showing the presence in the transplant of all the characteristic layers of the fascia dentata: gr. granule cell layer; h, hilus (CA4); m, molecular layer. × 30.

Fig. 11. Adjacent Timm-stained section. Note the coarse dark staining in the outer part of the dentate molecular layer (m), and the presence of supragranular mossy fibers (sgr). × 30.

Fig. 12. High magnification of the interface between hippocampal and cerebellar tissue (at open arrow in Fig. 11). × 275.

Fig. 13. High magnification of the interface between hippocampal and cerebellar tissue (at open arrow in Fig. 11), as seen in Nauta silver staining. × 275.

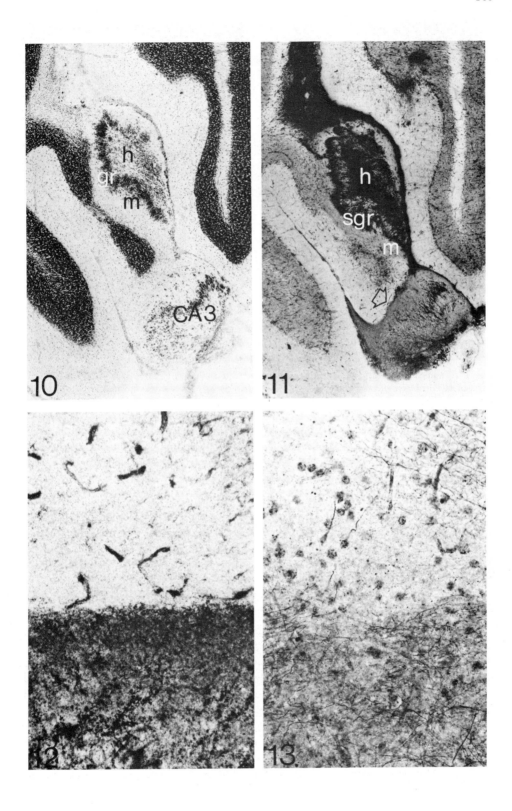

184

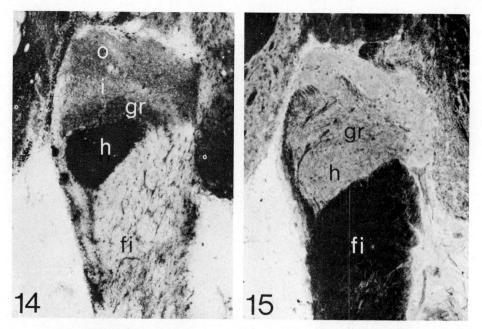

Figs. 14 and 15. Horizontal sections from a 2-month-old rat. showing a piece of dentate tissue transplanted into the fimbria from a littermate rat at postnatal day 1.

Fig. 14. Timm-stained section of the transplant. Note the presence of coarse dark staining in the outer parts of the dentate molecular layer (o), while the inner part (i) looks almost normal, without any supragranular mossy fibers. × 70.

Fig. 15. Nauta silver impregnated section, showing fibers extending from the fimbria through the hilus (h) and the granule cell layer (gr) to the molecular layer of the transplant. × 70.

Although disproving the existence of absolute specification, in the sense that anomalous connections would never form under any circumstances, the results just presented nevertheless indicate that (both normally and in transplants) there are preferences within the fascia dentata for the termination of different afferent systems. In the absence of the normal afferents, second-best choices are allowed, which choices might be determined by temporal factors and/or by proximity (Zimmer, 1974a; Zimmer and Hjorth-Simonsen, 1975).

(iv) The use of mutants or inbred strains

Studies using mutant 'reeler' mice have shown that, among several other brain areas (Sotelo, this volume), this mutation also affects the hippocampus. Due to a failure in migration, many of the developing neurons become malpositioned, as a result of which the cell layers become disorganized and wrinkled (Caviness, 1973). Despite the malposition of the target cells, however, the laminar distribution of the major afferent pathways is not much disturbed (Bliss and Chung, 1974; Bliss et al., 1976; Stanfield, 1977). As in the X-irradiation experiments (see above), this points to the afferent axons themselves as the factor chiefly responsible for afferent lamination.

Inbred strains of mice are also available which are useful for studying hippocampal development. Some of these strains differ significantly not only with regard to the number of neurons within the different parts of the hippocampus and fascia dentata (Wimer et al., 1976) but also with regard to the distribution of afferent systems, e.g. the infrapyramidal bundle of mossy fibers in CA3c (Barber et al., 1974; Fredens, personal communication). Recently, the relative lack of infrapyramidal mossy fibers in BALB/cJ mice in comparison with SM/J mice (or most other laboratory mice and rats) has been related to a difference in the way the CA3c pyramidal cells settle (Vaughn et al., 1977). Thus, the CA3c pyramidal cells in BALB/cJ mice settle in an *outside-in* sequence, while the pyramidal cells in the rest of CA3 (and in *all* of CA3 in other mice) settle in an *inside-out* sequence (asterisk in Fig. 3). Results of this kind strengthen the concept that the *timing* of arrival of afferent axons, in relation to a certain stage of differentiation of the target cell, is of great importance for the establishment and final distribution of the nervous connections.

The recent finding by Lauder and Mugnaini (1977) that rats treated with thyroxine during the first two weeks after birth develop excessive and aberrant infrapyramidal mossy fiber boutons in CA3ab may be interpreted in the same way, since thyroxine is known to interfere with cell proliferation and differentiation (e.g. Baláizs, 1976).

CONCLUDING REMARKS

As a tentative conclusion of this presentation, the following points will be made.

(i) The major afferent pathways to the hippocampus and fascia dentata become established within their appropriate laminae in the early postnatal period, or even earlier.

(ii) The development and differentiation of the afferent pathways tend to proceed along the general morphogenetic gradients of the region.

(iii) The afferent pathways to the fascia dentata normally have a preference for this structure and for their normal laminae within it. However, alien fiber systems are able to innervate the fascia dentata, or an abnormal lamina within it, if the normal afferents are not there. Absolute axonal-dendritic specification therefore does not exist in the fascia dentata.

(iv) The distribution of afferent systems *within* a given lamina, or following invasion into a denervated area, most likely depends upon proximity and temporal competition; in this way the innervation pattern would be determined by differences in the arrival of various afferents, in relation to the stage of differentiation of the target neurons.

(v) The segregation into laminae of the afferent systems seems to be a process which is promoted by the afferent axons rather than by the target neurons. During development, this process may involve stimulation by the afferent axons, of growth in specific parts of the target cell and/or mutual inhibition of axonal growth at the interface between different afferent systems (Diamond et al., 1976; Changeux and Danchin, 1976; Changeux and Mikoshiba, this volume).

ACKNOWLEDGEMENTS

The author gratefully acknowledges the help of Mrs. K. Christensen, Mrs. E. Kjær Hansen, Mr. A. Meier, Mr. T.A. Nielsen, Miss M. Sørensen and Miss K. Wiedemann. Thanks are also due to Dr. F.-M.S. Haug, and Drs. N.A. Sunde and B. Rasmussen, with whom the studies on the development of Timm staining and the transplants have been performed. Supported by the Danish Medical Research Council.

REFERENCES

Altman, J. and Das, G.D. (1965) Autoradiographic and histological evidence of postnatal hippocampal neurogenesis in rats, *J. comp. Neurol.*, 124: 319–336.

186

Angevine, J.B., Jr. (1965) Time of neuron origin in the hippocampal region. An autoradiographic study in the mouse, *Exp. Neurol.,* Suppl. 2: 1–70.

Angevine, J.B., Jr. (1975) Development of the hippocampal region, In *The Hippocampus. I: Structure and Development,* R.L. Isaacson and K.H. Pribram (Eds.), Plenum Press, New York, pp. 61–94.

Balázs, R. (1976) Hormones and Brain Development. In *Perspectives in Brain Research, Progr. Brain Res., Vol. 45,* M.A. Corner and D.F. Swaab (Eds.), Elsevier, Amsterdam, pp. 139–160.

Banker, G.A. and Cowan, W.M. (1977) Rat hippocampal neurons in dispersed cell culture, *Brain Res.,* 126: 397–425.

Barber, R.P., Vaughn, J.E., Wimer, R.E. and Wimer, C.C., (1974) Genetically-associated variations in the distribution of dentate granule cell synapses upon pyramidal cell dendrites in mouse hippocampus, *J. comp. Neurol.,* 156: 417–434.

Bayer, S.A. and Altman, J. (1974) Hippocampal development in the rat. Cytogenesis and morphogenesis examined with autoradiography and low-level X-irradiation, *J. comp. Neurol.,* 158: 55–80.

Bayer, S.A. and Altman, J. (1975) The effects of X-irradiation on the postnatally-forming granule cell population in the olfactory bulb, hippocampus, and cerebellum of the rat, *Exp. Neurol.,* 48: 167–174.

Blackstad, T.W. (1956) Commissural connections of the hippocampal region of the rat, with special reference to their mode of termination, *J. comp. Neurol.,* 105: 417–537.

Blackstad, T.W., Brink, K., Hem J. and Jeune, B., (1970) Distribution of hippocampal mossy fibers in the rat. An experimental study with silver impregnation methods, *J. comp. Neurol.,* 138: 433–450.

Bliss, T.V.P. and Chung, S.H. (1974) An electrophysiological study of the 'Reeler' mutant mouse, *Nature (Lond.),* 252: 153–155.

Bliss, T.V.P., Chung, S.H. and Stirling, R.V. (1974) Structural and functional development of the mossy fibre system in the hippocampus of the post-natal rat, *J. Physiol. (Lond.),* 239: 92–93P.

Bliss, T.V.P., Chung, S.H. and Stirling, R.V. (1976) Electrophysiological and anatomical observations on the hippocampus of the Reeler mouse, *Exp. Brain Res.,* Suppl. 1: 235–236.

Brown, J.W. (1966) Some aspects of the early development of the hippocampal formation in certain insectivorous bats, In *Evolution of the Forebrain,* R. Hassler and H. Stephan (Eds.), G. Thieme, Stuttgart, pp. 92–103.

Cajal, S. Ramón y, (1893) Estructura del asta de Ammon. *Anal. Soc. esp. Hist. Nat. Madr.,* 22: 53–114. English translation: *The Structure of the Ammon's Horn,* Thomas, Springfield, Ill., 1968, 78 pp.

Cajal, S. Ramón y (1911) *Histologie du Système de l'Homme et de Vertébrés, Vol. II,* A. Maloine, Paris, pp. 733–799.

Caviness, V.S., Jr. (1973) Time of neuron origin in the hippocampus and dentate gyrus of normal and reeler mutant mice: an autoradiographic analysis, *J. comp. Neurol.,* 151: 113–120.

Changeux, J.-P. and Danchin, A. (1976) Selective stabilisation of developing synapses as a mechanism for the specification of neuronal networks, *Nature (Lond.),* 264: 705–712.

Changeux, J.-P., and Mikoshiba, K. (1978) Genetic and 'epigenetic' factors regulating synapse formation in vertebrate cerebellum and neuromuscular junction, this volume.

Cotman, C.W., Taylor, D. and Lynch, G. (1973) Ultrastructural changes in synapses in the dentate gyrus of the rat during development, *Brain Res.,* 63: 205–213.

Crain, B., Cotman, C.W., Taylor, D. and Lynch, G. (1973) A quantitative electron microscopic study of synaptogenesis in the dentate gyrus of the rat, *Brain Res.,* 63: 195–204.

Danscher, G., Fjerdingstad, E.J., Fjerdingstad, E. and Fredens, K. (1976) Heavy metal content in subdivisions of the rat hippocampus (zinc, lead and copper), *Brain Res.,* 112: 442–446.

Danscher, G. and Zimmer, J. (1978) Improvements of the Timm sulphide silver method for light and electron microscopic localization of heavy metals in biological tissues, *Histochemistry,* 55: 27–48.

Das, G.D. (1975) Differentiation of dendrites in the transplanted neuroblasts in the mammalian brain. In *Physiology and Pathology of Dendrites, Advanc. Neurol., Vol. 12,* G.W. Kreutzberg (Ed.), Raven Press, New York, pp. 181–199.

Diamond, J., Cooper, E. and Macintyre, L. (1976) Trophic regulation of nerve sprouting, *Science,* 193: 371–377.

Euler, C. von (1962) On the significance of the high zinc content of the hippocampal formation, In *Physiologie de l'Hippocampe,* P. Passouant (Ed.) C.N.R.S., Paris, pp. 135–145.

Fricke, R. and Cowan, W.M. (1977) An autoradiographic study of the development of the entorhinal and commissural afferents to the dentate gyrus of the rat, *J. comp. Neurol.,* 173: 231–250.

Godina, G. e Barassa, A. (1964) Morfogenesi ed istogenesi della formazione ammonica, *Z. Zellforsch.*, 63: 327–355.

Gottlieb, D.I. and Cowan W.M. (1972) Evidence for a temporal factor in the occupation of available synaptic sites during the development of the dentate gyrus, *Brain Res.*, 41: 452–456.

Gottlieb, D.I. and Cowan, W.M. (1973) Autoradiographic studies of the commissural and ipsilateral association connections of the hippocampus and dentate gyrus of the rat. I. The commissural connections, *J. comp. Neurol.*, 149: 393–422.

Haug, F.-M.Š. (1967) Electron microscopical localization of the zinc in hippocampal mossy fiber synapses by a modified sulphide silver procedure, *Histochemie*, 8: 355–368.

Haug, F.-M.Š. (1973) Heavy metals in the brain. A light microscope study of the rat with Timm's sulphide silver method. Methodological considerations and cytological and regional staining patterns, *Advance Anat. Embryol. Cell Biol.*, 47: 1–71.

Haug, F.-M.Š. (1974) Light microscopical mapping of the hippocampal region, the pyriform cortex and the corticomedial amygdaloid nuclei of the rat with Timm's sulphide silver method. I Area dentata, hippocampus and subiculum , *Z. Anat. Entwickl.-Gesch.*, 145: 1–27.

Haug, F.-M.Š. (1975) On the normal histochemistry of trace metals in the brain, *J. Hirnforsch.*, 16: 146–158.

Haug, F.-M.Š. (1976) Laminar distribution of afferents in the allocortex, visualized with Timm's sulphide silver method for 'heavy' metals, *Exp. Brain Res.*, Suppl. 1: 177–178.

Haug, F.-M.Š., Blackstad, T.W., Simonsen, A.H. and Zimmer, J. (1971) Timm's sulfide silver reaction for zinc during experimental anterograde degeneration of hippocampal mossy fibers, *J. comp. Neurol.*, 142: 23–32.

Hine, R.J. and Das, G.D. (1974) Neuroembryogenesis in the hippocampal formation of the rat, *Z. Anat. Entwickl.-Gesch.*, 144: 173–186.

Hjorth-Simonsen, A. (1972) Projection of the lateral part of the entorhinal area to the hippocampus and fascia dentata, *J. comp. Neurol.*, 146: 219–232.

Hjorth-Simonsen, A. (1973) Some intrinsic connections of the hippocampus in the rat: an experimental analysis, *J. comp. Neurol.*, 147: 145–162.

Hjorth-Simonsen, A. and Jeune, B. (1972) Origin and termination of the hippocampal perforant path in the rat studied by silver impregnation, *J. comp. Neurol.*, 144: 215–232.

Hu, K.H. and Friede, R.L. (1968) Topographic determination of zinc in human brain by atomic absorption spectrophotometry, *J. Neurochem.*, 15: 667–685.

Humphrey, T. (1966) The development of the human hippocampal formation correlated with some aspects of its phylogenetic history. In *Evolution of the Forebrain*, R. Hassler and H. Stephan (Eds.), G. Thieme, Stuttgart, pp. 104–116.

Ibata, Y. and Otsuka, N. (1968) Fine structure of synapses in the hippocampus of the rabbit with special reference to dark presynaptic endings, *Z. Zellforsch.*, 91: 547–553.

Kaplan, M.S. and Hinds, J.W. (1977) Neurogenesis in the olfactory bulb and dentate gyrus of the adult rat: electron microscopic analysis of light radioautographs, *Anat. Rec.*, 187: 620.

Lauder, J.M. and Mugnaini, E. (1977) Early hyperthyroidism alters the distribution of mossy fibers in the rat hippocampus, *Nature (Lond.)*, 268: 335–337.

Laurberg, S. and Hjorth-Simonsen, A. (1977) Growing central axons deprived of normal target neurons by neonatal X-irradiation still terminate in a precisely laminated fashion, *Nature (Lond.)*, 269: 158–160.

LaVail, J.H. and Wolf, M.K. (1973) Postnatal development of the mouse dentate gyrus in organotypic cultures of the hippocampal formation, *Amer. J. Anat.*, 137: 47–66.

Lorente de Nó, R. (1934) Studies on the structure of the cerebral cortex. II. Continuation of the study of the Ammonic system, *J. Psychol. Neurol. (Lpz.)*, 46: 113–177.

Loy, R., Lynch, G. and Cotman, C.W. (1977) Development of afferent lamination in the fascia dentata of the rat, *Brain Res.*, 121: 229–243.

Lynch, G., Rose, G., Gall, C. and Cotman, C.W. (1975) The response of the dentate gyrus to partial deafferentation. In *Proc. Golgi Centennial Symposium*, M. Santini (Ed.), Raven Press, New York, pp. 305–317.

Maske, H. (1965) Uber den topochemischen Nachweis von Zinc im Ammonshorn verschiedener Säugetiere, *Naturwissenschaften*, 42: 424.

Matthews, D.A., Cotman, C. and Lynch, G. (1976) An electron microscopic study of lesion-induced synaptogenesis in the dentate gyrus of the adult rat. I. Magnitude and time course of degeneration, *Brain Res.*, 115: 1–21.

McWilliams, J.R., Lynch, G.S. and Cotman, C.W. (1975) Synaptic reinnervation in the inner molecular layer of the dentate gyrus following partial deafferentation: an electron microscope study in the rat, *Neurosci. Abstr.*, p. 517.

Minkwitz, H.-G. (1976a) Zur Entwicklung der Neuronenstruktur des Hippocampus während der prä- und postnatalen Ontogenese der Albinoratte. I. Mitteilung: Neurohistologische Darstellung der Entwicklung langaxoniger Neurone aus den Regionen CA3 und CA4, *J. Hirnforsch.*, 17: 213–231.

Minkwitz, H.-G. (1976b) Zur Entwicklung der Neuronenstruktur des Hippocampus während der prä- und postnatalen Ontogenese der Albinoratte. II. Mitteilung: Neurohistologische Darstellung der Entwicklung von Interneuronen und des Zusammenhanges lang- und kurzaxoniger Neurone, *J. Hirnforsch.*, 17: 233–253.

Minkwitz, H.-G. (1976c) Zur Entwicklung der Neuronenstruktur des Hippocampus während der prä- und postnatalen Ontogenese der Albinoratte. III. Mitteilung: Morphometrische Erfassung der ontogenetischen Veränderungen in Dendrittenstruktur und Spinebesatz an Pyramidenneuronen (CA1) des Hippocampus, *J. Hirnforsch.*, 17: 255–275.

Minkwitz, H.-G. und Holz, L. (1975) Die ontogenetische Entwicklung von Pyramidenneuronen aus dem Hippocampus (CA1) der Ratte, *J. Hirnforsch.*, 16: 37–54.

Purpura, D.P. and Pappas, G.D. (1968) Structural characteristics of neurons in the feline hippocampus during postnatal ontogenesis, *Exp. Neurol.*, 22: 379–393.

Rakic, P. (1977) Prenatal development of the visual system in rhesus monkey, *Phil. Trans. B,* 278: 245–260.

Schlessinger, A.R., Cowan, W.M. and Gottlieb, D.I. (1975) An autoradiographic study of the time of origin and the pattern of granule cell migration in the dentate gyrus of the rat, *J. comp. Neurol.*, 159: 149–176.

Schwartz, I.R., Pappas, G.D. and Purpura, D.P. (1968) Fine structure of neurons and synapses in feline hippocampus during postnatal ontogenesis, *Exp. Neurol.*, 22: 394–407.

Sotelo, C. (1978) Purkinje cell ontogeny: formation and maintenance of spines, this volume.

Stanfield, B. (1977) The morphogenesis of the hippocampus in the normal and the reeler mutant mouse, *Anat. Rec.*, 187: 721–722.

Stensaas, L.J. (1967) The development of hippocampal and dorsolateral pallial regions of the cerebral hemisphere in fetal rabbits. III. Twenty-nine millimeter stage, marginal lamina, *J. comp. Neurol.*, 130: 149–162.

Stensaas, L.J. (1968) The development of hippocampal and dorsolateral pallial regions of the cerebral hemisphere in fetal rabbits. VI. 90 mm stage, cortical differentiation, *J. comp. Neurol.*, 132: 93–108.

Steward, O. (1976) Topographical organization of the projections from the entorhinal area to the hippocampal formation of the rat, *J. comp. Neurol.*, 167: 285–314.

Steward, O. and Scoville, S.A. (1976) Cells of origin of entorhinal cortical afferents to the hippocampus and fascia dentata of the rat, *J. comp. Neurol.*, 169: 347–370.

Stirling, R.V. and Bliss, T.V.P. (1978) Mossy fiber development at the ultrastructural level, this volume.

Timm, F. (1958) Zur Histochemie der Schwermetalle. Das Sulfid-Silberverfahren, *Dtsch. Z. ges. gerichtl. Med.*, 47: 428–481.

Vaughn, J.E., Matthews, D.A., Barber, R.P., Wimer, C.C. and Wimer, R.E. (1977) Genetically-associated variation in the development of hippocampal pyramidal neurons may produce differences in mossy fiber connectivity, *J. comp. Neurol.*, 173: 41–52.

Voigt, E. (1959) Untersuchungen mit der Sulfidsilbermethode an menschlichen und tierischen Bauchspeicheldrüsen (unter besonderer Berücksichtigung des Diabetes mellitus und experimenteller Metalvergiftungen), *Virchows Arch. (Pathol. Anat.),* 332: 295–323.

Wimer, R.E., Wimer, C.C., Vaughn, J.E., Barker, R.P., Balvanz, B.A. and Chemow, C.R. (1976) The genetic organization of neuron number in Ammon's horn of house mice, *Brain Res.*, 118: 219–243.

Zimmer, J. (1971) Ipsilateral afferents to the commissural zone of the fascia dentata, demonstrated in decommissurated rats by silver impregnation, *J. comp. Neurol.*, 142: 393–416.

Zimmer, J. (1973a) Extended commissural and ipsilateral projections in postnatally deentorhinated hippocampus and fascia dentata demonstrated in rats by silver impregnation, *Brain Res.*, 64: 293–311.

Zimmer, J. (1973b) Changes in the Timm sulfide silver staining pattern of the rat hippocampus and fascia dentata following early postnatal deafferentation, *Brain Res.*, 64: 313–326.

Zimmer, J. (1974a) Proximity as a factor in the regulation of aberrant axonal growth in postnatally deafferented fascia dentata, *Brain Res.*, 72: 137–142.

Zimmer, J. (1974b) Long term changes of synaptic reorganization in rat fascia dentata deafferented at adolescent and adult stages: Observations with the Timm method, *Brain Res.*, 76: 336–342.

Zimmer, J. (1976) Postlesional remodelling of fiber connections in the hippocampus and fascia dentata. I. Observations on immature rats, *Exp. Brain Res.*, Suppl. 1: 191–196.

Zimmer, J. and Hjorth-Simonsen, A. (1975) Crossed pathways from the entorhinal area to the fascia dentata. II. Provokable in rats, *J. comp. Neurol.*, 161: 71–102.

Zimmer, J. and Laurberg, S. (1976) Postlesional formation of anomalous supragranular mossy fibers in the fascia dentata of adult rats, *Anat. Rec.*, 184: 570.

Zimmer, J. and Haug, F.-M.Š. (1978) Laminar differentiation of the hippocampus fascia dentata and subiculum in developing rats, observed with the Timm sulphide silver method, *J. comp. Neurol.*, in press.

DISCUSSION

SOTELO: Why do you use the Timm staining method instead of staining for acetylcholinesterase, or using a more classic histochemical method for the development of the hippocampus?

ZIMMER: One of the advantages of using the Timm method for studying hippocampal development is that the terminal field of all the major afferent systems are stained en bloc. By using only a few sections from different septotemporal levels of the hippocampal region, it is possible in this way to screen at the same time both for developmental gradients within each of these systems, and for the mutual distribution of all of the systems present.

CHANGEUX: What about the vascularization of your transplants? How does it take place?

ZIMMER: I do not know about the exact pattern or time-course of the vascularization. Certainly the transplants must get vascularized quite rapidly, since the survival is surprisingly good (about 90%). In this regard, one may ask the question why neonatal brain tissue is not rejected by an immunological reaction when transplanted into the brain of adult rats. The blood-brain-barrier may be of importance here. During ontogeny the barrier has formed at about the end of the first postnatal week, and following a lesion to an adult brain it repairs within one week or so. In the transplant situation, then, the transplant itself ought to have developed its blood-brain-barrier after one week, at which time also the lesion of the recipient's barrier should be repaired. Although the implantation of foreign tissue may initially stimulate the recipient's immunological apparatus, the time needed to raise the antibodies against this tissue to a critical level might be sufficient for the blood-brain-barrier to be formed or repaired, thus preventing any further immunological reaction from taking place.

Hippocampal Mossy Fiber Development at the Ultrastructural Level

R. VICTORIA STIRLING and T.V.P. BLISS

Dept. of Developmental Biology, National Institute for Medical Research, London (Great Britain)

INTRODUCTION

This appendix to the previous paper (i.e. Zimmer, this volume) describes preliminary findings on the postnatal maturation of the characteristic, highly invaginated giant terminals of the hippocampal mossy fiber axons (Blackstad and Kjaerheim, 1961; Hamlyn, 1962). It attempts to correlate their ultrastructural development with both the development of synaptic efficiency, as determined electrophysiologically (Bliss et al., 1974), and with the Timm staining pattern (see Zimmer, this volume; Zimmer and Haug, 1977). The basic description of the trends in development seen at 2, 5, 10, 15 and 27 days postnatally (where the day of birth is taken as postnatal day 1) are based on observations of at least three Sprague-Dawley rats in each age group. The quantitative data in this account is based on preliminary measurements made from one animal in each group with the aid of a computer. Observations were confined to the septal pole of the hippocampus, the level which is most accessible for physiological recording.

Animals were fixed with paraformaldehyde alone, or with gluteraldehyde added to the fixative after initial perfusion; blocks of tissue were postfixed in osmium tetroxide, and embedded in araldite. The correct area was located using toluidine blue-stained semi-thin sections. Ultra-thin sections were viewed with an AEI Corinth microscope after conventional staining with uranyl acetate and lead citrate (Reynolds, 1963). Micrographs at a magnification of 10,000 X were taken of terminals encountered on the apical dendrites just above the CA3b (Lorente de Nó, 1934) pyramidal cell bodies. The micrographs were printed at a magnification of 4.2 X, and the presynaptic profiles were marked with colored pens. The profiles were then traced around with a soft pencil on a conductive plate. Potentials applied across the plate defined the x and y coordinates for successive points, which were then stored on disc. The computer was programmed to analyze perimeter length, total enclosed area, and the proportion of perimeter occupied by synaptic and non-synaptic specializations (see Fig. 5).

THE ULTRASTRUCTURAL MATURATION OF THE MOSSY FIBER TERMINALS

The electron micrographs illustrating the development of the mossy fiber terminals in Figs. 1 and 2 are taken from a single 7-day postnatal animal. At this time, profiles showing various states of development can be seen; with advancing age the proportion of more mature profiles increases.

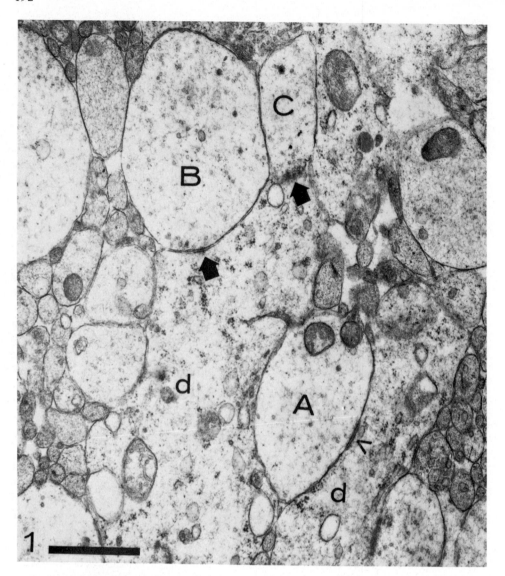

Fig. 1. Presynaptic profiles contacting apical dendrites (d) of CA3b pyramids in a 7-day postnatal rat. Profile A shows an immature contact, with symmetrical membrane specializations and no associated vesicles (arrowhead). In profile B there is a small cluster of vesicles above the presynaptic membrane (arrow). Profile C contains a larger cluster of vesicles in the synaptic region (arrow). Calibration bar 1 μm.

Fig. 2. Terminals in the mossy fiber zone, taken from the same rat as Fig. 1. The contact in profile A has few associated vesicles but displays well-developed presynaptic and postsynaptic membrane specializations (arrow). Profile B has a much more intimate relationship with its dendrite (d), invaginating into it (i), and being itself indented by a dendritic spine (s). Compare the Gray type-I contacts (arrows) with the presumed non-synaptic contacts (arrowheads) along the shaft of the dendrite. Calibration bar 1 μm.

Fig. 3. Mossy fiber terminal from a 15-day postnatal rat. Numerous dendritic spines (s) are clearly visible, with typical synaptic contacts (arrow), while non-synaptic contacts (arrowheads) are confined to the smooth dendritic shaft (d). Calibration as Fig. 2.

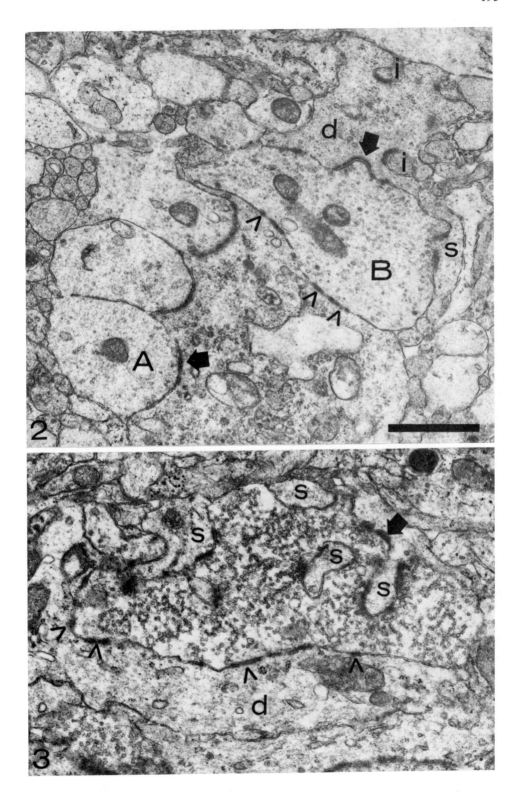

At postnatal day 2, the proximal portions of the apical dendrites of CA3b are surrounded by axon growth cones, small axon profiles and the large, ribosome-rich, proximal dendrites of the pyramidal cells. There is considerable intercellular space which is filled with a fine filamentous material. Contacting the dendrites are scattered profiles which seem to represent several stages in the maturation of presynaptic boutons. The most immature of these are large, round, clear profiles which contain only filamentous material, with no vesicles or neurotubules. Where these structures contact the dendrite there is a clear symmetrical membrane specialization, as shown in Fig. 1A. Other structures contacting the dendrites at this time contain a small number of vesicles clustered above Gray type-I (Gray, 1959), asymmetrical, membrane specializations (as in Fig. 1B, C). Rarely, more complex profiles can be found enclosing or invaginating into the postsynaptic dendrites (Fig. 2B).

At day 5, although the general shape of the profiles in the mossy fiber zone is similar to that found at two days (as in Fig. 1B, C), there are many more profiles which contain vesicles and distinct membrane specializations. The immature profiles containing no vesicles, and having symmetrical membrane thickenings, have become sparse, while the number of more mature terminals, which are sometimes invaginated into the dendrite, is greater than at two days. No characteristic mossy fiber terminals of the adult type are seen at this age in any position along Ammon's horn. It is striking that synapses of similar stages of development occur together in clusters, suggesting that axons from neighboring granule cells of the same age fasciculate as they pass from the dentate to the pyramidal cells. The weak synaptic activity which can be evoked by mossy fiber stimulation in some 5-day animals (Bliss, et al., 1974) reflects the immaturity of most of the terminals and, possibly, also the relatively few vesicles which they contain.

Synaptic depolarization of the CA3 pyramids can reliably be evoked in 10-day animals, but they do not fire consistently to each afferent volley (Bliss et al., 1974). The majority of the synaptic profiles now begin to resemble the mossy fiber terminals of adult animals, and no longer have a simple rounded shape. Terminals are often enclosed within the dendrite (Fig. 2, i) or, alternatively, enclose small dendritic spines (Fig. 3, s). The terminals are well filled with vesicles and also contain a few mitochondria. This increase in the complexity of the terminal-dendrite relationship is reflected in the sharp decrease in the 'shape factor' of presynaptic profiles between 5 and 10 days (Fig. 4B). (The shape factor of a profile is defined as the ratio of the area of the profile to the area of a circle having the same perimeter; it is thus a measure of the 'circularity' of the profile; the rounder the profile the closer its shape factor is to unity, whereas the more indented the profile the closer its shape factor is to zero.) At this time a second type of contact between the dendritic shaft and the mossy terminals can be seen (Figs. 2 and 3, arrow heads). Both the terminal and the dendritic membranes are thickened over a distance of 0.2–0.3 μm, with no associated vesicles or other cellular inclusions on either side of the contact. These contacts are very similar to the 'mechanical fixation points' described by Hamlyn (1962) in mossy fiber boutons of adult rabbits. They possibly serve to anchor the presynaptic bag onto the dendritic shaft as the terminal changes its configuration to form the highly invaginated structure characteristic of the adult animal.

The number of both these fixation points and of Gray type-I synaptic contacts increases after day 10, while their mean lengths decrease (Fig. 5). A similar break-up of membrane specializations into smaller, more numerous elements has been noted by Larramendi (1969) in developing cerebellar mossy fiber terminals. The synaptic contacts are found almost exclusively at the tips of the dendritic spines invaginating into the boutons, even in cases where these invaginations are no more than small bumps in the membrane. Whether these are the original synaptic contacts (which later become the apex of the invaginating spine) or whether membrane specializations migrate to the spine as it pushes into the terminal is a matter of conjecture.

Reliable generation of population spikes in CA3 pyramids to mossy fiber volleys is obtained by 15 days after birth (Bliss et al. 1974), at which time the terminals have an almost adult appearance (Fig. 3). Terminals invaginating into the postsynaptic dendrite are now rare. The histograms in Figs. 4 and 5 show that there is a much greater change in all the parameters measured between 5 and 15 days than between 15 and 27 days. The configurational changes seen at 10 days continues in older animals at a progressively slower rate as more profiles assume the adult shape and type.

THE LINK BETWEEN ULTRASTRUCTURE AND THE TIMM STAINING PATTERN

A number of factors make it difficult to correlate the development of the Timm staining pattern described by Zimmer (this volume) with the ultrastructural maturation of the mossy fiber terminals. In the first place, the ultrastructural analysis has dealt only with the complexity and specializations of the limiting presynaptic and postsynaptic membranes, while the Timm staining reaction is dependent upon heavy metals present in the cytoplasm of the terminal. Secondly, rats of slightly different ages and of different strains were used in the two studies.

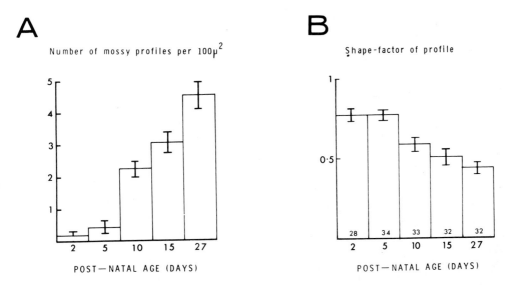

Fig. 4. A: histogram showing the increase during development of the areal density of presynaptic profiles terminating on proximal apical dendrites of CA3b pyramidal cells. Counts were made from random low power micrographs of this region, and are expressed as mean number (± standard error) per 100 μm^2. Terminals were defined as enclosed figures, containing at least one Gray type-I synaptic membrane specialization, and with one or more associated vesicles. The most dramatic rise in the number of terminals is between 5 and 10 days. Increases occurring later than this can partly be accounted for by the increase in the complexity of the terminals, allowing a single terminal to give rise to more than one enclosed profile. B: histogram showing the change in the mean shape factor (see text for definition) of presynaptic profiles in the mossy terminal zone during development. Measurements were made from 10 micrographs each covering an area of 360 μm^2, obtained from a single animal in each age group. The number of profiles measured is shown at the base of each column. Bars indicate standard error. Note that the major decrease in shape factor occurs between 5 and 10 days.

196

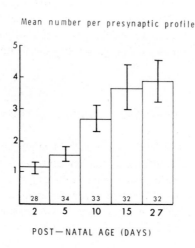

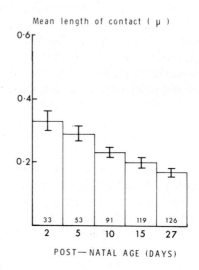

A

MATURE SYNAPTIC CONTACTS

Mean number per presynaptic profile

Mean length of contact (μ)

B

NON—SYNAPTIC CONTACTS

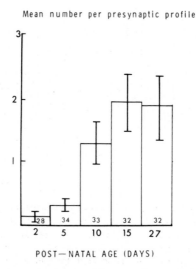

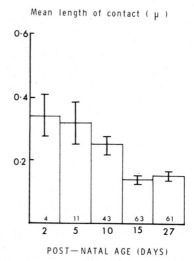

Mean number per presynaptic profile

Mean length of contact (μ)

Fig. 5. A. analysis of the number and mean lengths of mature synaptic contacts (clear Gray type-I contacts with associated vesicles) in the mossy fiber terminal zone of the developing hippocampus. B: number and mean length of non-synaptic contacts (more or less symmetrical membrane specializations without associated vesicles) in the same region. All histograms in this figure were constructed from measurements made on the same set of micrographs used to analyze changes in shape factor with development (Fig. 4B). The number of profiles or membrane specializations measured is shown at the base of each column. Bars indicate standard error.

Despite these objections, the findings do tie together reasonably well. The presence of a definite band of Timm staining on day 1 (and especially evident at day 3) suggests that, as soon as EM profiles develop into recognizable synaptic contacts, they also contain enough heavy metal to give a positive staining reaction. The individual scattered dense clumps of Timm's stain at day 3 may correspond to the more mature terminals. The narrow band of Timm stain seen at 3 days extends evenly over the whole suprapyramidal region of CA3, and this correlates with the lack of obvious differences in the maturity of synapses contacting the proximal apical dendrites of CA3a and CA3c pyramids. At day 5 the Timm staining is much heavier, which correlates with the increase in the vesicle content of the profiles at this stage.

The first signs of staining in the infrapyramidal mossy fibers from the granule cells of the medial blade of the dentate gyrus are seen at 5 days. At the ultrastructural level there are many fewer terminals contacting the basal dendrites of CA3c cells than the apical dendrites, and many of these are less well-developed than those in the suprapyramidal mossy fiber zone. However, the range of maturities present is similar at both sites, so that a direct quantitative comparison of the two regions would require the analysis of a large number of profiles. This variation in maturity of terminals may reflect the range of ages and differentiation of the parent dentate granule cells, which continue to be born into the third postnatal week (Altman and Das, 1965; Angevine, 1965; Schlessinger et al., 1975).

The clumps of heavy Timm staining in the mossy fiber zone of CA3a and CA3b in 7-day animals is noticeably less dense just above the cell bodies than it is more superficially. As with the 5-day animals, the wide range of profile development makes it difficult to find an ultrastructural correlate to this gradient within the mossy fiber layer. There is a tendency, however, for more mature profiles (as in Fig. 2), showing the beginnings of dendritic invaginations and evaginations, to be found more distally on the apical dendrites. A similar developmental gradient of maturity from superficial to deep within the suprapyramidal mossy fiber layer is also seen in Golgi material, where the first large mossy excrescenses on dendritic shafts (Cajal, 1911) are found some distance from pyramidal layer. The more proximally situated spines develop later, with those just above the cell somata first appearing reliably after day 12. These observations suggest that the sharp laminar segregation between the fibers of the mossy fiber zone and those lying more superficially in the stratum radiatum could, in part, be the result of the occupation of border sites by the earliest arriving mossy fibers, with later arriving axons filling in more proximally as the dendrites extend locally.

The Timm staining reaction of the mossy fiber layer goes through its final maturation from days 12—18. This correlates well with the start of the final ultrastructural maturation at day 10, and the almost adult appearance and function at day 15.

CONCLUSIONS

It is clear from a comparison of these two studies that the Timm method gives a broadly accurate picture of mossy fiber development. Ultrastructural analysis of the terminal profiles shows a wide range of maturity which gradually evens out by day 15, when the more primitive synapses have become extremely rare. These variations will not be obvious in the Timm staining, where the densest staining will tend to color the whole picture. It would be of interest to correlate changes in terminal structure with heavy metal content more directly, using X-ray diffraction techniques to estimate the contents of individual identified profiles. Similarly, after the 15th postnatal day (by which time pyramidal cells fire reliably in response to a mossy fiber volley) it is difficult to detect any further increase in synaptic efficiency using field potential analysis (Bliss et al., 1974).

It is interesting that synaptic potentials can be recorded in 5-day animals when the majority of the mossy fiber terminals have a far from adult appearance. The absence of recordable activity in 2-day-old animals may reflect both the scarcity of terminals and their low vesicle content. The presence of synapses at different stages of development (Figs. 1 and 2), side by side on the same dendrite, suggests that the formation of a post-synaptic specialization occurs when the presynaptic element immediately in contact with it has reached a critical level of development.

REFERENCES

Altman, J. and Das, G.D. (1965) Autoradiographic and histological evidence of post-natal hippocampal neurogenesis in rats, *J. comp. Neurol.*, 124: 319–336.

Angevine, J.B. (1965) Time of neuron origin in the hippocampal region, *Exp. Neurol.*, Suppl. 2: 1–70.

Blackstad, T.W. and Kjaerheim, A. (1961) Special axodendritic synapses in the hippocampal cortex. Electron and light microscopic studies on the layer of mossy fibres, *J. comp. Neurol.*, 117: 113–160.

Bliss, T.V.P., Chung, S.-H. and Stirling, R.V. (1974) Structural and functional development of the mossy fibre system in the hippocampus of the post-natal rat, *J. Physiol. (Lond.)*, 239: 92–93P.

Cajal, S. Ramón y (1911) *Histologie du Système Nerveux de l'Homme et des Vertébrés*, Vol. 2, A. Maloine, Paris.

Gray, E. G. (1959) Axosomatic and axodendritic synapses of the cerebral cortex: an electron microscope study, *J. Anat. (Lond.)*, 93: 420–443.

Hamlyn, L. H. (1962) The fine structure of the mossy fibre endings in the hippocampus of the rabbit, *J. Anat. (Lond.)*, 96: 112–120.

Larramendi, L.M.H. (1969) Analysis of synaptogenesis in the cerebellum of the mouse. In *Neurobiology of Cerebellar Evolution and Development*, R. Llinas (Ed.), Amer. Med. Assoc., Chicago, pp. 803–845.

Lorente de Nó, R. (1934) Studies on the structure of the cerebral cortex. II. Continuation of the study of the Ammonic system, *J. Psychol. Neurol. (Lpz.)*, 46: 113–177.

Reynolds, E.S. (1963) The use of lead citrate at high pH as an electron opaque stain in electron microscopy, *J. Cell Biol.*, 17: 208–212.

Schlessinger, A.R., Cowan, W.M. and Gottlieb, D.I. (1975) An autoradiographic study of the time of origin and the pattern of granule cell migration in the dentate gyrus of the rat, *J. comp. Neurol.*, 159: 149–176.

Zimmer, J. (1978) Development of the hippocampus and fascia dentata: morphological and histochemical aspects, this volume.

Zimmer, J. and Haug, F.-M.Š. (1977) Laminar differentiation of the hippocampus fascia dentata and subiculum in developing rats, observed with the Timm sulphide silver method, *J. comp. Neurol.*, in press.

Non-Ketotic Hyperglycinemia (NKH): An Inborn Error of Metabolism Affecting Brain Function Exclusively

C.J. de GROOT, V. BOELI EVERTS, B.C.L. TOUWEN and F.A. HOMMES

Departments of Pediatrics and Developmental Neurology, University Hospital, Groningen (The Netherlands)

INTRODUCTION

Non-ketotic hyperglycinemia (NKH) was first described in 1965 by Gerritsen et al. (1965), and up till now about 40 patients have been described. The inheritance is autosomal recessive. By adding *non-ketotic* to hyperglycinemia, Gerritsen et al. (1965) separated this type of hyperglycinemia (in which the hyperglycinemia is a primary and continuously present biochemical abnormality) from the earlier described cases of hyperglycinemia, where the raised plasma glycine concentration was not always present, and which were accompanied by other biochemical abnormalities. Most of the latter types of hyperglycinemia are presently known to be caused by enzymatic defects in the catabolic pathways of the branched chain amino acids (propionic acidemia, methylmalonic acidemia, isovaleric acidemia, etc.). Why these enzymatic defects are often accompanied by a rise in glycine concentration has not yet been established. There are studies (e.g. Kolvraa, 1977) which indicate that the products of branched chain amino acid metabolism, when present in abnormally high concentrations, may interfere with glycine metabolism.

In vivo (Ando et al., 1968) and in vitro (Yoshida et al., 1969; De Groot et al., 1970) studies have shown that the defect in NKH is due to an abnormality in the glycine cleavage reaction (Fig. 1). In the normal human infant, glycine cleavage is shown to occur in liver, kidney and brain (Perry et al., 1975). Furthermore, Revsin et al. (1976) showed that the fibroblasts of a

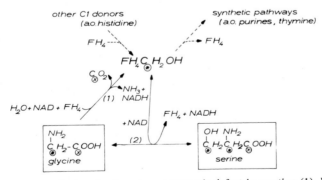

Fig. 1. In non-ketotic hyperglycinemia, there is an enzymatic defect in reaction (1). Reaction (2) might be indirectly involved when the normal C_1 supply via reaction (1) is interrupted.

NKH patient have a reduced transport capacity of glycine across the outer cell membrane. The glycine cleavage reaction is a complicated one, with at least four proteins participating in the enzymatic cleavage (Koch and Kikuchi, 1976). The exact nature of the enzymatic defect of NKH is not yet known, which is the reason why the purely descriptive name, 'non-ketotic hyperglycinemia', has now survived for more than ten years.

The clinical picture of NKH is surprisingly homogeneous, a consistent finding being the normal appearance at birth. Pregnancy, birth and the first hours of life are in fact described as 'normal' in most cases. Thereafter, signs of hypotonia, apathy and respiratory depression begin to appear. A definite, but only partial, recovery is observed if the infants survive this first period. Without exception, the children gradually progress into a state of severe mental deficiency, and show continuous low grade convulsions in addition.

The only biochemical abnormality observed is a rise in glycine concentration in various tissues, up to 5-fold the normal level in the plasma but 30—40-fold in the spinal fluid. Perry et al. (1975) pointed out that the clinical symptoms were closely correlated with the glycine concentration within the central nervous system, and not with the plasma glycine concentration.

Concerning the pathogenetic aspects, two mechanisms could be responsible for the neurological symptoms: (1) a *neurotoxicity* of glycine, and (2) a *deficiency* of 5,10-methylene tetrahydrofolic acid, or a combination of both. At this moment, clinical studies and animal experiments do not conclusively support either one or the other of these postulated pathogenetic principles. A neurotoxic action of glycine is plausible, however; particularly since Werman et al. (1968), Aprison and Werman (1965) and Curtis et al. (1967) have all shown that glycine acts as a neurotransmitter agent in certain inhibitory neurons of the spinal cord. Curtis et al. (1967) showed, furthermore, that strychnine was a rather specific antagonist for glycine, probably by competing with glycine for the receptor sites on the postsynaptic membrane.

Our studies were undertaken to investigate further this aspect of glycine neurotoxicity in patients with NKH, and in animal experiments, to study the potential of strychnine as an antidote for glycine neurotoxicity. Besides a systematic neurological examination of a newborn infant suffering from NKH, experiments will be described which aimed to simulate in animals the abnormal glycine concentration found in patients, and then to investigate the effect of strychnine administration.

CASE HISTORY AND CLINICAL INVESTIGATIONS

This particular case is especially instructive for its detailed study of the neurological abnormalities. Further, a unique longitudinal observation of the symptoms was available here.

A previous child of the family had died with the clinical and biochemical symptoms of NKH. A second child was born after a normal pregnancy of 40 weeks. Except for some weakness in crying, no abnormalities were noted at birth, and at the sixth hour of life a neurological examination revealed only some abnormal eye movements and vertical nystagmus. The infant deteriorated rapidly thereafter (Figs. 2 and 3), however, and in the period from the fourth to the eighth postnatal day was extremely hyptonic. There was almost no response to any type of external stimulus, and the respiration was shallow and irregular, with frequent periods of apneu (Table I shows the glycine concentration in plasma

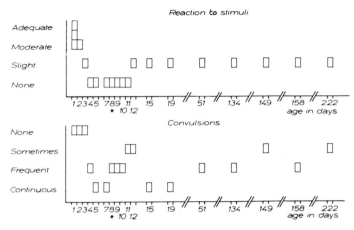

Fig. 2. Reaction to stimuli and convulsions per day. The figures on the horizontal axis denote days on which a neurological examination was carried out. The lower levels of scoring (vertical axis) indicate increasingly pathological reactions. From days 3 to 11 the patient hardly reacted to stimuli. On day 8 muscle and skin reactions were absent (demonstrated by an asterisk).

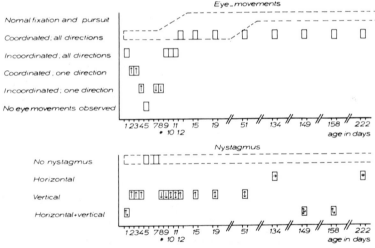

Fig. 3. Eye movements and occurrence of nystagmoid movements. The figures on the horizontal axis denote days on which a neurological examination was carried out. The scoring scale is given on the vertical axis. The stippled areas indicate expected normal responsiveness. The arrows indicate, respectively, the preponderant direction of eye movements and nystagmoid movements. A vertical nystagmus is abnormal at any age. The asterisk denotes the worst condition of the child (day 8).

and spinal fluid). She was expected to die, but from day 8 onward she showed a slight but definite recovery. She remained grossly neurologically abnormal, however, and at the age of five years is severely mentally retarded, with hypsarrhythmic convulsions occurring frequently.

TABLE I

Age	Plasma glycine (μmol/ml)	CFS-GLY (μmol/ml)	P/CFS
42 (hr)	0.72	0.17	4.2
4 (days)	0.76	0.24	3.2
12	0.91	0.21	4.3
35	1.08	0.17	6.3
102	1.09	0.13	8.4
118	0.76	0.09	8.4
Normal	0.16–0.28	0.005–0.01	>20

GLYCINE NEUROTOXICITY IN RATS OF DIFFERENT AGES

Rats were treated with a massive dose of glycine by subcutaneous injections (3 mg/g). Such a high dose was needed to reach concentrations of glycine in the forebrain comparable to that found in patients with NKH (Bachman et al. 1971; Perry et al., 1975). A control group of rats was treated with equimolar doses of serine. A characteristic sequence of abnormal behavior was observed in glycine-treated newborn rats, which was not seen in the serine-treated newborn rats (Table II). The symptoms of neurotoxicity observed were restricted to newborn and 8-day-old rats, no symptoms being observed in older rats with even higher forebrain glycine concentrations. (The ammonia levels were elevated to the same extent after both the serine and the glycine injections, so that this cannot be the factor responsible for the effects observed in the experimental group.) Administration of a relatively low dose of strychnine to the glycine-treated newborn rats clearly improved the survival rate (Table III). It was not possible to demonstrate the converse relationship between strychnine and glycine, i.e. whether strychnine toxicity would be mitigated by a high glycine concentration; the rigidity produced by strychnine was not any less when the animals were pretreated with different doses of glycine (Table IV).

TABLE II

THE NEUROTOXICITY OF GLYCINE IN RATS AT DIFFERENT AGES

(Subcutaneous injection of glycine, 3 mg per g weight.)

	Newborn	8 days	15 days	21 days
Glycine μmol/g (forebrain)	2–7	4–7	4–8	5–10
1–8′: rotatory behavior	+	–	–	–
7–14′: periods of prolonged standstill	+	–	–	–
11–30′: no spontaneous movements, convulsions	+	±	–	–
18–30′: respiratory depression, cyanosis	+	±	–	–
† at 30′	21/29	3/8	0/10	0/8

TABLE III

THE DIFFERENCE IN SURVIVAL RATE IN GLYCINE,
GLYCINE-STRYCHNINE AND STRYCHNINE TREATED
NEWBORN RATS

	Total	Survival	%
Glycine (3 mg/g)	29	8	28
Glycine + strychnine (0.2 μg/g)	30	27	90
Strychnine (0.2 μg/g)	24	23	96

TABLE IV

THE INFLUENCE OF GLYCINE AND SERINE ON THE DEVELOPMENT OF STRYCHNINE
RIGIDITY IN RATS

n.o.: not observed; +: weak rigidity; ++: stronger rigidity; +++: total rigidity (†); −: no rigidity.

Strychnine (μg/g weight)	Newborn				8 days			
	Gly 3 mg/g	Gly 4.5 mg/g	Ser 4.2 mg/g		Gly 3 mg/g	Gly 4.5 mg/g	Ser 4.2 mg/g
0.06	−	−	n.o.	n.o.	−	−	n.o.	−
0.1	−	n.o.	n.o.	n.o.	±	±	n.o.	±
0.2	−	−	−	n.o.	n.o.	n.o.	n.o.	n.o.
0.4	+	+	+	n.o.	+	+	n.o.	n.o.
0.8	+	n.o.	+	n.o.	+	+	n.o.	n.o.
2.0	++	++	++	++	++	++	n.o.	n.o.
4.0	++	++	++	n.o.				
8.0	+++	+++	+++	+++				

CONCLUSIONS AND SUMMARY

The neurological sequence of the patient described here is more in accordance with a glycine neurotoxicity than with a deficiency of some metabolic factor, both because of its sudden onset, and because the abnormalities could be simulated in newborn rats by injecting glycine. Moreover, the very rapid change seen in the infant is more likely the result of a toxic action than the expression of an abnormality in a synthetic process. The type of clinical abnormalities show that the toxicity is expressed as an extreme inhibition of both voluntary and involuntary movements. This is consistent with the idea that the glycine neurotransmission system is hyperactive. Whether it is glycine re-uptake from the synaptic cleft, or axonal transport which is altered by the defective mitochondrial glycine cleavage cannot be decided. Support for the former theory, i.e. that the glycine neurotransmission system is overactive, is provided by the animal experiments.

Noteworthy is the very characteristic rotatory behavior ('barrelling') appearing a few minutes after the glycine injection in the rats, which could be the analogue of the abnormal eye movements observed in the newborn infant. In the newborn rat, a glycine concentration in the forebrain comparable to the glycine concentration found in the cerebral cortex of NKH patients (postmortem assay), resulted in marked hypotonia, respiratory depression and convulsions. These symptoms were seen to a much lesser degree when serine was injected, nor were there any convulsive or barrelling movements. The mitigating action of strychnine supports the suggestion that glycine neurotransmission could be involved in the syndrome. The failure to observe any mitigating action of glycine on the appearance of strychnine rigidity, on the other hand, could be due to the stronger binding capacity of strychnine for postsynaptic receptor sites, as compared with glycine. Another possibility is that strychnine has additional actions than on glycine-sensitive receptors (see Sedláček, this volume).

A remarkable phenomenon is the decreased neurotoxicity of glycine with increasing age of the rats. In the patient, a slight recovery was observed which could not be attributed to a change in the glycine concentration of the spinal fluid. The age-dependent neurotoxicity could point to immaturity of the glycine synapses at birth, with a hyper-sensitivity of the postsynaptic membrane for glycine. This has been shown to be true for the noradrenergic system: rats in which the noradrenergic synapses had been damaged by 6-hydroxydopamine became extremely sensitive to low doses of noradrenaline (Woodward et al., 1971).

The question whether the severe mental deficiency observed in NKH patients is related to glycine neurotoxicity is impossible to answer by either the clinical observation or the animal experiments. The clinical syndrome is perhaps partly due to a disturbance of glycine neuro-transmission, and partly to a shortage of methylated groups which are normally supplied by glycine cleavage. It might well be that the physiological role of glycine cleavage within the CNS is to prevent a rise in glycine concentration, and so to protect glycine neurotransmission (but one wonders about the physiological role of this same reaction in liver and kidney, where an absence of glycine cleavage does not appear to be associated with any symptoms indicative of dysfunction).

REFERENCES

Ando, T., Nyhan, W.L., Gerritsen, T., Gong, L., Heiner, D.A. and Bray, P.F. (1968) Metabolism of glycine in the non-ketotic form of hyperglycinemia, *Ped. Res.*, 2: 254–291.

Aprison, M.H. and Werman, R. (1965) The distribution of glycine in cat spinal cord and roots, *Life Sci.*, 4: 2075–2083.

Bachman, C., Mihatsch, M.J., Baumgartner, R.E., Brechbuhler, T., Bühler, U.K., Olafsson, A., Ohnacker, A. und Wick, H. (1971) Nicht-ketotische hyperglyzinämie: perakuter Verlauf im Neugebornalter, *Helv. paediatr. Acta*, 26: 228–243.

Curtis, D.R., Hösli, L. and Johnston, G.A.R. (1967) The inhibition of spinal neurones by glycine, *Nature (Lond.)*, 215: 1502–1503.

De Groot, C.J., Troelstra, J.A. and Hommes, F.A. (1970) Non-ketotic hyperglycinemia: an in vitro study of the glycine-serine conversion in liver of three patients and the effect of dietary methionine, *Ped. Res.*, 4: 238–243.

Gerritsen, Th., Kaveggia, E. and Waisman, H.A. (1965) A new type of idiopathic hyperglycinemia with hypo-oxaluria, *Pediatrics*, 36: 882–891.

Kochi, H. and Kikuchi, K. (1976) Mechanism of reversible glycine cleavage reaction in *Arthrobacter globiformis*. *Arch. Biochem. Biophys.*, 173: 71–81.

Kolvraa, S. (1977) Inhibition of the glycine cleavage system by branched chain aminoacid metabolites, *Abstract, S.S.I.E.M. Meeting*, Copenhagen, in press.

Morel, P. (1976) *L'Hyperglycinémie sans Cetose*, Thesis, Lille.

Perry, T.L., Urquhart, N., MacLean, J., Evans, M.E., Hansen, S., Davidson, A.G.F., Applegarth, D.A., MacLeod, P.J. and Lock, J.E. (1975) Non-ketotic hyperglycinemia: glycine accumulation due to absence of glycine cleavage in brain, *New Engl. J. Med.*, 292: 1269–1273.

Revsin, B. and Morrow, I.I.I. (1976) Glycine transport in normal and non-ketotic hyperglycinemic human diploid fibroblasts, *Exp. Cell Res.*, 100: 95–103.

Sedláček, J. (1978) The development of supraspinal control of spontaneous motility in chick embryos, this volume.

Werman, R., Didoff, R. and Aprison, M.H. (1968) Inhibitory action of glycine on spinal neurones in the cat, *J. Neurophysiol.*, 31: 81–95.

Woodward, D.J., Hoffer, B.J., Siggins, G.R., Bloom, F.E. (1971) The autogenetic development of synaptic junctions, synaptic activation and responsiveness to neurotransmittor substances in rat cerebellar Purkinje cells, *Brain Res.*, 34: 73–97.

Yoshida, T., Kikuchi, G., Tada, K., Narisawa, K. and Arakawa, T. (1969) Physiological significance of glycine cleavage system in the human liver as revealed by the study of a case of hyperglycinemia, *Biochem. biophys. Res. Commun.*, 35: 577–583.

Note added in proof.

Gitzelmann et al. recently treated a boy of 6.5 months with NKH for 12 months with oral strychnine with remarkable results (*Helv. paediat. Acta* (1978) 32: 517–525).

DISCUSSION

CORNER: Is there anything known about the distribution and the compartmentation of the glycine in the brain at stages during which it *is* very toxic in the rat, as compared to stages when it does not seem to have this toxicity?

DE GROOT: We have not made any studies of this kind. About the glycine distribution in the CNS, it is known that the glycine concentration is higher in spinal cord and brain stem than in the midbrain and cortical structures. The glycine cleavage reaction, on the contrary, is known to be more active in the cortical structures than in the lower parts of the CNS. As far as I know, there are no data available in animals for glycine distribution at stages where it is toxic. In patients, Perry et al. and Morell do mention some data about glycine concentration in the brain.

MEISAMI: The 8th postnatal day is a rather interesting day because, in the rat, the blood-brain-barrier develops at about that age. Could the development of the neurotoxic effect be actually a problem of the maturity of the blood-brain-barrier?

DE GROOT: That is what we thought at first, but it seemed not to be the case in our experiments. The glycine concentration in the forebrain was not lower in the older animals; in fact, we measured higher concentrations (up to 10 μmol/g) in the older animals, whereas the symptoms of acute toxicity diminished (see Table II).

MEISAMI: Did you observe this high glycine level in the CSF of mature animals as well, after injection?

DE GROOT: We did not measure the glycine level in the CSF. In the young animals we could not get enough cerebrospinal fluid for reliable measurements. All measurements were made in forebrain tissue (Table II).

ZIMMER: From your slides I saw that you started taking blood samples from 0 hours. How did you know that this particular child was going to be sick?

DE GROOT: It is a recessive disorder, and the child had a sister who has the disease. In fact, we had already measured amniotic fluid levels of glycine, because we knew there was a 25% chance that another child in the family might have the same disease. The amniotic fluid glycine concentration was absolutely normal.

MURPHEY: It is well known that high levels of one amino acid will affect the transport and uptake of others. In your human studies, did you measure amino acid concentrations, (e.g. other short-chain neutroaminoacids), to see if your high glycine concentration was in fact affecting concentrations of other amino acids in the brain?

DE GROOT: Yes, we measured many other amino acids in the cerebrospinal fluid of patients (lysine, histidine, threonine, serine, glutamic acid, glutamine, asparagine, alanine, valine, isoleucine, leucine, tyrosine, phenylalanine) and we could not find any differences in concentrations of these amino acids as compared with normal. In some of our rats we measured these amino acids as well, and here too there was no significant difference from controls. As far as the pathogenesis of NKH is concerned, I would also like to say that the change of condition in patients is so dramatic and rapid that it is unlikely that this is due to a secondary competition of transport of the other amino acids, particularly because the glycine concentration in the plasma of patients with NKH is only 3–5 times higher.

BLOW: Could it be that glycine is interfering with brain development only in a certain 'critical' stage of development?

DE GROOT: Yes, our working hypothesis is that the glycine synapse is developing around that period, and that what we are seeing in our rats could be the period of extremely high sensitivity during the final stages of development of this synapse, when the postsynaptic membrane is already there and is very sensitive for glycine. The reason for this could be that the synapse is not fully mature, and that glycine from the environment is more easily coming into contact with the postsynaptic membrane.

BLOM: Is the EEG pattern different from the normal developmental pattern, and do you have any neuropathological data on these children?

DE GROOT: Well, what you see in many of these infants are spike- and wave-patterns. The EEG very often has the characteristics of hypsarrhythmia. In some other reported children a postmortem examination was done but nothing specific was found in these infants. It is indeed very remarkable, compared with the severe clinical picture, that most reports show no specific abnormalities in the brain. But the investigations which have been made so far are not very sophisticated.

BERRY: Dr. Dobbing, I would like you to make a comment on the comparability of the newborn rat and the newborn human being, with respect to the relative maturation of the brain.

DOBBING: Well, you are making guesses when you try and match them up. We think we have reason for believing that a newborn human is approximately equivalent to the 5- or 6-day-old rat. But a newborn rat is somewhere around mid-pregnancy in the human. However, this does not tell us very much because you don't know that, if you were to have a prematurely born baby, you might not have had these changes at that stage just as readily.

DE GROOT: Speculating further, you could postulate either that in the rat the glycine synaptic system appears relatively early in development, or that in the newborn infant the glycine synaptic system appears relatively late. Why the fetus is so free from symptoms is the real question. The blood-brain-barrier is (for glycine at least) already present before birth. Taking into account the altered ratio between glycine concentration of blood and brain, and also the fact that the glycine-splitting reaction is already active before birth, you would expect to find a high glycine concentration in the spinal fluid and brain of NKH-patients prior to birth.

DOBBING: I don't understand what you mean by: the glycine blood-brain-barrier is there at such and such a time.

DE GROOT: What I mean by the glycine blood-brain-barrier is the difference between the plasma glycine concentration and the glycine concentration in the brain or CSF, without attempting to indicate the location of the barrier. When you measure CSF levels of glycine and the ratio of blood to CSF, you will find a much higher ratio for glycine than for glucose or lactate, for instance.

DOBBING: Another therapeutic possibility is that if only you could protect that brain from getting too much glycine until the time of insensitivity, then your protection could probably persist without any further disability over the age of 18 months or 2 years, just as with many of the inborn errors.

DE GROOT: I agree with you that it seems most important to protect the brain, at least during the first 2 years. It remains to be seen, however, whether or not glycine accumulation in the brain after that period is harmless.

SECTION IV

SENSORY INFLUENCES UPON NEUROGENESIS

Influence of Early Anosmia
on the Developing Olfactory Bulb

ESMAIL MEISAMI

Institute of Biochemistry and Biophysics, University of Tehran, P.O. Box 314-1700, Tehran (Iran)

The older conception of ontogeny as a process of construction of a machine which, after construction is completed, begins to function, seems less and less satisfactory as our knowledge advances. Living protoplasm is functioning at all times and development is a process of functional construction, that is beginning with a given structure and function, the continuance of function modifies the structural substratum, and this in turn modifies further function and so on (Child, 1921).

INTRODUCTION

Although the relative shares of nature and environment in the development of the individual's brain and behavior has always been an engaging subject among the philosophers, serious experimental work on this subject started only by the end of the nineteenth century. The famous embryologist, W. Roux, by 1895 had proposed a theory stating that the development of the nervous system consists of an early stage of intrinsic growth and self differentiation, followed by a later period when neural development depends on functional activity of its structural constituents (Roux, 1895). An early experiment often cited by reviewers was that of H. Berger (1900); he studied the effects of closure of eyelids of young puppies and kittens on the development of cortical visual areas, and found shrinkage of the visual cortex accompanied by increased cell crowding and reduced Nissl substance. Berger's own conclusion is a good summary of the whole case of the neurobiologist with environmentalist convictions:

> These investigations have demonstrated that the brain which has received stimulation is significantly different in a material way from brain which has not received any. Also, these findings have their major significance in so far as they reveal that the external stimulation leaves lasting changes in the brain – the organ of the psyche.

Throughout the twentieth century and up to the present time there have been numerous experiments in this area (for reviews see: Riesen, 1966; Globus, 1975; Meisami, 1975), nearly all of which utilized the visual system as their model, and most of which supported either in substance or in theory the generalization made by Berger. Searching for more universal verification of this generalization, investigators have occasionally turned their attention to other sensory modalities as a model system. An example can be found in the work of Van der Loos and Woolsey (1973), who observed in mice that, following removal at birth of mystacial hairs in the vibrissal pads, massive structural and functional alterations occur in the corresponding cell assemblies ('barrels') of the somatosensory cortex.

It is time that developmental neurobiology, in its quest for finding the mechanisms of sensory influences on brain development, pays due attention to the variety of long neglected senses; in fact some of these senses, such as the above mentioned vibrissal pads of the rodents and carnivores and the olfactory sense of rodents (see below), may be of much more general significance in the early life of these animals than the visual system which, incidentally, begins functioning at a relatively late stage in brain development. In this paper, through a preliminary discussion of the merits of the developing olfactory system, followed by presentation and discussion of some experimental findings, we wish to suggest that the olfactory system of the rat possesses most of the requirements for a suitable model system for the study of the influence of sensory receptors in general, and their functional activity, on central sensory structures during the postnatal phase of brain development.

The rat is a macrosmatic animal with very well developed central olfactory structures. The two olfactory bulbs, being anatomically distinct from the rest of the brain and possessing a highly regular and well-laminated structure, lend themselves easily to detailed quantitative analysis of their morphological elements as well as of the neurochemical constituents. Thus, reliable and reproducible counts of the total number of mitral and tufted cells may be made without resort to the statistical extrapolations commonly exercised when similar procedures are carried out for a structure such as the cerebral cortex. Similarly, the ease with which one can isolate the entire bulb from the brain allows total DNA measurements in the whole bulb, which in turn may be used as a good measure of the total number of cells.

In the account given below we shall summarize some of our published and unpublished work on the effects of olfactory deprivation during the postnatal period on the morphological and neurochemical features of the developing rat olfactory bulb.

EXPERIMENTAL METHODS FOR PRODUCTION OF NEONATAL ANOSMIA

Unilateral olfactory deprivation

As was stated above, each olfactory bulb receives its entire afferent input solely from its ipsilateral olfactory mucosa. This anatomical situation provides an ideal system, where the effects of unilateral olfactory deprivation on the ipsilateral olfactory bulb may properly be compared with its control counterpart, i.e. the contralateral bulb. Under this condition, since the same animal serves as its own control, all statistical problems arising from inter-animal differences in the magnitude of the variables being measured can be bypassed.

Until recently no suitable method was available for producing unilateral olfactory deprivation. The olfactory mucosa is situated on a highly convoluted bony surface inside the posterior and upper parts of the ventral nasal cavity. Normally the stimulation of the olfactory mucosa is brought about by active sniffing of the inspiratory air containing the odorous substances. The most reasonable way to deprive the olfactory receptors of stimulation would, therefore, be to prevent the flow of inspiratory air into the nasal cavity. In the adult animal, whose skull and nasal cavities have reached mature size, one can use various mechanical stoppers inside or in front of the nares to prevent the flow of inspiratory air temporarily. However, such procedures are not practical for the growing rat pup, where the constant and rapid growth of the skull and nasal passages as well as the nursing activities of the animal prevent continuous use of a stopper. Furthermore, the soft tissues around the nare of the newborn are very sensitive and do not withstand excessive manipulation; they rupture very easily and cause excessive bleeding. We therefore devised a simple method for production of neonatal unilateral anosmia which would cause no direct mechanical or chemical damage to the olfactory mucosa, and which would prevent the inflow of inspiratory air to the nasal passages.

In our method, the tissue surrounding one of the external nares of the newborn or the young pup is cauterized. The damaged tissue soon regenerates and often forms a continous membrane over the external nare, producing a natural mechanical barrier against the flow of inspiratory air and odours. The appearance of this membrane a few days and a few weeks after the operation is shown in Fig. 1. The details of technical procedures and further discussions of this method may be found elsewhere (Meisami, 1976). Once such a condition of unilateral olfactory deprivation is produced, one can then proceed to study its effect on the developing olfactory bulb.

B

A

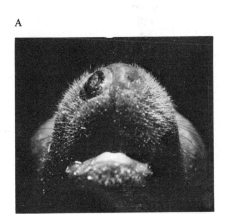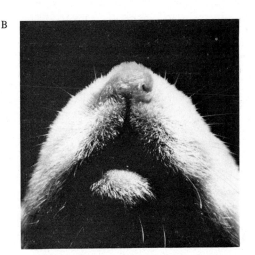

Fig. 1. Demonstration of the cauterized and normal nares of a 5-day-old (A) and a 25-day-old (B) rat. The right nare had been cauterized two days after birth. Formation of a membrane and consequent occlusion of the right nare is clearly evident in the 25-day-old animal.

Olfactory deafferentation

In addition to the milder and more physiological condition of olfactory deprivation, one can also study the effects of complete olfactory deafferentation on the developing bulb. The latter condition is admittedly a more severe case of sensory deprivation, involving pathological responses consequent to the complete withdrawal of the axons of the degenerating olfactory receptor cells. However, such a study is useful for the purpose of comparison and interpretation of the effects produced by the deprivation of olfactory stimulation alone.

Unlike the visual system, where deafferentation is a fairly simple operation, brought about by the removal of one or two eyes or sectioning of one or two of the optic nerves, deafferentation in the olfactory system is a difficult operation posing several serious practical problems. First and foremost, it is not possible to remove the entire mucosa by surgical procedures, since the highly convoluted bony surface makes complete deafferentation an impossible task. The surest way of causing complete olfactory deafferentation is to destroy the olfactory receptors by means of bathing the entire olfactory mucosa with a poisonous chemical solution such as zinc sulfate (Smith, 1938). Complete and irreversible degeneration of the olfactory neuroepithelium can be rapidly produced in rats by the application of a 1%

214

solution to the nasal cavities. The technique has been extensively used for the study of degeneration and regeneration phenomena in the olfactory mucosa (Mulvaney and Heist, 1971; Margolis et al., 1974; Schulz, 1960), although up till now only in the adult rat. In our studies we extend this procedure to the newborn animal (the details and problems of the technical procedure are given elsewhere: Meisami and Manochehri, 1977).

EFFECTS OF OLFACTORY DEPRIVATION OR DEAFFERENTATION ON THE GROWTH OF THE OLFACTORY BULB

Effects of unilateral olfactory deprivation

In order to observe the effects of unilateral olfactory deprivation on the growth of the olfactory bulb, several litters of albino rat pups were made unilaterally anosmic during the first two days after birth, according to the procedure outlined above. Observations of the central olfactory structures were made at days 10, 25 and 60, and in older rats. Visual examination of the olfactory structures revealed a distinct underdevelopment of the olfactory bulb and tract on the side ipsilateral to the closed nare, the effect being seen already at day 10 (Fig. 2). The mean weights of the normal and anosmic bulbs at various ages are shown in Fig. 3, and confirm the qualitative impressions. In addition, it appears that the greatest inhibitory effects are exerted during the first 3 weeks, when the bulb is showing its highest rate of growth.

Examination and comparison of a number of left and right bulbs in normal animals at various ages shows that there is no significant difference between the two bulbs (Fig. 4).

A

B

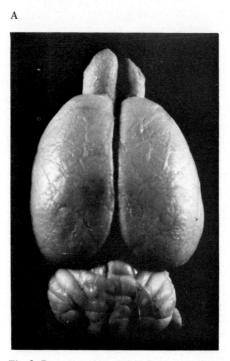
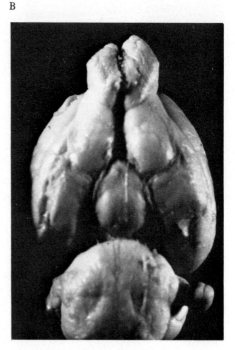

Fig. 2. Demonstration of the effects of unilateral olfactory deprivation on the appearance of the olfactory structures in a 30-day-old rat, (A: dorsal view; B: ventral view).

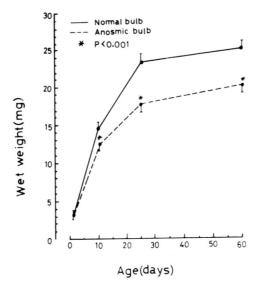

Fig. 3. Effects of neonatal unilateral anosmia on the growth of normal and anosmic olfactory bulbs. The anosmic bulb is that which is ipsilateral to the cauterized nare, whether it be on the right or left side. Each point is the mean weight of at least 18 bulbs. Vertical bars indicate standard error of the mean. *P* values are obtained using the *t*-test for paired sample means. (See Meisami, 1976.)

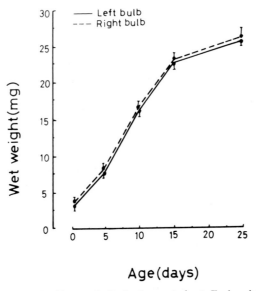

Fig. 4. Growth of the right and left olfactory bulbs in the normal rat. Each point is the mean weight of at least 12 bulbs. Vertical bars indicate the magnitude of the standard error of the mean. No significant difference between the mean weights are evident at any age.

Further, comparison of the mean weight of normal bulbs in experimental animals with the mean weight of either the left or right bulbs in normal animals (Table I) reveals no significant difference. These results rule out the possibility that the observed effects are the result of hypertrophy of the control bulb in experimental animals, rather than an inhibitory effect

TABLE I

COMPARISON OF THE WEIGHTS OF INDIVIDUAL OLFACTORY BULBS IN
NORMAL AND UNILATERALLY ANOSMIC 25-DAY-OLD RATS

	Normal animal		Unilaterally anosmic animal	
	Left bulbs	Right bulbs	Normal bulbs	Anosmic bulbs
Weight (mg)	25.5 ± 1.1*	25.6 ± 0.8	23.8 ± 0.9	17.8 ± 1.1
% Difference		–	(25%)**	

*Mean ± S.E.M; each value is the mean of at least 20 bulbs.
**$P < 0.01$, based on the t-test.

TABLE II

EFFECTS OF NEONATAL UNILATERAL OLFACTORY DEPRIVA-
TION ON THE DIMENSIONS OF THE OLFACTORY BULBS

	Dimension (microns)		
	Length	Width	Height
Normal bulbs	3018 ± 91*	2491 ± 30	2685 ± 79
Anosmic bulbs	2482 ± 98**	2247 ± 82	1902 ± 94**
% Difference	18%	10%	29%

*Mean ± S.E.M; each value is the mean of 4 measurements. Length and
height measurements were made on sagittal sections and width on
frontal sections.
**$P < 0.05$, based on the t-test.

on the anosmic bulb. We have made similar observations with regard to other neurochemical
and anatomical parameters (see below). Growth inhibition was naturally manifested also in
the *size* of the anosmic bulbs; in 25-day-old unilaterally anosmic animals, the length, width
and height of the anosmic bulbs were 18, 10 and 29% smaller, respectively (Table II).

Effects of bilateral olfactory deafferentation

In the bilaterally deafferented animals similar results were obtained. Fig. 5 shows the
extent of growth retardation in the olfactory bulbs of the deprived rats; it is clear that the
effect of actual deafferentation is more severe than with unilateral deprivation. As expected
the effect is more severe in the deafferented group than in the olfactory deprived group,
because while olfactory deprivation is thought to be a state of relative absence of function
in the presence of structure (olfactory receptor neuron and its axon), deafferentation is the
state of absence of structure and function. Yet, even though part of this severity is due to
massive transneuronal degeneration, it must be stated that animals made completely anosmic
at birth suffer considerable overall growth retardation (by 22%) as a result of undernutrition
(Meisami and Manochehri, 1977; Shafa et al., 1976). In fact, the mean weight of the cerebellum in anosmic animals (which obviously could not be directly affected by olfactory
deafferentation) was 10% lower than in the control group.

The response seen in our deafferented bulb experiments is apparently not limited to the
developing animal, nor is it species-specific; a similar, but milder, weight loss has been

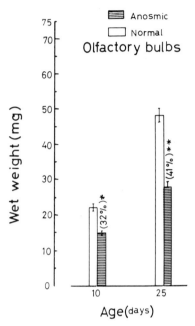

Fig. 5. Mean weights of olfactory bulbs in normal and bilaterally deafferented (anosmic) rats at 10 and 25 days of age. Each point is the mean of at least 14 pairs of bulbs. Vertical bars indicate S.E.M. *$P < 0.05$ **$P < 0.01$. (From Meisami and Manochehri, 1977.)

reported in the adult mouse by Margolis and coworkers (1974). It has also been observed in young (but weaned) rabbits (Powell, 1967) and dogs (Klosovsky and Kosmarskaya, 1963) that the olfactory bulbs become smaller after destruction of the olfactory mucosa. Interestingly, similar findings had been noted by Gudden (1870) a century ago: suturing one of the nostrils, or surgical removal of the mucosa, in newborn rabbits led to the underdevelopment of central olfactory structures 6—8 weeks after the operation.

SOME NEUROCHEMICAL CORRELATES OF OLFACTORY DEPRIVATION AND DEAFFERENTATION IN THE OLFACTORY BULB

Having observed the effects of olfactory deprivation and deafferentation on the growth of the bulb, we attempted to investigate the underlying metabolic and neurochemical causes of the underdevelopment. We wished to know whether the observed biochemical effects would show a general pattern of underdevelopment of various neurochemical parameters of the olfactory bulb, or rather some selective and specific effects on a particular neuronal system or component.

We measured protein, RNA and DNA content in the bulb, as well as the activity of two brain enzymes, *Na,K-ATPase* and *acetylcholinesterase*. Protein and RNA measurements would indicate the general metabolic state of the normal versus anosmic bulb, while DNA content is a standard method for estimating the total cell number. Na,K-ATPase is a well known marker for synaptic membranes, and acetylcholinesterase an index of cholinergic or cholinoreceptive neuronal system.

Unpublished work from our laboratory has shown that during the first month after birth, the total protein, RNA and DNA in the bulb increase 12-, 5- and 6-fold, respectively. Part of the increase in DNA is no doubt due to proliferation of glial cells, but neurogenesis in the postnatal bulb has also been demonstrated by thymidine autoradiography (Bayer and Altman, 1975). Our studies indicate that bulbar Na,K-ATPase activity is practically absent at birth, but that some acetylcholinesterase activity is present. However, both of these enzymes show extremely large increases in activity during the first postnatal month.

In order to observe the biochemical consequences of unilateral olfactory deprivation in the developing bulb, we rendered the newborn rats unilaterally anosmic as shown above. At day 25 (i.e. just after weaning) the bulbs were carefully and rapidly removed, frozen in liquid nitrogen and assayed later on for the above chemical constituents. The total protein content and concentration of protein in the normal and anosmic bulbs were determined at other ages as well, and the results are depicted in Fig. 6. The data for DNA, cell number and RNA are depicted in Table III, for Na,K-ATPase in Table IV and for acetylcholinesterase in Table V.

Effects on DNA, RNA and protein

Examinations and comparison of the data in Tables III–V, and in Fig. 6 reveals that neonatal olfactory deprivation leads to a state of chemical underdevelopment in the anosmic bulb. Thus, while our measurements show no difference between the two bulbs in the normal animal, the mean total content of DNA, RNA and protein of the anosmic bulb in experimental animals are lower by 20, 34 and 31%, respectively (as compared with the normal bulb).

The fact that the anosmic bulb contains 20% less DNA than does the normal bulb indicates a smaller number of cells, which could be due to either one or both of the following causes: (a) an inhibitory effect on postnatal cell proliferation; (b) extensive cell death as a result of anosmia. If cell death is in fact occurring, then it is of course impossible from the DNA data alone to determine which population of bulbar cells are dying. The histologic results to be presented below indicate that a considerable percentage of the *macroneurons* drop out in the anosmic bulb. However, since the proportion of these cells is very small,

TABLE III

EFFECTS OF NEONATAL UNILATERAL OLFACTORY DEPRIVATION ON THE CONCENTRATION AND TOTAL CONTENT OF DNA AND RNA IN THE OLFACTORY BULBS OF 25-DAY-OLD RATS*

		Normal bulb	Anosmic bulb	% Change
DNA concentration	(μg/mg wet wt.)	3.0 ± 0.2**	3.0 ± 0.2	–
DNA content	(μg/bulb)	70.7 ± 3.0	56.3 ± 2.1	20[§]
Total number of cells***	(no./bulb)	10.1×10^6	8.0×10^6	20[§]
RNA concentration	(μg/mg wet wt.)	3.2 ± 0.3	2.8 ± 0.2	12
RNA content	(μg/bulb)	88.6 ± 6.8	59.4 ± 2.6	33[§]

*DNA and RNA were measured according to Burton's (1956) and Cerrioti's (1955) procedures, respectively, as modified in our laboratory.

**Mean ± S.E.M.; each value is the mean of measured values from at least 6 bulbs, each bulb being measured in duplicate and independently.

***This value was computed by dividing the total content of DNA by 7 pg, the estimated amount of DNA per nerve cell.

[§]$P < 0.05$, based on the t-test.

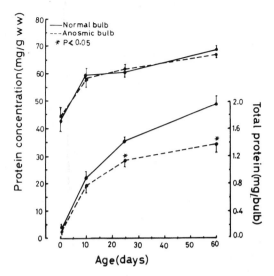

Fig. 6. Effects of neonatal unilateral anosmia on protein concentration (top) and total protein content (bottom) of normal and anosmic olfactory bulbs. The anosmic bulb is that which is ipsilateral to the cauterized and occluded nare. Each point is the mean of at least 20 independent determinations from 10 bulbs. Vertical bars indicate the magnitude of the standard error of the mean. Protein determination was carried out in duplicate using homogenates of single bulbs, according to the method of Lowry et al. with lyzozyme as the standard. P values are obtained using the t-test for paired sample means. (See Meisami, 1976.)

the considerable amount of DNA lost must mostly be due to the death of either glial cells or smaller (granular) neurons.

The significantly lower total contents of RNA and protein in the anosmic bulb (34 and 31%, Table III) could also be the sum of two different causes: (a) loss of cells from the bulb; (b) loss of metabolic vigor in the remaining cells due to decreased olfactory stimulation. The latter possibility is suggested by the fact that RNA and protein levels in the anosmic bulb are both reduced by about 30%, which exceeds the reduction observed for DNA by more than 10%.

That the concentration of all three substances is the same in both normal and anosmic bulbs indicates that postnatal olfactory deprivation does not affect any one of these substances specifically.

Effects on Na,K-ATPase

NA,K-ATPase is an enzyme abundant in plasma and in synaptic membranes (de Robertis, 1969). Functionally, the enzyme is thought to be intimately associated with the operation of the Na–K pump of the plasma membrane, essential for the maintenance of membrane potentials in excitable cells (Skou, 1965). This fact, plus the demonstration that the activity of the enzyme appears after birth and increases profoundly during the postnatal period, has led to the use of this enzyme as a marker for biochemical differentiation of the neuronal membranes and synapses during the postnatal period of brain development.

In our experiments we measured the activity of Na,K-ATPase in the olfactory bulbs of normal, of bilaterally deolfacted, and of unilaterally anosmic animals. The two latter groups had been made anosmic a few days after birth and the activity measurements were carried out at day 25. It is clear from examination of the results in Table IV that complete

TABLE IV

EFFECTS OF NEONATAL UNILATERAL OLFACTORY DEPRIVA-
TION AND NEONATAL BILATERAL OLFACTORY DEAFFEREN-
TATION ON THE ACTIVITY OF Na,K-ATPase IN THE OLFACTORY
BULBS OF 25-DAY-OLD RATS*

Na,K-ATPase activity (nmoles Pi/min/mg wet wt.)			
Unilateral olfactory deprivation		Bilateral olfactory deafferentation	
Normal bulb	Anosmic bulb	Normal bulbs	Anosmic bulbs
36.8 ± 3.3**	24.2 ± 2.4 §	27.8 ± 2.9	19.2 ± 2.1
	(35%)		(30%)

*Na,K-ATPase was assayed according to Meisami and Timiras (1974);
phosphate was assayed according to Eibl and Land (1969).
**Mean ± S.E.M.; each value is the mean activity of at least 8 samples,
each assayed in duplicate and independently. Values in parentheses indicate per cent change from the normal value.
§$P < 0.05$, based on the t-test.

olfactory deafferentation, as well as unilateral olfactory deprivation, retards the postnatal
increases in the specific activity of the enzyme. Thus, it is concluded that postnatal
membranogenesis and synaptogenesis in the olfactory bulb are partly dependent upon the
presence of olfactory input during the early life of the animal. It is interesting that we
found similar results in the visual system of dark-reared rats (Meisama and Timiras, 1974).

Effects on acetylcholinesterase

The second enzyme investigated was acetylcholinesterase, which is generally considered
to be a good index of cholinergic and/or cholinoreceptive neurons in nervous tissue. Our
unpublished observations indicate that, in the rat olfactory bulb, the specific enzyme activity
present at birth is less than 10% of that found in the adult. The great rise of activity during
postnatal development presumably reflects both the formation of new cholinergic neurons,
or synapses, and the continued maturation of the already existing ones.

TABLE V

EFFECTS OF NEONATAL UNILATERAL OLFACTORY
DEPRIVATION ON THE ACTIVITY OF ACETYL-
CHOLINESTERASE IN THE OLFACTORY BULBS OF 25-
DAY-OLD RATS*

	Acetylcholinesterase activity	
	Normal bulb	Anosmic bulb
Specific activity**	5.8 ± 0.8	5.5 ± 0.3
Total activity***	146.0 ± 7.0	129.0 ± 7.3

*Acetylcholinesterase activity was determined according to
Ellman et al. (1961).
**nmoles ACh hydrolyzed/min/mg wet wt.
***nmoles ACh hydrolyzed/min/bulb.

Our purpose in measuring acetylcholinesterase activity in the anosmic bulb was to investigate the possible role of olfactory stimulation on the maturation of cholinergic neurons. Our results (Table V) revealed that, while the total activity of acetylcholinesterase in the anosmic bulb is lower than that found in the normal bulb, the *specific* activity of this enzyme in the anosmic bulb (whether expressed per unit fresh weight or per unit protein) shows no significant difference from the values found in the normal bulb. It thus appears that lack of olfactory stimulation has no specific effect on cholinergic neurons during the postnatal period, but rather a general loss of cells in the bulb, including the cholinergic ones.

These results further indicate that the primary olfactory neurons are probably not cholinergic because, if they were, the specific activity of acetylcholinesterase in the bulb ought to show a decline in the absence of functional activity of these cells. Margolis and coworkers (1974) working with adult deolfacted mice, reached the same conclusion. The absence of a specific effect upon bulbar acetylcholinesterase by olfactory deprivation is in contrast with the marked lowering of the activity of this enzyme in subcortical visual structures following visual deprivation in the rat (Maletta and Timiras, 1976).

EFFECTS OF UNILATERAL ANOSMIA ON THE TOTAL NUMBER OF MITRAL AND TUFTED CELLS AND OLFACTORY GLOMERULI

Having established that neonatal olfactory deprivation results in a considerable amount of cell loss in the olfactory bulb (see above), we then directed our attention to the quantitative anatomic study of the normal and anosmic olfactory bulbs. Although cell counting has long been used by neuroanatomists, it has always faced great difficulties in determining the *total* number of cells in neural structures when the volume of the structure cannot be easily determined. Estimates of cell density are then usually made, which may be quite misleading in view of the contribution of the neuropil. Such estimates become even more problematic when an experimental situation is compared with the normal case.

In a structure such as the olfactory bulb, where the cell layers are distinctly separate and the anatomical boundaries can be clearly delineated, one has relatively little difficulty in making reliable determinations of the total number of a particular class of cells or cell groups. In our study we therefore chose to count the number of mitral and tufted cells, i.e. the principle cell types of the olfactory bulb which receive direct input from the olfactory receptor neurons, and would thus seem to be the principle targets of any transneuronal effects of olfactory deprivation.

We also attempted to count the total number of olfactory glomeruli, which are the most distinct morphologic feature of the olfactory bulb. Since the olfactory glomeruli are the locus of synaptic relay between the primary olfactory neurons, on the one hand, and mitral and tufted cells on the other, measurement of the diameter and total number of glomeruli would give a general indication of what was happening at these loci under the influence of olfactory deprivation. The glomeruli are particularly interesting in this regard, because according to our recent work the formation of periglomerular cell assemblies is largely a postnatal event.

To count the total number of mitral cells, tufted cells and glomeruli, normal and anosmic bulbs from 25-day-old rats that had been made unilaterally anosmic after birth were prepared with a Nissl stain (thionin). Typical appearance of the layers of the normal and anosmic bulbs, as well as the appearance of mitral cells and glomeruli at higher magnifications, are shown in Figs. 7 and 8. Mitral cells located on, or in the vicinity of, the mitral cell layer were

222

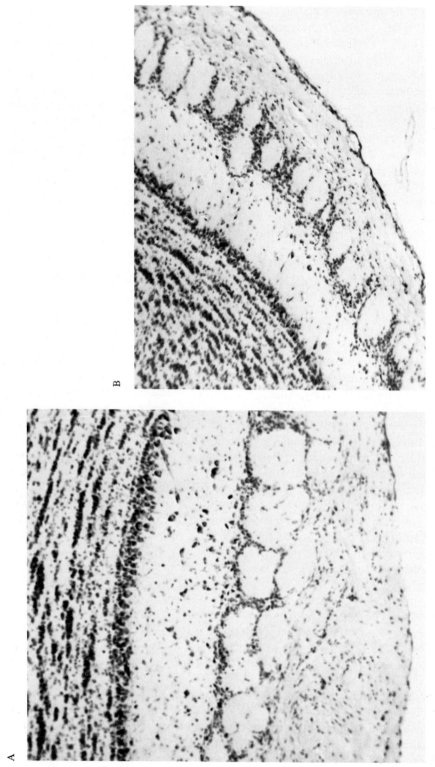

Fig. 7. Partial cross-sections of olfactory bulb in *normal* (A) and *anosmic* (B) 25-day-old rats. Thionin staining (× 200). All the typical layers of the bulb are present in both bulbs and no gross deformity due to anosmia can be detected. A reduction in the thickness of the external plexiform layer and relative absence of large cells in this layer is evident in the anosmic bulb (B).

A

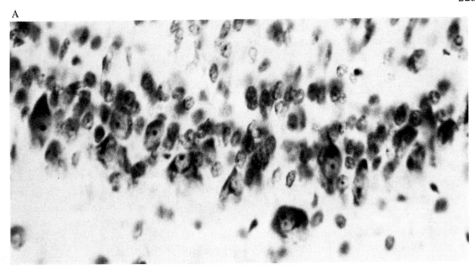

B

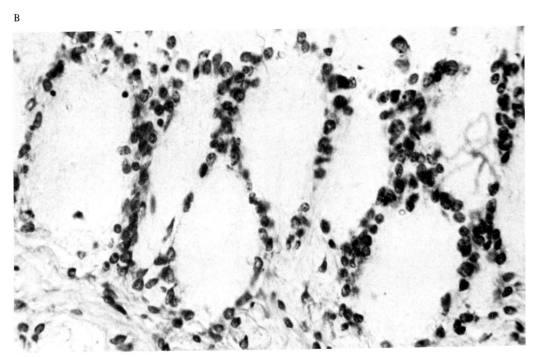

Fig. 8. The appearance of mitral cells and glomeruli in the normal olfactory bulb of a 25-day-old rat. Thionin staining (× 500).

counted when they showed at least one distinctly visible nucleolus as well as the special miter shape, thus minimizing the possibility of counting a cell twice. Tufted cells were considered as any large neuron occurring below the midline of the external plexiform layer, i.e. in or near the glomerular layer.

Counts of mitral and tufted cells were made mostly on sections 50 μm apart. In sagittal sections, however, there exists a plane of mitral cells giving very high counts; around this

224

plane the counts were made on every other section. Each count was added with the next one, divided by two and multiplied by the number of sections in between, giving the total number of cells in that interval. The sum total of these segmental total counts gives, of course, the total number of cells per bulb.

To count the glomeruli, first the average glomerular diameter of each bulb was obtained by measuring the average diameter of all the glomeruli in three, randomly selected sections from various locations in the bulb. Assuming that the glomeruli are spheres packed tightly around the bulb within the glomerular layer, and starting with the first section showing the glomeruli, serial sections approximately one average diameter apart were counted for number of glomeruli. Each count was then corrected by multiplying with a coefficient obtained by dividing the average glomerular diameter by the thickness of the interval between the layers counted. The sum of all corrected counts would give the total number of glomeruli in the bulb.

In order to obtain graphic distribution profiles of the cells and glomeruli, the counts in the various sections were then plotted against the width of the bulb in sagittal sections and length of the bulb in frontal sections. Next, to make an average curve of the various distribution profiles, the length or width of each bulb was normalized on a percentile basis; all the counts from each 4% segment for the mitral and tufted cells, and each 5% segment for the glomeruli, were added together and an average obtained. Plotting of these values against the per cent of length or width of the bulb provides normalized and average distribution profiles for histological constituents of the bulbs in the same groups of animals.

Typical average distribution profiles obtained in this manner for olfactory bulbs (cut frontally) in normal 25-day-old rats are shown in Fig. 9. Naturally, the shape of this average curve resembles closely that of the distribution curves for individual bulbs. Fig. 9 also shows that the mode of distribution for all three constituents, mitral cells, tufted cells and glomeruli, is identical, confirming the classical thesis that the above anatomic features constitute the basic structural and functional unit of the olfactory bulb. As will be seen below, such an averaging technique would be a useful method for comparing the effects of

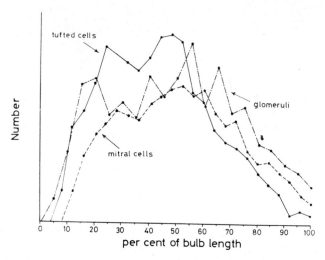

Fig. 9. Normalized average distribution profiles of mitral and tufted cells and glomeruli along the length of the normal olfactory bulbs; each curve is the average of four curves. Frontal sections. Since the scale is different for each curve, no absolute units are designated on the ordinate.

anosmia, or of any other experimental procedure, on the number and distribution of histological parameters in the bulb.

Comparison of the histologic appearance of the normal versus the anosmic bulb (Fig. 7) shows that neonatal olfactory deprivation does not cause any obvious deformation of the basic structure and layering of the bulb, except for a visible reduction in the thickness of the external plexiform and granular layers. Counts of the total number of mitral and tufted cells and of glomeruli in the normal and anosmic bulbs were carried out on eight 25-day-old animals that had been made unilaterally anosmic after birth. The mean total counts of mitral and tufted cells and of glomeruli of normal and anosmic bulbs are depicted in Table VI, and their average distribution profiles are shown in Fig. 10.

TABLE VI

EFFECTS OF NEONATAL UNILATERAL ANOSMIA ON THE TOTAL NUMBER OF MITRAL AND TUFTED CELLS AND GLOMERULI IN NORMAL AND ANOSMIC BULBS

	Normal bulb	Anosmic bulb	% Change
Mitral cells	82,218 ± 7119*	60,135 ± 4151	26**
Tufted cells	160,153 ± 2638	86,779 ± 1199	46**
Glomeruli	2727 ± 113	2718 ± 113	—

*Mean ± S.E.M.; each value is the mean of 8 counts, made on 8 olfactory bulbs, 4 cut sagittally and 4 frontally. Tufted cells were counted on 4 frontally sectioned bulbs.
**$P < 0.01$, based on the t-test.

It is clear from these results that the anosmic bulbs contain a significantly lower number of mitral and tufted cells (26 and 46%, respectively) but nearly the same number of glomeruli as in the controls. Each anosmic bulb invariably showed a lower total number than did its matched control, regardless of whether the total count was high or low in that particular animal. It is also interesting that the tufted cells, which are smaller than the mitrals, possess shorter dendrites and are located nearer to the glomeruli, seem to be more susceptible to the effects of olfactory deprivation. Another noteworthy point is that a specific population of mitral cells, amounting on the average to no more than 30% of the total, seems to be affected by neonatal olfactory deprivation. More recent studies on older anosmic animals suggest that the magnitude of the mitral cell loss does not increase appreciably with further prolongation of anosmia.

Since both mitral and tufted cells are embryonic macroneurons formed very early in bulbar development (Hinds, 1968), their lowered numbers indicate atrophy and death due to transneuronal effects of olfactory deprivation. Similar effects were suspected by Powell (1967) and by Klosovsky and Kosmarskaya (1963), working with older deolfacted rabbits and dogs, respectively. Also atrophy and loss of retinal ganglion cells in visually deprived animals had been observed earlier (Globus, 1975; Chow et al., 1957). However, demonstration of massive cell loss due directly to the lack of sensory stimulation has not been reported before.

The withdrawal of the mitral and tufted cells and their dendrites has a clear effect on the thickness of the external plexiform layer of the anosmic bulb, which is 30% thinner on the

226

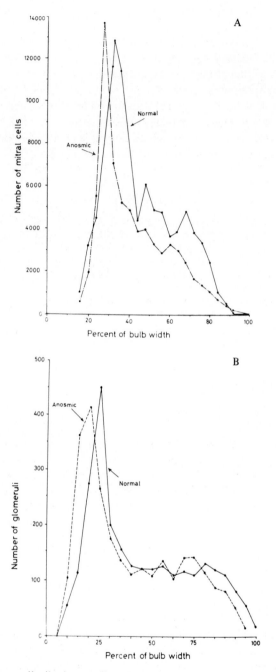

Fig. 10. Normalized average distribution profiles of *mitral cells* (A) and *glomeruli* (B) along the width of normal and anosmic olfactory bulbs, going from the medial to the lateral border of the bulb (sagittal sections). Each curve is the average of four bulbs. In A, each point is the sum of mitral cells present in the 4% segment corresponding to the location indicated on the abscissa. In B, each point is the sum of glomeruli present in the 5% segment corresponding to the location indicated (abscissa).

average than in the normal bulb (the thickness of the whole bulb is reduced only by 10%). The loss of the axons of mitral and tufted cells could also account for the visible under-development of the lateral olfactory tract on the anosmic side (see above).

In these studies, an unexpected finding was the absence of any effect of olfactory deprivation on the total number and average size of the glomeruli (Table VI; Fig. 10). It is puzzling that the withdrawal of dendrites of mitral and tufted cells in the anosmic bulb has no effect on the average size of the glomeruli: the mean diameter of the glomeruli in the anosmic bulbs was 68.0 μm against 70.2 μm in the normal bulb. It seems probable that glial processes take over the empty spaces left by the withdrawing dendrites. Examination of the average distribution profiles of glomeruli in the normal and anosmic bulbs (Fig. 10) shows that the profile is shifted somewhat to the left in the anosmic bulb, i.e. the average plane of the glomeruli in sagittal sections is nearer to the medial edge of the bulb. This could indicate a thinning of the olfactory nerve layer as a consequence of anosmia, perhaps after some of the olfactory receptors degenerate.

GENERAL CONCLUSIONS

It is clear from the data presented in this paper that normal anatomical and chemical development of the olfactory bulb during the early phase of postnatal development depends upon the presence of intact olfactory receptors. It is not known whether the trophic effects of the receptors are exerted on the bulb through the neural activity associated with normal sensory function, or whether through some other mechanism. Neither is it clear to what extent the observed chemical and morphologic effects influence the functional activity and capacities of the olfactory bulb. It would be interesting to see how much recovery could occur in the bulb after reopening of the closed nare. In general, the olfactory system of the developing rat promises to be a very rewarding and suitable model for the study of the effects of early sensory influences on brain development, an area which hitherto has been dominated by studies on the visual system.

SUMMARY

In this paper, it is first argued that the developing olfactory bulb of the rat is a suitable model for studies on the central neural correlates of early sensory deprivation. Then it is shown that early olfactory deprivation in this animal, whether produced by unilateral neonatal closure of one nostril or by bilateral chemical destruction of olfactory receptor neurons, leads to marked reduction in the growth of the olfactory bulb, accompanied by a state of chemical underdevelopment and anatomic atrophy. Specifically, early olfactory deprivation causes significant reductions in: weight, total protein, DNA, RNA, and Na,K-ATPase and acetylcholinesterase activities, as well as a marked reduction in the total number of mitral and tufted cells. It is suggested that during postnatal development, the presence of olfactory receptor activity is necessary for the proper development of the olfactory bulbs.

228

ACKNOWLEDGMENTS

The work presented in this paper was supported by grants from the Iranian Ministry of Science and Higher Education and from the University of Tehran. The author wishes to acknowledge the cooperation and invaluable assistance of Ms. R. Mousavi for biochemistry and experimental anosmia, Mr. L. Safari and Ms. F. Azimi for histology, counts and computations, and Mr. M. Navvab for histology and photography. The author is also grateful to Dr. F. Shafa for critical discussions of the subject.

REFERENCES

Altman, J. (1969) Autoradiographic and histological studies of postnatal neurogenesis. IV. Cell proliferation and migration in the anterior forebrain, with special reference to persisting neurogenesis in the olfactory bulb, *J. comp. Neurol.*, 137: 433–458.

Barlow, H.B. (1975) Visual experience and cortical development, *Nature (Lond.)*, 258: 199–204.

Bayer, S.A. and Altman, J. (1975) The effects of X-irradiation on the postnatally-forming granule cell populations in the olfactory bulb, hippocampus, and cerebellum of the rat, *Exp. Neurol.*, 48: 167–174.

Berger, H. (1900) Experimentall-anatomische Studien uber die durch den Mangel optischer Reize veranlassten Entwicklungschemmungen im Occipittallappen des Hundes und der Katze, *Arch. Psychiat.*, 33: 521–567.

Burton, K. (1956) A study of the conditions and mechanisms of the diphenylamine reaction for colorimetric estimation of dioxyribonucleic acid, *Biochem. J.*, 62: 315–323.

Ceriotti, G. (1955) Determination of nucleic acids in animal tissues, *J. biol. Chem.*, 214: 59–70.

Child, C.M. (1921) *The Origin and Development of the Nervous System: a Physiological Viewpoint*, University of Chicago Press.

Chow, K.L., Riesen, A.H. and Newell, F.W. (1957) Degeneration of retinal ganglion cells in infant chimpanzees reared in darkness, *J. comp. Neurol.*, 107: 24–42.

DeRobertis, E. (1967) Ultrastructure and cytochemistry of the synaptic region, *Science*, 156: 907–914.

Eibl, H. and Land, W.M. (1969) A new, sensitive determination of phosphate, *Analyt. Biochem.*, 30: 51–57.

Ellman, G.L., Courtney, D.K., Anders, V. and Featherstone, R.M. (1961) A new and rapid colorimetric determination of acetylcholinesterase activity, *Biochem. Pharmacol.*, 7: 88–95.

Globus, A. (1975) Brain morphology as a function of presynaptic morphology and activity. In *The Developmental Neuropsychology of Sensory Deprivation*, A.H. Riesen (Ed.), Academic Press, New York, pp. 9–92.

Gudden, (1870) *Arch. Psychiat. Nervenkr.*, 11: 693.

Hinds, J.W. (1968) Autoradiographic study of histogenesis in the mouse olfactory bulb. I. Time of origin of neurons and neuroglia, *J. comp. Neurol.*, 134: 287–304.

Hinds, J.W. and Ruffett, T.L. (1973) Mitral cell development in the mouse olfactory bulb: reorientation of the perikaryon and maturation of the axon initial segment, *J. comp. Neurol.*, 151: 281–306.

Hinds, J.W. and Hinds, P.L. (1976) Synapse formation in the mouse olfactory bulb, *J. comp. neurol.*, 169: 15–39.

Klosovsky, B.N. and Kosmarskaya, E.N. (1963) *Excitatory and Inhibitory States of the Brain*, National Science Foundation, Washington, D.C.

Lowry, O., Rosebrough, N., Farr, A. and Randall, R. (1951) Protein measurement with the Folin phenol reagent, *J. biol. Chem.*, 193: 265–275.

Margolis, F.L., Roberts, N., Ferriero, D. and Feldman, J. (1974) Denervation in the primary olfactory pathway of mice: biochemical and morphological effects, *Brain Res.*, 81: 469–483.

Meisami, E. (1975) Early sensory influences on regional activity of brain ATPases in developing rats. In *Growth and Development of the Brain*, M.A.B. Brazier (Ed.), Raven Press, New York, pp. 51–74.

Meisami, E. (1976) Effects of olfactory deprivation on postnatal growth of the rat olfactory bulb utilizing a new method for production of neonatal unilateral anosmia, *Brain Res.*, 107: 437–444.

Meisami, E. and Timiras, P.S. (1974) Influence of early visual deprivation on regional activity of brain ATPases in developing rats, *J. Neurochem.*, 22: 725–729.

Meisami, E. and Shafa, F. (1977) Postnatal structural development of the rat olfactory bulb and its functional significance. In *Proc. Sixth Int. Symp. Olfaction and Taste*, Paris.

Meisami, E. and Manochehri, S. (1977) Effects of early bilateral chemical destruction of olfactory receptors on postnatal growth, Mg-ATPase and Na,K-ATPase activity of olfactory and non-olfactory structures of the rat brain, *Brain Res.*, 128: 170–175.

Maletta, G.J. and Timiras, P.S. (1967) Acetylcholinesterase activity in optic structures after complete light deprivation from birth, *Exp. Neurol.*, 19: 513–518.

Mulvaney, B.D. and Heist, H.E. (1971) Regeneration of rabbit olfactory epithelium, *Amer. J. Anat.*, 131: 241–252.

Powell, T.P.S. (1967) Transneuronal cell degeneration in the olfactory bulb shown by the Golgi method, *Nature (Lond.)*, 215: 425–426.

Riesen, A.H. (1966) Sensory deprivation. In *Progress in Physiological Psychology, Vol. 1,* E. Stellar and J.M. Sprague, (Eds.), Academic Press, New York, pp. 117–142.

Roux, W. (1895) Einleitung, *Arch. Entwickl.*, 1: 1–42.

Samson, F.E. and Quinn, D.J. (1967) Na-K-activated ATPase in rat brain development, *J. Neurochem.*, 14: 421–427.

Scheibel, M.E. and Scheibel, A.B. (1975) Dendrite bundles, central programs and olfactory bulbs, *Brain Res.*, 95: 407–421.

Schultz, E.W. (1960) Repair of the olfactory mucosa, *Amer. J. Pathol.*, 37: 1–19.

Shafa, F., Meisami, E. and Mousavi, R. (1976) The role of olfaction in the nutrition of rat neonate, *Neurosci. Abstr.*, 2: 162.

Silver, A. (1974) *The Biology of Cholinesterases*, North-Holland, Amsterdam.

Skou, J.C. (1965) Enzymatic basis for active transport of Na^+ and K^+ across cell membrane, *Physiol. Rev.*, 45: 496–517.

Smith, C.G. (1938) Changes in the olfactory mucosa and the olfactory nerves following intranasal treatment with one percent zinc sulphate, *Canad. med. Assoc. J.*, 39: 138–140.

Van Der Loos, H. and Woolsey, T.A. (1973) Somatosensory cortex: structural alterations following early injury to sense organs, *Science*, 179: 395–397.

DISCUSSION

AXELRAD: In the anosmic animals the nasal cavity is still in contact with the throat. Do odors not come into the nasal cavity from behind, and so against the mucosa? In the second place, I noticed in the cell counts which you presented that there were no cells, but only fibers, in the first few millimeters. Is it correct that in the normal and the anosmic animals this distance, and thus the thickness of the fiber layer, was the same?

MEISAMI: To answer your first question: the very fact that the animal usually has to sniff actively means that it needs to generate quite some force in order to have the odoriforous molecules reach the olfactory area. Such a force cannot be expected from the backward flow, besides which there are very few odoriforous compounds in the expired air. Nevertheless, some influence of the backward flow cannot be completely ruled out. The answer to your second question is that there *is* in fact a difference in the first part of the curves. The glomeruli of the anosmic bulb are found sooner in the sections, and in fact the overall curve shows a shift to the left. This probably indicates that the thickness of the olfactory nerve layer is somewhat diminished in the anosmic olfactory bulb. Since this is a crucial problem, it needs to be investigated critically before any firm conclusion can be reached.

STIRLING: When are the mitral cells born, and do you expect them to die due to the operation?

MEISAMI: The mitral cells and the tufted cells are both born at day 12 of pregnancy in the rat, i.e. 8–9 days before birth. They die after the operation, presumably due to the deprivation of stimulation. In the normal situation the mitral cells do not start to show spontaneous cell death until the second year, and in 2.5-year-old animals the cell loss is about 20%. It is interesting that the total amount of cell loss among the mitral cells due to early anosmia is about the same as that normally lost due to aging (i.e. 20–25%).

CHANGEUX: Is this spontaneous cell death during development taking place in a particular cell layer or category of cells? Also, is there any kind of compensatory effect in the contralateral bulb in the long-lasting experiments, and what about the DNA?

MEISAMI: Besides what we know about the mitral and tufted cells, we have no idea about other cell types or layers because it is extremely time-consuming to make such cell counts. We intend to try this in the next few years, however. The growth curves of the normal bulb in the unilaterally anosmic animal has practically the same shape as does the curve for the right and left bulb in the normal animals. The DNA content is also the same. There is apparently no appreciable hyperplasia, or any other form of excessive development in the bulb contralateral to the anosmic bulb.

BEDI: In the methods that you used, did you make serial sections and count the number of cells of each section?

MEISAMI: In some parts of the bulb, such as the region near the medial border, where a vertical plane of mitral cells gives very high counts, we counted every other 5 sections, and rarely were we forced to count every successive section.

BEDI: In the cases where you counted the numbers of cells in each successive section, did you section some cells twice? And how did you correct for this?

MEISAMI: This would have been practically impossible in our procedure, since the mitral cells have an average diameter of about 10 μm. Furthermore, we counted the cells only if we could clearly visualize the nucleolus, which effectively eliminates the possibility of counting any cell twice.

Ontogenesis of the Visual Cortex of Rabbits and the Effects of Visual Deprivation

G. VRENSEN

The Netherlands Ophthalmic Research Institute, c/o Wilhelmina Gasthuis, Amsterdam-1013
(The Netherlands)

INTRODUCTION

The problem of innate versus experiential factors as the determinants of human and animal behavior and knowledge has deep historical roots, not only in neurobiology and sensory physiology but also in philosophy and psychology (see Lippe, 1976). The 'innate ideas' of Descartes and the 'a priori knowledge' of Kant were based on the assumption that the conscious mind had built-in associative mechanisms. In contrast, Hume, Locke and Berkely considered the human mind as a 'blank paper' or 'tabula rasa' which is molded by experience. These nativist and empiricist points of view greatly influenced early psychological thinking. Gestalt psychology is closely connected with the ideas of Kant and Descartes, and considers the ability to perceive, for example, spatial aspects of the environment as inborn. The ideas of Hume, Locke and Berkely have their counterparts in behaviorism, which considers that the spatial aspects of the environment such as form, size and depth must be learned. Early sensory physiological studies also displayed this dichotomous outlook. Thus, Hering thought that the retina was equipped with inborn local signs for depth perception, whereas Helmholtz was thinking of depth perception as depending upon learned cues.

Due to the pioneering work of neuroembryologists such as Harrison, Weiss, Sperry and Hamburger, along with the psychologist Hebb, the gap between these opposing points of view has been narrowed. At present it is generally accepted that both environmental and inborn factors interact during the functional and structural organization of the brain and mind (Lippe, 1976; Hamburger, 1975). The 'nature-nurture question', as it is often called, can now be reformulated as follows.

At what level of the organization and functioning of the brain does the interaction between innate and experiential factors take place, and what is the relative contribution of both in the molding of the mature brain?

The visual system is the most widely used in this kind of study because its natural input can easily be regulated without destruction of its neurological substrate. We will restrict this review to ontogenetic and deprivation aspects of the visual system. The effects of extra stimulation will be treated in separate papers in this symposium (Parnavelas; Uylings, Kuypers and Veltman).

PRESENT CONCEPTS ON THE INTERACTION BETWEEN INNATE AND EXPERIENTIAL FACTORS IN BRAIN MATURATION

For our purpose the central questions in the nature-nurture debate are most clearly stated by Eccles (1973) and Changeux and Danchin (1976) respectively. The general assumptions of these authors can be summarized in two opposing points of view, (Fig. 1).

From the basic statements made two most relevant morphological questions can be extracted:

(1) In Changeux's view, redundancy and degeneration are highly important factors for the maturation of the nervous system. This implies that, during certain ontogenetic stages, more neurons and synapses are present than in the adult animal, and that these redundant structures stabilize and degenerate in relation to the onset or alteration of the sensory input (or under the influence of *spontaneous* neuronal activity).

(2) Changes at the ultrastructural and ultrafunctional level are the most important factors for experiential alterations in the view of Eccles. This implies that changes at the synaptic level must take place during ontogenesis, and that these changes are affected by alteration of the visual input.

Before starting the description of some aspects of ontogenesis of the visual system and the effects of visual deprivation, it may be convenient to make a distinction between three levels of organization of the visual system (Fig. 2). As emphasized by Van Hof (1974) and by Cragg (1974), visual input restriction may act either at the level of the *wiring diagram*

Innate and Experiential Factors in Brain Maturation

Eccles (1973)	Changeux and Danchin (1976)
Brain Morphology	
a. Highly specific	Partly specific
b. Precisely precoded	Roughly precoded
c. Non-random network at all stages	Random network at some stages
d. No redundancy of neurons and synapses	Redundancy of neurons and synapses
Preponderance of Innate Factors	Balanced Interaction of Innate and Experiential Factors
Brain Plasticity	
Subtle alterations at the ultra-functional / ultrastructural level	Selective stabilization and degeneration at the synaptic and neuronal level

Fig. 1. The points of view summarized here are most clearly stated by Eccles (1973) and Changeux and Danchin (1976).

Organizational Level	Key-words
1. Macrostructural	Central representation of retina, (lateral geniculate nucleus, visual cortex, colliculus superior, pretectal nuclei, pulvinar), Retinotopic representation.
2. Microstructural	Laminar Organization, Columnar Organization, Wiring diagram, topology of neurons and synapses, Dendritic Organization, Receptive fields.
3. Ultrastructural	Fine structure of neurons, Fine structure of synapses, contact zones, synaptic vesicles, Chemical transmission, relation of structure and biochemical events.

Fig. 2. Levels of organization of the visual system.

(level 2), by changing the number or topology of the interconnections, or at the *synaptic* level (level 3), by changing the efficacy of the individual synapses.

ONTOGENETIC STUDIES

It is evident that subtle changes at the micro- and ultrastructural level or changes in the number of neurons and synapses are questions which can be answered only by using quantitative histological methods. The methods we have used not only in our descriptive ontogenetic but also in our deprivation studies are summarized in Fig. 3 (for more details see Vrensen and De Groot: 1973, 1974 and 1977). The compiled results of these quantitative analyses in visual and motor cortex of the rabbit are summarized in Figs. 4—9. More detailed descriptions, including statistical treatment of the data and distinctions between the different areas studied, are given elsewhere (Vrensen et al., 1977; De Groot and Vrensen, 1978). It is important to know that in the rabbit natural eye opening occurs (on the average) at day 10, and ranges from day 8 to 12 postnatally.

The maturation of neuronal organization is indicated by, for example, neuron density, neuronal volume, nuclear/cytoplasmic ratio and gray/cell coefficient. In the rabbit, neuron density per unit volume matures rapidly from birth up to one month with the most prominent decline in the first 10 postnatal days (Fig. 4). Simultaneously, neuronal volume increases (Fig. 5), nuclear/cytoplasmic ratio drops and the gray/cell coefficient increases (Vrensen et al., 1977). Careful observation of the histological sections did not reveal any sign of degenerating neurons during the first postnatal month. It can also be concluded (Figs. 4 and 5) that at birth the motor cortex is more mature with respect to these neuronal parameters. These observations agree well with the observations of Brizzee and Jacobs (1959) and of Cragg (1972, 1975) in the cerebral cortex of the cat. It is emphasized by

234

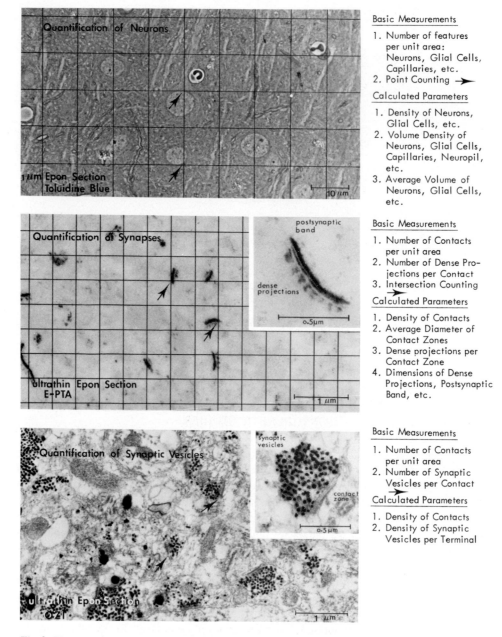

Basic Measurements

1. Number of features
   per unit area:
   Neurons, Glial Cells,
   etc.
2. Point Counting ⟶

Calculated Parameters

1. Density of Neurons,
   Glial Cells, etc.
2. Volume Density of
   Neurons, Glial Cells,
   Capillaries, Neuropil,
   etc.
3. Average Volume of
   Neurons, Glial Cells,
   etc.

Basic Measurements

1. Number of Contacts
   per unit area
2. Number of Dense Pro-
   jections per Contact
3. Intersection Counting
   ⟶

Calculated Parameters

1. Density of Contacts
2. Average Diameter of
   Contact Zones
3. Dense projections per
   Contact Zone
4. Dimensions of Dense
   Projections, Postsynaptic
   Band, etc.

Basic Measurements

1. Number of Contacts
   per unit area
2. Number of Synaptic
   Vesicles per Contact
   ⟶

Calculated Parameters

1. Density of Contacts
2. Density of Synaptic
   Vesicles per Terminal

Fig. 3. The stereological methods indicated in this figure are described in more detail by Vrensen and De
Groot, (1973, 1974) and by Vrensen et al. (1977).

Cragg (1975), and it can be inferred from the present results, that the rapid decrease in
neuron density is mainly caused by 'dilution'. That is, the volume of the cortex increases
due to outgrowth of cell bodies, dendrites and axons, and ingrowth of afferent axons,
thereby causing the density per unit volume to decline.

In an elegant study, Elgeti et al. (1976) investigated the postnatal development of the
neuron density and the volume of the lateral geniculate nucleus of the cat. They came to

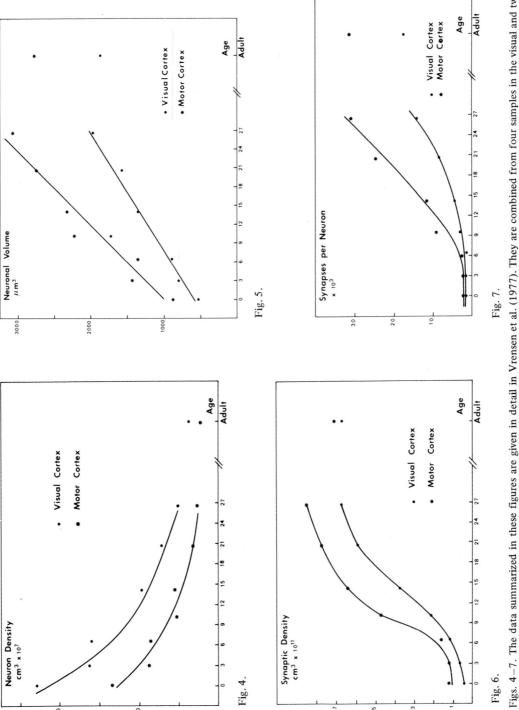

Fig. 5.

Fig. 4.

Fig. 7.

Fig. 6.

Figs. 4–7. The data summarized in these figures are given in detail in Vrensen et al. (1977). They are combined from four samples in the visual and two samples in the motor cortex (see Fig. 10). The age is in days (adults are seven months old).

236

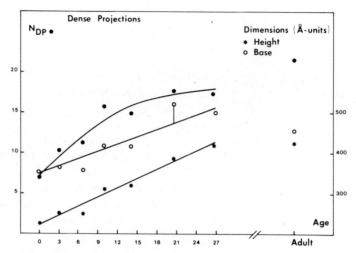

Fig. 8. The number of dense projections per contact zone (N_{DP}) and their dimensions are measured in visual area I in the left hemisphere (see Fig. 10). Age in days.

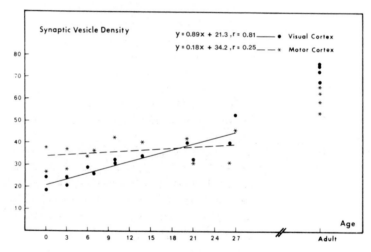

Fig. 9. Synaptic vesicle density is expressed as the number of synaptic vesicles per contact zone, as seen in ultrathin sections. Age in days.

the conclusion that the decline in neuron density can be completely explained by the increase in volume of the geniculate body itself, and that there is no question of significant cell loss. Harel et al. (1972) have shown that in the cerebrum of the rabbit there is a rapid increase in total DNA content, with a prominent growth spurt between birth and day 10. This growth spurt must be ascribed to proliferation of oligodendroglial cells. No signs of an extensive cell loss were observed in this biochemical study. The conclusions of this section are that neuronal development is quite rapid prior to eye opening, and that redundancy and degeneration are certainly not important factors in the visual system of mammals. Moreover, it can be inferred that there are significant regional differences in the postnatal maturation of the cerebral cortex.

Changes in synaptic density, which are to some extent indicative for the development of the cortical wiring diagram, start at days 6—10 and are most prominent between day 10 and day 21 (Fig. 6). As illustrated in Figs. 6 and 7, synaptic density and synapses per neuron in the motor cortex exceed that in the visual cortex. Moreover, the synaptic density at day 27 is in excess of the density in the motor cortex, but also in some areas of the visual cortex of 7-month-old animals. (Vrensen et al., 1977). Our analysis is in good agreement with the observations of Valverde (1971) in mice, of Aghajanian and Bloom (1967), Armstrong-James and Johnson (1970) and Kristt and Molliver (1976) in rats and of Cragg (1972, 1974, 1975) in cats. The observations in these postnatally developing animals differ from the observations in the prenatally developing guinea-pigs (Jones et al., 1974) in which the most prominent increase in synaptic density occurs shortly before birth.

We have also studied quantitatively the development of the synaptic grid and the density of synaptic vesicles. As illustrated in Fig. 8 both the number of dense projections per contact zone and the dimensions of the dense projections gradually increase during postnatal maturation. The same holds true for the intercleft line and postsynaptic band, (De Groot and Vrensen, 1978). As indicated in Fig. 9, the average number of synaptic vesicles per contact zone gradually increases during postnatal development in the visual cortex, but no age relation is observed in the motor cortex. These quantitative observations of the development of the fine structural components of the synapse agree with most of the descriptive studies devoted to this problem, (for references see De Groot and Vrensen, 1978). Jones et al. (1974) have observed a similar increase in the dimensions of dense projections in synapses of guinea-pigs after birth; however, without a simultaneous increase of the mean number of dense projections. Our observation of the absence of an age relation in the development of synaptic vesicles in the motor cortex of the rabbit is opposite to the observation of Armstrong-James and Johnson (1970) in the rat. In that animal a rapid increase in synaptic vesicles per unit area of terminal could be observed during postnatal development.

It can be concluded from this short section on synaptic development that the maturation of the wiring diagram, at least as far as is indicated by the increase in synaptic density, starts shortly before natural eye opening, and is most prominent during the two weeks after the onset of visual input. In some areas the number of synapses per unit volume is in excess of the adult number at a certain developmental stage. As emphasized by Cragg (1975), however, this 'overshoot' is most likely not a true redundancy but rather the 'dilution effect' referred to earlier. Cragg observed a later growth of glial cells, meaning that the cortical volume is still increasing during later phases and that, consequently, the number of synapses per unit volume decreases. The synaptic substructures all mature following natural eye opening, and thus could be affected by visual experience.

DEPRIVATION STUDIES

In addition to the ontogenetic aspects of the visual and motor cortex, we have studied in our laboratory the effects of dark-rearing and of monocular deprivation on the synaptic organization of the visual cortex, the superior colliculus and the motor cortex in rabbits (Vrensen and De Groot, 1974, 1975, 1977). The results of these studies are summarized in Figs. 10—13.

As was already pointed out, synaptic density can, to some extent, be considered as an indication of the completeness of the wiring diagram. Dark-rearing for 7 months has no effect on the synaptic density, in either the visual and motor cortices (Fig. 10) or in the

238

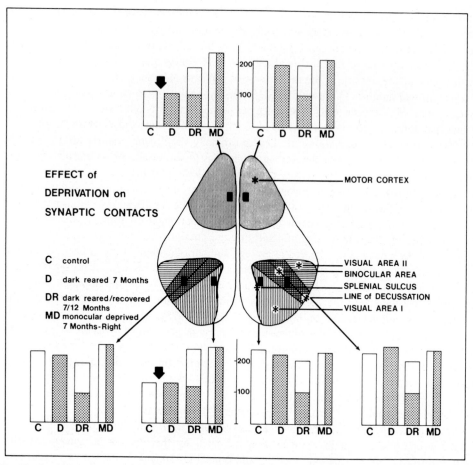

Fig. 10. Synaptic density is expressed as the number of contact zones in ultrathin sections of E-PTA stained tissue, per 1000 μm². For details see Vrensen and De Groot (1974, 1975).

Synapses in the Colliculus Superior of Control and Dark Reared Rabbits

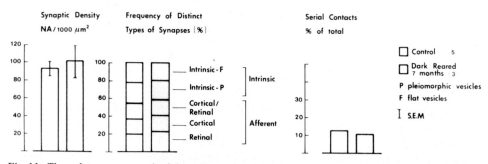

Fig. 11. These data are summarized from Vrensen and De Groot (1977). The distinction between the 4 types of synapses are based both on data given in the literature, and on ultrastructural features. NA, number of synapses per 1000 μm²; Intrinsic-F, intrinsic terminals with flat vesicles; Intrinsic-P, intrinsic terminals with pleiomorphic vesicles; Cortical/Retinal, in some instances, retinal and cortical terminals cannot be distinguished on the basis of their fine structure.

EFFECT of DEPRIVATION on SYNAPTIC VESICLES

	VISUAL CORTEX			MOTOR CORTEX		
	Vesicles/ Terminal	Change	t–test	Vesicles/ Terminal	Change	t–test
CONTROL (6)	71.3 ± 7.0	-	-	57.2 ± 5.3	-	-
DARK REARED (6) 7 months	43.7 ± 5.5	-39%	p < .01	44.9 ±10.5	-22%	p > .10
DARK REARED/RECOVERED 7/12 months (6)	43.4 ± 6.6	-39%	p < .01	42.8 ± 5.7	-25%	p < .05
MONOCULAR DEPRIVED 7 months–right						
NON DEPRIVED CORTEX (9)	64.3 ± 3.6	-	-	54.2 ± 4.0	-	-
DEPRIVED CORTEX (9)	53.7 ± 2.9	-17%	p < .025	55.7 ± 4.0	+3%	n.s.

Fig. 12. Vesicles per terminal indicate number of synaptic vesicles as seen in micrographs of ultrathin sections. For details see Vrensen and De Groot (1974, 1975).

Synaptic Vesicles in the Colliculus Superior of Control and Dark Reared Rabbits

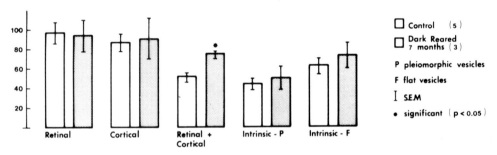

Fig. 13. Number of synaptic vesicles per synaptic contact zone as seen in ultrathin sections. For details see Vrensen and De Groot (1977).

superior colliculus (Fig. 11). In the visual cortex of the left hemisphere, there is an area close to the midline that has significantly fewer synapses than its right counterpart. A similar right hemispheric dominance is observed in the medial motor area used in our studies. This right dominance in synapses is already present during early ontogenesis (Vrensen et al., 1977). Monocular deprivation (*right* eye sutured) and recovery from dark-rearing give rise to a higher synaptic density, both in visual and in motor cortex, in the medial samples of the left hemisphere.

The conclusions to be drawn from these observations are the following:

(1) dark-rearing has no long-lasting effects on synaptic density;

(2) monocular deprivation of the right eye gives rise to a higher synaptic density in restricted areas of the visual and motor cortex of the contralateral side;

(3) the recovery experiments show that the visual and motor cortex possess synaptic plasticity even after 7 months.

In the superior, colliculus 4 types of terminals can be distinguished on the basis of their fine structural organization. They have a specific origin and a specific localization (Vrensen and De Groot, 1977). We have studied the relative frequency of these terminals, the serial contacts, and their specific location in control and dark-reared animals. No significant changes were observed (Fig. 11).

Synaptic vesicles are important for synaptic transmission (Akert, 1973), and it has been shown that there is some relationship between the number of vesicles and the excitatory postsynaptic potential (Heuser and Reese, 1974; Ceccarelli and Hurlbut, 1974). We have investigated the effects of dark-rearing and monocular deprivation on synaptic vesicles in the visual and the motor cortex (Fig. 12), and in the superior colliculus (Fig. 13). In the visual cortex of dark-reared animals the vesicle density is about 40% less than in control animals. The diminution is about 17% in the deprived hemisphere of monocular raised animals, both changes being significant. In the motor cortex, on the other hand, the changes are either much less pronounced or absent altogether. In the superior colliculus no changes in synaptic vesicle density could be observed in either the retinal, the cortical or the two types of intrinsic terminals.

The size and fine structure of the synaptic contact zones are important for the transmission of nerve impulses. Until now we have not observed any significant changes in the size of the synaptic contacts after light deprivation. This does not necessarily mean, however, that deprivation is ineffective at this level of synaptic organization. The quantitative procedures used in our studies up to now are based on test-line systems (Fig. 3) as described by Weibel (1969), and have the inherent disadvantage of giving only *mean* values of length, surface area and volume of all the specific structures present in a series of micrographs. Therefore, small changes in the size distribution of synaptic contacts cannot be detected. At present we are developing new procedures which are more sensitive for the detection of small changes in size.

Our investigations have shown that, in the rabbit, light deprivation has little effect on the quantitative aspects of the synaptic organization in the visual cortex and the superior colliculus. A highly relevant question is whether deprivation affects the topology of the wiring diagram, i.e. the proper location of the synapses (Van Hof, 1974; Cragg, 1974). Using the same animals as investigated by us, Van Hof (1974) and Van Hof and Kobayashi (1972) showed that the visual evoked responses in dark-reared animals are smaller than, but qualitatively identical to, those in control animals. After some weeks, the evoked potentials become completely normal. Visual discrimination performance is, after a period of recovery, completely normal in dark-reared and in monocular deprived animals, although visual acuity is permanently decreased. Collewijn (1977) has shown that optokinetic nystagmus and vestibulo-ocular performance are qualitatively alike in both control and dark-reared rabbits, and that the amplitude differences disappear within a few weeks. These observations are strong indications that neither has the wiring diagram been changed qualitatively nor has the topology of the synapses been significantly altered. This is indirectly supported by our observations in the superior colliculus, where no changes in frequencies and locations of the distinct types of terminals could be found after rearing in the dark.

The unmistakably lower synaptic vesicle density observed after dark-rearing and monocular deprivation in rabbits is in agreement with observations of Garey and Pettigrew (1974) in the cat. They also observed a lower vesicle density in the visual cortex of dark-reared cats, and showed that visual stimulation given within the critical period can restore the control level.

There exists a vast amount of literature regarding the effects of sensory input restriction on the visual system of mammals. Both Chow (1973) and Globus (1975) have recently reviewed this literature, and there is no need to repeat it at present. We have considered the results of these investigations only with respect to the question of quantitative changes in neuron and synaptic density, Except for the observations of Fifková and Hassler (1969) and Fifková (1970) in the lateral geniculate nucleus and in the visual cortex of rats after monocular deprivation, no changes in neuron density have been observed in the central visual stations. Hubel et al. (1976) have recently studied this for area 17 of the macaque monkey, and did not observe any changes in the density, volume or position of neurons after monocular deprivation. A phenomenon generally observed after deprivation, especially in the lateral geniculate nucleus, is shrinkage of the neurons. This shrinkage is often accompanied by a decrease in RNA and protein syntheses, along with changes in enzyme activity.

Valverde (1971) and Fifková (1970) have observed lower spine densities in the visual cortices of rats and mice. Most other investigations either failed to observe such changes or presented conflicting data. The lower spine density observed by Valverde (1971) in mice following dark-rearing is often taken as definite proof that restricted sensory input reduces the number of connections in the visual system. Careful analysis of the data, however, reveals that the spine reduction is only temporary, and is no longer apparent at 50–60 days of age. The conclusion could be that Valverde's observations have shown that dark-rearing causes a delay in normal development. This would be in agreement with the conception of Grobstein and Chow (1976), which was based upon anatomical and physiological observations in the rabbit.

SUMMARY AND CONCLUSIONS

In the visual cortex of largely postnatal developers such as rats, cats, mice and rabbits, neuronal maturation and maturation of the laminar organization start around birth and show their main growth spurts prior to natural eye opening. This means that the driving factor for this development cannot be the normal visual input, and that it is therefore unlikely that visual input has an important molding effect on the microstructural organization (Fig. 2) of the central visual brain regions. The fact that no, or only very few, degenerating neurons are seen during postnatal development, and that the normally occurring decrease in neuron density can be accounted for by the increased volume of the various brain structures strengthens this conclusion. This does not mean, however, that there is no redundancy at all during the growth of the nervous system. It may well be that neuroblasts are in excess during the prenatal proliferation phase and that some of them degenerate. Furthermore, there is good evidence that, in the peripheral nervous system, cell degeneration really does occur, and is guided by the lack of sufficient synaptic sites (e.g. Changeux and Danchin, 1976). We only intend to say that cell degeneration induced by functional verification is unlikely to be a general phenomenon in the nervous system, and almost certainly not in central visual brain regions.

Evidence supporting this point of view comes from studies on sensory input restriction. At present there is no proof that light deprivation leads to significant cellular losses. What has been observed is that dark-rearing and monocular deprivation give rise to a decrease in cell volume and in the activities of certain metabolic processes. These observations may indicate a corresponding decrease in the functional capabilities of these cells, arising as a consequence of the absence of visual input during ontogeny. The development of synaptic connections is most prominent after natural eye opening in rabbits, cats, mice and rats. This

242

suggests that the organization of the wiring diagram (microstructural level: Fig. 2) could be susceptible to a degree of guidance by sensory input. Studies concerning the effects of deprivation on spine or synaptic density do not support this theoretical vulnerability, however.

Our own studies in rabbits have shown that there are no long-term effects of dark-rearing on synaptic density in the visual cortex. Monocular deprivation studies have revealed density changes in a restricted area, but no changes in the colliculus are observed. Data from the literature are conflicting, and no conclusive proof for degeneration of synapses in central visual stations has been presented up till now. The most we can say at this time is that deprivation leads to a delay in the normal development of spines or synapses. The few clear instances of apparent synaptic excess during a certain developmental stage must be ascribed to an increase in later stages of the total volume of the visual area concerned. Changes in the topology of the connections, i.e. proper location in the wiring diagram, can hardly be verified using present day morphological methods. Electrophysiological and visual discrimination studies in deprived animals, however, did not show any qualitative changes in either the evoked responses or the visual performance, which indicates that the wiring diagram probably has not changed very dramatically.

Investigations at the ultrastructural level (see Fig. 2) are scarce. Both synaptic vesicles and synaptic contact zones develop after eye opening, and are at least theoretically susceptible to visual input modulation. Both Garey and Pettigrew (1974) and the present author have shown that in cats and rabbits definite irreversible changes in the synaptic vesicle population occur in the visual cortex, which changes can be reversed by sensory input during a critical period. (No decrease in synaptic vesicles occurs in the colliculus.) It may be postulated that the decrease reflects a diminution of the efficacy of synaptic transmission, but, it is evident that such an idea needs far more verification.

If we now return to the 'nature-nurture problem', as formulated in the introduction to this paper, we can now give an answer to the two questions raised.

(1) There is very little conclusive evidence for the visual system, that light deprivation affects the macrostructural and microstructural organization of this system. It seems likely, therefore, that this organization is quite specifically genetically precoded.

(2) Changes in the ultrastructural organization of the neurons and their synapses have been observed. This may indicate that the plasticity of the nervous system, so evident from behavioral and electrophysiological studies, finds its origin at the ultrafunctional level.

ACKNOWLEDGEMENT

I am greatly indebted to Miss D. de Groot and Mr. J. Nunez Cardozo for their invaluable technical assistance during the last several years. I greatly acknowledge the useful advice and stimulating discussions of Prof. Dr. M.W. Van Hof and his coworkers. The practical work included in this paper was carried out in the Dept. of Electron Microscopy of the Mental Hospital 'Endegeest', Oegstgeest, (The Netherlands), and was partly supported by the Foundation for Medical Research FUNGO (Grant 13-14-24), which is subsidized by the Netherlands Organization for the Advancement of Pure Research (Z.W.O.). I thank Miss M. Korpershoek for drawing the figures and Mrs. H. Fopma-Bonnes for typing the manuscript.

REFERENCES

Aghajanian, G.K. and Bloom, F.E. (1967) The formation of synaptic junctions in developing rat brain: a quantitative electron microscopic study, *Brain Res.*, 6: 716–727.

Akert, K. (1973) Dynamic aspects of synaptic ultrastructure, *Brain Res.*, 49: 511–518.

Armstrong-James, M. and Johnson, R. (1970) Quantitative studies of postnatal changes in synapses in rat superficial motor cerebral cortex, *Z. Zellforsch.*, 110: 559–568.

Brizzee, K.R. and Jacobs, L.A. (1959) Postnatal changes in volumetric and density relationships of neurons in cerebral cortex of cat, *Acta anat. (Basel)*, 38: 291–303.

Ceccarelli, B. and Hurlbut, W.P. (1975) Transmitter release and the vesicle hypothesis. In *Golgi Centennial Symposium*, M. Santini, (Ed.), Raven Press, New York, pp. 529–545.

Changeux, J.P. and Danchin, A. (1976) Selective stabilisation of developing synapses as a mechanism for the specification of neuronal networks, *Nature (Lond.)*, 264: 705–712.

Chow, K.L. (1973) Neuronal changes in the visual system following visual deprivation. In *Handbook of Sensory Physiology, Vol. VII/3A*, R. Jung, (Ed.), Springer, Berlin, pp. 599–627.

Collewijn, H. (1977) Optokinetic and vestibulo-ocular reflexes in dark-reared rabbits, *Exp. Brain Res.*, 27: 287–300.

Cragg, B.G. (1972) The development of synapses in cat visual cortex, *Invest. Ophthal.*, 11: 377–386.

Cragg, B.G. (1974) Plasticity of synapses. *Brit. med. Bull.*, 30: 141–145.

Cragg, B.G. (1975) The development of synapses in the visual system of the cat, *J. comp. Neurol.*, 160: 147–166.

De Groot, D. and Vrensen, G. (1978) Postnatal development of synaptic contact zones in the visual cortex of rabbits, *Brain Res.*, in press.

Eccles, J.C. (1973) *The Understanding of the Brain*, McGraw-Hill, New York.

Elgeti, H., Elgeti, R. and Fleischhauer, K. (1976) Postnatal growth of the dorsal lateral geniculate nucleus of the cat, *Anat. Embryol.*, 149: 1–13.

Fifková, E. (1970) The effect of unilateral deprivation on visual centers in rats, *J. comp. Neurol.*, 140: 431–438.

Fifková, E. and Hassler, R. (1969) Quantitative morphological changes in visual centers of rats after unilateral deprivation, *J. comp. Neurol.*, 135: 167–178.

Garey, L.J. and Pettigrew, J.D. (1974) Ultrastructural changes in kitten visual cortex after environmental modification, *Brain Res.*, 66: 165–172.

Globus, A. (1975) Brain morphology as a function of presynaptic morphology and activity. In *The Developmental Neuropsychology of Sensory Deprivation*, A.H. Riesen, (Ed.), Academic Press, New York, pp. 9–91.

Grobstein, P. and Chow, K.L. (1976) Receptive field organization in the mammalian visual cortex: the role of individual experience in development. In *Neural and Behavioral Specificity*, G. Gottlieb, (Ed.), Academic Press, New York, pp. 155–193.

Guillery, R.W. and Casagrande, V.A. (1977) Studies of the modifiability of the visual pathways in midwestern Siamese cats, *J. comp. Neurol.*, 174: 15–46.

Hamburger, V. (1975) Changing concepts in developmental neurobiology, *Perspect. Biol. Med.*, 18: 162–178.

Harel, S., Watanaba, K., Linke, I. and Schain, R.J. (1972) Growth and development of the rabbit brain, *Biol. Neonate*, 21: 381–399.

Heuser, J.E. and Reese, T.S. (1974) Morphology of synaptic vesicle discharge and reformation at the frog neuromuscular junction. In *Synaptic Transmission and Neuronal Interaction*, M.V.L. Bennett, (Ed.), Raven Press, New York, pp. 59–85.

Hubel, D.H., Wiesel, T.N. and LeVay, S. (1976) Functional architecture of area 17 in normal and monocularly deprived macaque monkeys, *Cold Spr. Harb. Symp. quant. Biol.*, 40: 581–589.

Jones, D.G., Dittmer, M.M. and Reading, L.C. (1974) Synaptogenesis in guinea-pig cerebral cortex: a glutaraldehyde-PTA study, *Brain Res.*, 70: 245–259.

Kristt, D.A. and Molliver, M.E. (1976) Synapses in newborn rat cerebral cortex: a quantitative ultrastructural study. *Brain Res.*, 108: 180–186.

Lippe, W.R. (1976) Innate and experiential factors in the development of the visual system: historical basis of current controversy. In *Neural and Behavioral Specificity*, G. Gottlieb, (Ed.), Academic Press, New York, pp. 5–24.

Parnavelas, J. (1978) Influence of stimulation on cortical development, this volume.

Uylings, H.B.M., Kuijpers, K. and Veltman, W.A.M. (1978) Environmental influences on the neocortex in later life, this volume.

Valverde, F. (1971) Rate and extent of recovery from dark rearing in the visual cortex of the mouse, *Brain Res.*, 33:1–11.

Van Hof, M.W. (1974) Retinal input and early development of the visual system. *Docum. Ophthal. (Den Haag) Proc. Ser.*, 4: 466–471.

Van Hof, M.W. and Kobayashi, K. (1972) Pattern discrimination in rabbits deprived of light for 7 months after birth, *Exp. Neurol.*, 35: 551–557.

Vrensen, G. and De Groot, D. (1973) Quantitative stereology of synapses: a critical investigation. *Brain Res.*, 58: 25–35.

Vrensen, G. and De Groot, D. (1974) Osmium-zinc iodide staining and the quantitative study of central synapses, *Brain Res.*, 74: 131–142.

Vrensen, G. and De Groot, D. (1974) The effect of dark rearing and its recovery on synaptic terminals in the visual cortex of rabbits: a quantitative electron microscopic study. *Brain Res.*, 78: 263–278.

Vrensen, G. and De Groot, D. (1975) The effect of monocular deprivation on synaptic terminals in the visual cortex of rabbits: a quantitative electron microscopic study, *Brain Res.*, 93: 15–24.

Vrensen, G., De Groot, D. and Nunes-Cardozo, J. (1977) The postnatal development of neurons and synapses in the visual and motor cortex of rabbits: a quantitative light and electron microscopic study, *Brain Res. Bull.*, 2:405–416.

Vrensen, G. and De Groot, D. (1977) Quantitative aspects of the synaptic organization of the superior colliculus in control and dark-reared rabbits, *Brain Res.*, 134: 417–428.

Weibel, E.R. (1969) Stereological principles for morphometry in electron microscopic cytology. *Int. Rev. Cytol.*, 26: 235–320.

DISCUSSION

SPEKREIJSE: Why would you have expected to see a variation in the synaptic density after visual deprivation, since in one of the first slides you showed that there was a monotonic increase in synaptic density with age: there was no inflection in the curve around, for example, the period of eye-opening. A second question is: do you think that your conclusions are restricted to rabbits, and that you may not extrapolate them to animals with a more complicated visual behavior?

VRENSEN: With respect to the first question: we counted synaptic density because there were a number of studies — especially the work of Valverde is often cited as being conclusive — showing that the density of spines decreases because of visual deprivation. When you look at his data closely, however, you will see that the effect lasts for just a short period of time: after 30 days the number of spines is indeed lower, but at 65 days (the longest time at which he measured) the number of spines is quite normal. This is what has brought Chow and Grobstein to the conclusion that deprivation merely *delays* the formation of synapses; it does not alter or change the formation of synapses. As regards your second question: there are very few quantitative studies in this field, and extrapolation is therefore dangerous.

BERRY: It would be important to obtain some clarification of the apparent rabbit anomaly in this situation, since if you dark-rear a *cat* beyond the age of eye-opening, permanent visual blindness results.

VRENSEN: I think you have to be careful in saying that there is a difference between the rabbit, on the one hand, and the rat, the cat and the mouse, on the other hand. In the work of Valverde to which I referred, you can see that the changes in spine density on the apical dendrites of the visual cortex in the mouse are only temporary; they have disappeared by day 60. For the cat one of the few deprivation studies at the electron microscopic level is that of Garey and Pettigrew (in *Brain Res.*, 1974). In this study it is shown that the synaptic vesicle density is lower in deprived animals as compared with control animals. This is in line with our observations in the rabbit. Moreover, they have shown that the lower synaptic vesicle density can be abolished by providing visual input during the critical period. These few examples show that species differences are probably not as striking as is often thought, although they almost certainly do exist. However, the main causes of the apparently conflicting data are: (a) the type of deprivation used, and (b) the quantitative methods used.

BERRY: Were your animals blind during the recovery period? I ask this question because you say that the connections in the visual cortex (at least as far as synaptic numbers are concerned) were not altered by dark-rearing. If the animals can't see, then the kind of synapses that they form obviously have nothing to do with visual functioning.

VRENSEN: That is quite unlikely, for when the light-deprived rabbits come out of their cages (which is why the behavioral experiments are so interesting in this respect) they just need, let's say, one week to get accustomed to the light. After one or two weeks they were used for visual discrimination tests, and they behaved quite well. I can't see how these animals could have had a normal visual performance after such a short time if the neuronal connections had not been properly made. Furthermore, this recovery also holds true for visual-evoked potentials measured directly after the dark-rearing period.

STIRLING: Did you see any difference in the *length* of the synaptic contacts during maturation, as I have found in the hippocampal mossy fibers?

VRENSEN: When we analyzed the lengths of synaptic contact zones during maturation in random sections, using the stereological methods mentioned, no change in length was observed. However, detailed analysis of the contact zones has revealed an increase in the number of dense projections, and also in their dimensions, thus suggesting an increase in synaptic size. This apparent contradiction between the overall values and the detailed analysis can be explained by the fact that many *small* synapses are formed during maturation. This means that, at a certain developmental stage, new small synapses are mixed up with old large ones. Because of this, the mean values of the contact zones does not change, but we are, nevertheless, pretty sure that there is some increase in size such as you have found in hippocampal terminals.

CHANGEUX: Using this EPTA-technique, one may miss the very early stages of synaptogenesis. This being said, there is another stage (just taking the neuromuscular junction as an example) where, once the subsynaptic membrane has differentiated, you have a redundancy of the nerve endings on a given subsynaptic membrane. Maybe your counts of synaptic vesicles in fact showed exactly the same thing. I don't know if you can really say that you have not had any change in the number of nerve terminals.

VRENSEN: I realize quite well that with the EPTA-, and also with the OZI-method used, we only visualize morphologically well-differentiated synaptic terminals, and that we are not able to detect non-occupied receptor sites on the subsynaptic membrane. So it may be that we have indeed missed undifferentiated redundant nerve terminals. On the other hand, we are pretty sure that once the synapse has become established morphologically (and probably functionally) it does not disappear. No signs of cortical degeneration have been observed up to one month postnatally, and also not in the adult rabbit either.

Influence of Stimulation on Cortical Development

JOHN G. PARNAVELAS*

Department of Anatomy, University College London, London (Great Britain)

BACKGROUND

In 1964 Sharpless, reviewing the changes in neuronal connections found to result from excessive use or disuse, argued against the excessive use theory as an explanation for the strengthening of functional connections which may be occurring in learning. He drew heavily upon data from experiments on the effects of disuse, primarily in the peripheral nervous system. Since then, a variety of studies of increased neuronal activity in the central nervous system (for a recent review see Cragg, 1972) suggest that the excessive use theory should not be abandoned. Stimulation and environmental manipulation have been used to study the changes in the properties of neurons and synapses produced by use in an effort to understand the ways in which these changes are induced. Many of these studies, which belong to one of two categories, involve increased sensory input to the cerebral cortex. The first paradigm consists of raising animals from birth inside a cage containing toys and learning experiences (enriched environment); this condition is then compared with one which is devoid of these things (impoverished environment) (Krech et al., 1960). The second paradigm involves experiments of forced activity or overstimulation; the majority of such experiments reported in the literature involves either direct electrical stimulation or increased stimulation by means of light.

I have used constant light as a means of producing an environment of continuous visual stimulation (Parnavelas, 1976a, b; Parnavelas and Globus, 1976a, b). It is now well established that continuous illumination causes damage of the photoreceptors in the retina of rats and other animals (Noell et al., 1966; Noell and Albrecht, 1971; O'Stein and Anderson, 1972). This condition, therefore, provides an additional advantage by creating a model of the retina for the investigation of interrelationships among cell types within the retina and the visual system. In this chapter I will review changes in certain morphological parameters (dendritic branching of non-pyramidal neurons and spine density of pyramidal neurons) and electrophysiological parameters (evoked potentials) in the visual cortex (area 17) of rats reared under continuous illumination from birth to 80 days, as compared with the same area of cortex in control animals reared in a similar environment but on a 12-hr light-dark cycle. The details of the rearing procedure have been published elsewhere (Parnavelas and Globus, 1976a). These experiments were designed to test the hypothesis that certain postsynaptic structures might respond to an increase in the amount of sensory information by increasing the number of available synaptic sites. This is feasible in view of evidence, derived from developmental studies, which shows that the development and maturation of dendrites and

*Now at Dept. of Cell Biology, University of Texas, Health Science Center at Dallas, Texas 75235, U.S.A.

synapses in the mammalian brain occurs to a considerable extent postnatally (Cajal, 1960; Morest, 1969; Molliver and Van der Loos, 1970; Krist and Molliver, 1976). Moreover, studies of environmental manipulation suggest that the structural and functional maturation of visual system components depend partly upon visual experience (see Globus, 1975; Blakemore and Van Sluyters, 1975). The findings to be reported here will be examined in relation to other experiments of increased sensory stimulation produced by continuous illumination and by other means. Experiments which describe short-term synaptic modification in response to brief bursts of electrical stimulation (see Cragg, 1972; Chung, 1977) or hormonal effects on the growth of synapses (see Cragg, 1972) will not be included in this paper.

It is well known that retinal ganglion cells display continuous maintained activity under conditions of steady illumination or darkness. This implies that visual stimuli are transmitted by modulation of the ever-present activity (Kuffler et al., 1957). In this experiment of continuous illumination, it is assumed that the visual stimulus is provided by the contents of the cage (i.e. members of the litter, sawdust and food pellets on the floor, water bottle, light source and air circulation fans) and by the brief presence of the experimenter who provides a supply of food and water daily. It can also be assumed that this experimental condition, like all conditions of forced activity, is probably one of stress as well as of increased sensory input.

MORPHOLOGICAL AND PHYSIOLOGICAL RESULTS

Dendrite measurements on cortical non-pyramidal neurons

The dendrites of non-pyramidal cells in layer IV of the visual cortex were studied in experimental and control animals at 35 days of age. Using the Golgi-Cox technique, preliminary measurements were made on 12–15 non-pyramidal cells of the spine-free and spinous varieties (Parnavelas et al., 1977a) from each animal of each of 6 littermate pairs. A three-dimensional automated system for tracing and quantification of neuronal processes developed by Coleman and coworkers (Coleman et al., 1977) was used for the measurements. Information obtained from each cell included a list of all dendrite segments as well as their order and length. A branch emanating from the soma was defined as first order, both branches after the first bifurcation were defined as second order, the two branches past the second bifurcation as the third order, and so forth (Fig. 1a).

Analysis of the measurements showed that the mean number of branches of all orders for animals reared in continuous light from birth was not statistically different from their littermate controls (one-tailed Mann Whitney U-test and Student's t-test) (Fig. 2). In addition, there was no systematic pattern related to rearing conditions in differences of mean total dendritic length per neuron for the 6 littermate pairs of rats. The mean dendritic length per non-pyramidal cell of the continuous light group of animals (1126.5 μm) was not statistically different from that of the control group (1145.1 μm) (Table I).

Spine counts in cortical pyramidal neurons

Using the rapid Golgi technique, spines on the dendrites of pyramidal cells were counted in layers IV and V of the visual cortex in animals 8–80 days of age (Fig. 1b). A higher density of spines was found in animals reared in constant light than in controls. A significant increase was first observed along the proximal two-thirds of the apical shafts at 16 days of age. It became generalized over the entire dendritic field at day 20, and persisted at least until day 80 (Fig. 3; also see Tables I–IV in Parnavelas and Globus, 1976b). Counts on dendrites of layer IV pyramidal cells in the frontal cortex, an area which receives no direct

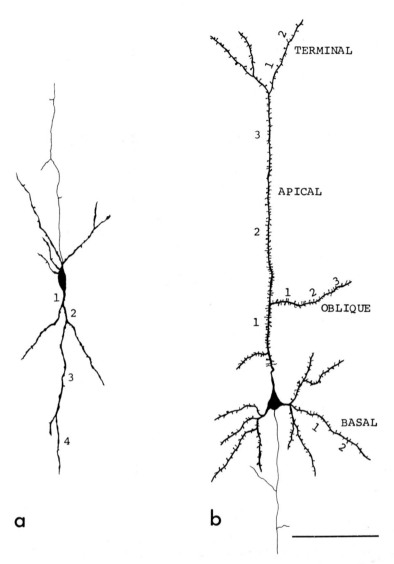

Fig. 1. a: camera lucida drawing of a non-pyramidal cell in layer IV of rat visual cortex. The numbers refer to the order of the dendritic segments. b: camera lucida drawing of a pyramidal cell in layer IV of rat visual cortex showing the spine counting stations on the apical, oblique, terminal and basal dendrites. Scale: 100 μm.

visual input, did not show any statistically significant differences in the number of spines for any part of the dendritic field between experimental and control animals at 35 days of age (Table II).

Visual evoked responses

Visual evoked responses were recorded from area 17 of rats reared in constant light from birth to 35, 45 and 80 days as well as from controls of the same ages. A minimum of four averaged responses, each to 50 flashes of light, were obtained from every animal (for details of the experimental procedure see Parnavelas, 1976b). In the analysis of the averaged responses, peak-to-peak amplitudes from $P_1–N_1$, $N_1–P_2$, and $P_2–N_2$ were measured (Fig. 4A).

250

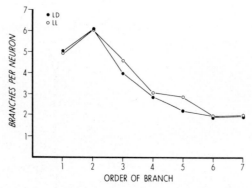

Fig. 2. Plot of the mean number of dendritic branches of each order per non-pyramidal neuron from 6 littermate pairs. LD, control illumination; LL, continuous illumination.

TABLE I

TOTAL DENDRITIC LENGTH IN MICROMETERS

Littermate pair	LD	LL
1	1152.3 ± 99.4*	1137.9 ± 104.1
2	969.6 ± 102.4	891.6 ± 50.9
3	1275.6 ± 170.8	1196.9 ± 108.6
4	1163.6 ± 79.5	1123.6 ± 92.2
5	1041.0 ± 118.3	994.7 ± 92.5
6	1268.8 ± 82.2	1414.5 ± 103.5

* Standard error of the mean.
LD, control illumination; LL, continuous illumination.

Analysis of the recorded potentials showed that all three components had a significantly higher amplitude in rats reared in continuous illumination for 35 days than in control animals (Fig. 4A; Table III). The responses obtained from the 45-day experimental animals were similar to those recorded from control animals except that they had a slightly lower amplitude (Fig. 4B). Finally, the evoked responses recorded from experimental rats at 80 days displayed all primary components, but were reduced considerably in amplitude (Fig. 4C).

SIGNIFICANCE OF THE RESULTS

Morphological changes

Analysis of dendritic branching patterns has been found useful in elucidating the principles of neuronal interaction (Sholl, 1953). Only recently have careful and systematic analyses of the branching patterns of neurons in various parts of the central nervous system appeared in the literature (Hollingworth and Berry, 1975; Uylings et al., 1975). These methods of analysis have been facilitated by automated measuring systems such as the one used in this study (see Coleman et al., 1977).

In the present study, the effects of exposing rats to constant light from birth were sought in measurements of dendritic branching and length of layer IV non-pyramidal neurons in the visual cortex. There was no significant difference in either the branching pattern or the total

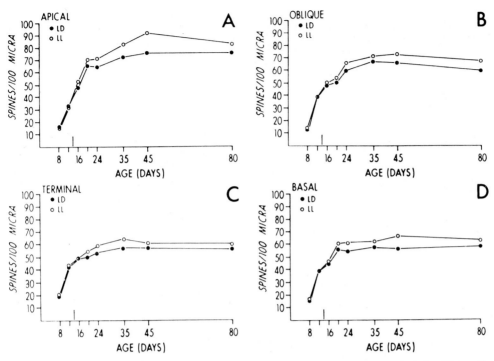

Fig. 3. Changes with age in the mean density of spines counted at station 1. A: apical; B: oblique; C: terminal and D: basal dendrites. Line on day 14 indicates the approximate time of opening of the animals' eyes. LD, control illumination; LL, continuous illumination.

TABLE II

FRONTAL CORTEX: DENDRITIC SPINES PER MICROMETER

		LD	LL	P*
Apical:	1	0.75 ± 0.011**	0.75 ± 0.008	n.s.
	2	0.75 ± 0.007	0.76 ± 0.012	n.s.
	3	0.66 ± 0.011	0.65 ± 0.013	n.s.
Oblique:	1	0.67 ± 0.010	0.68 ± 0.010	n.s.
	2	0.64 ± 0.012	0.64 ± 0.008	n.s.
	3	0.62 ± 0.009	0.63 ± 0.008	n.s.
Basal:	1	0.63 ± 0.009	0.62 ± 0.011	n.s.
	2	0.60 ± 0.011	0.61 ± 0.010	n.s.
Terminal:	1	0.56 ± 0.012	0.56 ± 0.013	n.s.
	2	0.46 ± 0.011	0.47 ± 0.013	n.s.

*Student t-test; n.s. = not significant.
** Standard error of the mean.
LD, control illumination; LL, continuous illumination.

dendritic length of neurons between the experimental and control rats at 35 days. Therefore, continuous illumination and the degenerative changes in the retino-geniculate pathway after day 20 due to degeneration of photoreceptors (only one-half of the normal number of

252

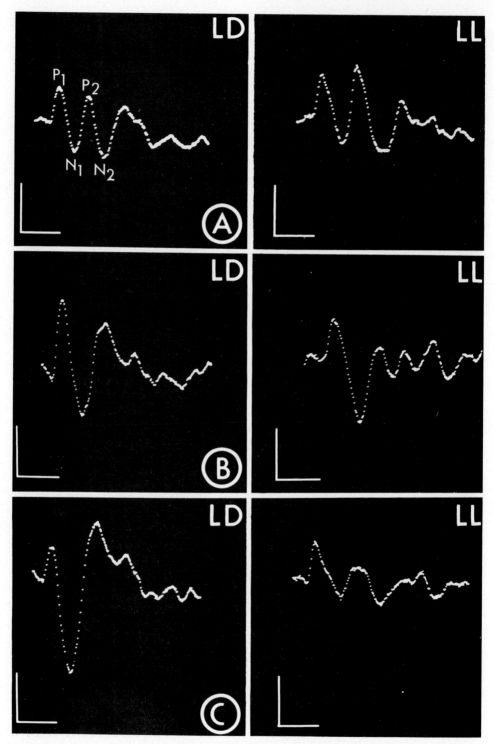

Fig. 4. Averaged visual evoked potentials recorded from control (LD) and experimental (LL) rats to 50 flashes of light at: A, 35 days; B, 45 days and C, 80 days of age. Calibrations: 50 msec and 200 μV.

TABLE III

MEAN AMPLITUDE OF VISUAL EVOKED RESPONSE COMPONENTS IN
MICROVOLTS

	P_1-N_1	N_1-P_2	P_2-N_2
LD	321.8 ± 19.8*	307.1 ± 25.1	253.0 ± 19.5
LL	443.7 ± 36.4	424.5 ± 47.7	353.9 ± 43.3
$P**$	<0.005	<0.005	<0.005

*Standard error of the mean.
** Student's t-test.
LD, control illumination; LL, continuous illumination.

photoreceptors are present in the retinae of the 35-day experimental animals; Parnavelas and Globus, 1976a) do not appear to alter the dendritic field of layer IV non-pyramidal neurons at 35 days of age, although ultrastructural studies suggest that these neurons are recipients of at least some of the geniculo-cortical axons (Peters and Feldman, 1976, 1977).

The present findings differ from results of experiments involving rats reared in an enriched environment. These experiments have shown an increase in the branching of non-pyramidal cells in the visual cortex of enriched animals as compared to impoverished rats (Volkmar and Greenough, 1972). Inconsistent findings have been reported concerning the response of non-pyramidal neurons to lack of visual stimulation (Coleman and Riesen, 1968; Globus and Scheibel, 1967a; Valverde, 1968; Borges and Berry, 1976), although these differences could be due to species and/or methodological differences. However, it might still be that experiments involving environmental manipulation are inadequate to determine precisely the ways in which non-pyramidal cell dendrites are affected by stimuli.

Increased branching has been reported for the basal dendrites of pyramidal cells in layers II, III and IV of young rats reared in an enriched environment (Greenough and Volkmar, 1973). Increased branching and length of the terminal segments has also been observed in basal dendrites of layer II and III pyramids in adult rats exposed to an enriched environment for 30 days (Uylings et al., 1978). In a different experiment, which involved electrical stimulation of the suprasylvian gyrus of adult cats every day for several weeks, Rutledge and coworkers (Rutledge et al., 1974; Rutledge, 1976) reported that pyramidal cells of layers II and III in the cortex contralateral to the side of stimulation developed more branches in the terminal portion of the apical dendrites. On the basis of these few studies, it appears that stimulation increases the branching of cortical pyramidal neurons.

A variety of types of stimulation seem to increase the number of dendritic spines in cortical neurons. In the present study, a greater density of spines was found on the dendrites of cortical pyramidal cells in animals reared in constant light than in control littermates reared on a 12-hr light-dark cycle. This increase appeared prior to the onset of the photoreceptor degeneration, although it is possible that degeneration commenced earlier but was not detected with the light microscope. Dendritic spines in the cerebral cortex receive almost exclusively excitatory synapses (Gray, 1959; Parnavelas et al., 1977b). It appears, therefore, that continuous illumination produces an increase in the number of excitatory connections, which might reflect increased demand for processing of information in the visual cortex.

The increased number of spines along the apical shafts of pyramidal neurons was observed shortly after the time of eye opening, presumably as a direct result of excess visual stimulation transmitted by the primary visual pathway. This finding lends support to the results of some investigators suggesting that the apical dendrites of pyramidal neurons whose perikarya are situated in the deeper cortical layers are the sites of termination of geniculo-cortical fibers (Globus and Scheibel, 1967b: Winfield and Powell, 1976), although recent studies by Peters and colleagues (e.g. Peters and Feldman, 1977) suggest that most neuronal elements in layer IV which are capable of forming asymmetric synaptic junctions are potential recipients of the geniculo-cortical afferents. As for the increase in spine density in the remaining portion of the dendritic field (i.e. basal, oblique and terminal dendrites) of the layer IV and V pyramidal neurons, it might be due to influence(s) exerted by other pyramidal neurons via intracortical connections from the ipsilateral and contralateral cortex. This is consistent with the findings of Globus (1971) following cortical lesions in rabbits. The fact that no differences in spines were observed in pyramidal cells of frontal cortex suggests that the effects of continuous illumination are restricted to the visual system and related areas.

It has been suggested that enhanced visual stimulation is the cause of the increase in number of spines observed in the visual cortex connected to the undeprived eye of rats with monocular eye closure, compared to undeprived controls (Fifková, 1974). In another study of stimulation, Schapiro and Vukovich (1970) reported an increase in the density of spines, although sparse at the stage of development studied, in pyramidal cells of 8-day-old rats subjected to a variety of sensory stimuli from birth. Rutledge et al. (1974) also reported higher density of spines on the dendrites of pyramidal cells in the suprasylvian gyrus of adult cats after long-term electrical stimulation of the contralateral side. Finally, in rats reared in an enriched environment for 30 days after weaning, the density of spines was found to be higher along the basal, oblique and terminal dendrites of layer V pyramids of the visual cortex compared to impoverished animals (Globus et al., 1973).

There have also been reported changes in overall dimensions, in cell numbers and in cell morphology and chemistry in animals exposed to various forms of stimuli. Quantitative measurements of the thickness of the visual cortex have been made in mice reared in continuous light from birth to 51 days and in animals reared in normal lighting conditions. No difference was observed in the thickness of cortex between the two groups of animals (Egert, 1975). Enriched environment results in an increase in cortical weight and thickness over that of animals reared in an impoverished environment, with the increase being greatest in the occipital area (Bennett et al., 1964; Rosenzweig et al., 1972). This effect, which can also be induced in adult rats, does not appear to be solely the result of visual stimulation. For example, it has been reported that environmentally enriched but blinded rats showed an increased weight of visual cortex relative to impoverished animals (Krech et al., 1963). The possibility still remains that this increase in cortical weight and thickness is due to some hormonal influence, and not due to increased visual stimulation.

There are only a few studies which have examined changes in cell numbers in the cerebral cortex as a result of stimulation. The number of glial cells (astrocytes and oligodendrocytes) is increased in animals exposed to an enriched environment, while the number of neurons remains unchanged (Diamond et al., 1966; Szeligo and Leblond, 1977). In adult rats reared in an enriched environment from weaning there is increased proliferation of glial cells in the cortex, and particularly in the cortical radiation and corpus callosum (Altman and Das, 1964), relative to animals reared in an impoverished environment. In a pilot study, nerve cell proliferation was reported to be increased in the neocortex as well as in the cerebellum and hippocampus of rats handled daily, from day 2 to 11 (Altman et al., 1968). Handling of rats has also been found to produce cortical enlargement and an increase in the number of astrocytes (Szeligo and Leblond, 1977).

A variety of perikaryal changes have been reported in the cortex of animals as a result of stimulation. Intense light stimulation for 3 hr produced no changes in protein metabolism in the visual cortex of adult rabbits (Gomirato and Boggio, 1962). In rats exposed to visual stimulation for 3 hr following dark rearing, an increase was observed in visual cortex acetyl-cholinesterase (Sinha and Rose, 1976). Talwar et al. (1966) reported an increase in the incorporation of radioactive precursors into protein in the visual cortex of adult rabbits which were kept in the dark but stimulated daily by flickering light. These authors also reported that protein content increased markedly in the developing visual cortex of rabbits after opening of the eyes. In a similar study, Rose (1977) reported increased incorporation of radioactive lysine in the visual cortex, lateral geniculate nucleus and retina of rats reared in the dark from birth to 50 days, and subsequently exposed to controlled illumination. In another experiment of stimulation, Kocher (1916) subjected a variety of mammals to forms of forced activity including shock, electrical and chemical stimulation. By using a modification of the Nissl method, he observed no quantitative changes in neurons of the cerebrum, cerebellum and spinal cord. Finally, in rats exposed to an enriched environment, neuronal perikarya in the cortex were larger in diameter, compared to those of animals reared in an impoverished environment (Diamond, 1967).

Physiological changes

Visual evoked responses recorded from rats reared in continuous light had primary components of higher amplitude at 35 days as compared with potentials recorded from animals reared on a 12 hr light-dark cycle. The increased amplitude of the evoked response, an unexpected result in view of the findings in the retina which show that approximately one-half of the photoreceptors have degenerated in these experimental animals (Parnavelas and Globus, 1976a), is presumably due to either increased cortical connectivity or decreased inhibition of cortical neurons. This effect, which was the opposite of that recorded from rats reared in darkness from birth to 35 days (Spencer et al., 1974), was principally in amplitude and not latency, implying that the transmission rate through the system had not changed.

In a similar study of continuous illumination, O'Steen and Anderson (1971) recorded visual evoked potentials from adult rats which had been exposed to constant light for 4 to 30 days. Their results, which show potentials of lower amplitude and longer latency in the experimental animals, are inconsistent and disagree with the findings reported in the present paper. My findings, however, are in agreement with results of other experiments involving continuous illumination or other forms of cortical stimulation. Rose and Gruenau (1973), for instance, reported an increase in the components of the visual evoked response recorded from cats reared in continuous illumination from birth to 8 months as compared with normal controls. Although these investigators did not examine the retinae of these cats, by extrapolation from the findings in other species (Lauber et al., 1961; Siss et al., 1970; Lawwill, 1973; Tso, 1973; Parnavelas 1976a; Parnavelas and Globus, 1976a) it may be assumed that the retinae were at least partially degenerated, but that photoreceptors were present in sufficient numbers to evoke a response in the visual cortex.

The strength of the visual stimulus necessary to produce a cortical response might be critical, as suggested by the evoked potentials of reduced amplitude recorded from animals reared in constant light from birth to 45 and to 80 days. Although these animals had a greater number of spines in the visual cortex, their retinae were so severely damaged that they appeared to be completely devoid of photoreceptors at 80 days (Parnavelas and Globus, 1976a). Enucleation at 80 days abolished the response totally, indicating the presence of photoreceptors in the eyes of these experimental rats (Parnavelas, 1976b). Survival of some photoreceptor cells, particularly cones, has indeed been demonstrated by electron microscopy in the retinae of rats following long-term exposure to continuous illumination (LaVail, 1976).

Other studies of excess stimulation during ontogeny have also shown an increase in cortical electrical activity. Visual evoked potentials of higher amplitude were recorded in rabbits reared in an environment of intermittent light stimulation from birth to 6 months (Fourment and Cramer, 1961). In a similar study, the EEG recorded from rats presented constantly with clicks and flashes of light at a frequency of 5 per second from birth to adult displayed spindle-shaped bursts of high amplitude activity in the visual cortex and subcortical matter (Heron and Anchel, 1964). Enhanced evoked responses were also recorded from the cortex of cats as a result of conditional stimulation of the contralateral homotopic area (Rutledge, 1965). Finally, visual evoked responses to photic stimulation were of shorter latency in rats reared in an enriched environment than in control animals, or in rats whose environment was devoid of visual stimuli (Mailloux et al., 1974).

CONCLUSION

The findings of this study show that stimulation of the visual pathway by means of continuous illumination enhances the growth of receptive portions of pyramidal neurons and, therefore, increases the opportunity for neuronal interaction in the visual cortex. This, and the numerous studies reviewed in this paper, indicates clearly that the growth of neural receptive surface in the cerebral cortex can be increased under conditions of enhanced function.

ACKNOWLEDGEMENTS

I wish to thank Drs. A.R. Lieberman and H.B.M. Uylings for helpful critcisms, Dr. P.D. Coleman for allowing me to use his dendrite tracking system, and Liza Rosser for the typing.

REFERENCES

Altman, J. and Das, G.D. (1964) Autoradiographic examination of the effects of enriched environment on the rate of glial multiplication in the adult rat brain, *Nature (Lond.)*, 204: 1161–1163.

Altman, J., Das, G.D. and Anderson, W.J. (1968) Effects of infantile handling on morphological development of rat brain: an exploratory study, *Develop. Psychobiol.*, 1: 10–20.

Bennett, E.L., Diamond, M.C., Krech, D. and Rosenzweig, M.R. (1964) Chemical and anatomical plasticity of brain, *Science*, 146: 610–619.

Blakemore, C. and Van Sluyters, R.C. (1975) Innate and environmental factors in the development of the kitten's visual cortex, *J. Physiol. (Lond.)*, 248: 663–716.

Borges, S. and Berry, M. (1976) Preferential orientation of stellate cell dendrites in the visual cortex of the dark-reared rat, *Brain Res.*, 112: 141–147.

Cajal, S.R. (1960) *Studies on Vertebrate Neurogenesis,* translated by L. Guth. Charles C. Thomas, Springfield, Ill.

Chung, S.-H. (1977) Synaptic memory in the hippocampus, *Nature (Lond.)*, 266: 677–678.

Coleman, P.D. and Riesen, A.H. (1968) Environmental effects on cortical dendritic fields. I. Rearing in the dark, *J. Anat. (Lond.)*, 102: 363–374.

Coleman, P.D., Garvey, C.F., Young, J.H. and Simon, W. (1977) Semiautomatic tracking of neuronal processes. In *Computer Analysis of Neuronal Structures*, R.D. Lindsay (Ed.), Plenum Press, New York, pp. 91–110.

Cragg, B.G. (1972) Plasticity of synapses. In *The Structure and Function of Nervous Tissue, Vol. 4*, G.H. Bourne (Ed.), Academic Press, New York, pp. 1–60.

Diamond, M.C. (1967) Extensive cortical depth measurements and neuron size increases in the cortex of environmentally enriched rats, *J. comp. Neurol.*, 131: 357–364.

Diamond, M.C., Law, F., Rhodes, H., Lindner, B., Rosenzweig, M.R., Krech, D. and Bennett, E.L. (1966) Increases in cortical depth and glial numbers in rats subjected to enriched environment, *J. comp. Neurol.*, 128: 117–126.

Egert, M. (1975) Quantitativ-architektonische Veränderugen der Schrinde von Mäusen bei unterschiedlichen Lichteinwirkungen auf das Sehorgan, *J. Hirnforsch.*, 16: 15–36.

Fifková, E. (1974) Plastic and degenerative changes in visual centers. In *Advances in Psychobiology, Vol. 2*, G. Newton and A.H. Riesen (Eds.), Wiley, New York, pp. 59–131.

Fourment, A. et Cramer, H. (1961) Résponses électrocorticales visuelles du Lapin soumis durant son développement á une surstimulation lumineuse, *Rev. Neurol. (Paris)*, 105: 196–197.

Globus, A. (1971) Neuronal ontogeny: its use in tracing connectivity. In *Brain Development and Behavior*, M.B. Sterman, D.J. McGinty and A.M. Adinolfi (Eds.), Academic Press, New York, pp. 253–263.

Globus, A. (1975) Brain morphology as a function of presynaptic morphology and activity. In *The Developmental Neuropsychology of Sensory Deprivation*, A.H. Riesen (Ed.), Academic Press, New York, pp. 9–91.

Globus, A. and Scheibel, A.B. (1967a) The effect of visual deprivation on cortical neurons: a Golgi study, *Exp. Neurol.*, 19: 331–345.

Globus, A. and Scheibel, A.B. (1967b) Synaptic loci on visual cortical neurons of the rabbit: the specific afferent radiation, *Exp. Neurol.*, 18: 116–131.

Globus, A., Rosenzweig, M.R., Bennett, E.L. and Diamond, M.C. (1973) Effects of differential experience on dendritic spine counts in rat cerebral cortex, *J. comp. physiol. Psychol.*, 82: 175–181.

Gomirato, G. and Baggio, G. (1962) Metabolic relations between the neurons of the optic pathway in various functional conditions, *J. Neuropath, exp. Neurol.*, 21: 634–644.

Gray, E.G. (1959) Axo-somatic and axo-dendritic synapses of the cerebral cortex: an electron microscope study, *J. Anat. (Lond.)*, 93: 420–433.

Greenough, W.T. and Volkmar, F.R. (1973) Pattern of dendrite branching in occipital cortex of rats reared in complex environments, *Exp. Neurol.*, 40: 491–504.

Hollingworth, T. and Berry, M. (1975) Network analysis of dendritic fields of pyramidal cells in neocortex and Purkinje cells in the cerebellum of the rat, *Phil. Trans. B*, 270: 227–264.

Heron, W. and Anchel, H. (1964) Synchronous sensory bombardment of young rats: effects on the electroencephalogram *Science*, 145: 946–947.

Kocher, R.A. (1916) The effect of activity on the histological structure of nerve cells, *J. comp. Neurol.*, 26: 341–358.

Krech, D., Rosenzweig, M.R. and Bennett, E.L. (1960) Effects of environmental complexity and training on brain chemistry, *J. comp. physiol. Psychol.*, 53: 509–519.

Krech, D., Rosenzweig, M.R. and Bennett, E.L. (1963) Effects of complex environment and blindness on rat brain, *Arch. Neurol. (Chic.)*, 8: 403–412.

Krist, D.A. and Molliver, M.E. (1976) Synapses in newborn rat cerebral cortex: a quantitative ultrastructural study, *Brain Res.*, 108: 180–186.

Kuffler, S.W. Fitzhugh, R. and Barlow, H.B. (1957) Maintained activity in the cat's retina in light and darkness, *J. gen. Physiol.*, 40: 683–702.

Lauber, J.K., Shutze, J.V. and McGinnis, J. (1961) Effects of exposure to continuous light on the eye of the growing chick, *Proc. Soc. exp. Biol. (N.Y.)*, 106: 871–872.

LaVail, M.M. (1976) Survival of some photoreceptor cells in albino rats following long-term exposure to continuous light, *Invest. Ophthal.*, 15: 64–70.

Lawwill, T. (1973) Effects of prolonged exposure of rabbit retina to low-intensity light, *Invest. Ophthal.*, 12: 45–51.

Mailloux, J.G., Edwards, H.P., Barry, W.F., Rowsell, H.C. and Achorn, E.G. (1974) Effects of differential rearing on cortical evoked potentials of the albino rat, *J. comp. physiol. Psychol.*, 87: 475–480.

Molliver, M.E. and Van der Loos, H. (1970) The ontogenesis of cortical circuitry: the spatial distribution of synapses in somesthetic cortex of newborn dog, *Ergebn. Anat. Entwickl.-Gesch.*, 42(4): 1–53.

Morest, D.K. (1969) The growth of dendrites in the mammalian brain, *Z. Anat. Entwickl.-Gesch.*, 128: 290–317.

Noell, W.K. and Albrecht, R. (1971) Irreversible effects of visible light on the retina: role of vitamin A, *Science,* 172: 76–80.

Noell, W.K., Walker, V.S., Kang, B.S. and Berman, S. (1966) Retinal damage by light in rats, *Invest. Ophthal.,* 5: 450–473.

O'Stein, W.K. and Anderson, K.V. (1971) Photically evoked responses in the visual system of rats exposed to continuous light, *Exp. Neurol.,* 30: 525–534.

O'Steen, W.K. and Anderson, K.V. (1972) Photoreceptor degeneration after exposure of rats to incandescent illumination, *Z. Zellforsch.,* 127: 306–313.

Parnavelas, J.G. (1976a) The electroretinogram of rats reared in continuous illumination, *Exp. Neurol.,* 51: 648–652.

Parnavelas, J.G. (1976b) Photically evoked responses from the visual cortex of rats reared under continuous illumination, *Exp. Neurol.,* 52: 110–118.

Parnavelas, J.G. and Globus, A. (1976a) The damaging effects of continuous illumination on the morphology of the retina of the rat, *Exp. Neurol.,* 51: 171–187.

Parnavelas, J.G. and Globus, A. (1976b) The effect of continuous illumination on the development of cortical neurons in the rat: a Golgi study, *Exp. Neurol.,* 51: 637–647.

Parnavelas, J.G., Lieberman, A.R. and Webster, K.E. (1977a) Organization of neurons in the visual cortex, area 17, of the rat, *J. Anat. (Lond.),* 124: 305–322.

Parnavelas, J.G., Sullivan, K., Lieberman, A.R. and Webster, K.E. (1977b) Neurons and their synaptic organization in the visual cortex of the rat: Electron microscopy of Golgi preparations. *Cell Tiss. Res.,* 183: 499–517.

Peters, A. and Feldman, M. (1976) The projection of the lateral geniculate nucleus to area 17 of the rat cerebral cortex. I. General description, *J. Neurocytol.,* 5: 63–84.

Peters, A. and Feldman, M.L. (1977) The projection of the lateral geniculate nucleus to area 17 of the rat cerebral cortex. IV. Termination upon spiny dendrites. *J. Neurocytol.,* 6: 669–689.

Rose, S.P.R. (1977) Early visual experience, learning, and neurochemical plasticity in the rat and chick. *Phil. Trans. B,* 278: 307–318.

Rose, G.H. and Gruenau, S.P. (1973) Alterations in visual evoked responses and behavior in kittens reared under constant illumination, *Develop. Psychobiol.,* 6: 69–77.

Rosenzweig, M.R., Bennett, E.L. and Diamond, M.C. (1972) Chemical and anatomical plasticity of brain: Replications and extensions. In *Macromolecules and Behavior,* 2nd ed., J. Gaito (Ed.), Appleton-Century-Crofts, New York, pp. 205–278.

Rutledge, L.T. (1965) Facilitation: electrical response enhanced by conditional excitation of cerebral cortex, *Science,* 148: 1246–1248.

Rutledge, L.T. (1976) Synaptogenesis: effects of synaptic use. In *Neural Mechanisms of Learning and Memory,* M.R. Rozenzweig and E.L. Bennett (Eds.), The MIT Press, Cambridge, Mass., pp. 329–339.

Rutledge, L.T., Wright, C. and Duncan, J. (1974) Morphological changes in pyramidal cells of mammalian neocortex associated with increased use, *Exp. Neurol.,* 44: 209–228.

Schapiro, S. and Vukovich, K.R. (1970) Early experience effects upon cortical dendrites: A proposed model for development, *Science,* 167: 292–294.

Sharpless, S.K. (1964) Reorganization of function in the nervous system – use and disuse, *Ann. Rev. Physiol.,* 26: 357–388.

Sholl, D.A. (1953) Dendritic organization in the neurons of the visual and motor cortices of the cat, *J. Anat. (Lond.),* 87: 387–406.

Sinha, A.K. and Rose, S.P.R. (1976) Dark rearing and visual stimulation in the rat: Effect on brain enzymes, *J. Neurochem.,* 27: 921–926.

Sisson, T.R.C., Glauser, S.C., Glauser, E.M., Tasman, W. and Kuwabara, T. (1970) Retinal changes produced by phototherapy, *J. Pediat.,* 77: 221–227.

Spencer, R.F., Parnavelas, J.G. and Coleman, P.D. (1974) Effect of light deprivation on the electroretinogram and the visual evoked response in the rat. In *Soc. Neurosci., Fourth Annu. Meet.,* abstract, p. 433.

Szeligo, F. and Leblond, C.P. (1977) Response of the three main types of glial cells of cortex and corpus callosum in rats handled during suckling or exposed to enriched, control and impoverished environments following weaning, *J. comp. Neurol.,* 172: 247–264.

Talwar, G.P., Chopra, S.P., Goel, B.K. and D'Monte, B. (1966) Correlation of the functional activity of the brain with metabolic parameters – III. Protein metabolism of the occipital cortex in relation to light stimulus, *J. Neurochem.,* 13: 109–116.

Tso, M.O.M. (1973) Photic maculopathy in rhesus monkey. A light and electron microscopic study, *Invest. Ophthal.*, 12: 17–34.

Uylings, H.B.M., Kuypers, K. and Veltman, W.A.M. (1978) Environmental influences on cortical development in later life, this volume.

Uylings, H.B.M., Smit, G.J. and Veltman, W.A.M. (1975) Ordering methods in quantitative analysis of branching structures of dendritic trees. In *Physiology and Pathology of Dendrites, Advances in Neurology, Vol. 12,* G.W. Kreutzberg (Ed.), Raven Press, New York, pp. 247–254.

Valverde, F. (1968) Structural changes in the area striata of the mouse after enucleation, *Exp. Brain Res.*, 5: 274–292.

Volkmar, F.R. and Greenough, W.T. (1972) Rearing complexity affects branching of dendrites in the visual cortex of the rat, *Science*, 176: 1445–1447.

Winfield, D.A. and Powell, T.P.S. (1976) The termination of thalamo-cortical fibres in the visual cortex of the cat, *J. Neurocytol.*, 5: 269–281.

DISCUSSION

VRENSEN: You have talked about a condition of increased visual stimulation, produced by means of continuous illumination. The animals reared in this condition showed severe degenerative changes in the outer segments of the photoreceptors, and they eventually lost their photoreceptors. The question then of course arises, whether you really have a condition of increased stimulation at all, and not in fact one of *decreased* visual stimulation. The input to the visual cortex must surely be changed as a result of degeneration of the photoreceptors.

PARNAVELAS: We studied the retina and visual cortex in rats reared in constant light from birth to 80 days. A significantly higher density of spines was found to be present on the dendrites of cortical pyramidal neurons of these animals compared to controls, and this increase in spines appeared *before* the photoreceptors began to degenerate. A full description of the pathophysiology of animals exposed to continuous illumination is not yet available. The degeneration of photoreceptors in the retina indeed must result in changes of transmission of information from the retinal ganglion cells to the lateral geniculate nucleus. Studies involving enucleation or visual deprivation have shown a loss of spines on the dendrites of pyramidal cells in the visual cortex, while studies involving augmented light stimulation have shown an increase in the number of spines in the same cortical area. Because of these findings in the visual cortex, it is difficult to accept the idea (at least for the time-span between birth and 80 days) that the demonstrated degeneration of photoreceptors is similar to visual deprivation or degeneration. In fact, on the basis of these results, the effects of increased visual stimulation by means of continuous illumination are *opposite* to those of visual deprivation and degeneration.

BERRY: I wonder what the repercussions of the degeneration of photoreceptors are in the lateral geniculate body and in the visual cortex. Have cell counts been done of various layers, and how does this measure up against the hypothesis of increased activity?

PARNAVELAS: We did not do any cell counts in the lateral geniculate body or in the visual cortex. In Nissl preparations the two structures appeared indistinguishable in experimental and control animals. However, measurements of dendrites of relay neurons in the dorsal lateral geniculate nucleus at 35 days showed increased branching and dendritic length in the continuous light animals, when compared with control littermates.

BLOM: I wonder what the latencies of the components of the evoked potentials are, because they are probably more important than the amplitude differences which you measure.

PARNAVELAS: There were no differences in the latencies of the components of the visual evoked potentials between the two groups of animals.

Environmental Influences
on the Neocortex
in Later Life

HARRY B.M. UYLINGS, KAREL KUYPERS and WIM. A.M. VELTMAN

Netherlands Institute for Brain Research, Amsterdam (The Netherlands)

INTRODUCTION

It has been assumed for a long time that no neuronal growth occurs in adult mammals. Cajal (1914), for example, thought that regeneration of axons and dendrites in fully mature nerve centers is irrevocable, since the nerve paths would be fixed by adulthood. However, he did not completely reject the possibility that future research could alter this view (Cajal, 1914, p. 391). It was not until recently that it became accepted that some degree of regeneration of neurites can occur in adult mammals (e.g. Stenevi et al., 1973; Kerr, 1975). Dendrites of hypoglossal neurons in adult rats were found by Sumner and Watson (1971) to regenerate following either transection of the hypoglossal nerve or injection of botulinum toxin into the tongue.

Dendritic outgrowth in adult mammals can occur not only after degeneration but also be induced by electrical stimulation. Thus, Rutledge et al. (1974) observed additional outgrowth of apical dendrites in the cortex of adult cats after longterm electrical stimulation (twenty 2-sec trains per day for about 80 days) applied to the left suprasylvian gyrus. After this period, the apical dendrites of layer II and III pyramidal neurons were shown to have significantly more dendritic branches and spines in the cortex contralateral and homotopic to the stimulated side. They interpreted this as evidence that increased use of specific pathways to and within the cerebral cortex of adult cats can induce postsynaptic growth (Rutledge, et al., 1974; Rutledge, 1976).

The above-mentioned increase in dendritic branching and spines, however, was artificially induced by experimental intervention directly within the neuronal system. It was therefore important to examine the question of whether or not *environmental* conditions can induce additional growth of nerve cell processes in adult mammalian brain. In addition, this would provide some data concerning the question of extrinsic versus intrinsic factors influencing the shaping of neuronal organization (e.g. Tanzi, 1893; Cajal, 1937, pp. 457–460; Jacobson, 1974; Rakic, 1974; Berry et al., this volume; Changeux and Mikoshiba, this volume; Sotelo, this volume).

In this paper, we will focus especially upon the effects of differential environmental experience on dendrites of cortical pyramidal cells in *adult* rats (Uylings, 1977; Uylings et al., 1978). In addition, the results of other studies on environmental influences on the cortex of adult rats will be critically considered. For the effects of increased stimulation or of light deprivation during early development, we refer to the papers of Parnavelas, Berry et al., and of Vrensen, all in this volume.

262

ENVIRONMENTAL CONDITIONS

The conditions commonly used in the differential environmental experience paradigm are the following three. (1) The 'enriched condition' (EC), in which 12 rats of the same sex are housed in a large cage (70 cm × 70 cm × 46 cm), exposed daily to a new set of 6 or more toys, and placed for about a half hour each day in a Hebb-Williams maze apparatus (75 cm × 75 cm). (2) The 'social' or 'standard condition' (SC), in which 3 rats of the same sex are housed in a standard laboratory cage (32 cm × 20 cm × 28 cm) without any toys or exploration of the Hebb-Williams apparatus. (3) The 'isolated condition' (IC), in which a single rat is housed in a cage similar in size to SC cages, and without toys, and which is placed in a quiet and dimly illuminated room. In all three conditions the rats are fed ad libitum (e.g. (Rosenzweig et al., 1972; Greenough, 1976). While the 'enriched condition' is enriched relative to the 'standard' and 'isolated' condition, it probably provides less stimulation than does the natural environment of wild rats. Recently, however, a new 'super-enriched' environmental condition has been introduced by Kuenzle and Knüsel (1974) and by Davenport (1976), in which 45 or more rats live together in a large living-training apparatus.

In our experiment we used the 'enriched condition' and the 'standard condition', since we were interested in studying the effects of *increased* experience on adult rats. Sets of 3 male littermates of Berkeley S_1 rats were housed in standard laboratory cages from weaning until day 112. At this age, each set was distributed in such a way that one member of a littermate set was sacrificed to provide baseline material for 112-day-old rats (B group), another was assigned to an EC group, and the third rat was assigned to a SC group. The SC and EC rats were exposed to their new environments for 30 days (i.e. until day 142), at which time they were sacrificed for histological examination. The dendrites of layer II and III pyramidal neurons were measured in 150 μm coded sections, stained with the Golgi-Cox technique (Fig. 1).

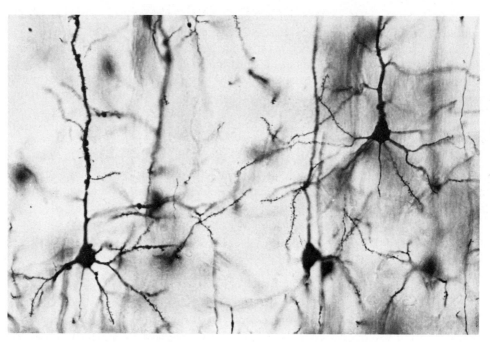

Fig. 1. A photomicrograph of a portion of the neocortex of an SC rat (142 days) stained with the Golgi-Cox method.

A semi-automatic tracking system (Coleman et al., 1977) was used for the measurements. The reasons for selecting layer II and III pyramidal neurons and details of the analysis methods are given elsewhere (Uylings, 1977; Uylings et al., 1978).

ENVIRONMENTAL EFFECTS ON DENDRITES OF CORTICAL PYRAMIDAL NEURONS

To select the best cortical area for making dendritic analyses, the thickness of several neocortical areas was measured by M.C. Diamond (University of California, Berkeley). The exact location of the examined cortical areas is described in Diamond et al. (1972) The results reported in Uylings et al. (1978) are summarized in Fig. 2; they show that, with only one exception, there are no significant differences in *cortical thickness* between the SC group and the B group. In the EC rats, on the other hand, the motor and visual cortices are significantly thicker than in the B rats, the difference being larger in the visual cortex (7%). The dendrites of the pyramidal neurons were therefore investigated in area 17 of Krieg.

PERCENTAGE DIFFERENCES IN CORTICAL THICKNESS

Cortical area		$(100 \times \frac{EC-B}{B})$ %	$(100 \times \frac{SC-B}{B})$ %
M	B	3***	−1
	C	2	0
	B	3	−2
S	C	3	−1
	D	3	2
	B	7***	0
V	C	4*	0
	D	0	−3*
	E	0	−3

*) p < .05; ***) p < .001 (according paired t-test, df 10).

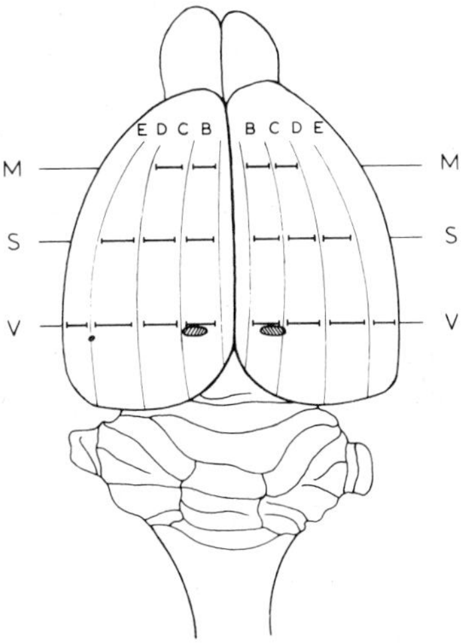

Fig. 2. A dorsal view of the rat brain, indicating the cortical areas examined for cortical thickness. The M, S and V represent sections taken from, respectively, the motor, somesthetic and occipital cortices. Each section is divided into dorsal and dorsolateral strips (B and C) and into lateral strips (D and E) of cortex. See Diamond et al. (1972) for specific localization. On the figure the lines closed with vertical bars show the positions of cortical thickness measurements, and the hatched areas the positions of dendritic measurements.

The mean *number of segments* of the basal dendrites versus order are given in Fig. 3. Ordering was done by denoting the segments arising directly from the cell body as order-*one*, and then raising the segmental order number by one after each branching point (Uylings et al., 1975). The number of first order segments appeared to be the same for all the three groups (EC, SC and B) which is equivalent to the statement that the mean number of basal dendrites per neuron did not change in any of the three groups. The higher order segment counts, however, showed significantly higher values in both the EC group and the SC group than in the B group. Moreover, the EC group showed slightly higher values for all higher orders than did the SC group. By counting the total number of segments per neuron irrespective of order, a significantly higher branching frequency was found in the EC than in the SC group.

264

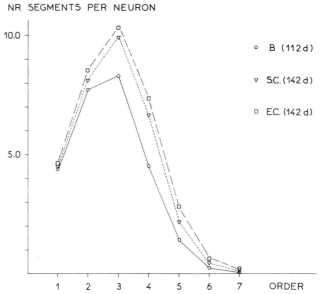

Fig. 3. Mean number of segments per superficial pyramidal cell (layer II and III) versus order. B, baseline group of rats housed in a 'standard colony' until day 112; SC, group of rats housed in a 'standard colony' until day 142 (they were recaged at day 112); EC, group of rats housed in a 'standard colony' until day 112, and thereafter under 'enriched conditions' until day 142.

The difference between the EC group and the SC group was most pronounced, however, in the *length of terminal segments* of basal dendrites (Figs. 4 and 5 and Table I). The difference in length between the EC and the SC groups was in fact larger than the difference between the SC and the B groups (Fig. 5). In contrast to the terminal segments, the length of intermediate segments of all orders of the basal dendrites (except for order-1) did not differ significantly among the three environmental groups. The first-order intermediate segments were significantly longer in the EC than in the SC rats, which in turn were significantly longer than in the B group (Uylings et al., 1978).

The length of the intermediate segments of the *apical main shaft* (Fig. 4) also did not differ significantly among the three environmental groups (Table II). The only exceptions were in order-2 between the EC and the B groups, and in order-4 between the SC and B groups. For the *oblique* dendrites (Fig. 4) we have preliminary data which suggest that, here too, the length of terminal segments is larger in the EC group than in the SC group, and larger in the SC than in the B group (Table III). Greenough (1976), in a preliminary study, also reported increased branching in apical dendrites of layer V pyramidal neurons in cortical areas 17 and 18 of young adult rats, trained on a series of Hebb-Williams maze problems for water reward. He and his collaborators found a significant increase in the frequency of intersection with superimposed concentric circles, by those parts of the apical dendrites which were located more than 250 μm away from the cell body. The differences were less pronounced in the apical dendrites of layer IV pyramidal neurons, while in the basal dendrites no consistent differences could be detected.

The differences in segment lengths observed in our experiment were also reflected in the *radial distance* of terminal dendritic tips from the cell center. For basal dendrites we found that the radial distance was significantly larger in the EC group than in the B or SC groups (Table IV). Furthermore, unlike the B and the SC group, the mean terminal distance in the

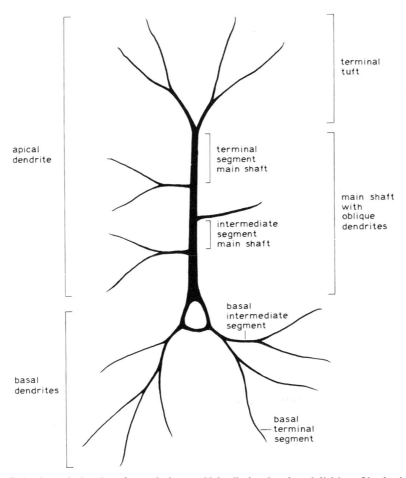

Fig. 4. A schematic drawing of a cortical pyramidal cell, showing the subdivision of its dendrites.

TABLE I

LENGTH TERMINAL SEGMENTS OF BASAL DENDRITES

| Order | B | | | SC | | | EC | | | Students t-test | | P value < |
	mean (μm)	S.E.M. (μm)	No.	mean (μm)	S.E.M. (μm)	No.	mean (μm)	S.E.M. (μm)	No.	EC > B	SC > B	EC > SC
1	128	15	10	134	18	8	171	13	10	0.05	n.s.	0.05
2	115	4	113	122	5	110	141	4	112	0.001	n.s.	0.01
3	104	3	253	115	3	303	126	3	288	0.001	0.01	0.01
4	101	3	162	107	3	262	113	3	269	0.01	n.s.	n.s.
5	84	5	60	101	4	103	105	4	112	0.001	0.01	n.s.
6	93	8	13	93	8	28	106	11	18	n.s.	n.s.	n.s.
7	–	–	0	–	–	3	–	–	4	–	–	–

EC condition was approximately equal, irrespective of order (Table IV; Fig. 6). The mean radial distance from the cell center to bifurcation points was considerably smaller for all orders than was the distance to the terminal tips, irrespective of order (Fig. 6). The analysis

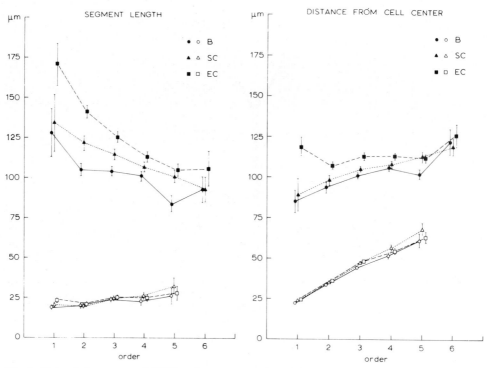

Fig. 5. Plots of the mean and S.E.M. values, versus order, of lengths of intermediate segments (open figures) and terminal segments (closed figures).

Fig. 6. Plots of the mean and S.E.M. values, versus order, of the distances from the cell centers to bifurcation points (open figures) and terminal tips (closed figures).

TABLE II

LENGTH INTERMEDIATE SEGMENTS OF APICAL MAIN SHAFT

Order	B			SC			EC			Mann-Whitney U-test		P value <
	mean (μm)	S.E.M. (μm)	No.	mean (μm)	S.E.M. (μm)	No.	mean (μm)	S.E.M. (μm)	No.	EC vs B	SC vs B	EC vs SC
1	27.3	1.3	103	26.7	1.5	102	24.3	1.3	106	n.s.	n.s.	n.s.
2	27.7	1.8	94	25.8	1.7	94	23.0	1.7	100	0.05	n.s.	n.s.
3	29.2	2.1	81	30.1	2.4	69	28.4	2.6	89	n.s.	n.s.	n.s.
4	41.9	5.5	58	26.7	2.4	53	37.2	3.9	75	n.s.	0.05	n.s.
5	50.3	6.9	32	31.7	3.7	30	35.3	3.9	34	n.s.	n.s.	n.s.
6	50.3	7.9	14	48.5	8.3	18	49.6	11.1	16	n.s.	n.s.	n.s.
7	–	–	3	–	–	5	–	–	5	–	–	–

of the *bifurcation angles* (see Smit and Uylings, 1975; Uylings and Smit, 1975; Uylings and Veltman, 1975) revealed that the environmental conditions did not influence this parameter (Uylings, 1977).

Quantitative analysis of dendrites thus indicates that the pyramidal neurons in visual cortex layers II and III of adult EC and SC rats had undergone a lengthening of the terminal

TABLE III

OBLIQUE DENDRITES

Order	B			SC			EC		
	mean (μm)	S.E.M. (μm)	No.	mean (μm)	S.E.M. (μm)	No.	mean (μm)	S.E.M. (μm)	No.
Length intermediate segments									
1	23.7	1.4	122	24.4	1.3	131	28.1	1.7	170
2	24.7	2.7	52	26.4	3.5	43	24.8	2.5	68
3	30.1	5.5	16	–	–	6	19.6	3.4	13
4	–	–	2	–	–	0	–	–	2
Length terminal segments									
1	97	4	70	122	5	65	124	5	79
2	94	5	57	91	5	64	101	4	98
3	79	8	31	83	7	25	105	6	46
4	84	15	11	–	–	2	–	–	8
5	–	–	1	–	–	0	–	–	4

TABLE IV

DISTANCE BASAL DENDRITIC END POINTS FROM CELL CENTER

Order	B			SC			EC			Mann-Whitney U-test		P value <
	mean (μm)	S.E.M. (μm)	No.	mean (μm)	S.E.M. (μm)	No.	mean (μm)	S.E.M. (μm)	No.	EC > B	SC > B	EC > SC
1	85	7	10	89	10	8	119	6	10	–	–	–
2	94	3	113	98	3	110	107	2	112	0.001	n.s.	0.01
3	101	2	253	105	1	303	113	2	283	0.001	0.05	0.001
4	106	2	162	108	2	262	113	2	269	0.01	n.s.	0.05
5	102	3	60	113	3	103	112	2	112	0.01	0.01	n.s.
6	122	8	13	119	5	28	126	7	18	n.s.	n.s.	n.s.
7	–	–	0	–	–	3	–	–	4	–	–	–

segments, and an increase in branching, relative to the adult B animals (especially in the basal dendrites). Compared with the group B rats, the branching was predominantly on terminal segments but at a considerable distance from the tips (Uylings, 1977; Uylings et al., 1978). This mode of growth is not different from the mode of growth of basal dendrites during normal development. As reported by Berry and his coworkers (Hollingworth and Berry, 1975; Berry and Bradley, 1976a, b), terminal growth occurs in basal dendrites of layer V cortical pyramidal cells, and also in the developing dendrites of Purkinje cells in the cerebellum. Furthermore, Ten Hoopen and Reuver (1971) deduced that, during development, branching of basal dendrites must be occurring predominantly at a considerable distance from the terminal tips.

Given the increased extension of the basal dendrites, and assuming that the thickness of the dendrites is not reduced, it can be stated that the enriched condition produces an increase in the dendritic surface area of cortical pyramidal neurons in adult rats. This provides such neurons with additional area for possible new synaptic connections with other nerve cells. It may be assumed that new spine synapses were indeed formed in the new portions of dendrites, since no spineless terminal segments were observed in the EC rats.

Jacobson (1974) has postulated that Golgi type I cells 'develop deterministically' and 'have invariant structure and functions which are genetically predetermined'. However, the present findings suggest that the dendritic pattern of cortical pyramidal neurons can be changed in adult rats by environmental influences, just as Greenough and Volkmar (1973) had shown in *developing* rats. For a further discussion of Jacobson's theory, we refer to the paper of Berry et al. (this volume).

Rats of the SC as well as of the EC group showed an increase in dendritic area at day 142 relative to the B group (i.e. day 112). The possibility cannot be excluded, however, that recaging and increased social exploration after day 112 were the factors primarily responsible for the increase in dendritic length in the SC rats, 142 days of age.

In the literature, growth cones – i.e. structures found on growing dendrites and axons in *developing* animals (e.g. Morest, 1969) – have never been reported for *adult* cerebral cortex. Although we have found evidence for dendritic growth in adult rats, no structures resembling growth cones were observed in our Golgi-Cox-stained material. Thus, the failure to observe growth cones in Golgi preparations does not exclude the possibility of further dendritic outgrowth. This is also indicated by Rutledge (1976) and by Parnavelas et al. (1977.)

ENVIRONMENTAL EFFECTS IN ADULTHOOD

Several effects of differential environmental experience will be reviewed below, as far as they bear upon adult rats. Data about influences of enriched experience upon the *cortical thickness* of (young) adult rats are only to be found in Diamond et al. (1972). They reported that the cortex of rats, raised in EC and SC from 60 to 90 days, was significantly thicker only in the frontal and in the occipital cortex (by 2–3% and 5%, respectively). The same authors also examined the differences between the EC and IC rats at two different ages. For rats 'enriched' from 60 to 90 days, the cortex was significantly thicker in the frontal, parietal and occipital areas (3%, 4% and 7%, respectively). For rats 'enriched' from 105 to 185 days, however, the cortex was significantly thicker (5%) only in the occipital area. This difference is a little smaller than in the cortical measurements reported here.

In 1964, Altman and Das reported that the rate of *glial multiplication* in the neocortex of adult rats, housed in an enriched environment from weaning to about 4.5 months, was increased relative to that in adult IC rats. This increase was greater in some cortical areas than in others, and was especially pronounced in the occipital cortex (more than double the control value).

Also in 1964, Bennett et al. reported that adult rats subjected to EC from 105 to 185 days had both a significantly higher *cortical weight* (especially in the occipital area: 10.9%) and a higher *acetylcholinesterase activity* than rats under IC (also 105 to 185 days). Riege (1971) also showed that cortical weight (again, especially of the *occipital* cortex) increased in adult rats living under EC, relative to rats under SC and IC; in this case the experimental conditions started on day 285 and lasted, respectively, 30, 60 and 90 days. Only in the occipital region (and only in the 90-day experimental group) was a significant increase found in the activities of acetylcholinesterase and cholinesterase in the EC rats.

Adult EC rats, furthermore, learned faster in the Lashley III maze than did their IC agemates (Riege, 1971). An improvement of certain *learning capacities* in adult rats subjected to enriched environments was also found by Doty (1972). Rats placed for 360 days in an enriched environment at 300 days of age performed better on discrimination reversal and passive avoidance problems (but not on active avoidance problems) than did the control rats. Other studies on effects of differential experience on learning can be found in Davenport (1976).

Finally, the *ratio of RNA to DNA* increased significantly in the occipital cortex of EC rats (relative to IC rats) when the rats were placed for 30 days in their respective environments starting at 110, 210 and 260 days of age. The increases were 5.5%, 10.5% and 5%, respectively (Bennett, personal communication).

No studies are known to us concerning the *persistence* of brain effects induced by enriched experience started in adulthood. In this connection, brain effects induced by enrichments beginning at weaning seem to dissipate when the rats are then placed in the 'isolated' condition, although a residual effect can still be detected 45 days after terminating the EC (Bennett et al., 1974). Furthermore, Denenberg et al. (1968) found significantly better performance in rats solving Hebb-Williams maze problems more than 300 days after exposure to the pre- and postweaning enriched conditions. Also Davenport (1976) and Walsh and Cummins (1976) found lasting, although decreasing, effects upon both maze performance and cortex morphology after terminating the 'enrichment'. Mandel (1975) reported that the effects upon brain (presumably its enzymatic activity) eventually disappeared, but he provided no details. In conclusion, we may expect that environmentally induced brain effects in adulthood will decline after termination of the enrichment period. The extent and the rate of reduction would depend, among other things, on the duration and type of the enriched condition, and on the difference between the enriched environment and the environment into which the animals are placed afterwards.

From the various reported influences of differential experience upon brain and behavior, it is clear that cortical plasticity is not limited to a particular period in a rat's life. This implies that a properly enriched environment could be beneficial for partial compensation of the effects of brain damage caused by a variety of factors. Will et al. (1976), and Will and Rosenzweig (1976), showed that enrichment-therapy indeed leads to improvement of problem-solving behavior in lesioned rats (bilateral occipital cortex lesions, carried out either neonatally or at 120 days of age). Other evidence supporting the proposition that recovery (at least partial) following brain damage is possible under the influence of experiential factors has been recently reviewed by Greenough et al. (1976), as well as by Walsh and Cummins (1976). In addition, certain learning deficits in hypothyroid rats can be reduced by enriched environment therapy (Davenport, 1976; Eayrs, 1955); this includes deficits found in maze-learning, -acquisition and -retention, and in bar-pressing extinction (Davenport, 1976). Similarly, there are indications (e.g. Winick et al. 1975; Barnes, 1976) that retardation effects caused by malnutrition in humans can be alleviated to some extent by rearing the undernourished children in a specially enriched environment. The therapeutic potential of this category of treatments, therefore, warrants systematic research into the mechanisms which ultimately determine its success or failure.

CONCLUSION

Environmental influences are indeed capable of affecting cortical structure and function in rats. An increase in branching and in length of dendritic processes in pyramidal neurons in the visual cortex of adult rats can be induced by an enriched environment. This additional dendritic outgrowth in adulthood has been found to occur in a fashion similar to that observed in the rat cortex during normal development. Whether or not such outgrowth in adulthood is limited to the visual cortex still needs to be investigated. Other reported changes which are not limited to early stages are in: cortical weight, cortical thickness, certain learning capabilities, enzymatic activities, and ratio of RNA to DNA. Although the effects of experience appear to be most pronounced in the occipital cortex, visual stimuli are not necessary in the differential experience paradigm (Rosenzweig et al., 1969; Krech et al., 1963). The persistence of brain effects induced by enriched environmental experience, as well as the potential therapeutic applications, are important issues for further research.

ACKNOWLEDGEMENTS

We are indebted to Dr. M.C. Diamond (Berkeley, California) for supplying the rat brains of the different rat groups, to Dr. P.D. Coleman (Rochester, New York) for the use of his dendritic tracking system, to Mrs. S.W. Lust-Bosboom for typing this paper, and to Dr. J.G. Parnavelas for his critical reading of the manuscript. H.B.M.U. was supported by a fellowship of the Netherlands Organization for the Advancement of Pure Research (Z.W.O.).

REFERENCES

Altman, J. and Das, G.P. (1964) Autoradiographic examination of the effects of enriched environment on the rate of glial multiplication in the adult rat brain, *Nature (Lond.)*, 204: 1161–1163.

Barnes, R.H. (1976) Dual role of environmental deprivation and malnutrition in retarding intellectual development. *Amer. J. clin. Nutr.*, 29: 912–917.

Bennett, E.L., Diamond, M.C., Krech, D. and Rosenzweig, M.R. (1964) Chemical and anatomical plasticity of brain, *Science*, 146: 610–619.

Bennett, E.L., Rosenzweig, M.R., Diamond, M.C., Morimoto, H. and Hebert, M. (1974) Effects of successive environments on brain measures, *Physiol. Behav.*, 12: 621–631.

Berry, M. and Bradley, P.M. (1976a) The growth of dendritic trees of Purkinje cells in cerebellum of the rat, *Brain Res.*, 112: 1–35.

Berry, M. and Bradley, P.M. (1976b) The applications of network analysis to the study of branching patterns of large dendritic fields, *Brain Res.*, 109: 111–132.

Berry, M., Bradley, P.M. and Borges, S. (1978) Environmental and genetic determinants of connectivity in the central nervous system – an approach through dendritic field analysis, this volume.

Changeux, J.P. and Mikoshiba, K. (1978) Genetic and 'epigenetic' factors regulating synapse formation in vertebrate cerebellum and neuromuscular junction, this volume.

Coleman, P.D., Garvey, C.F., Young, J.H. and Simon, W. (1977) Semiautomatic tracking of neuronal processes. In *Computer Analysis of Neuronal Structures*, R.D. Lindsay (Ed.), Plenum Press, New York, pp. 91–109.

Davenport, J.W. (1976) Environmental therapy in hypothyroid and other disadvantaged animal populations. In *Environments as Therapy for Brain Dysfunction, Advance Behav. Biol., Vol. 17*, R.N. Walsh and W.T. Greenough (Eds.), Plenum Press, New York, pp. 71–114.

Denenberg, V.H., Woodcock, J.M. and Rosenberg, K.M. (1968) Long-term effects of preweaning and postweaning free-environments experience on rats' problem solving behavior, *J. comp. physiol. Psychol.*, 66: 533–535.

Diamond, M.C., Rosenzweig, M.R., Bennett, E.L., Lindner, B. and Lyon, L. (1972) Effects of environmental enrichment and impoverishment on rat cerebral cortex, *J. Neurobiol.*, 3: 47–64.

Doty, B.A. (1972) The effects of cage environment upon avoidance responding of aged rats, *J. Gerontol.*, 27: 358–360.

Eayrs, J.T. (1955) The cerebral cortex of normal and hypothyroid rats, *Acta anat. (Basel)*, 25: 160–183.

Greenough, W.T. (1976) Enduring brain effects of differential experience and training. In *Neural Mechanisms of Learning and Memory*, M.R. Rosenzweig and E.L. Bennett (Eds.), M.I.T. Press, Cambridge, Mass., pp. 255–278.

Greenough, W.T. and Volkmar, F.R. (1973) Pattern of dendritic branching in occipital cortex of rats reared in complex environments, *Exp. Neurol.*, 40: 491–504.

Greenough, W.T., Fass, B. and De Voogd, T.J. (1976) The influence of experience on recovery following brain damage in rodents: hypotheses based on development research. In *Environments as Therapy for Brain Dysfunction, Advanc. Behav. Biol., Vol. 17*, R.N. Walsh and W.T. Greenough (Eds.), Plenum Press, New York, pp. 10–50.

Hollingworth, T. and Berry, M. (1975) Network analysis of dendritic fields of pyramidal cells in the neocortex and Purkinje cells in the cerebellum of the rat, *Phil. Trans. B*, 270: 227–262.

Jacobson, M. (1974) A plentitude of neurons. In *Aspects of Neurogenesis*, G. Gottlieb (Ed.), Academic Press, New York, pp. 151–166.

Kerr, F.W.L. (1975) Structural and functional evidence of plasticity in the central nervous system, *Exp. Neurol.*, 48: 16–31.

Krech, D., Rosenzweig, M.R. and Bennett, E.L. (1963) Effects of complex environment and blindness in rat brain, *Arch. Neurol. (Chic.)*, 8: 403–412.

Kuenzle, C.C., and Knüsel, A. (1974) Mass training of rats in a superenriched environment, *Physiol. Behav.*, 13: 205–210.

Mandel, P. (1975) Biochemical correlates of the genetic and environmental determinism of some behaviors. In *Growth and Development of the Brain: Nutritional, Genetic and Environmental Factors*, M.A.B. Brazier (Ed.), Raven Press, New York, pp. 203–218.

Morest, D.K. (1969) The growth of dendrites in the mammalian brain, *Z. Anat. Entwickl.-Gesch.*, 128: 290–317.

Parnavelas, J.G. (1978) Influence of stimulation on cortical development, this volume.

Parnavelas, J.G., Mounty, E.J., Bradford, R. and Lieberman, A.R. (1977) The postnatal development of neurons in the dorsal lateral geniculate nucleus of the rat: a Golgi study, *J. comp. Neurol.*, 171: 481–500.

Rakic, P. (1974) Intrinsic and extrinsic factors influencing the shape of neurons and their assembly into neuronal circuits. In *Frontiers in Neurology and Neuroscience Research*, P. Seeman and G.M. Brown (Eds.), University of Toronto Press, Toronto, pp. 112–132.

Ramón y Cajal, S. (1914) *Estudios sobre la Degeneración y Regeneración del Sistema Nerviosa*, Tomo II, Imprenta de Hijos de Nicholas Moya, Madrid.

Ramón y Cajal, S. (1937) *Recollections of my Life*, (Transl. E.H. Craigie), American Philosophical Society, Philadelphia.

Riege, W.H. (1971) Environmental influences on brain and behavior of year-old rats, *Devel. Psychobiol.*, 4: 157–167.

Rosenzweig, M.R., Bennett, E.L. and Diamond, M.C. (1972) Chemical and anatomical plasticity of brain: replications and extensions. In *Macromolecules and Behavior*, 2nd ed., Gaito, J. (Ed.), Appleton-Century-Crofts, New York, pp. 205–278.

Rosenzweig, M.R., Bennett, E.L., Diamond, M.C., Wu, S., Slagle, R.W. and Saffran, E. (1969) Influences of environmental complexity and visual stimulation on development of occipital cortex in rat, *Brain Res.*, 14: 427–445.

Rutledge, L.T. (1976) Synaptogenesis: effect of synaptic use. In *Neural Mechanisms of Learning and Memory*, M.R. Rosenzweig and E.L. Bennett (Eds.), The M.I.T. Press, Cambridge, Mass., pp. 329–339.

Rutledge, L.T., Wright, C. and Duncan, J. (1974) Morphological changes in pyramidal cells of mammalian neocortex associated with increased use, *Exp. Neurol.*, 44: 209–228.

Smit, G.J. and Uylings, H.B.M. (1975) The morphometry of the branching pattern in dendrites of visual cortex pyramidal cells, *Brain Res.*, 87: 41–53.

Sotelo, C. (1978) Purkinje cell ontogeny: formation and maintenance of spines, this volume.

Stenevi, U., Björklund, A. and Moore, R.Y. (1973) Morphological plasticity of central adrenergic neurons, *Brain Behav. Evol.*, 8: 110–134.

Sumner, B.E.H. and Watson, W.E. (1971) Retraction and expansion of the dendritic tree of motor neurones of adult rats induced in vivo, *Nature (Lond.)*, 233: 273–275.

Tanzi, E. (1893) I fatti e le induzioni nell'odierna istologia del sistema nervosa, *Riv. Sperim. Freniat.*, 19: 419–472.

Ten Hoopen, M. and Reuver, H.A. (1971) Growth patterns of neuronal dendrites — an attempted probabilistic description, *Kybernetik*, 8: 234–239.

Uylings, H.B.M. (1977) *A Study on Morphometry and Functional Morphology of Branching Structures*, *with Applications to Dendrites in Visual Cortex of Adult Rats under Different Environmental Conditions,* Doctoral dissertation, University of Amsterdam.

Uylings, H.B.M. and Smit, G.J. (1975) Three-dimensional branching structure of pyramidal cell dendrites, *Brain Res.,* 87: 55–60.

Uylings, H.B.M. and Veltman, W.A.M. (1975) Characterizing a dendritic bifurcation, *Neurosci. Lett.,* 1: 127–128.

Uylings, H.B.M., Smit, G. J. and Veltman, W.A.M. (1975) Ordering methods in quantitative analysis of branching structures of dendritic trees. In *Physiology and Pathology of Dendrites, Advanc. Neurol. Vol. 12,* G.W. Kreutzberg, (Ed.), Raven Press, New York. pp. 247–254.

Uylings, H.B.M., Kuypers, K., Diamond, M.C. and Veltman, W.A.M. (1978) Effects of differential environments on dendrites of cortical pyramidal neurons in adult rats, submitted for publication.

Vrensen, G. (1978) Ontogenesis of the visual cortex of rabbits and the effects of visual deprivation, this volume.

Walsh, R.N. and Cummins, R.A. (1976) Neural responses to therapeutic sensory environments. In *Environments as Therapy for Brain Dysfunction, Advanc. Behav. Biol., Vol. 17,* R.N. Walsh and W.T. Greenough (Eds.), Raven Press, New York, pp. 171–200.

Will, B.E. et Rosenzweig, M.R. (1976) Effets de l'environnement sur la récupération fonctionelle après lésions cérébrales chez les rats adultes, *Biol. Behav.,* 1: 5–15.

Will, B.E. Rosenzweig, M.R. and Bennett, E.L. (1976) Effects of differential environments on recovery from neonatal brain lesions, measured by problem-solving scores and brain dimensions, *Physiol. Behav.,* 16: 603–611.

Winick, M., Meyer, K.K. and Harris, R.C. (1975) Malnutrition and environmental enrichment by early adoption, *Science,* 190: 1173–1175.

DISCUSSION

CHANGEUX: In all these environmental manipulation experiments, as well as in those on sensory deprivation, could you not imagine that humoral factors are involved which may have a *general* effect on growth, rather than to enhance a specific class of neurons?

UYLINGS: This question has not been investigated in adult animals. However, viewing the results of Volkmar and Greenough (1972), obtained from immature animals living under the same experimental conditions, I can imagine that other classes are affected too, such as the non-pyramidal neurons in layer IV. As regards humoral factors, they have not yet been extensively examined. Rosenzweig et al. (1972), however, found a reduction in 'enriched' experimental effects after hypophysectomy, so it might well be that these effects are mediated by humoral factors. On the other hand, it appears from the cortical thickness measurements of Dr. Diamond, and from other investigations reviewed in our paper, that such environmental experiments preferentially influence specific parts of the neocortex.

BERRY: It is interesting in these results that presumably the *terminal* growth mechanisms are still open to these adult animals, while *interstitial* growth mechanisms are not available for the basal dendrites. However, I would like to ask what sort of information you think that layer II and III pyramidal cells are receiving.

UYLINGS: I don't know exactly, but besides input of a visual modality they must receive input of other modalities too, as is indicated by the experiments, for instance, of Rosenzweig et al. (1969) with blinded and dark-reared animals.

PURPURA: What could be the electrophysiological implications of a 15–20% increase in length of terminal segments, and an 8% increase in the number of basal dendrite segments? Does this influence the core-conductive properties of the dendritic 'cables', the electrotonic input to the soma? I suspect that the changes that you see in the terminals and the dendritic growth have very little physiological significance. Even changes in dendrite diameters are not necessarily indications for physiological changes.

UYLINGS: There are no experimental data on the electrophysiological effects of the increase of the terminal part of the dendritic field induced by differential experience. We can therefore only speculate on this matter, especially since we deal with *basal* dendrites, for which no theoretical model is available to describe the voltage and conductance changes (Rall and Rinzel, 1974). Rall and Rinzel (1974), however, did show theoretically that the terminal parts of the motoneuron dendrites are not without significance. In their neuron model, the synaptic input (transient EPSP) at the terminal tip of a dendrite causes a conductance change at the soma which is 1/7 that of a somatic input. Furthermore, the total amount of charge dissipated by the soma (i.e. the time-integral of the current across the soma) during synaptic activation on a terminal dendrite is almost one-half the charge dissipated when the same degree of synaptic activation is applied directly to the soma (Rinzel, 1975).

Concerning your point about dendrite diameters, Rall (1974) has made theoretical studies about the role of spines on the dendrites. One of the most interesting points is that changes in size of spine-head or spine-stem are less effective than are changes in diameter of the trunk itself. A change at a spine affects only the immediate vicinity, whereas a change in diameter of the dendrite affects the electrotonic conduction of synaptic input at *all* spines on that particular trunk. Besides these theoretical model considerations, there could also be some interneuronal interactions between parts of dendrites and other neurites involved in a so-called *local neuronal circuit*. Changes in dendrites could alter the functional connectivity properties characteristic of these local neuronal circuits. I therefore believe that the dendritic increase must have some functional significance, but of course this still needs to be shown empirically.

REFERENCES

Rall, W. (1974) Dendritic spines, synaptic potency and neuronal plasticity. In Ch. D. Woody, K.D. Brown, T.J. Crow and J.D. Knispel (Eds.), *Cellular Mechanisms Subserving Changes in Neuronal Activity*, B.I.S., UCLA, pp. 13–21.

274

Rall, W. and Rinzel, J. (1973) Branch input resistance and steady attenuation for input to one branch of a dendrite neuron model, *Biophys. J.,* 13: 648–688.

Rinzel, J. (1975) Voltage transients in neuronal dendritic trees, *Fed. Proc.,* 34: 1350–1356.

Rosenzweig, M.R., Bennett, E.L., Diamond, M.C., Wu, S., Hagle, R.W. and Saffran, E. (1969), see references this paper.

Rosenzweig, M.R., Bennett, E.L. and Diamond, M.C. (1972) see references this paper.

Volkmar, F.R. and Greenough, W.T. (1972) Rearing complexity affects branching of dendrites in the visual cortex of the rat, *Science,* 176: 1445–1447.

SECTION V

HORMONAL REGULATION
OF BRAIN MATURATION

Fetal Neuroendocrine Mechanisms
in Development and Parturition

D.F. SWAAB, G.J. BOER, K. BOER, J. DOGTEROM, F.W. VAN LEEUWEN and M. VISSER

Netherlands Institute for Brain Research and (M.V.) Wilhelmina Gasthuis, Department of Obstetrics and Gynaecology, University of Amsterdam, Amsterdam (The Netherlands)

INTRODUCTION

The study of the factors influencing intrauterine growth and labor might contribute towards the understanding of disturbances in these processes and so towards the reduction of perinatal mortality and brain traumata that are caused by these disturbances (e.g. Roberts and Thomson, 1976; Alberman, 1976). Recent investigations make it probable that, of the various factors involved in intrauterine growth and parturition, the fetus itself plays an important role by means of neuroendocrine mechanisms.

In some species, for example in birds, there is no question about the importance of the fetus itself in such processes. The chick fetal brain and pituitary are stimulating growth (for references see Thommes et al., 1973), while the forebrain controls the final stage of hatching (Corner et al., 1973; Sohal, 1976). But not in all species are fetal factors so clearly separated by an egg-shell from maternal and environmental factors. In mammals, where environmental, maternal, placental and fetal factors are strongly intermingled and inter-related, the importance of the fetal component cannot be defined easily. In order to study to what extent the human fetal brain is involved in the control of fetal growth and parturition, observations were performed in anencephaly and other congenital brain anomalies. Although these studies suffer from all the drawbacks inherent in pathological material, it is the only available means of obtaining data on this subject in man. Therefore, hypotheses arising from these observations are tested experimentally in rat, while mechanisms found by such experiments are in turn examined for their presence in man. The evidence for fetal neuroendocrine mechanisms in intrauterine growth and birth in man and rat are reviewed in the present paper.

THE FETAL BRAIN AND INTRAUTERINE GROWTH

Human congenital brain anomalies and intrauterine growth

Jost (e.g. 1954) has emphasized that the fetal brain and pituitary are not of importance in intrauterine growth because growth does not stop in human anencephalics and in fetuses of various other species after decapitation. This is only partly true because, generally, a decreased growth rate is observed after such lesions (Honnebier and Swaab, 1973; Swaab and Honnebier, 1973, 1974) (Fig. 1a, d).

Normal fetal growth in man shows an S-shaped course with an acceleration of the growth

278

rate at about 20 weeks of pregnancy (e.g. Swaab et al., 1977b). This 'growth spurt' is dependent on the integrity of the fetal brain, as appears from (1) the low birth weight in cases of spontaneous decapitation during the first trimester (Liggins, 1974) and (2) of anencephaly (Honnebier and Swaab, 1973) (Fig. 1a), (3) from clinical data on growth arrears in anencephalics (Swaab and Honnebier, 1974) and (4) from the low birth weight of microcephalics in which the hypothalamus was absent (Janigan et al., 1962). In addition, (5) a normal birth weight was observed in one case of hydranencephaly which had an absent cerebrum but intact brain stem (Liggins, 1974). All these data point to the importance of an intact hypothalamus for normal intrauterine growth in man.

The difference at 40 weeks of pregnancy between the mean anencephalic birth weight and the normal mean (i.e. the 50th percentile line) in our material is considerable: about 1000 g on a total corrected normal birth weight of 3000 g (Fig. 1a). The difference in lean body weight might even be greater since the anencephalics have an increased mass of subcutaneous fat (e.g. Bearn, 1971). The decreased body weight in anencephalics of 1000 g is an important difference as compared with, for example, the well-known serious fall in body weight observed in very severe undernutrition. The decrease in birth weight during the Dutch famine (1944–1945) was 200 g, and during the second world war siege of Leningrad the birth weight decrease was 400 g (Winick, 1976). The growth impairment in anencephaly cannot be explained by the fact that all kinds of congenital anomalies are growth retarded, since the reduction of body weight in other kinds of serious congenital anomalies was much less extreme than that in anencephalics (Swaab and Honnebier, 1974). Data strikingly similar to ours in anencephalic children (Fig. 1a) were obtained by Kittinger (1977) in the

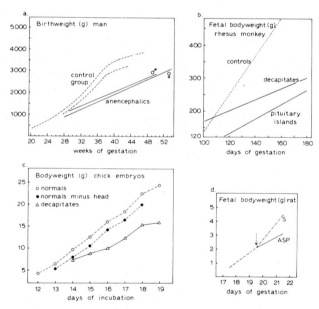

Fig. 1. Retarded intrauterine growth in the absence of the fetal brain in man (a), rhesus monkey (b), chick (c) and rat (d). a: upper broken line = 50th percentile line of the control group; lower broken line = same line after subtraction of the brain weight. The linear regression lines for male and female anencephalics are based on Honnebier and Swaab (1973). b: reproduced from Kittinger, 1977, with permission of the Ciba Foundation. c: body weights of normal and in stage 11–13 decapitated chick embryos (with permission after Case, 1952). d: body weight of rat fetuses which were sham operated (arrow) on day 19 (S) or brain-aspirated (ASP) on day 19 of pregnancy (data calculated from Swaab and Honnebier, 1973).

rhesus monkey (Fig. 1b). Following surgical encephalectomy or decapitation at about 75 days of gestation, fetal growth was delayed in a similar way as in anencephaly.

The fetal rat brain and pituitary in growth

Also in the rat the fetal brain is stimulating intrauterine growth. During normal intrauterine development fetal growth in rat shows a sudden acceleration at day 19 of pregnancy. This 'growth spurt' appeared to be absent in rat fetuses from which the brain and pituitary had been removed (Swaab and Honnebier, 1973) (Fig. 1d). After removal of the fetal brain and pituitary, fetal body weight is lower than after removal of the fetal brain alone (Table I).

The minor difference between these last two groups shows that the pituitary is to a high degree dependent on the fetal brain for the stimulation of intrauterine growth. Removal of the fetal brain and pituitary in this experiment (Table I) decreased the body weight 18% against more than 25% in earlier experiments (cf. Swaab and Honnebier, 1973). This difference in size of the effect might be due to compounds crossing from the intact fetuses to the operated ones in the present experiment, which was not possible in former experiments in which the entire litter was treated in the same way.

The hypothalamus seems to be an essential structure for normal fetal growth, since a reduction in fetal body weight has also been found after selective destruction of the fetal rat hypothalamus, but not after destruction of other brain areas (Fujita et al., 1970). Fujita's experiments showed, in addition, that such growth rate changes following brain lesions were not due to the duration of the surgical procedure, amniotic fluid loss or uterine damage as suggested by Rieutort and Jost (1976) since all these factors were the same in his experiments.

In order to test the possibility that humoral factors of hypothalamo-hypophysial origin play a role in the regulation of intrauterine growth in rat, pituitary hormones and hypothalamic extracts were injected directly into rat fetuses from which the brain and pituitary had been removed. No stimulation of intrauterine growth was obtained with any of the following compounds: growth hormone, $ACTH_{1-24}$, $ACTH_{4-10}$, TSH, prolactin, LH, FSH, HCG, oxytocin, hypothalamic extract (fraction C), insulin, placenta extract and cyclic AMP (Swaab and Honnebier, 1974; Honnebier and Swaab, 1974, Swaab et al., 1977b). The only factor which was found to stimulate intrauterine growth was the hormone of the intermediate lobe of the pituitary, α-MSH (Honnebier and Swaab, 1974; Swaab and Honnebier, 1974).

TABLE I

FETAL BODY WEIGHT IN RAT (IN PERCENTAGE (± S.E.M.) OF SHAM OPERATED CONTROLS) AFTER REMOVAL OF THE PITUITARY AND/OR THE BRAIN

In each of 7 rat litters the fetuses were divided at random at day 19 of pregnancy in operation group I, II or III (for operation procedures see Swaab and Honnebier, 1973). Body weight was determined at day 21 of pregnancy and expressed as a percentage of the sham-operated controls which had a mean weight of 4.49 ± 0.091 g. The absence of pituitary and/or brain was checked by means of a stereomicroscope on a midsagital section through the fetal head. In the entire group one fetus died and two could not be placed into one of the three groups. The differences between I and II and II and III are highly significant (Student's t-test = $P < 0.001$).

I	Sham operation (needle only stabbed into cerebrum)	(n = 30)	100	(± 1.23)%
II	Removal of the fetal brain (leaving the pituitary intact)	(n = 27)	85.3	(± 1.58)%
III	Removal of the fetal brain and pituitary	(n = 25)	81.9	(± 1.42)%

MSH and intrauterine growth

Evidence is accumulating that the growth promoting effect of α-MSH is indeed a physiological function of this hormone in the fetus. MSH is detectable by means of bioassay and immunofluorescence in the fetal rat pituitary from day 18 of pregnancy, i.e. one day before the intrauterine growth spurt starts (Swaab et al., 1976), while by means of radioimmunoassay α-MSH was found in the fetal pituitary and amniotic fluid already on day 17 of pregnancy (Thody, unpublished observations). Moreover, a significant negative correlation was found between the pituitary content of bioassayable MSH and fetal body weight on day 19 of pregnancy (Swaab and Visser, 1977), suggesting an earlier onset of hormone release in the heavier fetuses. That endogenous fetal α-MSH has indeed a function in stimulating intrauterine growth appeared, in addition, from the growth inhibition following injection of purified anti-α-MSH plasma directly into the fetuses on the day of the intrauterine growth spurt (Swaab et al., 1976; Swaab et al., 1978).

MSH and brain development

The body of evidence increases that those endogenous compounds which affect behavior in adult organisms are necessary for normal brain development. This holds true for the thyroid hormones (cf. Querido et al., 1978), sex hormones (cf. Van de Poll et al., 1978) and neurotransmitters (Lewis et al., 1977).

There are various arguments in support of a possible involvement of α-MSH in adult brain function. α-MSH and related compounds were found to have important behavioral effects (for review see Van Wimersma Greidanus, 1977). Such central effects are also reflected by the influence of MSH on the electrical activity of the nervous system (for references see Kastin et al., 1973). In addition, rat nervous tissue has been shown to contain MSH activity (Rudman et al., 1974) which was confirmed by us using a radioimmunoassay for α-MSH (unpublished observations). The compound present might be either α-MSH itself (Oliver et al., 1977) or an α-MSH-like compound which was found by means of immunofluorescence (Swaab and Visser, 1977) and, more recently, by an immunoperoxidase technique (unpublished observations) to be localized throughout the rat nervous system. It has also been suggested that both related compounds are present (Vaudry et al., 1976). Since the α-MSH-like compound remains measurable (Vaudry et al., 1977) and visualizable (Swaab and Visser, 1977) after hypophysectomy, it is more likely to be synthetized in the nervous system itself than in the intermediate lobe of the pituitary. Because of the neurotropic effects of α-MSH in adults and its involvement in fetal body growth, the involvement of this hormone in brain development is currently being investigated. Injection of anti-α-MSH subcutaneously into the rat fetus induced not only a decrease in fetal body weight, but also a decrease in brain wet- and dry weights, protein and lipid contents, while brain DNA remained unaffected (Swaab et al., 1978). These data point to a role of α-MSH in nerve cell differentiation rather than in multiplication.

MSH in human development

In order to see whether a growth promoting role for α-MSH might exist in man, a study is currently being carried out in the human fetus. By means of immunofluorescence microscopy, α-MSH was indeed found in the intermediate and anterior lobe of all 6 normal fetuses that have been studied so far between 15 and 20 weeks of pregnancy (Visser and Swaab, 1977). This agrees with the data of Silman et al. (1976) who assayed α-MSH radioimmunologically after chromatographic isolation. No intermediate lobe is present in the majority of anencephalics (Angevine, 1938). In the two anencephalics that we have examined until now by means of immunofluorescnece, no α-MSH could be demonstrated in the anterior pituitary (the only part of the hypophysis that was present in these newborns) (Visser and Swaab, 1977). Since anencephalics show a lower intrauterine growth rate (Honnebier and Swaab, 1973), and have probably lower MSH levels in blood (Honnebier and Swaab, 1975), α-MSH might well play a role in intrauterine growth also in man. The absence of α-MSH in the pituitary of human anencephalics and its presence in normal human fetuses would, moreover, point to the fetal brain as the structure which is necessary for the appearance of the intermediate lobe and α-MSH in development.

THE HYPOTHALAMO-NEUROHYPOPHYSIAL SYSTEM (HNS) IN DEVELOPMENT

The fetal HNS and water balance

A second neuroendocrine system which might be of importance during development in the fetus is the HNS. Neurohypophysial hormones are already present before term. In rat neurohypophysis axons appear between day 17 (Galabov and Schiebler, 1978) and 18 (Paull, 1973) of pregnancy, while oxytocin and arginine vasopressin (AVP) were found by radioimmunoassay in the fetal pituitary from day 17 of pregnancy (Forsling, 1973). In the human fetal pituitary AVP was found radioimmunologically from 12 weeks of pregnancy (Skowsky and Fisher, 1973), while quantitative bioassay estimates of oxytocin and vasopressin activity became possible at 16 weeks of pregnancy (Dicker and Tyler, 1953). Immunofluorescence was found using either unpurified or purified antibodies against oxytocin and vasopressin in the human fetal neurohypophysis from 15–16 weeks of pregnancy (Fig. 2).

Characteristic for the fetal neurohypophysis in all species studied to date is the high vasopressor to oxytocic ratio. According to Perks and Vizsolyi (1973), this might indicate that the supraoptic nucleus becomes active earlier in development than does the paraventricular nucleus. This hypothesis, however, is based upon the assumption that the supraoptic nucleus would synthetize mainly vasopressin and the paraventricular nucleus mainly oxytocin; this has been proven not to be the case. In the adult rat, both nuclei show the

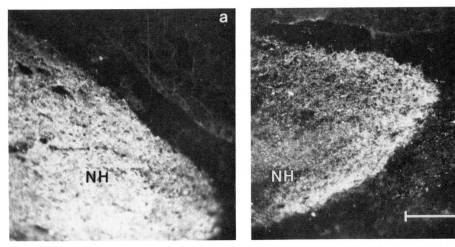

Fig. 2. Immunofluorescence in the neurohypophysis (NH) of a human fetal pituitary of 16 weeks of pregnancy (code B), using unpurified anti-vasopressin (# 126) (a) and anti-oxytocin (# 02D) (b) (for technical details see Swaab and Pool, 1975). The horizontal bar represents 100 μm.

same ratio of oxytocin- to vasopressin-containing cells (Swaab et al., 1975). In their study on the nature of fetal seal neurohypophysial hormones, Perks and Vizsolyi (1973) found a principle with high frog bladder activity. Together with the amino acid analysis, this finding made it most probable that the fetal neurohypophysis contained, as a third hormone, arginine-vasotocin (AVT), a peptide hitherto thought to be confined to lower vertebrates (Heller and Pickering, 1960; Sawyer, 1966). AVT was reported also to be present in the pituitary of the fetal sheep (Vizsolyi and Perks, 1976; Skowsky and Fisher, 1973), the human fetus (Skowsky and Fisher, 1973) and the rat fetus at term (Swaab et al., 1977b).

New observations make it improbable, however, that the compound that was measured in the fetal rat pituitary is indeed AVT. Recently we have produced antibodies against AVT that permit a sensitive (up to 0.25 pg) and specific radioimmunoassay for this peptide, and we are currently repeating the various observations on this peptide reported in the literature. No AVT has been found until now with this assay, in Wistar rat pituitaries and in brains from day 17 of pregnancy until postnatal day 6, in two midpregnancy sheep pituitaries (kindly donated by Dr. P.W. Nathanielsz) or in human midpregnancy amniotic fluid (Table II). These data make us doubt the importance, and even the existence, of arginine-vasotocin in the fetus. The presence of AVT in the fetal pituitary would also not go together with ideas (cf. Sawyer, 1966; De Wied, 1978) about the molecular evolution of neurohypophysial peptides. If AVT were indeed the 'ancestral peptide' that was changed during phylogeny by amino acid substitution, it is hard to imagine how this mutation process could be repeated in each generation anew during ontogeny.

The physiological role of the fetal neurohypophysial hormones in early pregnancy remains to be determined. Neurohypophysial hormones were reported to have only a very slight effect on urinary concentration in the human newborn (Heller, 1944). This relative insensitiveness to AVP cannot be attributed to a lack of collecting tube responsiveness to the hormone, but rather to the poorly developed osmotic gradient in the renal medulla (Abramov and Dratwa, 1974). Neurohypophysial hormones could also affect water balance of the fetus by acting on the fetal urinary bladder, skin or the extraembryonic membranes (for review see Challis et al., 1976). Perks and Vizsolyi (1973) have speculated that the neuro-

TABLE II

NEUROHYPOPHYSIAL HORMONE LEVELS IN MAN (pg/ml) ± S.E.M.

	Oxytocin	Vasopressin	Vasotocin
Midpregnancy amniotic fluid n = 3	< 4	< 1	< 1
Maternal plasma at term n = 16	20.6 ± 3.1	< 2	< 2
Maternal plasma immediately postterm n = 5	28.7 ± 6.2	< 2	< 2
Umbilical cord plasma n = 5	68.1 ± 18.4	75.8 ± 50.6	< 2

hypophysial hormones pass via the fetal urine into the amniotic fluid and cause water uptake into the amniotic cavity. Oxytocin, AVP and AVT were not detectable in amniotic fluid at midpregnancy, however (Table II). In addition, the high frequency of hydramnios in anencephalics (Honnebier and Swaab, 1973), together with the absence of the fetal neurohypophysis in the majority of these children (Angevine, 1938), makes it unlikely that this mechanism is of primary importance for the formation of amniotic fluid.

As a possible explanation for hydramnios in anencephaly, a disturbed swallowing of amniotic fluid or an increased fetal urine output because of the observed kidney changes and AVP deficiency have been mentioned (Nakano, 1973; Potter and Craig, 1975), but both possibilities are doubtful (Taussig, 1927; Ferm and Saxon, 1971; Honnebier and Swaab, 1973). Another, perhaps additional, mechanism could be that hydramnios is due to an overproduction of cerebrospinal fluid directly into the amnion (cf. Taussig, 1927), since structures resembling the intact choroid plexus are prominent in anencephaly (Potter and Craig, 1975). In this context it seems of importance that AVP has been demonstrated to be present in the cerebrospinal fluid of adult organisms (Dogterom et al., 1978), while a related peptide was found in the choroid plexus (Rudman and Chawla, 1976). AVP is thought to reduce cerebrospinal fluid production (for references see Brownfield and Kozlowski, 1977). The latter authors described (in adult rat) neurosecretory fibers stained for neurophysins that innervated the choroid plexus. Recently we have shown that such fibers do indeed contain neurohypophysial hormones (Fig. 3).

Although all these data have still to be confirmed in the fetus, hydramnios in anencephaly might thus be due to increased cerebrospinal fluid production directly into the amniotic fluid by the exposed choroid plexus in the absence of vasopressin.

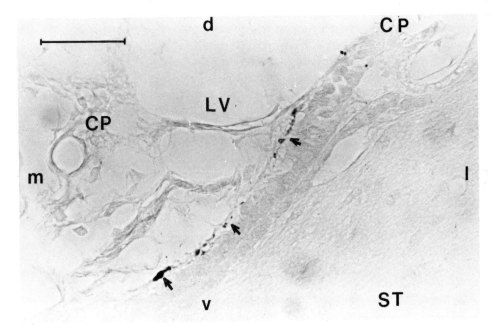

Fig. 3. A neurosecretory fiber (arrows) running into the choroid plexus (CP) of the lateral ventricle (LV) of an adult Wistar rat. The staining was performed by M. Everts using unpurified anti-vasopressin (# 125) 1:800 according to the unlabeled antibody enzyme technique of Sternberger (for details see Buijs et al., 1977). d, dorsal; l, lateral; v, ventral; m, medial; ST, stria terminalis. The horizontal bar indicates 50 μm.

The fetal brain and the onset of parturition

A wealth of data shows that, in sheep, the fetal hypothalamus is primarily responsible for the sequence of events that results in birth. Since this sequence involves fetal pituitary ACTH, an ACTH releasing factor seems to be *the* hypothalamic stimulus initiating labor (for recent reviews see Liggins et al., 1977b; Nathanielsz et al., 1977). There is some evidence that AVP might be this hypothalamic factor (e.g. Challis and Thorburn, 1976). Intravenous infusion of AVP into the sheep fetus results in increased ACTH release (Jones and Rurak, unpublished observations, mentioned in Challis et al., 1976). A rise in fetal plasma AVP has been reported during the last few days before birth in the lamb (Alexander et al., 1974) but was not confirmed in later studies, in which AVP was found to rise only during the last hours of pregnancy (Stark, 1977). It remains questionable, therefore, whether fetal AVP is indeed of any physiological importance for the initiation of labor in sheep. It is certainly not such a factor in rats since fetal brain aspiration does not prolong gestation length in this species (Swaab et al., 1977a) while homozygous Brattleboro rats with a homozygous litter have even a shorter gestation length than do heterozygous animals (Boer, unpublished observations).

The initiation of labor in man has appeared to be less dependent on the fetal brain and pituitary than in sheep. Data such as increased cortisol levels in the human amniotic fluid and umbilical cord during pregnancy and labor indicated a role of the human fetus in the onset of parturition similar to that of the sheep (Challis and Thorburn, 1976). Yet, in contrary to the general opinion expressed in the literature (e.g. Potter and Craig, 1975), we found the mean gestation length in human anencephalics without hydramnios to be the same as that of the controls. However, a high percentage of both pre- and post-mature labors were found in anencephaly (Honnebier and Swaab, 1973) (Fig. 4 left). A similar distribution of births was found in rhesus monkeys: the majority of the experimental anencephalics delivered either pre- or post-term (Novy, 1977) (Fig. 4 right).

Additional data arguing against a crucial role of the fetal brain in the initiation of labor are the few reported cases of acephaly (cf. Liggins, 1974), pituitary aplasia (cf. Swaab and Honnebier, 1974) and microcephaly, accompanied by absence of the hypothalamus (Janigan et al., 1962) in man, which on the average did not deliver post-term. All these facts show that the fetal pituitary in the primate does not play the same triggering role in the initiation of labor as it does in sheep, but rather is involved in the precision of control of the initiation of labor within close limits around the species mean. It is not known whether the mechanisms by which the brain effectuates this 'timing' mechanism in man is also the fetal hypothalamo-hypophysial-adrenal system which initiates labor in sheep. Arguing in favor of this possibility is the finding that either corticosteroid or ACTH administration in the human fetus initiated labor in postmature pregnancies (Mati et al., 1973; Nwosu et al., 1976), and did not induce labor at term (Gamissans et al., 1975, 1976). Moreover, a tendency towards prolongation of pregnancy length was reported following betamethasone treatment of premature labors (Liggins and Howie, 1972).

The fetal brain and the course of labor

The integrity of the fetal brain appears to be necessary for a normal course of delivery in man and rat. In human anencephalics without hydramnios, expulsion of the fetus took twice as long as in controls, and the average time between birth of the fetus and birth of the placenta was nearly three times longer in the anencephalic group. In addition, in the anencephalics 10% of the placenta had to be removed manually, while the overall mean in the university clinic of Amsterdam was only 2% (Swaab et al., 1977a). In this respect it is of

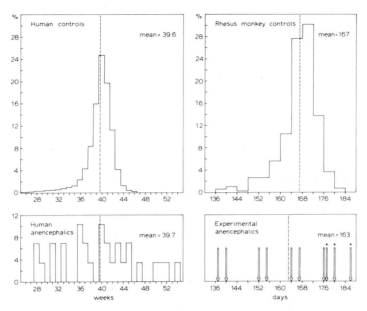

Fig. 4. The influence of anencephaly on the distribution of birth in man (left) and rhesus monkey (right). Left: frequency distribution of gestation length for a control group (n = 49,996) and for spontaneous birth of anencephalic fetuses (n = 29) without hydramnios, omitting those who had stillborn fetuses with third degree maceration, fetuses which were given intrauterine injections, twins and those in whom labour was induced, (from Honnebier and Swaab, 1973). Right: frequency distribution of gestation length in a group of 310 rhesus monkeys which produced live-born infants and after experimental anencephaly (based upon Novy, 1977, with permission of the Ciba Foundation). Each arrow indicates the birth of one anencephalic fetus. * = delivered by Caesarean section. Note the huge scatter of anencephalic births and the normal mean in both groups.

interest that in the group of children who died during pregnancy (1968–1972: n = 143), a high number of placentas (8.4%) had to be removed manually (Huidekoper and Kloosterman, personal communication). All these data point to an active involvement of the fetus in the course of its own delivery, and in the delivery of its placenta.

In the rat a protracted course of labor was found after brain aspiration (Swaab et al., 1977a). Since a prolonged course of labor was also found in Brattleboro rats as compared to normal Wistars, the fetal neurohypophysis may play a role in the acceleration of the course of labor (Swaab et al., 1977a). Such a role of fetal oxytocin was already suspected in 1938 by Bell and Robson, who found appreciable amounts of oxytocin in fetal pig and sheep pituitaries. This possibility is reinforced by the finding that uterine contractions could effectively be evoked in sheep (Nathanielsz et al., 1973) and in man (Honnebier et al., 1974) by injection of posterior lobe hormones into the fetal compartment, despite the conceptual difficulties in postulating the route which the fetal hormones should take to the myometrium (cf. Liggins et al., 1977a). Furthermore, fetal rat pituitary extracts had the potency to induce uterine contractions (Swaab and Boer, 1978). In addition, high levels of these hormones are present in umbilical cord blood (Chard et al., 1977 and Table II) that rise during the last hours of pregnancy in man (Chard et al., 1977) and in sheep (Forsling et al., 1975; Stark, 1977). The fetus thus appears to have the means to stimulate the uterus and, so, the course of labor by increasing its neurohypophysial hormone release.

AVT was found to be oxytocic in the rat at term (Swaab et al., 1977a). Whether this hormone (if indeed present) or related peptides play a role in the acceleration of the course of labor from the fetal side, is the subject of current investigations.

SUMMARY AND CONCLUSIONS

The fetal hypothalamus is active in stimulating intrauterine growth. In man this appears from the low birth weight found in congenital anomalies in which the fetal hypothalamus was absent, i.e. acephaly, anencephaly and certain cases of microcephaly. In rat, fetal growth was impaired after removal of the fetal pituitary and/or brain, or destruction of the hypothalamus. The intermediate lobe hormone, α-MSH, was found to stimulate fetal growth in rat. Although this hormone was also found to be present in the human fetus during the intrauterine growth spurt while absent in human anencephalics, its relation to intrauterine growth has still to be confirmed.

The fetal brain in man is not involved in the initiation of labor in the same way as found in the sheep, but rather plays a role in the exact timing of the moment of birth around the species mean pregnancy length. Neurohypophysial hormones are present in very high concentrations in umbilical blood, and these fetal hormones are thought to accelerate the course of labor. This hypothesis is supported by the protracted course of labor found in human anencephalics, and brainless rat fetuses. The fetus itself plays thus an active role in its own intrauterine growth and parturition by means of neuroendocrine mechanisms.

ACKNOWLEDGEMENT

The authors are greatly indebted to the Foundation for Medical Research FUNGO for additional financial support.

REFERENCES

Abramow, M. and Dratwa, M. (1974) Effect of vasopressin on the isolated human collecting duct, *Nature (Lond.)*, 250: 492–493.

Alberman, E. (1976) Factors influencing perinatal wastage. In *Fetal Physiology and Medicine*, R.W. Beard and P.W. Nathanielsz (Eds.), Saunders, London, pp. 415–432.

Alexander, D.P., Bashore, R.A., Britton, H.G. and Forsling, L. (1974) Maternal and fetal arginine vasopressin in the chronically catheterized sheep, *Biol. Neonate*, 25: 242–248.

Angevine, D.M. (1938) Pathologic anatomy of hypophysis and adrenals in anencephaly, *Arch. Pathol.*, 26: 507–518.

Bearn, J.G. (1971) The role of the foetal pituitary in organogenesis. In *Hormones in Development*, M. Hamburgh and E.J.W. Barrington (Eds.), Appleton-Century-Crofts, New York, pp. 121–134.

Bell, G.H. and Robson, J.M. (1938) The oxytocin content of the foetal pituitary, *Quart. J. exp. Physiol.*, 27: 205–208.

Brownfield, M.S. and Kozlowski, G.P. (1977) The hypothalamo-choroidal tract. I. Immunohistochemical demonstration of neurophysin pathways to telencephalic choroid plexuses and cerebrospinal fluid, *Cell Tiss. Res.*, 178: 111–127.

Buijs, R.M., Swaab, D.F., Dogterom, J. and Van Leeuwen, F.W. (1977) Intra- and extrahypothalamic vasopressin and oxytocin pathways in the rat, *Cell Tiss. Res.*, 186: 423–433 (1978)

Case, J.F. (1952) Adrenal cortical-anterior pituitary relationships during embryonic life, *Ann. N.Y. Acad. Sci.*, 55: 147–158.

Challis, J.R.G. and Thorburn, G.D. (1976) The fetal pituitary-adrenal axis and its functional interactions with the neurohypophysis. In *Fetal Physiology and Medicine*, R.W. Beard and P.W. Nathanielsz (Eds.), Saunders, London, pp. 233–250.

Challis, J.R.G., Robinson, J.S., Rurak, D.W. and Thornburn, G.D. (1976) The development of endocrine function in the human fetus. In *The Biology of Human Fetal Growth*, D.F. Roberts and A.M. Thomson (Eds.), Taylor and Francis, London, pp. 149–194.

Chard, T., Silman, R.E. and Rees, R.H. (1977) The fetal hypothalamus and posterior pituitary in the initiation of labour. In *The Fetus and Birth, Ciba Foundation Symp. No. 47*, J. Knight and M. O'Connor (Eds.), Elsevier, Amsterdam, pp. 359–378.

Corner, M.A., Bakhuis, W.L. and Van Wingerden, C. (1973) Sleep and wakefulness during early life in the domestic chicken, and their relationship to hatching and embryonic motility. In *Studies on the Development of Behavior and the Nervous System, Vol. 1. Behavioral Embryology*, G. Gottlieb (Ed.), Academic Press, New York, pp. 245–279.

De Wied, D. (1978) The modulation of memory processes by vasotocin, the evolutionary oldest neurosecretory principle, this volume.

Dicker, S.E. and Tyler, C. (1953) Vasopressor and oxytocic activities of the pituitary glands of rats, guinea pigs and cats and of human foetuses, *J. Physiol. (Lond.)*, 121: 206–214.

Dogterom, J., Van Wimersma Greidanus, Tj.B. and Swaab, D.F. (1978) Evidence for the release of vasopressin and oxytocin into cerebrospinal fluid: measurements in plasma and CSF of intact and hypophysectomized rats, *Neuroendocrinology*, 24: 108–118 (1977).

Ferm, V.H. and Saxon, A. (1971) Amniotic fluid volume in experimentally induced renal agenesis and anencephaly, *Experientia (Basel)*, 27: 1066–1068.

Forsling, M.L. (1973) In *Endocrine Factors in Labour, Mem. Soc. Endocrinology No. 20*, A. Klopper and J. Gardner (Eds.), Cambridge University Press, London, p. 174 (figure).

Forsling, M.L., Jack, P.M.B. and Nathanielsz, P.W. (1975) Plasma oxytocin concentrations in the foetal sheep, *Horm. Metab. Res.*, 7: 197.

Fujita, T., Eguchi, Y., Morikawa, Y. and Hashimoto, Y. (1970) Hypothalamic-hypophysial adrenal and thyroid systems: observations in fetal rats subjected to hypothalamic destruction, brain compression and hypervitaminosis A, *Anat. Rec.*, 166: 659–672.

Galabov, P. and Schiebler, T.M. (1978) On the development of the principles in the neural lobe of the rat. In *Neural Hormones and Reproduction*, D.E. Scott, G.P. Koslowski and A. Weindl (Eds.), Karger, Basel, pp. 57–66.

Gamissans, O., Pujol-Amat, P., Davi, E., Pérez-Picanol, E. and Wilson, G.R. (1975) The effect of intraamniotic administration of β-metasone on the onset of labour in human pregnancy, *Acta endocr. (Kbh.)*, Suppl. 199: 95.

Gamissans, O., Davi, E., Pérez-Picanol, E., Pujol-Amat, P. and Wilson, G.R. (1976) Effect of ACTH administration into the fetus, on onset of labour and on maternal plasma steroid levels. In *Research on Steroids, Vol. 7*, A. Vermeulen (Ed.), Elsevier/North-Holland Biomedical Press, Amsterdam.

Heller, H. (1944) The renal function of newborn infants, *J. Physiol. (Lond.)*, 102: 429–440.

Heller, H. and Pickering, B.T. (1960) Identification of a new neurohypophysial hormone, *J. Physiol. (Lond.)*, 152: 56P–57P.

Honnebier, W.J. and Swaab, D.F. (1973) The influence of anencephaly upon intrauterine growth of fetus and placenta and upon gestation length, *J. Obstet. Gynaecol.* 80: 577–588.

Honnebier, W.J. and Swaab, D.F. (1974) Influence of α-melanocyte-stimulating hormone (α-MSH), growth hormone (GH) and fetal brain extracts on intrauterine growth of fetus and placenta in the rat, *J. Obstet. Gynaecol.*, 81: 439–447.

Honnebier, W.J. and Swaab, D.F. (1975) Regulation of growth velocity by the foetus, *Acta endocr. (Kbh.)*, Suppl. 199: 97.

Honnebier, W.J., Jöbsis, A.C. and Swaab, D.F. (1974) The effect of hypophysial hormones and human chorionic gonadotrophin (HCG) on the anencephalic fetal adrenal cortex and on parturition in the human, *J. Obstet. Gynaecol.*, 81: 423–438.

Janigan, D.T., Smith, O.D. and Nichols, J. (1962) Observations on the central nervous system, pituitary and adrenal in two cases of microcephaly, *J. clin. Endocr. Metab.*, 22: 683–687.

Jost, A. (1954) Hormonal factors in the development of the fetus, *Cold Spr. Harb. Symp. quant. Biol.*, 19: 167–181.

Kastin, A.J., Miller, L.H., Nockton, R., Sandman, C.A., Schally, A.V. and Stratton, L.O. (1973)

288

Behavioral aspects of melanocyte-stimulating hormone (MSH). In *Drug Effects on Neuroendocrine Regulation, Progress in Brain Research, Vol. 39*, E. Zimmerman, W.H. Gispen, B.H. Marks and D. de Wied (Eds.), Elsevier, Amsterdam, pp. 461–470.

Kittinger, G.W. (1977) The endocrine regulation of fetal development and its relation to parturition in the rhesus monkey. In *The Fetus and Birth, Ciba Foundation Symp. No. 47*, J. Knight and M. O'Connor (Eds.), Elsevier, Amsterdam, pp. 235–257.

Lewis, P.D., Patel, A.J., Béndek, G. and Balázs, R. (1977) Do drugs acting on the nervous system affect cell proliferation in the developing brain?, *Lancet*, 1: 399–401.

Liggins, G.C. (1974) The influence of the fetal hypothalamus and pituitary on growth. In *Size at Birth, Ciba Foundation Symp. No. 27*, K. Elliott and J. Knight (Eds.), Elsevier, Amsterdam, pp. 165–183.

Liggins, G.C. and Howie, R.N. (1972) A controlled trial of antepartum glucocorticoid treatment for prevention of the respiratory distress syndrome in premature infants, *Pediatrics*, 50: 515–525.

Liggins, G.C., Forster, C.S., Grieves, S.A. and Schwartz, A.L. (1977a) Control of parturition in man, *Biol. Reprod.*, 16: 39–56.

Liggins, G.C., Fairclough, R.J., Grieves, S.A., Forster, C.S. and Knox, B.S. (1977b) Parturition in the sheep. In *The Fetus and Birth, Ciba Foundation Symp. No. 47*, J. Knight and M. O'Connor (Eds.), Elsevier, Amsterdam, pp. 5–30.

Mati, J.K.G., Horrobin, D.F. and Bramley, P.S. (1973) Induction of labour in sheep and humans by single doses of corticosteroids, *Brit. med. J.*, 2: 149–151.

Nakano, K.K. (1973) Anencephaly: a review, *Develop. Med. Child Neurol.*, 15: 383–400.

Nathanielsz, P.W., Comline, R.S. and Silver, M. (1973) Uterine activity following intravenous administration of oxytocin to the foetal sheep, *Nature (Lond.)*, 243: 471–472.

Nathanielsz, P.W., Jack, P.M.B., Krane, E.J., Thomas, A.L., Ratter, S. and Rees, L.H. (1977) The role and regulation of corticotropin in the fetal sheep. In *The Fetus and Birth, Ciba Foundation Symp. No. 47*, J. Knight and M. O'Connor (Eds.), Elsevier, Amsterdam, pp. 73–98.

Novy, M.J. (1977) Endocrine and pharmacological factors which modify the onset of labour in rhesus monkeys. In *The Fetus and Birth, Ciba Foundation Symp. No. 47*, J. Knight and M. O'Connor (Eds.), Elsevier, Amsterdam, pp. 259–295.

Nwosu, U.C., Wallach, E.E. and Bolognese, R.J. (1976) Initiation of labor by intra-amniotic cortisol instillation in prolonged pregnancy, *Obstet. Gynecol.*, 47: 137–142.

Oliver, C., Barnea, A., Warberg, J., Eskay, R.L. and Porter, J.C. (1977) Distribution, characterization, and subcellular localization of MSH in the brain. In *Melanocyte Stimulating Hormone: Control, Chemistry and Effects*, F.J.H. Tilders, D.F. Swaab and Tj.B. Van Wimersma Greidanus (Eds.), Karger, Basel, pp. 162–166.

Paull, W.K. (1973) *A Light and Electronmicroscopic Study of the Development of the Neurohypophysis of the Fetal Rat*, Doctoral dissertation, Univ. South. California, U.S.A.

Perks, A.M. and Vizsolyi, E. (1973) Studies of the neurohypophysis in foetal mammals. In *Foetal and Neonatal Physiology, Proc. Sir Joseph Barcroft Centenary Symposium*, K.S. Comline, K.W. Cross, G.S. Dawes and P.W. Nathanielsz (Eds.), Cambridge University Press, London, pp. 430–438.

Potter, E.L. and Craig, J.M. (1975) *Pathology of the Fetus and the Infant*, Yearbook Medical Publishers, Chicago.

Querido, A., Bleichrodt, N. and Djokomoeljanto, R. (1978) Thyroid hormones and human mental development, this volume.

Rieutort, M. and Jost, A. (1976) Growth hormone in encephalectomized rat fetuses, with comments on the effect of anesthetics, *Endocrinology*, 98, 1123–1129.

Roberts, D.F. and Thomson, A.M. (1976) (Eds.) *The Biology of Human Fetal Growth, Symposia Society for the Study of Human Biology, Vol. 15*. Taylor and Francis, London.

Rudman, D. and Chawla, R.K. (1976) Antidiuretic peptide in mammalian choroid plexus, *Amer. J. Physiol.*, 230: 50–55.

Rudman, D., Scott, J.W., Del Rio, A.E., Houser, D.H. and Sheen, S. (1974) Melanotropic activity in regions of rodent brain, *Amer. J. Physiol.*, 226: 682–686.

Sawyer, W.H. (1966) Biological assays for neurohypophysial principles in tissues and in blood. In *The Pituitary Gland, Vol. 3*, G.W. Harris and B.T. Donovan (Eds.), Butterworths, London, pp. 288–329.

Silman, R.E., Chard, T., Lowry, P.J., Smith, I. and Young, I.M. (1976) Human foetal pituitary peptides and parturition, *Nature (Lond.)*, 260: 716–718.

Skowsky, R. and Fisher, D.A. (1973) Immunoreactive arginine vasopressin (AVP) and arginine vasotocin (AVT) in the fetal pituitary of man and sheep, *Clin. Res.*, 21: 205.

Sohal, G.S. (1976) Effects of reciprocal forebrain transplantation on motility and hatching in chick and duck embryos, *Brain Res.*, 113: 35–43.

Stark, R. (1977) In *The Fetus and Birth, Ciba Foundation Symp. No. 47*, J. Knight and M. O'Connor (Eds.), Elsevier, Amsterdam, discussion p. 371.

Swaab, D.F. and Boer, K. (1977) The role of the fetal brain and pituitary in intrauterine growth and parturition. In *Proc. Vth Int. Symp. Obstet. Gynaecol.*, Barcelona, in press.

Swaab, D.F. and Honnebier, W.J. (1973) The influence of removal of the fetal rat brain upon intrauterine growth of the fetus and the placenta and on gestation length, *J. Obstet. Gynaecol.*, 80: 589–597.

Swaab, D.F. and Honnebier, W.J. (1974) The role of the fetal hypothalamus in development of the feto-placental unit and in parturition. In *Integrative Hypothalamic Activity, Progress in Brain Research, Vol. 41*, D.F. Swaab and J.P. Schadé (Eds.), Elsevier, Amsterdam, pp. 255–280.

Swaab, D.F. and Pool, C.W. (1975) Specificity of oxytocin and vasopressin immunofluorescence, *J. Endocr.* 66: 263–272.

Swaab, D.F. and Visser, M. (1977) A function for α-MSH in fetal development and the presence of an α-MSH-like compound in nervous tissue. In *Melanocyte Stimulating Hormone: Control, Chemistry and Effects*, F.J.H. Tilders, D.F. Swaab and Tj.B. Van Wimersma Greidanus (Eds.), Karger, Basel, pp. 170–178.

Swaab, D.F., Nijveldt, F. and Pool, C.W. (1975) Distribution of oxytocin and vasopressin in the rat supra-optic and paraventricular nucleus, *J. Endocr.*, 67: 461–462.

Swaab, D.F., Visser, M. and Tilders, F.J.H. (1976) Stimulation of intrauterine growth by α-MSH, *J. Endocr.* 70: 445–455.

Swaab, D.F., Boer, K. and Honnebier, W.J. (1977a) The influence of the fetal hypothalamus and pituitary on the onset and course of parturition. In *The Fetus and Birth, Ciba Foundation Symp. No. 47*, J. Knight and M. O'Connor (Eds.), Elsevier, Amsterdam, pp. 379–400.

Swaab, D.F., Van Leeuwen, F.W., Dogterom, J. and Honnebier, W.J. (1977b) The fetal hypothalamus and pituitary during growth and differentiation, *J. Steroid Biochem*, 8: 545–551.

Swaab, D.F., Visser, M. and Boer, G.J. (1978) The fetal brain and intrauterine growth. In *Proc. Fifth Unigate Paediatric Workshop: Paediatrics and Growth, Symposium Paediatrics and Growth, London, 1977*, D. Barltrop (Ed.), in press.

Taussig, F.J. (1927) The amniotic fluid and its quantitative variability., *Amer. J. Obstet. Gynecol.*, 14: 505–517.

Thommes, R.C., Hajek, A.S. and McWhinnie, D.J. (1973) The influence of 'hypophysectomy' by means of surgical decapitation on skeletal growth in the developing chick embryo, *J. Embryol. exp. Morph.*, 29: 503–513.

Van de Poll, N.E., De Bruin, J.P.C., Van Dis, H. and Van Oyen, H. (1978) Sex hormones in behavioral development, this volume.

Van Wimersma Greidanus, Tj.B. (1977) Effects of MSH and related peptides on avoidance behavior in rats. In *Melanocyte Stimulating Hormone: Control, Chemistry and Effects*, F.J.H. Tilders, D.F. Swaab and Tj.B. Van Wimersma Greidanus (Eds.), Karger, Basel, pp. 129–139.

Vaudry, H., Oliver, C., Vaillant, R. and Kraicer, J. (1976) Bioactive and immunoreactive αMSH in the rat brain. In *Proc. Vth Int. Congr. Endocr.*, Hamburg, Abstract No. 667.

Vaudry, H., Vaillant, R., Trochard, M.C. and Kraicer, J. (1977) MSH-like peptides in the brain of hypophysectomized rats. In *Proc. XXVIIth Int. Congr. Physiol. Sci.*, Paris, Abstract p. 781.

Visser, M. and Swaab, D.F. (1977) α-MSH in the human pituitary. In *Melanocyte Stimulating Hormone: Control, Chemistry and Effects*, F.J.H. Tilders, D.F. Swaab and Tj.B. Van Wimersma Greidanus (Eds.), Karger, Basel, pp. 42–45.

Vizsolyi, E. and Perks, A.M. (1976) Neurohypophysial hormones in fetal life and pregnancy. II. Chromatographic studies in the sheep (*Ovis aries*), *Gen. comp. Endocr.*, 29: 41–50.

Winick, M. (1976) (Ed.) *Malnutrition and Brain Development*, Oxford University Press, New York.

DISCUSSION

ZIMMER: You mentioned that the course of labor was protracted in the case of anencephalic babies. Could not this be a structural effect in the sense that, not having the normal shape of the head, they have more difficulties in adjusting in the right position? Do anencephalics not have a higher frequency of breech presentations?

SWAAB: Indeed, a high percentage of abnormal presentations is found in anencephalic labor (Honnebier and Swaab, 1973). Of course, clinical material is always difficult to interpret: it can be a source of inspiration but never a proof for any mechanism. That was the reason why we used the rat fetus to check the various clinical phenomena. After brain aspiration in the rat fetus we also found a protracted course of labor, although in those fetuses the head has the same shape as in the control fetuses. Concerning the anencephalic labor you can, however, not state the same for the placenta, which has the same shape in anencephaly as in normal children, while the delivery is very much protracted in anencephalics: three times longer than in matched controls.

McEWEN: Did you look for α-MSH in the brain itself?

SWAAB: Yes, there is a lot of α-MSH-like material present in the adult rat brain. High concentrations of α-MSH-like peptides were found both by means of bioassay (Rudman et al., 1974; Rudman and Scott, 1975) and radioimmunoassay (Vaudry et al., 1977, and our own unpublished observations). Since hypophysectomy does not alter the concentrations of these compounds in the brain (Rudman et al., 1974; Vaudry et al., 1977; Swaab and Visser, 1977), it seems to be produced in the nervous system rather than in the pituitary.

McEWEN: And what is the relative deficiency in the Brattleboro rat for oxytocin and vasopressin?

SWAAB: There is no biologically or radioimmunologically active vasopressin present in the homozygous rats. The cells that should produce vasopressin in these Brattleboros are present, however, and if you look with enzymatic parameters they seem to be in a high state of synthesizing activity (Swaab et al., 1973), but apparently it is not vasopressin what they produce. Oxytocin is found in 50% of the normal quantity in the neurohypophysis of the homozygous Brattleboro rats. This is not because they synthesize less, but because there is increased release. The level of circulating oxytocin in homozygous Brattleboro rats is 5 times the normal value (Dogterom et al., 1977).

REFERENCES

Dogterom, J., Van Wimersma Greidanus, Tj.B. and Swaab, D.F. (1977) Evidence for the release of vasopressin and oxytocin into cerebrospinal fluid: measurements in plasma and CSF of intact and hypophysectomized rats *Neuroendocrinology*, 24: 108–118 (1977).

Honnebier, W.J. and Swaab, D.F. (1973) The influence of anencephaly upon intrauterine growth of fetus and placenta and upon gestation length, *J. Obstet. Gynaec. Brit. Cwlth.*, 80: 577–588.

Swaab, D.F. and Visser, M. (1977) A function for α-MSH in fetal development and the presence of an α-MSH-like compound in nervous tissue. In D.F. Swaab and Tj.B. Van Wimersma Greidanus (Eds.), *Melanocyte Stimulating Hormone: Control, Chemistry and Effects*, Karger, Basel, pp. 170–178.

Swaab, D.F., Boer, G.J. and Nolten, J.W.L. (1973) The hypothalamo-neurohypophysial system (HNS) of the Brattleboro rat, *Acta endocr. (Kbh.)*, Suppl. 177: 80.

Rudman, D. and Scott, J.W. (1975) Melanotropic-lipolytic peptides of the pineal gland and other CNS regions. In M.D. Altschule (Ed.), *Frontiers of Pineal Physiology*, MIT Press, Cambridge, pp. 44–53.

Rudman, D., Scott, J.W., Del Rio, A.E. and Sheen, S. (1974) Melanotropic activity in regions of rodent brain, *Amer. J. Physiol.*, 226: 682–686.

Vaudry, H., Vaillant, R., Trochard, M.C. and Kraicer, J. (1977) MSH-like peptides in the brain of hypophysectomized rats. *Proc. Int. Union Physiol. Sci.*, 12: 781.

Sexual Maturation and Differentiation:
The Role of the Gonadal Steroids

BRUCE S. McEWEN

The Rockefeller University, New York, N.Y. 10021 (U.S.A.)

INTRODUCTION

The development of the neuroendocrine system involves not only the maturation of the individual components (brain, pituitary and target glands) and their abilities to produce hormones, but also the acquisition of the functional capacity of the brain and pituitary to be influenced by target gland hormones (thyroid hormone, adrenal and gonadal steroids). During development, target gland hormones may exert permanent organizational effects on development of brain function, besides exerting their reversible activational actions on neuro-endocrine function and behavior. These multiple actions of target gland hormones are perhaps best illustrated by the gonadal steroids, and this article will examine the ontogeny of hypothalamo-hypophyseal-gonadal function in the laboratory rat in relation to the development of sexual behavior, neuroendocrine feedback systems and the process of sexual differentiation.

TIME OF ORIGIN OF HYPOTHALAMIC AND PREOPTIC AREA NUCLEI

The technique of labeling cells with [^{3}H] thymidine prior to their final cell division has been used to identify 'birth dates' for neurons of the major nuclei of hypothalamus and pre-optic area of the rat. Laterally placed nuclei were found to have birth dates distributed around day 14 of gestation, while medially placed nuclei arise later, around day 16 (Table I) (Ifft, 1972). Because the final cell division is followed by differentiation of neuronal characteristics, it is not surprising that nerve fibers containing granular vesicles first appear in the median eminence of the rat around day 16 of gestation (Fink and Smith, 1971), and at least one hypothalamic hormone, gonadotropin-releasing-hormone (GnRH), is detectable in the hypothalamus as early as day 17 of gestation, and increases rapidly in amount in the ensuing weeks (Fig. 1) (Chiappa and Fink, 1977).

HYPOTHALAMO-HYPOPHYSEAL INTERACTION BEFORE AND AFTER BIRTH

That the hypothalamic GnRH may influence the pituitary before birth is supported by the existence of blood vessels in the mesenchyme between hypothalamus and pituitary as early as fetal day 15 (Fink and Smith, 1971). The fetal rat pituitary at term responds to

TABLE I

GESTATIONAL DAY OF ORIGIN OF HYPOTHALAMIC NUCLEI
IN THE RAT

Adapted from Ifft, 1972.

Day of origin	Nucleus
14	Preopticus lateralis
	Lateral
	Supraopticus
	Paraventricularis magnocellularis
	Supraopticus diffusus
	Ventromedialis anterior
	Ventromedialis lateralis
	Ventromedialis posterior et centralis
	Dorsomedialis dorsalis
	Posterior
	Perifornicalis
	Premamillaris ventralis
	Mamillaris lateralis
16	Preopticus medialis
	Periventricularis preopticus
	Suprachiasmaticus
	Anterior
	Paraventricularis parvocellularis
	Arcuatus
	Ventromedialis medialis
	Dorsomedialis ventralis
	Premamillaris dorsalis
	Supramamillaris
	Mamillaris medialis medialis
	Mamillaris medialis lateralis
	Mamillaris posterior

GnRH (Schafer and McShan, 1974). LH and FSH are detectable in fetal pituitary between days 17 and 20 of gestation (Chowdhury and Steinberger, 1976; Chiappa and Fink, 1977), while secretory granules (not identified as to hormone content) are detectable in anterior pituitary cells by day 17 of fetal life.

Nevertheless, the loops of the primary hypothalamo-hypophyseal plexus do not develop until postnatal day 4 or 5 (Fink and Smith, 1971), and catecholamine fluorescence increases markedly in the external layer of the median eminence around day 5 (Smith and Simpson, 1970). The first postnatal week of life is in fact accompanied by large increases in pituitary LH and FSH as well as hypothalamic GnRH content (Chiappa and Fink, 1977).

OPERATION OF THE NEGATIVE FEEDBACK SYSTEM IN THE INFANT RAT

Secretion of LH and FSH and of estrogens, androgens and progestins in the rat varies as a function of postnatal age and sex (Meijs-Roelofs et al., 1973, 1975; Ojeda et al., 1975; Dohler and Wuttke, 1975), but a detailed analysis of much of this information is beyond the scope of this article. However, it is important to consider the 'feedback' effects which indicate the operation of the entire system: hypothalamus → pituitary → gonad → hypothalamus/pituitary.

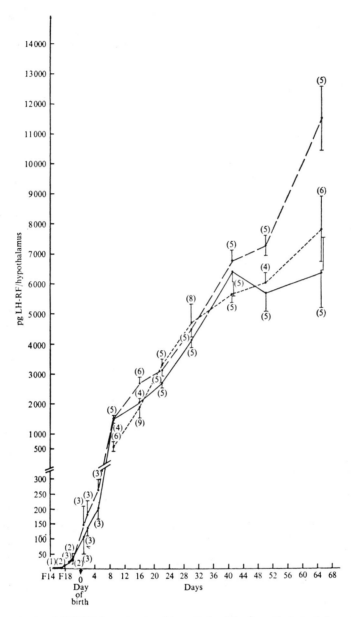

Fig. 1. Mean contents of LH-RF in extracts of hypothalami (pg/hypothalamus) from female (——), androgenized female (---) and male (– –) rats. Standard errors are indicated by the vertical bars, while the number of pools (foetal (F) day 15 to postnatal day 5; 7–23 hypothalami/group) or samples from individual rats are shown in parentheses. (Reprinted from Chiappa and Fink, 1977, by permission.)

One indication of this is the compensatory hypertrophy of the remaining ovary (COH) after unilateral ovariectomy. COH has been observed on postnatal day 10 after hemiovariectomy on day 1 (Dunlap and Gerall, 1973). Another indication of functional activity of the hypothalamo-pituitary-gonadal axis is the increase in both plasma LH and FSH levels after ovariectomy (OVX), and the suppression of these levels by exogenous steroids. Ovariectomy on day 1 has been reported to result in increased LH and FSH levels on days 9–10 (Caligaris et al., 1972, 1973). Estradiol benzoate (EB) produced some suppression of FSH and LH levels in female and male rats 5–10 days of age, but the inter-animal variations in LH were large, especially in females, so as to preclude a clearcut conclusion (Goldman and Gorski, 1971). In infant rats, OVX at day 9 or 25 resulted in elevated LH and FSH, but the response was faster and larger in the older rats; injections of EB reversed these elevations but were more effective in doing so in older rats (Ojeda et al., 1975). Thus, while ovarian feedback occurs before day 10, and negative feedback by estrogen is well-developed in 3–4-week-old rats, estradiol feedback is only marginal in 1–2-week-old animals. One reason for this is the existence in newborn rats of an estradiol-binding plasma protein, α-fetoprotein, which disappears by day 25. The role of this factor will be considered below. It has also been suggested that the ovarian products primarily responsible for negative feedback effects in 1–2-week-old rats may not be estrogens but, rather, steroids like 5α-dihydrotestosterone (DHT) and progesterone (Ojeda et al., 1977). Exogenous DHT is known to be effective in newborn male and female rats in suppressing both COH and the postcastration increases in FSH and LH (McDonald and Doughty, 1972; Korenbrot et al., 1975; Ojeda et al., 1977).

MATURATION OF OTHER COMPONENTS OF REPRODUCTIVE FUNCTION IN THE FEMALE RAT

During normal development of the female rat, vaginal opening (around day 37) precedes the display of the first sexual receptivity (around day 41) and of regular ovarian cyclicity (Södersten, 1975). As shown in Fig. 2, treatment of immature female rats with EB results in precocious lordosis displays to manual stimulation by the experimenter (100% responding by day 19), and also ear-wiggling displays somewhat earlier, but such precocious responses do not advance the development of behavioral cyclicity (Södersten, 1975). Likewise, EB treatment of immature female rats at 25–28 days of age is capable of triggering the first ovulation (Holweg effect, Holweg, 1934), and it advances the age of vaginal opening but does not advance the onset of regular, spontaneous ovarian cyclicity (Ramirez and Sawyer, 1965; Smith and Davidson, 1968; Ying and Greep, 1971; Caligaris et al., 1972; Döcke and Dörner, 1974). The ultimate limiting factor in the case of premature ovulation is the competence of the ovaries to release ova in response to gonadotropin, a property which appears around 17–18 days of age (Zarrow and Wilson, 1961).

MATURATION OF STEROID RESPONSIVE MECHANISMS OF RAT BRAIN

Some insight into developmental aspects of gonadal steroid feedback on brain and pituitary may be gained by considering (1) the ontogeny of two key enzymes involved in the transformation of testosterone, 5α-reductase and the aromatizing enzyme system (Fig. 3), and (2) the development of receptor mechanisms for estrogens and androgens. The full significance of androgen metabolism will become clearer below when we consider brain differentiation.

The aromatizing enzyme system (aromatase) of newborn rat brain, which is capable of generating estradiol from testosterone (Lieberburg and McEwen, 1975; Lieberburg et al., 1977; Westley and Salaman, 1976), is detectable one day before birth in male and female hypothalamus and in male limbic structures, but is practically undetectable in female limbic

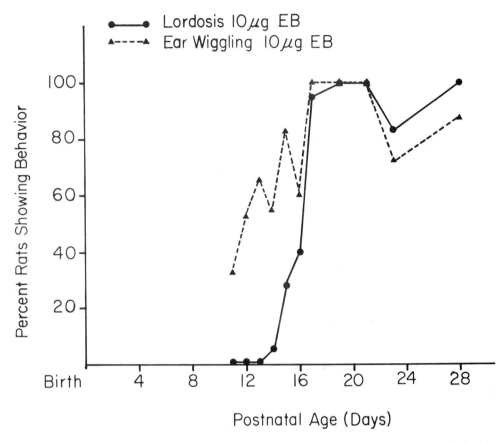

Fig. 2. Ontogeny of estrogen-stimulated proceptivity (ear wiggling) and receptivity (lordosis) in female rats. EB, estradiol benzoate. (Data taken from Södersten, 1975.)

structures and in cerebral cortex (Fig. 4; Reddy et al., 1974). Aromatase appears by *postnatal* day 1 in female limbic brain structures. Aromatase activity in neonatal rat hypothalamus is higher than that which is found in adult rat hypothalamus (Reddy et al., 1974; Weisz and Gibbs, 1974a). Aromatizing enzyme activity is practically undetectable at any age in rat cerebral cortex in vitro and in vivo, and is not found in pituitary either (Reddy et al., 1974; Weisz and Gibbs 1974a; Lieberburg and McEwen, 1975, 1977).

The 5α-reductase, capable of forming DHT from testosterone, is present on postnatal day 1 in pituitary and brain, and is at or near its highest activity between this age and day 5 in brain tissue, thereafter showing a gradual decline as the rats attain maturity (Denef et al., 1974; Massa et al., 1975). In contrast to the aromatizing enzyme system, which is regionally localized, DHT formation has a widespread distribution throughout the neonatal and adult brain (Denef et al., 1973, 1974; Massa et al., 1975). Pituitary DHT formation is higher in female than in male rats before puberty, and a peak of DHT formation in females coincides with an elevation of pituitary FSH content around day 14 (Fig. 5) (Denef et al., 1974; Massa et al., 1975).

Androgen receptors are present (but difficult to measure) in the neonatal rat brain, and have been described in brains of newborn mice, where they appear to have properties comparable to androgen receptors of the adult brain (Attardi and Ohno, 1976). Though detectable

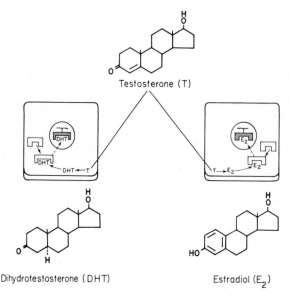

Fig. 3. Conversion of a 'prohormone' testosterone (T) to 5α-dihydrotestosterone (DHT) and estradiol (E$_2$) and interaction of these steroids with intracellular receptors.

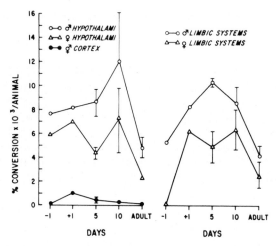

Fig. 4. In vitro aromatization by rat brain tissues. Single data points represent single experiments, bars represent the range of two experiments with the average per cent conversion (× 10^3) shown as the data point for that age. (Reprinted from Reddy et al., 1974, by permission.)

at birth in the mouse brain, using [^{3}H] DHT as ligand, they undergo a 2- to 3-fold increase during the first three postnatal weeks of life (Attardi and Ohno, 1976).

Estrogen receptor sites are barely detectable on day 20 of fetal life in the hypothalamus (Maclusky, unpublished), and this is consistent with the notion that estrogen receptors begin to emerge as differentiation proceeds, after the final cell divisions of hypothalamic neurons have been completed on days 14–16 (Ifft, 1972). Quite marked increases of estrogen receptor levels are seen within the first 12 hr of postnatal life, and are followed by

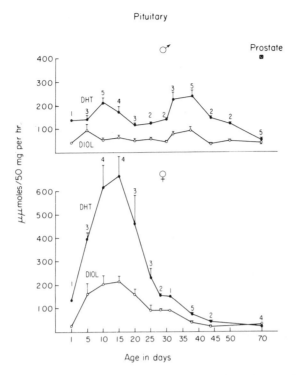

Fig. 5. Development of pituitary 5α-dihydrotestosterone (DHT) and 3α-androstanediol (DIOL) formation in male and female rats. Testosterone-1,2,H³ was incubated in vitro with intact pituitaries. Values are means ± S.E.M. of a number of incubations given above each time point. For one incubation, 3 to 4 pituitaries were pooled at days 1, 5 and 10; 2 to 3 pituitaries were pooled at day 15 to 30; and only 1 pituitary per incubation was used at later ages. A value for DHT obtained in adult prostate slices is also given. t-tests: male vs female, day 15: DHT and DIOL, $P < 0.005$; day 39: DHT, $P < 0.001$ and DIOL, $P < 0.005$. Males, DHT, day 10 vs day 20: $P < 0.025$; day 20 vs day 33: $P < 0.02$; day 38 vs days 45 and 50: $P < 0.01$. Females, DHT, day 5 vs day 15: $P < 0.05$; day 15 vs day 25: $P < 0.01$; DIOL, day 15 vs day 25: $P < 0.02$. (Reprinted from Denef et al., 1974, by permission.)

somewhat more gradual increases out to postnatal days 10–12 (Maclusky, unpublished). On postnatal day 3, the regional distribution of estrophilic cells in hypothalamus, preoptic area (Fig. 6B) and amygdala, as determined by autoradiography, resembles that found in the adult rat brain (Sheridan et al., 1974a, b; Gerlach and McEwen, unpublished), although the absolute number of receptors is smaller in newborn rats.

The principal topographic difference between estrophilic cells in baby and adult rat brains is the presence in the neonatal rat cerebral cortex of substantial numbers of estrogen receptors, which increase in parallel with hypothalamic receptors in the first two postnatal weeks, and which then disappear during the third postnatal week of life (Presl et al., 1971; Barley et al., 1974; McEwen et al., 1975; Maclusky et al., 1976; Westley and Salaman, 1976, 1977). From autoradiography it appears that many of the cortical estrophilic cells are located in the anterior cingulate cortex (Fig. 6A). Their function is unknown, but it is unlikely that they respond to testosterone-derived estradiol since, as noted above, the cortex lacks aromatizing enzyme activity.

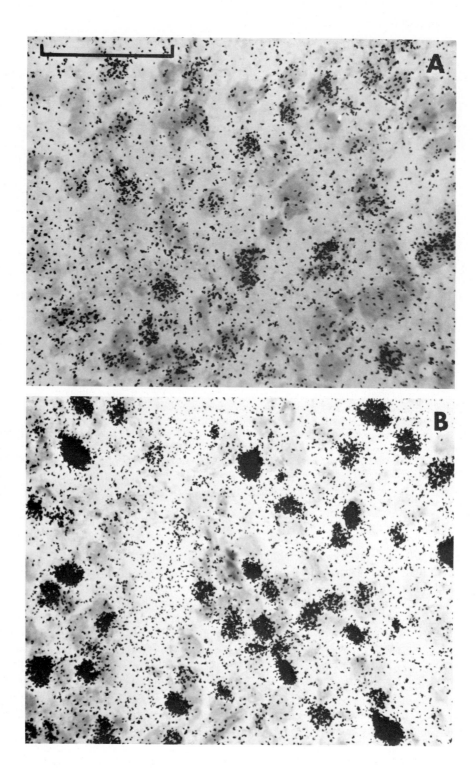

POSTNATAL DISAPPEARANCE OF α-FETOPROTEIN IN RAT

While estrogen receptor levels in the rat brain are increasing from birth, the level of another estrogen-binding protein, the α-fetoprotein, is declining (Table II) (Raynaud et al., 1971). Besides in serum, the α-fetoprotein is found in soluble extracts of neonatal rat brain (Fig. 7) (Plapinger et al., 1973) and in the uterus (Aussel et al., 1974); in the former case it appears to be a constituent of the cerebrospinal fluid. The predominant view of α-fetoprotein's role, with respect to estradiol, is that it retards by mass action the interaction of estradiol with intracellular estrogen receptors. (It should be noted that α-fetoprotein's lower affinity for estradiol, relative to intracellular estrogen receptors, is offset by its extremely high concentration in plasma – Table II.) It is conceivable that declining levels of α-fetoprotein may account for the age-related increase in sensitivity of the infant rat to negative feedback effects of estradiol, as well as for the age-related increase in sensitivity of the reproductive tract to estradiol (E_2) (see Ojeda and Ramirez, 1973/74; Raynaud, 1973). It is also possible that the decline of α-fetoprotein may be part of the explanation for the onset of estrogen-inducible lordosis behavior and ovulation between days 19 and 25, although neurological maturation undoubtedly plays the predominant role. As noted above, the ovary appears able to release ova in response to exogenous gonadotropin as early as 17–18 days of age. Finally, it is possible that the high titers of α-fetoprotein in late fetal and early neonatal life protect the brain and reproductive tract against the potentially deleterious effects of circulating estradiol (Plapinger and McEwen, 1977). We shall next consider the sexual differentiation of the developing reproductive tract and brain in the rat, and the role of estrogen receptors in the latter organ.

TABLE II

LEVELS OF α-FETOPROTEIN IN RAT PLASMA

From Raynaud et al. (1971).

Age (days)	Concentration of estrogen binding sites (μM)	
	Male*	Female*
Fetus (20)	70 ± 50	85 ± 20
Neonate (5)	40 ± 6	22 ± 8
Immature (20)	4 ± 1	5 ± 1
Immature (30)	0	0

*Mean ± S.E.M.

SEXUAL DIFFERENTIATION

Around day 14 of gestation, a genetically controlled signal related to the presence of the Y chromosome imposes testicular organogenesis on a presumptive gonad, which would otherwise become an ovary (Jost, 1970). Leydig cells of the testes show two distinct phases of activity, the first commencing in the rat around the 16–17th day of gestation and ending in

Fig. 6. Autroadiograms illustrating in vivo binding and retention of the synthetic steroidal estrogen, [³H]-11β-methoxy-17α-ethynylestradiol ([³H]RU2858), to neurons in the cingulate cortex (A) and medial preoptic area (B) in brains of 3-day-old, intact, female rats injected 2 hr earlier. Autoradiograms were prepared from unfixed, unembedded 2 μm frozen sections, exposed for 350 days, and stained lightly with methyl green-pyronin Y. Bar indicates 50 μm. (For details see Gerlach and McEwen, 1972.)

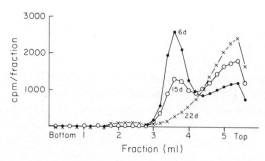

Fig. 7. Developmental time course of neonatal estradiol-binding activity in the brain. Density gradient representation of levels of labeled estradiol bound in vitro to neonatal binding sites of HPAMB cytosol, from female rats at different times after birth. Closed circles, 6-day-old HPAMB cytosol; open circles, 15-day-old; crosses, 22-day-old. (Reprinted from Plapinger et al., 1974, by permission.)

the second postnatal week, and the second beginning in the third postnatal week and continuing into adulthood (Niemi and Ikonen, 1963; Lording and De Kretser, 1972). The ability of the testes to produce testosterone can be detected as early as the 16th day of gestation, and this ability parallels the Leydig cell activity (Warren et al., 1973; Smeaton et al., 1975; Payne et al., 1977). That the brain may be controlling this early phase of testicular secretion in the rat is indicated by decreases in Leydig cell volume following decapitation of fetuses (Eguchi et al., 1975). Testosterone levels in blood and testes are elevated at birth in the rat, and decline, as does Leydig cell activity, during the first and second postnatal weeks (Resko et al., 1968).

According to Jost (1970), the process of masculine differentiation of body sex is imposed by testicular secretions on developing tissues which would otherwise acquire the feminine phenotype. This process consists of two components: (a) regression of the Mullerian ducts, and (b) masculinization of the Wolffian ducts, of the urogenital sinus, and of the urogenital tubercle and swelling. All of this occurs in the rat from approximately the 16th postnatal day until the first or second day after birth.

Brain sexual differentiation in the rat occurs while differentiation of the reproductive tract is well underway, and consists of at least three separable components: (1) induction of anovulatory sterility; (2) reduction of the capacity to show lordosis; and (3) enhancement of the capacity to show male-like mounting behavior. The first two components, which are separable from each other on the basis of dose responses to injected testosterone propionate (see Plapinger and McEwen, 1978, for references), are effects of 'defeminization', whereas the third is an effect of 'masculinization'.

Defeminization and masculinization can be distinguished from each other in a number of ways (see Goy and Goldfoot, 1975, for discussion). For example, low to moderate doses of androstenedione given to neonatally castrated male rats results in animals which display lordosis in adulthood, and also mounting, intromission and ejaculatory behavior (Goldfoot et al., 1969). Moreover, some anatomical separation of the masculinizing and the defeminizing effects of steroids has been obtained with steroid implants: T or E_2 implants in the preoptic area of newborn female rats masculinize with respect to mounting behavior, but do not defeminize, while T or E_2 implants in ventromedial hypothalamus do not masculinize, but produce defeminization with respect to ovulation and lordosis (Christiansen and Gorski, 1978).

The critical period of defeminization occurs postnatally within the first 4 or 5 days of life, whereas the critical period for masculinization may begin even before birth (see McEwen,

1978, for references). There are some interesting observations concerning which steroids are effective in masculinizing and defeminizing the rat brain. As noted above, both T and E_2 are effective agents for rat brain sexual differentiation. Androgens with the A-ring reduced, such as DHT, are generally reported to be ineffective in defeminizing female rats (Luttge and Whalen, 1970; McDonald and Doughty, 1972; Whalen and Rezek, 1974; Korenbrot et al., 1975), although one report indicates that there may be some slight effect of DHT (Gerall et al., 1976). With respect to masculinization, day-1 castrated male rats are responsive to a combined treatment on days 1 to 5 of DHT plus RU2858, a synthetic estrogen (Booth, 1977b). Separately, DHT and RU2858 at the particular dose chosen are relatively ineffective. Related studies on the hamster indicate that diethylstilbestrol, a synthetic estrogen, is by itself very effective in masculinizing female hamsters (Paup et al., 1972, 1974).

The discovery by Naftolin, Ryan and coworkers of brain enzymes capable of converting androstenedione or T in vitro to estrone or E_2, respectively, raised the possibility that the 'aromatization' process may be obligatory, or at least significantly involved, in sexual differentiation (Naftolin et al., 1975). The demonstration of aromatization in vitro established that this process is intrinsic to developing brain tissue, besides occurring in steroid-producing glands and the placenta (Reddy et al., 1974). Furthermore, as noted above, we now know that aromatization occurs in vivo in the neonatal rat brain (Weisz and Gibbs, 1974b; Lieberburg and McEwen, 1975).

Several kinds of evidence point to the involvement of aromatization in the sexual differentiation of the rat brain. First of all, there is the aforementioned conversion of [7-^{3}H]-testosterone to [^{3}H]estradiol and the retention of this steroid by cell nuclei in the hypothalamus and limbic areas of the neonatal rat's brain. Hypothalamic estrogen receptors of the 4-day-old male rat are partially occupied by androgen-derived estradiol (Westley and Salaman, 1976, 1977). Second, there is the demonstration of cell nuclear and soluble estrogen receptors in brains of newborn rats. These receptors have a specificity which parallels the action spectrum of steroids, in so far as it is presently known, in inducing brain sexual differentiation.

Proof that aromatization actually plays a significant role in brain sexual differentiation requires that one prevent the effect of exogenous T in females, and of endogenous T in males, by agents which either block aromatization or which prevent access of estrogen to intracellular receptor sites. With respect to inhibitors of aromatization, Clemens (1974) has reported some success in blocking the masculinizing effects of T given to castrated, newborn hamsters by means of pentobarbital and SKF 525A, which may decrease aromatization by competing for microsomal hydoxylating enzymes. More definitive results have recently been obtained using a steroid inhibitor of aromatization: androst-1,4,6-triene-3,17-dione (ATD). Implantation of silastic capsules of ATD into 4-day-old female rats reduces by more than 80% cell nuclear levels of [^{3}H]E_2 derived from an injection of [^{3}H]T. Tissue levels of [^{3}H]E_2 and [^{3}H]estrone are also reduced, indicating that aromatization is affected. Tissue and cell nuclear levels of [^{3}H]T and [^{3}H]DHT are unaltered by ATD treatment, nor did ATD interfere with cell nuclear retention of [^{3}H]diethylstilbestrol, indicating that it is neutral with respect to the estrogen receptor mechanism (Lieberburg et al., 1978). ATD treatment of newborn male rats feminized them with respect to their ability to display lordosis behavior as adults, while ATD treatment of females (also given T) blocked the defeminizing effects of T on lordosis behavior and on ovulation (McEwen et al., 1978). Similar results have been reported by Vreeburg et al. (1977) using ATD, and by Booth (1977a) using a related steroid, androst-4-ene-3,6,17-trione.

With respect to inhibitors of estrogen receptors, there have been reports of success in preventing defeminization of female rats by neonatal testosterone propionate (TP) using a non-steroidal estrogen antagonist, MER-25 (Doughty and McDonald, 1974). MER-25 also antagonizes the defeminizing action of a synthetic estrogen, RU2858, on brain sexual differentiation (Doughty et al., 1975). There have also been three reports of failures to obtain such antagonistic effects with MER-25 (Brown-Grant, 1974; Gottlieb et al., 1974; Hayashi, 1974), which may be explained by the poor solubility and limited effectiveness of this estrogen antagonist (Ruh and Ruh, 1974).

Recent experiments with a more potent anti-estrogen, CI628, support the successful MER-25 experiments: CI628 treatment of neonatal male rats feminized them with respect to lordosis display as adults. CI628 treatment of newborn females (in addition treated with TP) attenuated the defeminizing effects on lordosis behavior but did not prevent anovulatory sterility (McEwen et al., 1977). CI628 affords only partial protection against TP, and produces a weak effect on differentiation due to its own weak estrogenicity (McEwen et al., 1977). That CI628 may exert its effects by interfering with the action of estradiol derived from neural aromatization of T, is supported by work of Lieberburg et al. (1977) who found that levels of $[^3H]E_2$ derived from an injection of $[^3H]T$ into 5-day-old female rats were reduced by prior administration of CI628 on day 4. Tissue levels of $[^3H]E_2$ were unaltered by CI628, suggesting that aromatization was unaffected. Likewise unaltered were tissue and cell nuclear levels of $[^3H]T$ and $[^3H]DHT$.

As a result of sexual differentiation, the brain presumably acquires certain permanent characteristics which underlie the sex differences in behavioral responses and neuroendocrine function described above as 'masculinization' and 'defeminization'. That some of these characteristics may involve differences in brain structure is suggested by observations of sexually dimorphic brain structures in the rat preoptic area and hypothalamus (Gorski et al., 1977), and of sexually dimorphic patterns of synaptic (Raisman and Field, 1973) and dendritic (Greenough et al., 1977) organization in the preoptic area of rats and hamsters. These structural differences appear to arise in hypothalamus and preoptic area during the postnatal critical period, when the sexual differentiation of behavior and neuroendocrine function is taking place, and at a time after the final cell divisions of major cell groups has taken place (see Table I), although some limited proliferation of late-arising interneurons has not been absolutely excluded. Several possible mechanisms involving established neurons may be envisioned. Testicular secretion, presumably acting by way of estrogens formed within certain target cells, may influence the survival of cells (e.g. by causing destruction of cells, or by stabilization of cells which might otherwise die) and/or may influence the growth of axons and dendrites, leading to altered patterns of synaptic connections. The latter possibility is supported by recent studies of neonatal hypothalamic and preoptic tissue of mouse in tissue culture, in which marked stimulation of neurite outgrowth is reported to occur as a result of adding testosterone or estradiol to the culture medium (Toran-Allerand, 1976).

With regard to neuronal growth and maturation, there are studies with thyroid hormone which indicate that the 'critical period' for gonadal steroid action is related to the state of neural maturation. Hypothyroidism in the early postnatal period retards myelination and development of the neuropil, and also reduces synapse formation, although it does not cause a decrease in cell number; *hyper*thyroidism at birth decreases total cell number, facilitates myelinization, and transiently increases synapse formation (see McEwen, 1976, for references). With respect to sexual differentiation, hypothyroidism at birth prolongs the critical period of susceptibility of female rats to the defeminizing effects of TP (Kikuyama, 1969). *Hyper*thyroidism shortly after birth, on the other hand, shortens the critical period of susceptibility to TP (Phelps and Sawyer, 1976).

CONCLUSIONS

During the development of the rat brain in late fetal and early postnatal life, two major events are occurring with respect to reproductive function: sexual *maturation* and sexual *differentiation* (see Fig. 8). Sexual maturation is a result not only of neurological maturation, and of growth and maturation of the reproductive tract, gonads, pituitary, hypothalamic neurosecretory cells and hypothalamo-hypophyseal portal circulation, but also of acquisition of the competence of brain and pituitary to respond to the activating effects of gonadal steroids. We believe that this hormonal sensitivity consists of at least 3 components: (a) ontogeny of androgen metabolizing enzymes, which convert a 'prohormone', testosterone, to DHT or estradiol; (b) development of receptors for androgens and estrogens; and (c) disappearance of a plasma estrogen binding protein, α-fetoprotein, which retards estrogen (by mass action) from binding to the receptors. All of these components are present when the activational effects of gonadal steroids are first detected. The magnitude of the earliest of these, negative feedback, may be influenced by the presence of α-fetoprotein. The appearance of estrogen-inducible lordosis and of positive (ovulatory) feedback occur relatively late in the neonatal period (days 19–25), and are more easily explained by neurological maturation than by the continuing decline of the already low levels of α-fetoprotein.

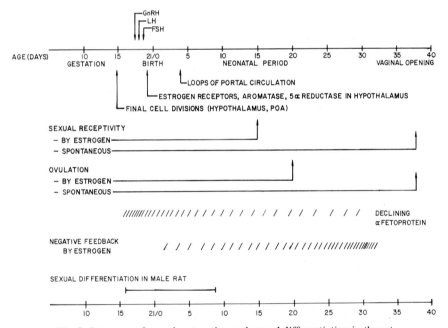

Fig. 8. Summary of sexual maturation and sexual differentiation in the rat.

Sexual differentiation of the rat brain takes place early in postnatal life, before sexual maturation has proceeded very far, but it takes place in a tissue which has acquired the ability to convert testosterone to estradiol or DHT and to bind estradiol or androgens to intracellular receptor sites. Present evidence favors the concept that, in the rat brain, it is the pathway involving estrogen production and estrogen receptors which is most important for testosterone action in producing brain sexual differentiation (although it would be premature

304

at this time to exclude a limited participation of androgen receptors). The fact that hormone-metabolizing enzymes and specific gonadal steroid receptors are present before sexual differentiation takes place implies that the action of the hormone is that of a trigger, in which testicular secretion precipitates certain aspects of differentiation in specific target neurons during a critical phase of their maturation. The triggering action of testosterone (or its metabolites) in the brain may be somewhat analogous to the action of an insect steroid hormone, ecdysone, in promoting the differentiation of the imaginal disks (Nöthiger, 1972). Ecdysone is responsible for triggering differentiation of different populations of imaginal disks into antennae, legs, compound eyes, or other structures of the exoskeleton. The determination of which structures will be formed occurs in the disks some time before they become competent to respond to ecdysone (Nöthiger, 1972).

Estrogen receptors in the developing rat brain may be involved in both permanent *organizational* and reversible *activational* effects of estradiol. From all the evidence so far accumulated, many of the estrogen receptors appear to be located in the same brain regions of newborn and adult rat brains, and the physical properties of neonatal and adult brain estrogen receptors appear to be identical. It will be interesting to find out what the critical maturational factors are which determine whether an estrogen-receptor complex will produce a permanent developmental effect or an adult-like activational action.

ACKNOWLEDGEMENTS

Research in the author's laboratory is supported by Research Grant NS07080 from the NIH and by an institutional grant for research in reproductive biology from the Rockefeller Foundation (RF70095).

The author wishes to acknowledge the essential contributions of his laboratory colleagues to the research described in this article: Mr. John Gerlach, Dr. Lewis Krey, Dr. Ivan Lieberburg, Dr. Neil Maclusky, and Dr. Linda Plapinger. He also expresses his appreciation to Ms. Freddi Berg for graphic work and editorial assistance.

REFERENCES

Attardi, B. and Ohno, S. (1976) Androgen and estrogen receptors in the developing mouse brain, *Endocrinology*, 99: 1279–1290.

Aussel, C., Uriel, J., Michel, G. and Baulieu, E.-E. (1974) Immunological demonstration of α-fetoprotein in uterine cytosol from immature rats, *Biochimie*, 56: 567–570.

Barley, J., Ginsburg, M., Greenstein, B.D., Maclusky, N.J. and Thomas, P.J. (1974) A receptor mediating sexual differentiation?, *Nature (Lond.)*, 252: 259–260.

Booth, J.E. (1977a) Effects of the aromatization inhibitor, androst-4-ene-3,6,17-trione on sexual differentiation induced by testosterone in the neonatally castrated rat, *J. Endocr.*, 72: 53P–54P.

Booth, J.E. (1977b) Sexual behavior of neonatally castrated rats injected during infancy with oestrogen and dihydrotestosterone, *J. Endocr.*, 72: 135–141.

Brown-Grant, K., (1974) Failure of ovulation after administration of steroid hormones and hormone antagonists to female rats during the neonatal period, *J. Endocr.*, 62: 683–684.

Caligaris, L., Astrada, J.J. and Taleisnik, S. (1972) Influence of age on the release of luteinizing hormone induced by oestrogen and progesterone in immature rats, *J. Endrocr.*, 55: 97–103.

Caligaris, L., Astrada, J.J. and Taleisnik, S. (1973) Development of the mechanisms involved in the facilitatory and inhibitory effects of ovarian steroids on the release of follicle-stimulating hormone in the immature rat, *J. Endocr.*, 58: 547–554.

Chiappa, S.A., and Fink, G. (1977) Releasing factor and hormonal changes in the hypothalamic-pituitary-gonadotrophin and adrenocorticotrophin systems before and after birth and puberty in male, female and androgenized female rats, *J. Endocr.*, 72: 211–224.

Chowdhury, M. and Steinberger, E. (1976) Pituitary and plasma levels of gonadotrophins in foetal and newborn male and female rats, *J. Endocr.*, 69: 381–384.

Christensen, L.W. and Gorski, R.A. (1978) Independent masculinization of neuroendocrine systems by intracerebral implants of testosterone or estradiol in the neonatal female rat, in preparation.

Clemens, L.G. (1974) Neurohormonal control of male sexual behavior. In *Reproductive Behavior*, W. Montagna and W.A. Sadler (Eds.), Plenum Press, New York, pp. 23–53.

Denef, C., Magnus, C. and McEwen, B.S. (1973) Sex differences and hormonal control of testosterone metabolism in rat pituitary and brain, *J. Endocr.*, 59: 605–621.

Denef, C., Magnus, C. and McEwen, B.S. (1974) Sex-dependent changes in pituitary 5α-dihydrotestosterone and 3α-androstanediol formation during postnatal development and puberty in the rat, *Endocrinol.*, 94: 1265–1274.

Docke, F. and Dorner, G. (1974) Oestrogen and the control of gonadotrophin secretion in the immature rat, *J. Endocr.*, 63: 285–298.

Dohler, K.D. and Wuttke, W. (1975) Changes with age in levels of serum gonadotropins, prolactin, and gonadal steroids in prepubertal male and female rats, *Endocrinology*, 97: 898–907.

Doughty, C. and McDonald, P.G. (1974) Hormonal control of sexual differentiation of the hypothalamus in the neonatal female rat, *Differentiation*, 2: 275–285.

Doughty, C., Booth, J.E., McDonald, P.G. and Parrott, R.F. (1975) Inhibition, by the anti-oestrogen MER-25, of defeminization induced by the synthetic oestrogen RU2858, *J. Endocr.*, 67: 459–460.

Dunlap, J.L. and Gerall, A.A. (1973) Compensatory ovarian hypertrophy can be obtained in neonatal rats, *J. reprod. Fert.*, 32: 517–519.

Eguchi, Y., Sakamoto, Y., Arishima, K., Morikawa, Y. and Hashimoto, Y. (1975) Hypothalamic control of the pituitary-testicular relation in fetal rats: measurement of collective volume of Leydig cells, *Endocrinology*, 96: 504–507.

Fink, G. and Smith, G.C. (1971) Ultrastructural features of the developing hypothalamo-hypophysial axis in the rat: a correlative study, *Z. Zellforsch.*, 119: 208–226.

Gerall, A.A., Dunlap, J.L. and Wagner, R.A. (1976) Effects of dihydrotestosterone and gonadotropins on the development of female behavior, *Physiol. Behav.*, 17: 121–126.

Goldfoot, D.A., Feder, H.H. and Goy, R.W. (1969) Development of bisexuality in the male rat treated neonatally with androstenedione, *J. comp. physiol. Psychol.*, 67: 41–45.

Goldman, B.D. and Gorski, R.A. (1971) Effects of gonadal steroids on the secretion of LH and FSH in neonatal rats, *Endocrinology*, 89: 112–115.

Gorski, R., Shryne, J., Gordon, J. and Christensen, L. (1977) Evidence for a morphological sex difference within the medial preoptic area (MPOA) of the rat, *Anat. Rec.*, 187: 591.

Gottlieb, H., Gerall, A.A. and Thiel, A. (1974) Receptivity in female hamsters following neonatal testosterone, testosterone propionate, and MER-25, *Physiol. Behav.*, 12: 61–68.

Goy, R.W. and Goldfoot, D.A. (1975) Neuroendocrinology: animal models and problems of human sexuality, *Arch. sex. Behav.*, 4: 405–420.

Greenough, W.T., Carter, C.S., Steerman, C. and DeVoogd, T. (1977) Sex differences in dendritic patterns in hamster preoptic area, *Brain Res.*, 126: 63–72.

Hayashi, S. (1974) Failure of intrahypothalamic implants of antiestrogen, MER-25, to inhibit androgen sterilization in female rats, *Endocr. jap.*, 21: 453–457.

Holweg, W. (1934) Veranderungen des Hypophysenvorderlappens und des Ovariums nach Behandlung mit grossen Dosen von Follikelhormon, *Klin. Wschr.*, 13: 92–95.

Ifft, J.D. (1972) An autoradiographic study of the time of final division of neurons in rat hypothalamic nuclei, *J. comp. Neurol.*, 144: 193–204.

Jost, A. (1970) Hormonal factors in the sex differentiation of the mammalian foetus, *Phil. Trans. B*, 259: 119–130.

Kikuyama, S. (1969) Alteration by neonatal hypothyroidism of the critical period for the induction of persistent estrus in the rat, *Endocr. jap.*, 16: 269–273.

Korenbrot, C.C., Paup, D.C. and Gorski, R.A. (1975) Effects of testosterone propionate or dihydrotestosterone propionate on plasma FSH and LH levels in neonatal rats and on sexual differentiation of the brain, *Endocrinology*, 97: 709–717.

Lieberburg, I. and McEwen, B.S. (1975) Estradiol-17β: a metabolite of testosterone recovered in cell nuclei from limbic areas of neonatal rat brains, *Brain Res.*, 85: 165–170.

Lieberburg, I., Wallach, G. and McEwen, B.S. (1977) The effects of an inhibitor of aromatization (1,4,6-androstatriene-3,17-dione) and an anti-estrogen (CI628) on in vivo formed testosterone metabolites recovered from neonatal rat brain tissues and purified cell nuclei. Implications for sexual differentiation of the rat brain, *Brain Res.*, 128: 176–181.

Lording, D.W. and De Kretser, D.M. (1972) Comparative ultrastructural and histochemical studies of the interstitial cells of the rat testis during fetal and postnatal development, *J. reprod. Fert.*, 29: 261–269.

Luttge, W.G. and Whalen, R.E. (1970) Dihydrotestosterone, androstenedione, testosterone: comparative effectiveness in masculinizing and defeminizing reproductive systems in male and female rats, *Horm. Behav.*, 1: 265–281.

Maclusky, N.J., Chaptal, C., Lieberburg, I. and McEwen, B.S. (1976) Properties and subcellular interrelationships of presumptive estrogen receptor macromolecules in the brains of neonatal and prepubertal female rats, *Brain Res.*, 114: 158–165.

McDonald, P.G. and Doughty, C. (1972) Comparison of the effect of neonatal administration of testosterone and dihydrotestosterone in the female rat, *J. reprod. Fert.*, 30: 55–62.

McEwen, B.S. (1978) Gonadal influences on the developing brain. In *Handbook of Biological Psychiatry*, H.M. Van Praag, M.H. Lader, O.J. Rafaelsen and E.J. Sachar (Eds.), Marcel Dekker, New York.

McEwen, B.S., Plapinger, L., Chaptal, C., Gerlach, J. and Wallach, G. (1975) Role of fetoneonatal estrogen binding proteins in the association of estrogen with neonatal brain cell nuclear receptors, *Brain Res.*, 96: 400–406.

McEwen, B.S., Lieberburg, I., Chaptal, C. and Krey, L.C. (1977) Aromatization: important for sexual differentiation of the neonatal rat brain, *Horm. Behav.*, 9: 249–263.

Massa, R., Justo, S. and Martini, L. (1975) Conversion of testosterone into 5-reduced metabolites in the anterior pituitary and in the brain of maturing rats, *J. steroid Biochem.*, 6: 567–571.

Meijs-Roelofs, H.M.A., Uilenbroek, J.Th.J., de Jongs, F.H. and Welschen, R. (1973) Plasma oestradiol-17β and its relationship to serum follicle-stimulating hormone in immature female rats, *J. Endocr.*, 59: 295–304.

Meijs-Roelofs, H.M.A., de Greef, W.J. and Uilenbroek, J.Th.J. (1975) Plasma progesterone and its relationship to serum gonadotrophins in immature female rats, *J. Endocr.*, 64: 329–336.

Naftolin, F., Ryan, K.J., Davies, I.J., Reddy, V.V., Flores, F., Petro, Z. and Kuhn, M. (1975) The formation of estrogens by central neuroendocrine tissues, *Rec. Progr. Horm. Res.*, 31: 295–315.

Niemi, M. and Ikonen, M. (1963) Histochemistry of the Leydig cells in the postnatal prepubertal testis of the rat, *Endocrinology*, 72: 443–448.

Nothiger, R. (1972) The larval development of imaginal disks. In *The Biology of Imaginal Disks*, H. Ursprung and R. Notiger (Eds.), Springer, Berlin.

Ojeda, S.R. and Ramirez, V.D. (1973/74) Short-term steroid treatment of plasma LH and FSH in castrated rats from birth to puberty, *Neuroendocrinology*, 13: 100–114.

Ojeda, S.R., Kalra, P.S. and McCann, S.M. (1975) Further studies on the maturation of the estrogen negative feedback on gonadotropin release in the female rat, *Neuroendocrinology*, 18: 242–255.

Ojeda, S.R., Jameson, H.E. and McCann, S.M. (1977) Developmental changes in pituitary responsiveness to luteinizing hormone-releasing hormone (LHRH) in the female rat: ovarian-adrenal influence during the infantile period, *Endocrinology*, 100: 440–451.

Paup, D.C., Coniglio, L.P. and Clemens, L.G. (1972) Masculinization of the female golden hamster by neonatal treatment with androgen or estrogen, *Horm. Behav.*, 3: 123–132.

Paup, D.C., Coniglio, L.P. and Clemens, L.G. (1974) Hormonal determinants in the development of masculine and feminine behavior in the female hamster, *Behav. Biol.*, 10: 353–363.

Payne, A.H., Kelch, R.P., Murono, E.P. and Kerlan, J.T. (1977) Hypothalamic, pituitary and testicular function during sexual maturation of the male rat, *J. Endocr.*, 72: 17–26.

Phelps, C.P. and Sawyer, C.H. (1976) Postnatal thyroxine modifies effects of early androgen on lordosis, *Horm. Behav.*, 7: 331–340.

Plapinger, L. and McEwen, B.S. (1977) Gonadal steroid-brain interactions in sexual differentiation. In *Biological Determinants of Sexual Behavior*, J. Hutchison (Ed.), Wiley, New York, in press.

Plapinger, L., McEwen, B.S. and Clemens, L.E. (1973) Ontogeny of estradiol-binding sites in rat brain. II. Characteristics of a neonatal binding macromolecule, *Endocrinology*, 93: 1129–1139.

Presl, J., Pospisil, J. and Horsky, J. (1971) Autoradiographic localization of radioactivity in female rat neocortex after injection of tritiated estradiol, *Experientia (Basel)*, 27: 465–467.

Raisman, G. and Field, P.M. (1973) Sexual dimorphism in the neuropil of the preoptic area of the rat and its dependence on neonatal androgen, *Brain Res.*, 54: 1–29.

Ramirez, V.D. and Sawyer, C.H. (1965) Advancement of puberty in the female rat by estrogen, *Endocrinology*, 76: 1158–1168.

Raynaud, J.P. (1973) Influence of rat estradiol binding plasma protein (EBP) on uterotrophic activity, *Steroids*, 21: 249–258.

Raynaud, J.P., Mercier-Bodard, C. and Baulieu, E.-E. (1971) Rat estradiol binding plasma protein (EBP), *Steroids*, 18: 767–788.

Reddy, V.V.R., Naftolin, F. and Ryan, K.J. (1974) Conversion of androstenedione to estrone by neural tissues from fetal and neonatal rats, *Endocrinology*, 94: 117–121.

Resko, J.A., Feder, H.H. and Goy, R.W. (1968) Androgen concentrations in plasma and testis of developing rats, *J. Endocr.*, 40: 485–491.

Ruh, T.S. and Ruh, M.F. (1974) The effect of anti-estrogens on the nuclear binding of the estrogen receptor, *Steroids*, 24: 209–224.

Schafer, S.J. and McShan, W.H. (1974) Gonadotropic hormone release from fetal and adult rat pituitary glands after in vitro exposure to synthetic LH-FSH-RH, *Neuroendocrinology*, 16: 332–341.

Sheridan, P.J., Sar, M. and Stumpf, W.E. (1974a) Autoradiographic localization of ^{3}H-estradiol or its metabolites in the central nervous system of the developing rat, *Endocrinology*, 94: 1386–1390.

Sheridan, P.J., Sar, M. and Stumpf, W.E. (1974b) Interaction of exogenous steroids in the developing rat brain, *Endocrinology*, 95: 1749–1753.

Smeaton, T.C., Arcondoulis, D.E. and Steele, P.A. (1975) The synthesis of testosterone and estradiol-17 by the gonads of neonatal rats in vitro, *Steroids*, 26: 181–192.

Smith, E.R. and Davidson, J.M. (1968) Role of estrogen in the cerebral control of puberty in female rats, *Endocrinology*, 82: 100–108.

Smith, G.C. and Simpson, R.W. (1970) Monoamine fluorescence in the median eminence of foetal, neonatal and adult rats, *Z. Zellforsch.*, 104: 541–556.

Sodersten, P. (1975) Receptive behavior in developing female rats, *Horm. Behav.*, 6: 307–317.

Toran-Allerand, C.D. (1976) Sex steroids and the development of the newborn mouse hypothalamus and preoptic area in vitro: implications for sexual differentiation, *Brain Res.*, 106: 407–412.

Vreeburg, J.T.M., van der Vaart, P.D.M. and van der Schoot, P. (1977) Prevention of central defeminization but not masculinization in male rats by inhibition neonatally of oestrogen biosynthesis, *J. Endocr.*, in press.

Warren, D.W., Haltmeyer, G.C. and Eik-Ness, K.B. (1973) Testosterone in the fetal rat testis, *Biol. Reprod.*, 8: 560–565.

Weisz, J. and Gibbs, C. (1974a) Conversion of testosterone and androstenedione to estrogen in vitro by the brain of female rats, *Endocrinology*, 94: 616–620.

Weisz, J. and Gibbs, C. (1974b) Metabolites of testosterone in the brain of the newborn female rat after an injection of tritiated testosterone, *Neuroendocrinology*, 14: 72–86.

Westley, B.R. and Salaman, D.F. (1976) Role of oestrogen receptor in androgen-induced sexual differentiation of the brain, *Nature (Lond.)*, 262: 407–408.

Westley, B.R. and Salaman, D.F. (1977) Nuclear binding of the oestrogen receptor of neonatal rat brain after injection of oestrogens and androgens; localization of sex differences, *Brain Res.*, 119: 375–388.

Whalen, R.E. and Rezek, D.L. (1974) Inhibition of lordosis in female rats by subcutaneous implants of testosterone, androstenedione or dihydrotestosterone in infancy, *Horm. Behav.*, 5: 125–128.

Ying, S.-Y. and Greep, R.O. (1971) Effect of age of rat and dose of a single injection of estradiol benzoate (EB) on ovulation and the facilitation of ovulation by progesterone (P), *Endocrinology*, 89: 785–790.

Zarrow, M.X. and Wilson, E.D. (1961) The influence of age on superovulation in the immature rat and mouse, *Endocrinology*, 69: 851–855.

DISCUSSION

UYLINGS: Although it is possible that sex differences are reflected in the shape of dendritic trees in the preoptic area (POA), I would like to comment on your reference to the work of Greenough and Carter. Their results are based on dendritic density values of the entire population of impregnated neurons in the POA. This type of study is very difficult and troublesome, due to the fact that the dendritic pattern varies with the location of cells within the POA, and also to problems arising when doing a Golgi impregnation using silver nitrate. This last can affect the analysis when the density of dendrites is determined within a large brain area, since the Golgi method stains only a small percentage of the neurons. So I think that Greenough's finding is only an indication, rather than conclusive evidence, that there are any sex differences in the dendritic patterns.

McEWEN: The first studies on this subject (by Raisman and Field) involved an incredibly time-consuming electron microscopic investigation, done double-blind. The second series of studies (the Greenough and Carter series) involved an equally time-consuming light microscopic study, with suggestive results. Most recently, Roger Gorski sat down and looked with the light microscope at Nissl sections, and found a sex difference in the size of the medial preoptic nucleus. It seems that, as people find the courage to look for sex differences in the brain, it becomes easier to find them, so that we don't have to depend exclusively on the dendritic tree story.

ZIMMER: Is it true that there now exist mice that have no steriod hormone receptors?

McEWEN: Mice having the androgen insensitivity syndrome called *testicular feminization* (TFM) lack androgen receptors. If androgen receptors mediated sexual differentiation, one would predict that TFM animals would be feminized but, in fact, a careful analysis of the TFM mutation in the rat indicates that the neuroendocrine-behavioral axis related to female sexual behavior and ovulation becomes *masculinized* (Shapiro et al., 1975; Beach and Buchler, 1977). This is consistent with the aromatization hypothesis that I presented.

SWAAB: You focused your attention upon the last part of the hypothalamo-hypophysial gonadal axis and, indeed, many effects of gonadal hormones on development are to be found. But, as you said already, the feedback loop is closed very early in development; this might mean that if levels of gonadal hormones change, the other level of the loop (hypothalamus and pituitary) are also changed. The possibility therefore exists that effects which are thought to be caused by sex-hormones are in fact indirectly caused by pituitary or hypothalamic hormones. Since LH-RH, for instance, has been shown to be present in various extrahypothalamic areas, and was found in addition to modify electrical activity and behavior, might it not be possible that this hormone is of much greater importance in the maturation of the brain than we thought before?

McEWEN: I agree with you that this may well be the case. I find it very difficult to think of an experiment to test it, however, because if the hormone *is* present in the brain there is not much you can do to get rid of it, especially if it is acting locally within the brain.

SWAAB: You could inject antibodies directed to LH-RH or other hormones that might be involved.

McEWEN: Antibodies – that is indeed a good idea, and I think that somebody should go and do it!

REFERENCES

Shapiro et al. (1975) *Endocrinology*, 97: 487–492.
Beach and Buchler (1977) *Endocrinology*, 109: 197–200.

Gonadal Hormones and the Differentiation of Sexual and Aggressive Behavior and Learning in the Rat

N.E. VAN DE POLL, J.P.C. DE BRUIN, H. VAN DIS and H.G. VAN OYEN

Netherlands Institute for Brain Research, Amsterdam (The Netherlands)

INTRODUCTION

Concerning the effects of sex hormones on the development of the central nervous system (CNS) and its functions in controlling behavior, an important distinction generally is made between 'organizational' effects, which take place in early life, and 'activational' effects occurring in adulthood. It has become more and more clear, however, that most of the 'organizational' effects can only be assessed by hormonal stimulation in adulthood. Because these two factors are highly interdependent, the present paper will deal with both effects of the hormones.

It was established quite some time ago that the differentiation of the embryonic gonads during early development into ovaries or testes, and the subsequent release of hormonal products from the testis in the male drastically affects the brain-pituitary-gonadal axis of the fetus, the newborn and the adult organism (Pfeiffer, 1936; Jost, 1970). On account of these effects upon somatic dimorphism and sexual differentiation of hypothalamic-pituitary functioning, some workers postulated that similar processes in the CNS would underlie sex differences in sexual behavior (Phoenix et al., 1959; Harris and Levine, 1962). These ideas stimulated a large amount of research into gonadal hormone-induced sexual differentiation of behavior. This particular history of the research on sex differences in behavior, however, led to biases in the formation of general concepts; we will deal briefly with these before discussing the current state of the field of sexual behavior, aggression and learning.

SEXUAL DIFFERENTIATION AND THE STUDY OF BEHAVIOR

Most behavioral research on influences of gonadal hormones during early development, for obvious reasons, was concentrated on *sexual* behavior. The original idea was that the behavioral effects would be dichotomous: an animal would either develop male or female behavioral characteristics, depending upon the perinatal presence or absence of testicular hormones. Beach (1971) stressed, however, the relativity of these behavioral effects by describing them in terms of increasing or decreasing probabilities of the occurrence of behavior in response to appropriate external stimulation. This view is of great importance because sex-reversals in behavioral terms are definitively left behind, which opens new perspectives for the involvement of these mechanisms in social adaptation. In addition, the importance of external stimuli for the occurrence of the behavior is emphasized, which facilitates the integration of sexual behavior into social behavior as a whole.

In most studies sexual behavior was considered to be a rather uncomplicated social interaction, readily described and quantified in terms of reproductive efficiency: behavior of the female in terms of *lordosis*, i.e. the facilitation of the male to reach intromission; and masculine behavior in terms of *ejaculatory* behavior. However, when studying the consequences of the presence of hormones on the development of the CNS and behavior, it is not easy to conceptualize sexual behavior — which is one of the fundamentals of social interaction — as occurring totally independent from, for instance, aggression, which appears also to be affected by the organizational effects of hormones (Edwards, 1969, 1970; Bronson and Desjardin, 1970). Sooner or later our questions will have to be reformulated in terms of which of the many aspects of functioning are changed, thus altering these specific classes of social behavior, instead of simply categorizing separate effects upon different kinds of behavior. In the study of hormonal effects on sexual behavior or aggression, very little attention has been paid thus far to the partner animal which, besides the hormonal stimulus, is very influential in determining the behavioral response of the test animal. Investigations, for instance aimed at determining the influence upon aggression of stimulus-properties of the partner, and of the motivational variables in the female as influenced by the presence of male partner, could give us valuable information about what aspects of behavior are affected by the presence or absence of hormones during development (see Meyerson et al., 1973; Leshner, 1975).

Lordosis in male rats

The inhibiting effect of early gonadal hormones on the occurrence of the feminine mating response, more specifically on lordosis, is the most clearcut effect on the development of sexual behavior. Females unaffected by male gonadal hormones during development are easily activated to show these responses during adulthood by administration of ovarian hormones (Boling and Blandau, 1939; Davidson et al., 1968). Males or females, injected neonatally with androgens, either loose this capacity completely or exhibit only very low levels of lordosis (Barraclough and Gorski, 1962; Aren-Engelbrektson et al., 1970). Neonatally castrated males (which are postnatally unaffected by testicular hormones) show female levels of lordosis (Feder and Whalen, 1965; Whalen and Edwards, 1966, 1967). The possibility of progesterone-facilitated lordosis behavior is generally thought to be present in the female rat but absent in the male (Davidson, 1969). To illustrate the relativity of these effects on lordosis, the percentage of responding animals and the mean lordosis quotients in groups of intact males, and also of males castrated in adulthood and treated with estrogen and progesterone, are given in Fig. 1. It is shown that treatment of intact male rats with a single dose of estrogen may result in substantial levels of lordosis. Moreover, the results suggest that the feminine mating pattern can even be *more* successfully induced in intact than in castrated males. Progesterone facilitated the occurrence of lordosis in castrated as well as in intact male rats. In comparison with sexually active males, animals which persistently failed to copulate showed lower levels of lordosis after treatment with estrogen and progesterone. These results therefore suggest the importance of additional factors in experimental animals, e.g. the level of masculine sexual activity, the presence of endogeneously produced testosterone, or the time schedule of hormone treatment (Van de Poll and Van Dis, 1977).

Effects on masculine sexual activity

The effect of perinatally present gonadal hormones on the development of masculine sexual behavior is more complicated. Although both sexes in the rat show masculine responses (i.e. the mounting of a receptive female) the behavioral pattern accompanying intromis-

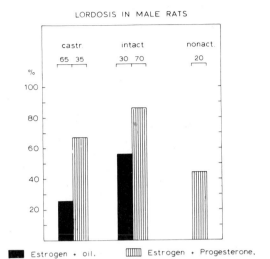

Fig. 1. Lordosis in male rats: estradiol benzoate (75 μg, i.m.) or estradiol benzoate + progesterone (1 mg, i.m.) treatment of *castrated* (n = 16 and N = 15 resp.), intact (n = 16 and N = 28 resp.) or *sexually inactive* (n = 9) male rats. The figures at the head of each column give the median lordosis quotient $\left(\frac{lordosis}{mounts} \times 100\right)$ of the responding animals. Estrogen was injected 44 hr, progesterone 8 hr before testing.

sion of the penis and ejaculation only occurs in normally developed intact males. Neonatally castrated males are in this respect like females, and thus readily mount receptive females but rarely ejaculate — when treated with hormones in adulthood (Beach and Holz, 1946; Grady et al., 1965). Androgenized females, especially when androgenization took place before birth, are reported to be capable of showing behavior which in the normal male accompanies intromission (Mullins and Levine, 1968; Ward and Renz, 1972). There apparently is a clearcut organizational effect of early present hormones on masculine responses. However, since both a peripheral source of stimulation and postnatal penis growth are essential for intromission and ejaculation, and since postnatal growth of the penis is affected by the early presence of gonadal hormones, absence of the ejaculatory pattern cannot be taken as sufficient evidence for a more centrally located effect (Beach et al., 1969). When trying to assess effects upon masculine sexual behavior, the percentage of *animals showing mounting* and the *number of mounts* are better parameters for comparing masculine sexual response tendencies in intact females, in intact males and in neonatally castrated males.

Fig. 2 represents data from an experiment in which neonatally castrated males and adult castrated males, both treated with testosterone, were compared under conditions in which the normally developed males show no ejaculation at all. This was accomplished by application of a mask to the vagina of the receptive (test) female, thus preventing intromission, and/or by applying an anesthetic unguent to the penis. From this figure it can be seen that males castrated either neonatally or in adulthood show considerable levels of mounting; in fact, in neonatally castrated groups there appeared to be relatively *more* mounts. The motivational aspects of masculine sexual behavior, as measured by the frequency of mounting, are thus apparently fully determined in the male at the moment of birth. Further *post*-natal organization can be conceived of as being an integration of peripheral input sources (also involving *inhibitory* mechanisms) into this behavioral system.

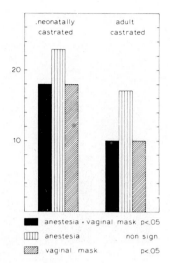

Fig. 2. Median number of mounts of neonatally castrated (n = 14) and adult castrated male rats (n = 11) treated with testosterone propionate (250 μg i.m.) for 6 weeks in three weekly tests of 10 min each. The animals were tested with receptive females under three experimental conditions which reduce tactile stimulation of the penis during sexual contact. Significance of the difference in number of mounts between both groups was tested with aid of the Mann-Whitney U-test for each condition.

Organizing effects upon the activation of sexual behavior by estrogen and testosterone

Systematic comparison of masculine and feminine sexual behavior in females, neonatally castrated males, males and androgenized females, treated in adulthood with either androgen or estrogen, has revealed early interactive effects of hormones with the activating effects of male and female sex hormones in adulthood. It was found that, regardless of hormonal manipulation at birth, males showed more mounting than did females (Whalen and Edwards, 1967). Moreover, feminization of male rats after neonatal castration was found to be independent of hormone treatment in adulthood (Pfaff and Zigmond, 1971). Our own results, however, favor a concept in which the response tendency to exhibit masculine or feminine mating patterns depends not only upon hormonal conditions during development but also upon the nature of the stimulating hormone in adulthood.

Testosterone appeared to activate mounting in adulthood when androgens were present, either before birth (the neonatally castrated males), after birth (the androgenized females) or both (the adult-castrated males). The very low levels of masculine responses in the females did not differ from those prior to activation, either in number or in percentage of responding animals. Lordosis was also activated by testosterone, but only in females and neonatally castrated males (indicating that postnatally present androgens diminish this response: Fig. 3).

Estrogen activated masculine responses in the four groups mentioned above, but in a pattern which did not show a distribution comparable to that following testosterone treatment. Highest levels occurred in the androgenized females, while the control females and the neonatally castrated males had much lower scores. Lordosis occurred in females and in neonatally castrated males to the same extent, whereas both of the other groups differed significantly from these two (Fig. 4). The perinatal presence of androgens thus seems to affect masculine and feminine sexual behavior in two ways: firstly, by facilitating or inhibiting the occurrence of feminine or masculine sexual behavior, and secondly, by changing the activating effects of hormones that can be elicited in adulthood.

The necessity of implicating the nature of the activating hormones in adulthood is also

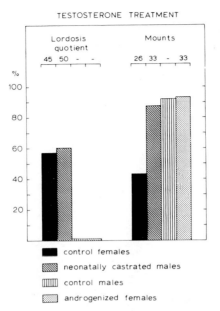

Fig. 3. Masculine and feminine responses in four groups of rats (n = 14, 15, 13 and 14, respectively) treated with 100 μg testosterone propionate i.m. for 14 days. Percentage of animals in each group showing *lordosis* (left) and *mounts* (right) are given. The figures ahead of each column give, respectively, the median lordosis quotient and number of mounts for the responding animals.

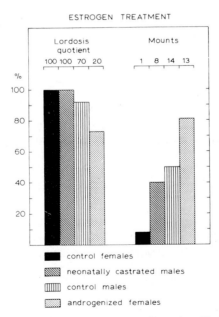

Fig. 4. Masculine and feminine responses in four groups of rats (n = 12, 10, 12 and 11, respectively) treated with 50 μg estradiol benzoate i.m. for 5 days. Percentage of animals in each group showing *lordosis* (left) and *mounts* (right) are given. The figure at the head of each column gives, respectively, the median lordosis quotient and number of mounts for the responding animals.

314

illustrated in the neonatally castrated male. Levels of feminine behavior comparable to those of normal females, and the absence of the ejaculatory pattern, together with the apparent capacity to show cyclic neuroendocrine functioning when ovarium grafts are implanted, has led to the generally accepted view that the central nervous system basically tends to show female characteristics. Fig. 5, however, makes it clear that this is only one part of the effect. Neonatally castrated males, when treated with estrogen or (even more so) with testosterone, do indeed show levels of lordosis comparable to those in females. However, masculine sexual behavior too is markedly facilitated when testosterone or estrogen is given, which makes these animals in some respects comparable to males rather than to females.

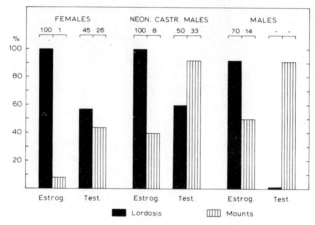

Fig. 5. Masculine and feminine responses in neonatally castrated male rats as compared to those of females and males gonadectomized in adulthood, under estrogen treatment (50 μg i.m. for 5 days) or testosterone treatment (100 μg i.m. for 14 days). Percentage of responding animals as well as the median lordosis quotients or number of mounts for the responding animals are given.

In order to conceptualize the changes brought about by early androgen treatment, two models were recently discussed by Whalen (1974). One of these was a linear model in which changes of sexual behavior take place along one axis, with 'pure' masculinity and femininity being opposite ends of the continuum. It will be clear that the results in neonatally castrated males (which show female sexual behavior comparable to females, but also masculine behavior comparable to that of the males) do not fit neatly into this model. Therefore, in accordance with other arguments given by Whalen, our results favor the *orthogonal* model, in which feminine and masculine sexual behavior can be influenced independently by the organizational effects and, possibly, at different stages of development.

Organizational effects of gonadal hormones and the neural substrate mediating sexual behavior
Processes of organization of the central nervous system, and subsequent changes in brain mechanisms underlying sex-dependent behavior, are poorly understood as yet. It will be clear that the activational and organizational effects of hormones on nervous tissue, as well as on enzyme systems metabolizing these hormones in the brain, will be good candidates for this effect (e.g. McEwen, 1978). Structural changes seem also to be involved in the process of sexual differentiation. In the preoptic area of the rat, Raisman and Field (1973) identified sex differences in the number of synaptic contacts on dendritic spines of non-amygdaloid origin. The effect of gonadal hormones during critical periods on these synaptic

contacts was well established. These data were interpreted in terms of an involvement of this structure in the cyclic regulation of gonadotrophin release occurring in females but not in males.

Only few studies attempting to localize the neural substrate underlying sexual behavior have thus far payed any attention to the bisexual character and the organizational aspects of sexual behavior. Mounting in female rats is inhibited both by preoptic lesions (Dörner et al., 1969) and by medial forebrain bundle lesions (Hitt et al., 1970). These data are in agreement with the extensive literature implicating these two structures in masculine sexual behavior in male animals (Heimer and Larsson, 1966/67; Davidson, 1966; Merari and Ginton, 1975).

Lordosis in males is facilitated by lesions in the preoptic anterior hypothalamic region (Dörner et al., 1969). The involvement of this area in feminine sexual behavior in the *female*, however, has not been well established (Law and Meagher, 1958; Singer, 1968; Powers and Valenstein, 1972). We have therefore studied masculine and feminine sexual behavior both in male and in female rats, with restricted lesions within the medial preoptic (mPOA) or anterior hypothalamic (AH) areas. It was found that masculine sexual behavior, in male as well as in female rats, was seriously affected by lesions in a small circumscribed area located at the transitional region of the mPOA and the AH (Figs. 6 and 7). Feminine sexual behavior, on the other hand, was affected differently in males and females: AH lesions slightly facilitated lordosis in males, but strongly reduced it in females. These findings,

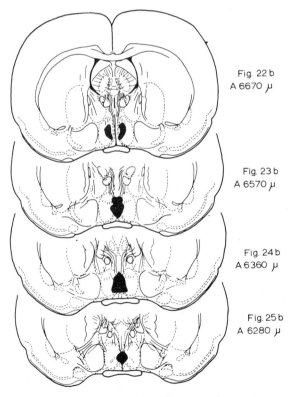

Fig. 22 b
A 6670 μ

Fig. 23 b
A 6570 μ

Fig. 24 b
A 6360 μ

Fig. 25 b
A 6280 μ

Fig. 6. Reconstruction on plates of König and Klippel (1963) of medial preoptic and anterior hypothalamic lesions common to 5 male rats showing a loss of all masculine sexual behavior after operation.

316

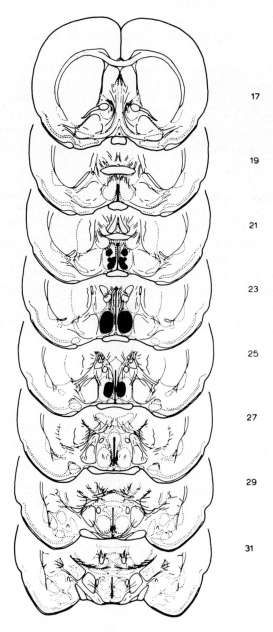

Fig. 7. Reconstruction on plates of König and Klippel (1963) of medial preoptic and anterior hypothalamic lesions common to two female rats showing a loss of all masculine sexual behavior after operation.

together with recent data on the role of gonadal hormones in the development of sex-dependent morphology of this part of the brain (discussed in Christensen et al., 1977), suggest that these sex differences are directly involved not only in neuroendocrine functioning but also in behavior.

AGGRESSIVE BEHAVIOR

Studies focussing upon the effects of hormones on aggressive behavior strongly suggest that gonadal hormones may predispose the animal to react more aggressively to conspecifics. Moreover, as in sexual behavior, the responsiveness to hormones in adulthood may be altered by the organizing effects of these hormones in development. Of the various kinds of aggressive behavior distinguished in the literature (Moyer, 1968), we have chosen to study aggressive behavior occurring ('spontaneously') between two conspecifics of the same sex. Sexual behavior and inter-male aggression are both influenced by hormones during development as well as in adulthood. Moreover, these two types of social behavior frequently occur in close temporal association. It therefore seems worthwhile to determine the behavioral mechanism which changes as a result of gonadal hormone action during development. Our research was therefore aimed at the interdependence of sex and aggression, and the influence on these behavioral patterns of gonadal hormones acting during development.

Aggressive behavior in female rats

Much research on aggression in rodents has thus far been done on laboratory *mice,* a species showing higher levels of inter-male aggressive behavior than do laboratory rats. As in most mammalian species, female mice are thought to exhibit a very low propensity for aggressive behavior. Treatment of female mice with testosterone propionate (TP) at birth appeared to predispose them to be more aggressive when this hormone was re-applied in adulthood, thus making them indistinguishable from males in this respect (Edwards, 1969; Bronson and Desjardin, 1970). In contrast, males castrated at birth were less responsive to androgen treatment in adulthood then were those castrated 10 days later (Edwards, 1969).

These effects are not completely analogous to perinatal hormonal influences on sexual behavior, however. Treatment of females on postnatal day 30 still affected aggressive behavior in adulthood, introducing some ambiguity about the duration and location of the so-called *critical period* (Edwards, 1970; Whitsett et al., 1972). Moreover, Svare et al. (1974), studying aggression in adult female mice, reported that aggressive behavior was increased by chronic exposure to TP in adulthood. As in males, this type of aggressive behavior was exclusively directed at males. These results are important for several reasons. First of all, it is again clear that the differences resulting from the presence of early gonadal hormones cannot be considered as absolute, but can be modified to a certain extent by gonadal hormones present during later stages in development (as was already concluded for sexual behavior). Secondly, by studying differences in terms of *response tendencies*, the importance of other factors affecting the response, e.g. the role of the social stimulus or of social experience, must be incorporated as well.

Most of the studies discussed so far were almost exclusively directed at the development either of sexual (masculine of feminine) or of aggressive behavior. In order to reveal the underlying behavioral mechanisms and the interaction between these two systems, we studied sexual and aggressive behavior in female rats — either non-treated or treated with TP, and tested with an untreated or with a testosterone-treated stimulus female. Subjects for these experiments were S-3 rats (Tryon Maze-Dull rats) chosen because of their somewhat higher level of intra-species aggression. The female was adapted to the test cage for one hour, and subsequently tested against a Wistar female. All animals were ovariectomized prior to behavioral testing. In this experiment, several parameters of *sexual* behavior (mounting, climbing and genital sniffing) and of *aggressive* behavior (lateral approach, fighting and boxing) were scored from videotape for the experimental as well as for the stimulus female. The results led to the following conclusions (Fig. 8).

318

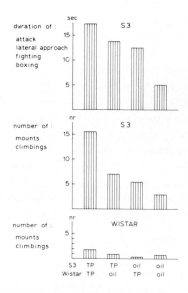

Fig. 8. Duration of aggressive encounters occurring in S-3 female rats (n = 12) tested against a female partner in four test conditions in which the animal was either treated with testosterone or was not. The occurrence of sexual behavior in the same tests of the S-3 as well as of the Wistar are presented in the lower part of the figure.

(1) Substantial levels of aggressive behavior occurred in each condition, even in the ovariectomized non-treated S-3 female tested against a non-treated Wistar female.

(2) Aggression appeared to depend upon hormonal treatment of the partner as well as of the experimental female. Thus, although testosterone treatment of the S-3 females increased their aggression against a non-treated stimulus (i.e. Wistar) female, even *oil*-treated S-3 females became more aggressive when tested against testosterone-treated stimulus females.

(3) When *both* animals were treated with testosterone, a general increase in social activity was seen: sexual behavior in both experimental and stimulus female was increased, but aggression increased also. Fig. 9 further illustrates the impact of TP treatment on social

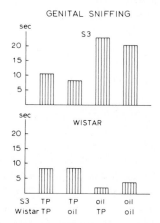

Fig. 9. Duration of genital sniffing occurring in S-3 female rats tested against a female partner in four test conditions in which the partner was either treated with testosterone or was not. Duration of genital sniffing of the Wistar in the same tests is presented in the lower part of the figure.

behavior, and the possible interaction of aggressive and sexual behavior: genital sniffing was exhibited more frequently by the S-3 animal than by the Wistar. It seems to be lowered by testosterone treatment in the dominant animal, but tends to increase in the Wistar when the S-3 animal is treated with TP.

In order to find further coherence between the different behavioral parameters, and to improve the scoring methods in the future, the results were subjected to a discriminant analysis. This statistical treatment of the data is aimed at combining the different parameters, and weighing them in such a way that differences among the four conditions are maximized. Although the results of this analysis indicated substantial levels of aggression in all four conditions, the parameters of sexual behavior of both S-3 and Wistar rats appeared to play the most prominent role in discriminating among the four conditions. Therefore, we strongly suggest the need, when studying the organizational effects of gonadal hormones on social behavior, to pay equal attention to aggressive and sexual behaviors.

LEARNING

This section, reviewing experiments which demonstrate effects of gonadal hormones on behavior development, deals with learning. Experiments investigating maze learning almost invariably point to a male superiority. This was interpreted as a reflection of the higher level of exploratory activity of females, since the sex difference is most prominent during the first few trials (Schenck and Slob, 1975). Others, however, considered these results to be an indication that the male's superiority in spatial abilities, well documented for humans, exists across species (Buffery and Gray, 1972; Gray and Buffery, 1971). Since the relative importance of olfactory, visual, auditive, and other possible cues for discrimination have hardly been investigated, interpretation of these results is difficult. Recent studies on maze learning show that the presence of androgens perinatally is of greater importance than are circulating gonadal hormones in adulthood (Stewart et al., 1975). In this section we will deal with learning and retention of two kinds of tasks, one based upon aversive motivation, the other based upon a positive reinforcer in the Skinner-box.

Various kinds of situations are commonly used with respect to learning based upon the effect of a *negative* stimulus. Females appear to be superior to males in the situation in which the animal has to perform a specific response in order to postpone or avoid an aversive event, the so-called active avoidance experiments (Levine and Broadhurst, 1963; Nakamura and Anderson, 1962). These sex differences have been shown to be related to the organization of the CNS by early gonadal hormones, although the parallel with sexual behavior is not complete: the effect of gonadal hormones on avoidance learning seems to take place before birth, since only before birth could the administration of *anti*-androgens induce a female level of active avoidance in male rats (Scouten et al., 1975). Neonatal administration of testosterone or estrogen to the female pups resulted only in masculine levels of avoidance if, as adults, they were ovariectomized and treated with testosterone (Beatty and Beatty, 1970).

In the passive avoidance situation the animal has to learn to avoid doing something that he was inclined to do beforehand. An interesting distinction was found in avoidance learning in active and passive avoidance tasks: males show longer latencies to perform the formerly punished activity, which points to a male superiority in retention in this respect (Beatty et al., 1973; Denti and Epstein, 1972). An aspect in which these tests differ logically is the specific way the experimenter manipulates the animal's propensity to execute a certain behavior. One test situation frequently used nowadays makes use of the predisposition of rats towards avoidance of a small illuminated elevated platform, in favor of a larger dark compartment (Ader et al., 1972). Fig. 10 gives the mean latency times with which males and females enter the compartment before being shocked; 24 and 48 hr after receiving a shock, significantly more females entered the box on the days following the aversive stimulation. No simple explanation can be given for these divergent results from studies of active and passive avoidance. It seems reasonable to suppose that the reported sex differences in *fear, activity* and *exploration* are all involved (Gray and Buffery, 1971).

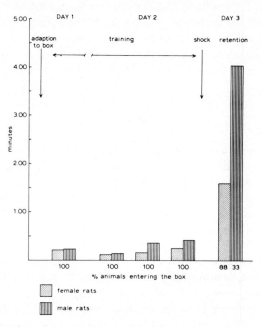

Fig. 10. Schematic presentation of the procedure and the results of a step-through passive avoidance test in which male (n = 16) and female rats (n = 16) are compared. The columns represent the mean latencies of both groups; the percentage of animals entering the box is given below. Retention was tested 24 hr after the shock (0.5 mA during 2 sec).

In a third category of learning experiments, learning is studied based on a positive rein-forcer obtained by responding to a manipulandum in the test situation, i.e. by pressing a lever in a Skinner-box to get a food pellet. The most important aspect of learning studied in the Skinner-box is the possibility of carefully manipulating the variables of the test situations and obtaining a variety of well controlled learning schedules. Sex differences were reported to be absent in schedules in which every response or every tenth response was reinforced (Beatty and O'Briant, 1973). When reinforcement depends upon the inhibition of low rate schedules, the females learned better (Beatty, 1973).

A series of experiments was recently started in our laboratory which seems to point to some other aspects of learning and retention that differ between the sexes. Rats in these experiments had to learn to press alternately the right and left lever (in a Skinner-box with two levers) in order to get a food reward. For rats this is a rather difficult task, as they have to learn to inhibit the most obvious response (which is pressing the lever that has just been rewarded). Learning curves of male and female rats in subsequent daily sessions are shown in Fig. 11. In these sessions each rat had to work until it made 60 correct responses.

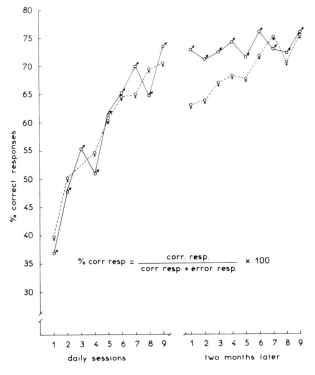

$$\% \text{ corr. resp} = \frac{\text{corr. resp.}}{\text{corr. resp.} + \text{error resp.}} \times 100$$

% CORRECT RESPONSES in male and female rats

Fig. 11. Percentage of correct responses of male (n = 9) and female (n = 10) rats (dotted line) in daily sessions in a Skinner-box. The animals had to alternatively press the left and right levers in order to be rewarded with a food pellet. Note that both groups started markedly below chance level in this procedure. The animals were kept at 85% of their body weight; during the two months in between both test series food was given ad libitum.

No sex differences exist in the changes in percentage of correct responses made during learning. A very remarkable and consistent difference was found in the time it took males and females to reach the criterion of 60 rewards: males responded much faster than females. When the animals were retested on retention of the task two months later, still another sex difference could be observed: the response accuracy of the males hardly differed from the final level in the first series of sessions, whereas the performance level of females had decreased significantly, and needed several days to reach previous levels.

Further results along this line of experimentation can be summarized as follows.

(1) Replication revealed the same sex differences, both in retention and in response rate.

(2) The sex differences in retention appears to be specific for the task left/right alternation; rats that learned to respond to a light-signalled lever, which had varied randomly across left and right, showed no sex differences either in retention or in response rate.

(3) When gonadectomized animals learned to respond in a signaled left/right alternation, and signalization was subsequently omitted, the backfall of the females was stronger than that of the males. This indicates that, under these conditions, the male's predisposition to specifically respond to spatial cues (also reflected by better retention in the first experiment) is not dependent upon circulating androgens. These results seem to point to a male superiority in the retention of learned behavior in which spatial cues are used, thus paralleling both the

well-documented finding that human males surpass females in spatial abilities (Maccoby and Jacklin, 1974), and the male rat's demonstrated superiority in maze learning, as was already discussed earlier in this paper. Further experimentation is aimed at establishing to what extent the organizing activity of gonadal hormones is involved in this difference between the sexes.

ORGANIZATIONAL EFFECTS OF GONADAL HORMONES ON THE NEURAL SUBSTRATE INVOLVED IN LEARNING AND AGGRESSION

Apart from establishing the diverse effects which gonadal hormones exert on behavior during development, and looking for the interrelation and common behavioral mechanisms of these effects, a large part of our research is being aimed at investigating the functional changes caused by these hormones in the brain structures which are presumably involved. Once having established that sexual behavior and aggression are influenced by the organizational activity of present gonadal hormones early in life, one of the worthwhile next steps is to look for the neural substrates involved in these behaviors. The septum, which seems to be generally involved in emotion (including aggression and sexual behavior), would be a possible site of action for this kind of hormonal effect and, indeed, some arguments can be found that this part of the limbic system differentiates under the control of gonadal hormones at critical stages in development (Phillips and Deol, 1973). A further specification of the relationship between aggressive and sexual behavior, and of the neural structures involved, would be a step forward in our understanding of the developing nervous system and the role played by hormonal and social stimuli.

Neural structures involved in the regulation of *aggressive* and *sexual* behavior are relatively well known, and speculation about which structures are affected by hormones during development therefore seem more promising than considering how and when changes in *memory* and *learning* could come into being. Some suggestions from the work of Gray and Buffery (1971), and also of Goldman (1976), lead to consideration of a possible specific role played by the prefrontal cortex in sexually dimorphic behavior. One of the several arguments given by Goldman (1976) will be dealt with in more detail, because a type of learning task in monkeys is involved which seems to correspond to that of our rats in the alternating-reinforcement learning situation. Goldman studied an object discrimination reversal task (a task involving training to discriminate between two objects, and then scoring errors during repeated reversals of the positive and negative objects).

In a second test, delayed spatial alternation, the monkey was required to alternate between left and right on successive trials, separated by a 5-sec interval. These tasks, like those of our rats, require the animal to remember the location of a stimulus over a very brief time interval. The ability to perform these tasks depends upon the integrity of the orbital prefrontal cortex in adult monkeys. Further work of Goldman (1976) revealed sex differences in the performance of this task in young animals (males performed better) which could be abolished by postnatal testosterone treatment of the females. Moreover, lesions in both males and androgenized females reduced performance levels to those of operated (c.q. unoperated) females, suggesting that this part of the cortex develops earlier in males than in females, and that gonadal hormones may play a role in the postnatal differentiation of the cortical mechanisms involved.

Of course, the step from monkeys to rats is a big one, not to mention the difficulties in comparing structure and function of parts of the prefrontal cortex in these two not closely related species. However, we believe that research aimed at investigating sexually dimorphic morphology and structure-function relationships of this part of the cortex would be worthwhile in the rat.

REFERENCES

Ader, R., Weijnen, J.A.W.M. and Moleman, P. (1972) Retention of a passive avoidance response as a function of the intensity and duration of electric shock, *Psychon. Sci.*, 26: 125–128.

Aren-Engelbrektsson, Larsson, K., Södersten, P. and Wilhelmsson, M. (1970) The female lordosis pattern induced in male rats by estrogen, *Horm. Behav.*, 1: 181–188.

Barraclough, C.A. and Gorski, R.A. (1962) Studies on mating behavior in the androgen-sterilized female rat in relation to the hypothalamic regulation of sexual behavior, *J. Endocr.*, 25: 175–182.

Beach, F.A. (1971) Hormonal differentiation and Ramstergig copulatory behavior. In *The Biopsychology of Development*, E. Tobach, L.R. Aronson and E. Shaw (Eds.), Academic Press, New York.

Beach, F.A. and Holz, A.M. (1946) Mating behavior in male rats castrated at various ages and injected with androgen, *J. exp. Zool.*, 101: 91–142.

Beach, F.A., Noble, R.G. and Orndoff, R.K. (1969) Effects of perinatal androgen treatment on responses of male rats to gonadal hormones in adulthood, *J. comp. physiol. Psychol.*, 68: 490–497.

Beatty, W.W. (1973) Effects of gonadectomy on sex differences in DRL behavior, *Physiol. Behav.*, 10: 177–178.

Beatty, W.W. and Beatty, P.A. (1970a) Effects of neonatal testosterone on the acquisition of an active avoidance responce in genotypical female rats, *Psychon. Sci.*, 19: 315–316.

Beatty, W.W. and Beatty, P.A. (1970b) Hormonal determinants of sex differences in avoidance behavior and reactivity to electric shock in the rat, *J. comp. physiol. Psychol.*, 73: 446–455.

Beatty, W.W., Beatty, P.A., O'Briant, D.A., Gregoire, K.C. and Dahl, B.L. (1973a) Factors underlying deficient passive-avoidance behavior by rats with septal lesions, *J. comp. physiol. Psychol.*, 85: 502–524.

Beatty, W.W., Gregoire, K.C. and Parmiter, L.L. (1973b) Sex differences in retention of passive avoidance behavior in rat, *Bull. Psychon. Soc.*, 2: 99–100.

Beatty, W.W. and O'Briant, D.A. (1973) Sex differences in extinction of food-rewarded approach responses, *Bull. Psychon. Soc.*, 2: 97–98.

Boling, J.L. and Blandau, R.J. (1939) The estrogen-progesterone induction of mating responses in the spayed female rat, *Endocrinology*, 25: 259–264.

Bronson, F.H. and Desjardins, C. (1970) Neonatal androgen administration and adult aggressiveness in female mice, *Gen. comp. Endocr.*, 15: 320–326.

Buffery, A.W.H. and Gray, J.A. (1972) Sex differences in the development of spatial and linguistic skills. In: *Gender Differences: Their Ontogeny and Significance,* C. Ounsted and D.C. Taylor (Eds.), Livingstone, London, pp. 123–157.

Christensen, L.W., Nance, D.M. and Gorski, R.A. (1977) Effects of hypothalamic and preoptic lesions on reproductive behavior in male rats, *Brain. Res. Bull.*, 2: 137–141.

Davidson, J.M. (1966) Activation of the male rat's sexual behavior by intracerebral implantation of androgen, *Endocrinology,* 79: 783–794.

Davidson, J.M. (1969) Effects of estrogen on the sexual behavior of male rats, *Endocrinology,* 84: 1365–1372.

Davidson, J.M., Smith, E.R., Rodgers, C.H. and Bloch, G.J. (1968) Relative thresholds of behavioral and somatic responses to estrogen, *Physiol. Behav.*, 3: 227–229.

Denti, A. and Epstein, A. (1972) Sex differences in the acquisition of two kinds of avoidance behavior in rats, *Physiol. Behav.*, 8: 611–615.

Dörner, G., Döcke, F. and Hinz, G. (1969) Homo- and hypersexuality in rats with hypothalamic lesions, *Neuroendocrinology,* 4: 20–24.

Edwards, D.A. (1969) Early androgen stimulation and aggressive behavior in male and female mice, *Physiol. Behav.*, 4: 333–338.

Edwards, D.A. (1970) Post-neonatal androgenization and adult aggressive behavior in female mice, *Physiol. Behav.*, 5: 465–467.

Edwards, D.A. (1970) Post-natal androgenization and adult aggressive behavior in female mice, *Physiol. Behav.*, 5: 465–467.

324

Feder, H.H. and Whalen, R.E. (1965) Feminine behavior in neonatally castrated and estrogen treated male rats, *Science*, 147: 306–307.

Goldman, P.S. (1976) Maturation of the mammalian nervous system and the ontogeny of behavior. *Advances in the Study of Behavior, Vol. 7*. Academic Press, New York.

Grady, K.L., Phoenix, Ch.H. and Young, W.C. (1965) Role of the developing rat testis in differentiation of the neural tissues mediating mating behavior, *J. comp. physiol. Psychol.*, 59: 176–182.

Gray, J.A. and Buffery, A.W.H. (1971) Sex differences in emotional and cognitive behavior in mammals including man: adaptive and neural bases, *Acta psychol.*, 35: 89–111.

Harris, G.W. and Levine, S. (1962) Sexual differentiation of the brain and its experimental control, *J. Physiol. (Lond.)*, 181: 379–400.

Heimer, L. and Larsson, K. (1966/67). Impairment of mating behavior in male rats following lesions in the preoptic-anterior hypothalamic continuum, *Brain Res.*, 3: 248–263.

Hitt, J.C., Hendricks, S.E., Ginsberg, S.I. and Lewis, J.H. (1970) Disruption of male, but not female, sexual behavior in rats by medial forebrain bundle lesions, *J. comp. physiol. Psychol.*, 73: 377–384.

Jost, A. (1970) Hormonal factors in the sex differentiation of the mammalian foetus. *Phil. Trans. B*, 259: 119–130.

König, J.F.R. and Klippel, R.A. (1963), *The Rat Brain*, Williams and Wilkins, Baltimore.

Law, T. and Meagher, W. (1958) Hypothalamic lesions and sexual behavior in the female rat, *Science*, 128: 1626–1627.

Leshner, A.I. (1975) (Theoretical review) A model of hormones and agonistic behavior, *Physiol. Behav.*, 15: 225–235.

Levine, S. and Broadhurst, P.L. (1963) Genetic and ontogenetic determinants of adult behavior in the rat, *J. comp. physiol. Psychol.*, 56: 423–428.

Maccoby, E.E. and Jacklin, C.N. (1974) *The Psychology of Sex Differences*, Stanford University Press.

McEwen, B.S. (1978) Sexual maturation and differentiation: the role of the gonadal steroids, this volume.

Merari, A. and Ginton, A. (1975) Characteristics of exaggerated sexual behavior induced by electrical stimulation of the medial preoptic area in male rats, *Brain Res.*, 86: 97–108.

Meyerson, B.J., Lindström, L., Nordström, E. and Agmo, A. (1973) Sexual motivation in the female rat after testosterone treatment, *Physiol. Behav.*, 11: 421–428.

Moyer, K.E. (1968) Kinds of aggression and their physiological basis. *Commun. Behav. Biol.*, 2: 65–87.

Mullins, R.F. Jr. and Levine, S. (1968) Hormonal determinants during infancy of adult sexual behavior in the female rat, *Physiol. Behav.*, 3: 333–338.

Nakamura, Ch.Y. and Anderson, N.H. (1962) Avoidance behavior differences within and between strains of rats, *J. comp. physiol. Psychol.*, 55: 740–747.

Pfaff, D.W. and Zigmond, R.E. (1971) Neonatal androgen effects on sexual and non-sexual behavior of adult rats tested under various hormone regimes, *Neuroendocrinology*, 7: 129–145.

Pfeiffer, C.A. (1936) Sexual differences of the hypophyses and their determination by the gonads, *Amer. J. Anat.*, 58: 195–225.

Phillips, A.G. and Deol, G. (1973) Neonatal gonadal hormone manipulation and emotionality following septal lesions in weanling rats, *Brain Res.*, 60: 55–64.

Phoenix, C.H., Goy, R.W., Gerall, A.A. and Young, W.C. (1959) Organizing action of prenatally administrated testosterone propionate on the tissues mediating mating behavior in the female guinea pig, *Endocrinology*, 65: 369–382.

Powers, B. and Valenstein, E.S. (1972) Sexual receptivity: facilitation by medial preoptic lesions in female rats, *Science*, 175: 1003–1005.

Raisman, G. and Field, P.M. (1973) Sexual differences in the neuropil of the preoptic area of the rat and its dependence on neonatal androgen, *Brain Res.*, 54: 1–29.

Schenck, P.E. and Slob, A.K. (1975) Sex differences and gonadal hormones in Hebb-Williams maze performance in adult rats, *J. Endocr.*, 64: 31–32.

Scouten, W., Groteleuschen, L.K. and Beatty, W.W. (1975) Androgens and the organization of sex differences in active avoidance behavior in the rat, *J. comp. physiol. Psychol.*, 88: 264–270.

Singer, J.J. (1968) Hypothalamic control of male and female sexual behavior in female rats, *J. comp. physiol. Psychol.*, 66: 738–742.

Stewart, J., Skvarenina, A. and Pottier, J. (1975) Effects of neonatal androgens and maze learning in the prepubescent and adult rat, *Physiol. Behav.*, 14: 291–295.

Svare, B., Davis, P.G. and Gandelman, R. (1974) Fighting behavior in female mice following chronic androgen treatment during adulthood, *Physiol. Behav.*, 12: 399–403.

Van de Poll, N.E. and Van Dis, H. (1977) Hormone induced lordosis and its relation to masculine sexual activity in male rats, *Horm. Behav.*, 8: 1–7.

Ward, I.L. and Renz, F.J. (1972) Consequences of perinatal hormone manipulation on the adult sexual behavior of female rats, *J. comp. physiol. Psychol.*, 78: 349–355.

Whalen, R.E. (1974) Sexual differentiation: models, methods and mechanisms. In *Sex Differences in Behavior*, R.C. Friedman, R.M. Richart and R.L. van de Wiele (Eds.), New York, pp. 467–481.

Whalen, R.E. and Edwards, A. (1966) Sexual reversibility in neonatally castrated male rats, *J. comp. physiol. Psychol.*, 62: 307–310.

Whalen, R.E. and Edwards, D.A. (1967) Hormonal determinants of the development of masculine and feminine behavior in male and female rats, *Anat. Rec.*, 157: 173–180.

Whitsett, J.M., Bronson, F.H., Peters, P.J. and Hamilton, T.H. (1972) Neonatal organization of aggression in mice: correlation of critical period with uptake of hormone, *Horm. Behav.*, 3: 11–21.

The Modulation of Memory Processes by Vasotocin, the Evolutionarily Oldest Neurosecretory Principle

D. de WIED and B. BOHUS

Rudolf Magnus Institute for Pharmacology, Medical Faculty, University of Utrecht, Utrecht
(The Netherlands)

INTRODUCTION

Neuropeptides are hormones which affect the nervous system. Various pituitary and hypothalamic hormones meet this definition, examples being adrenocorticotropic hormone (ACTH) and the related melanocyte stimulating hormone (α-MSH). The influence of these pituitary hormones on the nervous system is localized in a few amino acids of the molecule, and is thus independent of the classical endocrine effects of these hormones — which may act as prohormones (de Wied, 1969). Neuropeptides derived from ACTH and α-MSH ($ACTH_{4-7}$, $ACTH_{4-10}$, $ACTH_{7-16}$) affect motivational, learning and memory processes in the rat (de Wied, 1974) and motivation, attention and concentration in man (Kastin et al., 1975). Another example is the recent finding that pituitary β-LPH generates neuropeptides with opiate-like activity (Guillemin et al., 1976; Bradbury et al., 1976). Neuropeptides originating in the brain are releasing hormones like TRH and LRH (for review see Prange et al., 1977) and the neurohypophysial hormones vasopressin and oxytocin (van Wimersma Greidanus and de Wied, 1977).

The neurohypophysial hormones are formed predominantly in cell bodies of two hypothalamic nuclei, the supraoptic nucleus (SON) and the paraventricular nucleus (PVN) (for review see Knobil and Sawyer, 1974). Following their formation and storage in neurosecretory granules these peptide hormones are transported, together with their carrier proteins (neurophysins), within the axons to neurosecretory terminals where they are stored and released. The hormone producing cells have the essential characteristics of neurons, and a variety of stimuli can generate action potentials which are conducted along the axons, and which cause the release of stored material into the blood and so to the target organs. The most prominent stimuli which elicit the release of neurohypophysial hormones are changes in osmotic pressure or in blood volume, in the case of vasopressin, and suckling and manipulations of the genital tract, in the case of oxytocin.

Neurohypophysial hormones are also released into the portal vessel system. Zimmerman et al. (1973) demonstrated high vasopressin levels in hypophysial portal vessels of monkeys. They also showed the existence of neurosecretory nerve terminals in the capillary loops of hypophysial portal vessels in the median eminence, suggesting the expulsion of vasopressin into portal blood from neuronal terminals (Zimmerman, 1976). This suggests a role of neurohypophysial hormones in the regulation of anterior lobe function.

Neurohypophysial hormones may further use the cerebrospinal fluid (CSF) in addition to the bloodstream as a transport system for CNS action (Rodriguez, 1976). To achieve CNS effects these hormones may be released directly into the CSF via neurosecretory fibers originating from the magnocellular hypothalamic nuclei (Rodriguez, 1976; Nashold et al., 1963; Weindl et al., 1976; Vorherr et al., 1968; Goldsmith and Zimmerman, 1975). Another route which has been proposed for the transport of vasopressin and oxytocin to their central target sites is the peptidergic neurosecretory network ascending from the SON and the PVN to, in particular, limbic structures (Weindl et al., 1976; Sterba, 1974; Martin et al., 1975; Kozlowski et al., 1976). This may be an important channel for neurohypophysial hormones to modulate brain mechanisms. The presence of neurohypophysial hormones in the CSF (Heller et al., 1968; Vorherr et al., 1968; Pavel, 1970; Dogterom, 1977) indeed suggests an important role of these neuropeptides in brain functions.

PEPTIDES AND BEHAVIOR

The possibility that the pituitary might be involved in acquisition, consolidation and maintenance of learned behavior was first suggested by observations in partially and totally hypophysectomized rats. Whereas the extirpation of the anterior pituitary or the whole gland leads to an impairment in acquisition of a shuttle-box avoidance response (de Wied, 1964), the removal of the posterior pituitary does not materially affect acquisition but interferes with the maintenance of shuttle-box avoidance behavior (de Wied, 1965). These abnormalities could be readily corrected by treatment with various pituitary hormones such as ACTH, α-MSH, and vasopressin (de Wied, 1965). It subsequently appeared that fragments of these peptides which are practically devoid of classical endocrine effects of peripheral target organs are as effective in restoring the deficient behavior of the hypophysectomized rat (de Wied, 1969). Vasopressin improves shuttle-box avoidance learning of hypophysectomized rats and normalizes extinction of this kind of behavior in posterior lobectomized rats (de Wied, 1969). The influence of vasopressin is of a long-term nature since the behavioral effect persists without further exogenous supply of the peptide (Bohus et al., 1973). In intact rats vasopressin may affect acquisition of avoidance behavior, but extinction is a more sensitive parameter for the effect of vasopressin. The injection of relatively small amounts of vasopressin and related peptides increases resistance to extinction of shuttle-box and pole-jumping avoidance behavior. This effect is also of a long-term nature (de Wied and Bohus, 1966; de Wied, 1971). These observations led to the suggestion that vasopressin and related peptides influence memory processes (memory is defined here as the consolidation, retrieval and repression of newly acquired experience).

Further evidence for an effect of vasopressin on memory processes can be derived from studies on retrograde amnesia. Vasopressin and related peptides were found to protect against puromycin-induced amnesia in mice (Lande et al., 1972; Walter et al., 1975) and against amnesia for a passive avoidance response in rats induced by CO_2 inhalation or electro-convulsive shock (Rigter et al., 1974). These peptides do not affect the maintenance of a food running approach response in hungry rats (Garrud et al., 1974). However, vasopressin is active in sexually motivated approach behavior. Male rats, trained in a T-maze to run for a receptive female, choose the correct arm of the maze more frequently following treatment with DG-LVP than do saline-treated controls. Copulation reward is essential for this effect of the peptide (Bohus, 1977).

That vasopressin is physiologically involved in memory processes has been demonstrated in rats with hereditary hypothalamic diabetes insipidus. A homozygous variant of the Brattleboro strain lacks the ability to synthetize vasopressin (Valtin and Schroeder, 1964).

The heterozygous littermates have a relatively normal water metabolism while the other homozygous variant is completely normal in synthetizing vasopressin. Vasopressin is not detectable in the posterior pituitary of the homozygous Brattleboros. The oxytocin content of this part of the pituitary of the homozygous diabetes insipidus rats (HO-DI) is low. This is not caused by a defective synthesis but rather is a result of augmented release in plasma and CSF (Dogterom 1977). The animals also lack AVT in the pineal gland (Rosenbloom and Fisher, 1975). HO-DI rats are inferior in acquiring and maintaining active and passive avoidance behavior (Bohus et al., 1975). Extinction of shuttle-box and pole-jumping behavior is facilitated. Celestian et al. (1975) found that HO-DI rats are inferior in acquiring shuttle-box avoidance behavior. Only 30% of the rats in these studies achieved the learning criterion (80% or more avoidances). Retention of the response in the remaining rats was markedly enhanced, however.

Severe memory impairment can be observed when HO-DI rats are subjected to a step-through one-trial passive avoidance test (de Wied et al., 1975). Absence of passive avoidance behavior was found 24 hr or later after the learning trial even after exposing the animals to electric footshocks of high intensity and long duration. In contrast, heterozygous (HE-DI) or homozygous normal (HO-NO) rats exhibited passive avoidance behavior already after a much milder punishment. Treatment of HO-DI rats with AVP or DG-LVP facilitated passive avoidance behavior. Avoidance latencies of thus treated HO-DI rats were indistinguishable from those of the HE-DI and HO-NO rats. Restoration of memory function is therefore not related to normalization of water metabolism, since DG-LVP is practically devoid of antidiuretic activities while retaining its behavioral potency (de Wied et al., 1972). HO-DI rats do avoid without treatment if tested immediately, or within one hour, after the learning trial. These observations suggest that memory rather than learning processes are at fault in the absence of vasopressin. Essentially the same thing was found in intact rats treated intraventricularly with specific vasopressin antiserum (van Wimersma Greidanus et al., 1975).

Oxytocin also increases the resistance to extinction of pole-jumping avoidance behavior, but this peptide is less active than vasopressin (de Wied and Gispen, 1977). However, Schulz et al. (1976) found that oxytocin has the reverse effect of vasopressin and facilitates extinction of active avoidance behavior. Systemically administered oxytocin either had no effect or it increased resistance to extinction, depending on the dose used. This apparently depends on the route of administration. Oxytocin given intraventricularly immediately after each acquisition session tended to facilitate extinction of pole-jumping avoidance behavior (Bohus et al., 1977). Conversely, the injection of oxytocin antiserum after each acquisition session increased resistance to extinction of pole-jumping avoidance behavior. Thus, in our hands centrally administered oxytocin led to behavioral effects opposite to those of vasopressin.

Passive avoidance behavior was used in subsequent experiments to study the influence of neurohypophysial hormones in more detail, using a one-trial learning paradigm in a step-through type situation as described by Ader and de Wied (1972). Retention was tested at 24 and 48 hr after the learning trial. Materials were injected through a permanent polyethylene cannula in one of the lateral ventricles immediately after the learning trial, and the latency for entering the dark compartment was recorded up to 300 sec.

AVP caused a facilitation of passive avoidance behavior. Given systemically immediately after the learning trial, it was found that the more AVP was given the stronger, and of longer duration, was the facilitation of passive avoidance behavior. Injection of 1 μg per rat markedly increased avoidance latency not only on the first (24 hr) retention test but also on the second (48 hr) and third (72 hr) retention sessions. To determine the critical period of the effect of AVP, the hormone was administered intraventricularly at various intervals after the learning trial. Intracerebral administration of 10 ng of AVP immediately after the learning trial appeared to be the most effective. The effect of AVP was greatly reduced if administration was postponed until 3 hr after the learning trial, whereas treatment 6 hr after the trial had no effect. Thus, the first hours after the learning trial are essential for AVP in order to affect memory consolidation. This is in agreement with previous studies in the pole-jumping test (de Wied, 1971). If AVP was given 23 hr after the learning trial, e.g. 1 hr prior to the first retention trial, passive avoidance behavior again was facilitated. Thus, AVP not only affects the consolidation but also the retrieval of information.

Structure-activity studies following intraventricular administration revealed that the effect of vasopressin on consolidation is contained in the covalent ring structure, pressinamide (PA), as was also found in the studies with the pole-jumping test (de Wied, 1976). A second activity site might be present in the linear portion of the molecule, however, since PAG had a slight effect on passive avoidance behavior. Oxytocin given intraventricularly had an effect opposite to that of AVP. Passive avoidance behavior was attenuated following the injection of 0.1 and 1 ng oxytocin. This neuropeptide reduces the consolidation of information and may thus be regarded as an amnesic neuropeptide. The whole molecule is needed for this effect since the covalent ring structure of oxytocin, tocinamide (TA), in a dose of 0.1 ng had a slight inhibitory effect on passive avoidance behavior, but it markedly facilitated passive avoidance responding in a dose of 1 ng. It acted even stronger than AVP, in fact, whereas the C-terminal tripeptide prolyl-leucyl-glycinamide (PLG) was inactive. The related peptides, oxypressin and vasotocin, had an effect similar to that of, respectively, vasopressin and oxytocin. This is in accord with the previous findings, since oxypressin has the same covalent ring structure as does vasopressin, and vasotocin the same as oxytocin (Table I).

TABLE I

AMINO ACID SEQUENCES OF NEUROHYPOPHYSIAL HORMONES AND RELATED NEUROPEPTIDES

Arginine[8]-vasopressin (AVP)	H-Cys-Tyr-Phe-Gln-Asn-Cys-Pro-Arg-Gly-NH$_2$
Lysine[8]-vasopressin (LVP)	H-Cys-Tyr-Phe-Gln-Asn-Cys-Pro-Lys-Gly-NH$_2$
Pressinamide (PA)	H-Cys-Tyr-Phe-Gln-Asn-Cys-NH$_2$
Prolyl-argyl-glycinamide (PAG)	H-Pro-Arg-Gly-NH$_2$
Oxypressin (OXP)	H-Cys-Tyr-Phe-Gln-Asn-Cys-Pro-Leu-Gly-NH$_2$
Oxytocin (OXT)	H-Cys-Tyr-Ile-Gln-Asn-Cys-Pro-Leu-Gly-NH$_2$
Tocinamide (TA)	H-Cys-Tyr-Ile-Gln-Asn-Cys-NH$_2$
Prolyl-leucyl-glycinamide (PLG = MIF)	H-Pro-Leu-Gly-NH$_2$
Arginine[8]-vasotocin (AVT)	H-Cys-Tyr-Ile-Gln-Asn-Cys-Pro-Arg-Gly-NH$_2$

As mentioned before, vasopressin and related peptides protect against puromycin-induced amnesia of mice in a Y-maze (Lande et al., 1972; Walter et al., 1975) as well as against amnesia for a passive avoidance response induced by CO$_2$ inhalation or electroconvulsive shock in rats when injected immediately after the learning trial (Rigter et al., 1974). Interestingly, vasopressin is active in this respect but not oxytocin. However, the linear tripeptide of oxytocin, PLG, is highly effective in protecting against amnesia, in contrast to the ring structures of vasopressin and oxytocin. It is possible, therefore, that different brain structures are involved in memory formation and in memory loss. However, resistance to extinction and retrograde amnesia represent different memory processes. Retrograde amnesia is a temporary disturbance in retrieval of recently acquired information, while resistance to extinction of avoidance behavior concerns the consolidation of information. As we have seen, the covalent ring structures of vasopressin and oxytocin, PA and TA, facilitate the consolidation of information, whereas the C-terminal tripeptides PLG and PAG are the sites of the molecules which protect against amnesia. These parts of the molecules may therefore be involved in the retrieval of information, while the whole oxytocin or vasotocin molecule is needed for the repression of information.

CONCLUDING REMARKS

The different behavioral effects of the neurohypophysial hormones and their fragments suggest that they act as precursor molecules for neuropeptides which modulate memory processes. If this were true, one would expect that specific enzymes which generate the linear and the ring portion of these molecules would be present in the brain. It has been found that a membrane-bound hypothalamic exopeptidase is able to generate MIF (PLG) from oxytocin which inhibits the release of MSH (Celis et al., 1971). Such enzymes have not been detected for vasopressin. There are enzymes present in the brain which inactivate vasopressin by hydrolysis of peptide bonds in the acyclic position of the molecule (Walter et al., 1973) but no enzymes have been identified so far which remove the proline residue to yield pressinamide.

The ancestral molecule of the neurohypophysial hormones vasopressin and oxytocin, which generated these hormones during evolution, is arginine[8]-vasotocin (AVT). This peptide is found in the neurohypophysis of all non-mammalian vertebrates and in the pineal gland of mammals (Pavel, 1965; Rosenbloom and Fisher, 1975). AVT combines the physiological effects of AVP and oxytocin (Sawyer, 1977). During evolution a point mutation may have taken place in the base sequences of triplets which code for the incorporation of a particular amino acid into the peptide chain during the synthesis of neurohypophysial hormones (Vliegenthart and Versteeg, 1967). It has been postulated that vasopressin and oxytocin evolved after doubling of the gene which controlled the synthesis of vasotocin, which is thought to be the evolutionarily oldest peptide (Sawyer, 1964; Vliegenthart and Versteeg, 1965). In fact, vasotocin is found already in the Agnata (cyclostomata) while oxytocin occurs for the first time in the Halocephali (Chimeras). Vasopressin is present in mammals only.

The present experiments show that effects on consolidation, retrieval and amnesia (repression) are present in various parts of the oldest neurohypophysial principle, vasotocin. It is possible, therefore, that the nervous system of non-mammalian vertebrates possesses the enzymatic capacity to generate the N-terminal and C-terminal parts of vasotocin. This might enable these organisms to consolidate, retrieve or repress information. Mammals may have evolved a more versatile system by the synthesis of vasopressin and oxytocin, which then allowed a separation of the various memory functions mediated by vasotocin. This possibly caused a loss in the capacity to generate the ring structure and the linear tripeptide of vasopressin. This would also be in accord with our findings showing that (1) vasopressin is the most active of the neuropeptides which increase resistance to extinction (consolidation), (2) the entire oxytocin molecule is needed to induce repression of avoidance behavior, and (3) PLG and PAG protect against amnesia (retrieval). Experiments

332

on the degradation of vasotocin might critically test our hypothesis. In addition, studies in which the various memory functions of vasopressin, oxytocin, vasotocin and their fragments are determined in more detail in the various paradigms used may provide further information needed to test this hypothesis.

REFERENCES

Ader, R. and de Wied, D. (1972) Effects of lysine vasopressin on passive avoidance learning, *Psychon. Sci.*, 29: 46–48.

Bohus, B. (1977) Effect of desglycinamide-lysine vasopressin (DG-LVP) on sexually motivated T-maze behavior in the male rat, *Horm Behav.*, 8: 52–61.

Bohus, B., Gispen, W.H. and de Wied, D. (1973) Effect of lysine vasopressin and ACTH 4–10 on conditioned avoidance behavior of hypophysectomized rats, *Neuroendocrinology*, 11: 137–143.

Bohus, B., van Wimersma Greidanus, Tj.B. and de Wied, D. (1975) Behavioral and endocrine responses of rats with hereditary hypothalamic diabetes insipidus (Brattleboro strain), *Physiol. Behav.*, 14: 609–615.

Bohus, B., Urban, I., van Wimersma Greidanus, Tj.B. and de Wied, D. (1977) Opposite effects of oxytocin and vasopressin on avoidance behavior and hippocampal theta rhythm in the rat, *Neuropharmacology*, in press.

Bradbury, A.F., Smyth, D.G. and Snell, C.R. (1976) Biosynthetic origin and receptor conformation of methionine enkephalin, *Nature (Lond.)*, 260: 165–166.

Celestian, J.F., Carey, R.J. and Miller, M. (1975) Unimpaired maintenance of a conditioned avoidance response in the rat with diabetes insipidus, *Physiol. Behav.*, 15: 707–711.

Celis, M.E., Taleisnik, S. and Walter, R. (1971) Regulation of formation and proposed structure of the factor inhibiting the release of melanocyte-stimulating hormone, *Proc. nat. Acad. Sci. (Wash.)*, 68: 1428–1433.

Dogterom, J. (1977) *The Release and Presence of Vasopressin in Plasma and Cerebrospinal Fluid as Measured by Radioimmunoassay; Studies on Vasopressin as a Mediator of Memory Processes in the Rat*, Thesis, Utrecht.

Garrud, P., Gray, J.A. and de Wied, D. (1974) Pituitary-adrenal hormones and extinction of rewarded behavior in the rat, *Physiol. Behav.*, 12: 109–119.

Goldsmith, P.C. ano Zimmerman, E.A. (1975) Ultrastructural localization of neurophysin and vasopressin in the rat median eminence. In *Abstracts Fifty-Seventh Annu. Meet. Endocr. Soc.*, p. 239.

Guillemin, R., Ling, N. et Burgus, R. (1976) Endorphines, peptides d'origine hypothalamique et neurohypophysaire a activité morphinomimetique. Isolement et structure moleculaire d'α-endorphine, *C.R. Acad. Sci. (Paris)*, Série D, 282: 783–785.

Heller, H., Hasan, S.H. and Saifi, A.Q. (1968) Antidiuretic activity in the cerebrospinal fluid, *J. Endocr.*, 41: 273–280.

Kastin, A.J., Sandman, C.A., Stratton, L.O., Schally, A.V. and Miller, L.H. (1975) Behavioral and electrographic changes in rat and man after MSH. In *Hormones, Homeostasis and the Brain, Progress in Brain Research, Vol. 42*, W.H. Gispen, Tj.B. van Wimersma Greidanus, B. Bohus and D. de Wied (Eds.), Elsevier, Amsterdam, pp. 143–150.

Knobil, E. and Sawyer, W.H. (1974) *Handbook of Physiology, Section 7: Endocrinology, Vol. IV, The Pituitary Gland and its Neuroendocrine Control, Part 1.*

Kozlowski, G.P., Brownfield, M.S. and Hostetter, G. (1976) Neurosecretory supply to extrahypothalamic structures: choroid plexus, circumventricular organs, and limbic system. In *Evolutionary Aspects of Neuroendocrinology*, A.L. Polenov, W. Bangman and B. Scharrer (Eds.), Springer, Berlin, in press.

Lande, S., Flexner, J.B. and Flexner, L.B. (1972) Effect of corticotropin and desglycinamide[9]-lysine vasopressin on suppression of memory by puromycin, *Proc. nat. Acad. Sci. (Wash.)*, 69: 558–560.

Martin, J.B., Renaud, L.P. and Brazeau, P. (1975) Hypothalamic Peptides: new evidence for 'peptidergic' pathways in the CNS, *Lancet*, II: 393–395.

Nashold, B.S., Jr., Mannarino, E.M. and Robinson, R.R. (1963) Effect of posterior pituitary polypeptides on the flow of urine after injection in lateral ventricle of the brain of a cat, *Nature (Lond.)*, 197: 293.

Pavel, S. (1965) Evidence for the presence of lysine vasotocin in the pig pineal gland, *Endocrinology*, 77: 812–817.

Pavel, S. (1970) Tentative identification of arginine vasotocin in human cerebrospinal fluid, *J. clin. Endocr.*, 31: 369–371.

Prange, A.J., Jr., Nemeroff, C.B., Lipton, M.A., Breese, G.R. and Wilson, I.C. (1977) Peptides and the central nervous system In *Handbook of Psychopharmacology*, L.L. Iversen, S.D. Iversen and S.H. Snyder (Eds.), Plenum Press, New York, in press.

Rigter, H., van Riezen, H. and de Wied, D. (1974) The effects of ACTH and vasopressin analogues on CO_2-induced retrograde amnesia in rats, *Physiol. Behav.*, 13: 381–388.

Rodriguez, E.M. (1976) The cerebrospinal fluid as a pathway in neuroendocrine integration, *J. Endocr.*, 71: 407–443.

Rosenbloom, A.A. and Fisher, D.A. (1975) Radioimmunossayable AVT and AVP in adult mammalian brain tissue: comparison of normal and Brattleboro rats, *Neuroendocrinology*, 17: 354–361.

Sawyer, W.H. (1964) Vertebrate neurohypophysial principles, *Endocrinology*, 75: 981–990.

Sawyer, W.H. (1977) Evolution of neurohypophyseal hormones and their receptors, *Fed. Proc.*, 36: 1842–1847.

Schulz, H., Kovács, G.L. and Telegdy, G. (1976) The effect of vasopressin and oxytocin on avoidance behavior in rats. In *Cellular and Molecular Bases of Neuroendocrine Processes*. E. Endröczi (Ed.), Akadémiai Kiadó, Budapest, pp. 555–564.

Sterba, G. (1974) Das oxytocinerge neurosekretorische System der Wirbeltiere. Beitrag zu einem erweiterten Konzept, *Zool. Jahrb. Abt. Allg. Zool. Physiol. Tiere*, 78: 409–423.

Valtin, H. and Schroeder, H.A. (1964) Familial hypothalamic diabetes insipidus in rats (Brattleboro strain), *Amer. J. Physiol.*, 206: 425–430.

Vliegenthart, J.F.G. and Versteeg, D.H.G. (1965) Evolution of the vertebrate neurohypophysial hormones, *Gen. comp. Endocr.*, 5: 712.

Vliegenthart, J.F.G. and Versteeg, D.H.G. (1967) The evolution of the vertebrate neurohypophysial hormones in relation to the genetic code, *J. Endocr.*, 38: 3–12.

Vorherr, H., Bradbury, M.W.B., Hoghoughi, M. and Kleeman, C.R. (1968) Antidiuretic hormone in cerebrospinal fluid during endogenous and exogenous changes in its blood level, *Endocrinology*, 83: 246–250.

Walter, R., Griffiths, E.C. and Hooper, K.C. (1973) Production of MSH release-inhibiting hormone by a particulate preparation of hypothalami: mechanisms of oxytocin inactivation, *Brain Res.*, 60: 449–457.

Walter, R., Hoffman, P.L., Flexner, J.B. and Flexner, L.B. (1975) Neurohypophyseal hormones, analogs, and fragments: their effect on puromycinin-induced amnesia, *Proc. nat. Acad. Sci. (Wash.)*, 72: 4180–4184.

Weindl, A., Sofroniew, M.W. und Schinko, I. (1976) Psychotrope Wirkungen hypothalamischer Hormone: Immunohistochemische Identifikation extrahypophysärer Verbindungen neuroendokriner Neurone, *Arzneimittelforsch.*, 26: 1191–1194.

de Wied, D. (1964) Influence of anterior pituitary on avoidance learning and escape behavior, *Amer. J. Physiol.*, 207: 255–259.

de Wied, D. (1965) The influence of the posterior and intermediate lobe of the pituitary and pituitary peptides on the maintenance of a conditioned avoidance response in rats, *Int. J. Neuropharmacol.*, 4: 157–167.

de Wied, D. (1969) Effects of peptide hormones on behavior. In *Frontiers in Neuroendocrinology 1969*, W.F. Ganong and L. Martini (Eds.), Oxford University Press, London, pp. 97–140.

de Wied, D. (1971) Long term effect of vasopressin on the maintenance of a conditioned avoidance response in rats, *Nature (Lond.)*, 232: 58–60.

de Wied, D. (1974) Pituitary-adrenal system hormones and behavior. In *The Neurosciences, Third Study Program*, F.O. Schmitt and F.G. Worden (Eds.), MIT Press, Cambridge, Mass., pp. 653–666.

de Wied, D. (1976) Behavioral effects of intraventricularly administered vasopressin and vasopressin fragments, *Life Sci.*, 19: 685–690.

de Wied, D. and Bohus, B. (1966) Long term and short term effects on retention of a conditioned avoidance response in rats by treatment with long acting pitressin and α-MSH, *Nature (Lond.)*, 212: 1484–1486.

de Wied, D. and Gispen, W.H. (1977) Behavioral effects of peptides. In *Peptides in Neurobiology*, H. Gainer (Ed.), Plenum Press, New York, pp. 397–448.

de Wied, D., Greven, H.M., Lande, S. and Witter, A. (1972) Dissociation of the behavioral and endocrine effects of lysine vasopressin by tryptic digestion, *Brit. J. Pharmacol.*, 45: 118–122.

334

de Wied, D., Bohus, B. and van Wimersma Greidanus, Tj.B. (1975) Memory deficit in rats with hereditary diabetes insipidus, *Brain Res.*, 85: 152–156.

van Wimersma Greidanus, Tj.B. and de Wied, D. (1977) The physiology of the neurohypophysial system and its relation to memory processes. In *Biochemical Correlates of Brain Structure and Function*, A.N. Davison (Ed.), Academic Press, London, pp. 215–248.

van Wimersma Greidanus, Tj.B., Dogterom, J. and de Wied, D. (1975) Intraventricular administration of anti-vasopressin serum inhibits memory consolidation in rats, *Life Sci.*, 16: 637–644.

Zimmerman, E.A. (1976) Localization of hypothalamic hormones by immunocytochemical techniques. In *Frontiers in Neuroendocrinology, Vol. 4*, L. Martini and W.F. Ganog (Eds.), Raven Press, New York, pp. 25–62.

Zimmerman, E.A., Carmel, P.W., Husain, M.K., Ferin, M., Tannenbaum, M., Frantz, A.G. and Robinson, A.G. (1973) Vasopressin and neurophysin: high concentrations in monkey hypophyseal portal blood, *Science*, 182: 925–927.

DISCUSSION

VELTMAN: Consolidation of memory can probably be considered as a process in which many factors are involved. Would it, therefore, not be possible that vasopressin is only disturbing the equilibrium between these factors? This would mean that vasopressin would have an *effect* on memory consolidation, while it would not be possible to conclude a *function* for this hormone from such experiments.

DE WIED: There are various experiments that suggest a *function* for neurohypophysial hormones in memory consolidation. This can be shown, in the first place, by experiments in which specific vasopressin antiserum was injected intracerebro-ventricularly, which is assumed to neutralize vasopressin in the brain. Behavioral (van Wimersma Greidanus et al., 1975) and electro-physiological (Urban, 1977) data showed a marked reduction in the consolidation of avoidance behavior and changes in hippocampal theta activity. Secondly, homozygous Brattleboro diabetes insipidus rats, which lack vasopressin, have a marked disturbance in the consolidation of passive avoidance behavior (de Wied et al., 1975). The effect of vasopressin is exactly opposite to that of the effects of the antibodies (de Wied, 1976) and to the disturbances found in the Brattleboro rat (Bohus et al., 1975).

CHANGEUX: I will continue on the same question: did you see any side-effects which are not specially on memory, but on other behavioral processes, as in the open field situation?

DE WIED: If these animals are injected with 1–10 ng of vasopressin directly into the brain, there are no differences in open field behavior or other kinds of non-instrumental behavior. But if the intact vasopressin molecule is injected in doses above 10 or 30 ng, a syndrome may arise which indicates toxicity: the animals shows barrel rotation, a similar syndrome which is also seen with somatostatin (Kruse et al., 1977). This syndrome is, however, never found if the C-terminal is removed from the vasopressin molecule.

CHANGEUX: Are the behavioral effects you described specific for peptides?

DE WIED: There are some transmitters which may have similar kinds of effects (see, for review, van Ree et al., 1977). In addition, Tanaka et al. (1977a, b) and Versteeg et al. (1977) have determined the effect of a number of neurohypophysial hormones on the turnover of noradrenaline and dopamine in various discrete brain areas. They found that in various areas which may be the locus of action of these principles as derived from lesion studies (rostral septum, dorsal hippocampus) an increase in noradrenaline turnover was found following the injection of vasopressin. So I think that a transmitter is needed in order to induce that kind of behavior. But the peptides are of course more specific than the transmitters, because the peptides code for structure and receptor. Such changes in transmitter turnover may be the result of effects of neuropeptides on the cell membrane. It may also be possible that the action of neuropeptides is not mediated by neurotransmitter activity, but a direct effect on putative receptors may also be feasible.

STIRLING: During the jumping test Whishaw and Vanderwolf (1973) and Morris et al. (1976) looked at the theta rhythm and found that the theta frequency increased just before you jump. Do you find a difference in the theta activity in the hippocampus of animals after injection of peptides?

DE WIED: Yes, we see with vasopressin that there is a decrease in the higher frequencies and, with oxytocin, in hippocampal RSA during paradoxical sleep (Urban, 1977). But this was observed in a non-behavioral situation.

STIRLING: You have not tried these hormones on lower vertebrates, presumably. Do they have similar behavioral effects?

DE WIED: No, the lowest vertebrates we have in the laboratory are rats, rabbits and human beings.

K. BOER: Gray showed in the Brattleboro rats the same frequency shifts as you were mentioning now, but he found that hydration of the Brattleboro rat will reset the frequency band. This frequency shift might thus not be too relevant to the influence of vasopressin on behavior, but more related to water metabolism as such.

DE WIED: Desglycinamide lysine[8]-vasopressin (DG-LVP) has virtually no effect on water metabolism. It restores the behavioral effect in the Brattleboro rat as good as the whole vasopressin molecule. So the behavioral deficits in this animal cannot be due to the disturbed water metabolism.

K. BOER: It appeared from your results that an increasing amount of oxytocin did have less effect on memory consolidation. Do you have an explanation for this?

DE WIED: No, this is not correct. Systemic oxytocin in our hands increases resistance to extinction depending on the dose used. Intracerebrally it induces the opposite effect and reduces avoidance behavior. The covalent ring structure tocinamide facilitates passive avoidance behavior following intraventricular injection. I think that not enough oxytocin enters the brain in intact form after systemic injection and that it is therefore difficult to demonstrate the amnesic effect following this route. We are currently investigating this problem.

DISCUSSANT: Do peptides have the same effects on positively reinforced animals?

DE WIED: Not if you reinforce the rats with food (Garrud et al., 1974), but it does in sexually motivated behavior (Bohus, 1977) where copulation is, anthropomorphologically speaking, used as the reward.

REFERENCES

Bohus, B. (1977) Effect of desglycinamide-lysine vasopressin (DG-LVP) on sexually motivated T-maze behavior in the male rat, *Horm Behav.*, 8: 52–61.

Bohus, B., van Wimersma Greidanus, Tj.B. and de Wied, D. (1975) Behavioral and endocrine responses of rats with hereditary diabetes insipidus (Brattleboro strain), *Physiol. Behav.*, 14: 609–615.

Garrud, P., Gray, J.A. and de Wied, D. (1974) Pituitary-adrenal hormones and extinction of rewarded behaviour in the rat, *Physiol. Behav.*, 12: 109–119.

Kruse, H., van Wimersma Greidanus, Tj.B. and de Wied, D. (1977) Barrel rotation induced by vasopressin and related peptides in rats, *Pharmacol. Biochem. Behav.*, in press.

Morris, R.G.M., Black, A.H. and O'Keefe, J. (1976) Hippocampal EEG during ballistic movement, *Neurosci. Lett.*, 3: 102.

van Ree, J.M., Bohus, B., Versteeg, D.H.G. and de Wied, D. (1977) Neurohypophyseal principles and memory processes, *Life Sci.*, in press.

Tanaka, M., de Kloet, E.R., de Wied, D. and Versteeg, D.H.G. (1977a) Arginine[8]-vasopressin affects catecholamine metabolism in specific brain nuclei, *Life Sci.*, 20: 1799–1808.

Tanaka, M., Versteeg, D.H.G. and de Wied, D. (1977b) Regional effects of vasopressin on rat brain catecholamine metabolism, *Neurosci. Lett.* 4: 321–325.

Urban, I.J.A. (1977) *Electrophysiological Correlates of Behaviorally Active Neuropeptides: Influence on Hippocampal Theta Rhythm and Paradoxical Sleep.* Thesis, Utrecht.

Versteeg, D.H.G., Tanaka, M., de Kloet, E.R., van Ree, J.M. and de Wied, D. (1977) Prolyl-leucyl-glycinamide (PLG): regional effects on α-MPT-induced catecholamine disappearance in rat brain, *Brain Res.*, in press.

Whishaw, I.Q. and Vanderwolf, C.H. (1973) Hippocampal EEG and behaviour: changes in amplitude and frequency of RSA (theta rythm) associated with spontaneous and learned movement patterns in rats and cats, *Behav. Biol.*, 18: 461–484.

de Wied, D. (1976) Behavioral effects of intraventricularly administered vasopressin and vasopressin fragments, *Life Sci.*, 19: 685–690.

de Wied, D., Bohus, B. and van Wimersma Greidanus, Tj.B. (1975) Memory deficit in rats with hereditary diabetes insipidus, *Brain Res.*, 85: 152–156.

van Wimersma Greidanus, Tj.B., Dogterom, J. and de Wied, D. (1975) Intraventricular administration of anti-vasopressin serum inhibits memory consolidation in rats, *Life Sci.*, 16: 637–644.

Thyroid Hormones and Human Mental Development

A. QUERIDO, N. BLEICHRODT and R. DJOKOMOELJANTO

Department of Medicine, University of Leiden, Leiden, Department of Industrial and Organizational Psychology and Test Development, Free University of Amsterdam, Amsterdam (The Netherlands) and Department of Medicine, Diponegoro University, Semarang (Indonesia)

INTRODUCTION

There is abundant experimental evidence that thyroid deficiency in the neonatal period causes impaired development of the central nervous system. The studies were mainly done in rats, and especially the work of Eayrs and of Balázs deserves to be mentioned (e.g. Eayrs, 1971; Balázs, 1976). The techniques applied were histological, biochemical and behavioral, while EEG studies were also carried out. Biochemically, attention was given to nucleic acids, to various enzymes, and to the deposition of the myelin sheath. Interpreting these data in terms of the human situation is difficult, however, in part because of the differences in the state of brain development at birth between experimental animals and humans.

There are also a few studies available on primates, such as those reported by Holt et al. (1973) using the macaque as the animal model for study. Thyroidectomy was done through injection of radioactive iodine halfway through pregnancy (days 71—88). The authors concluded that overall RNA and protein synthesis is depressed in the fetal brain in the absence of thyroid hormone. Even with the monkey, however, there is still a large difference from the human in the timing of the period of rapid brain development relative to the moment of birth.

Before going into detail about what is known about the relationships between thyroid function and mental development in the human, a few basic facts should be mentioned. The thyroid in the human fetus is considered to start functioning around 10—12 weeks. According to Dobbing (1974, 1975) neuronal multiplication in humans occurs mainly from 10 to 18 gestational weeks. Transfer of thyroid hormones from the mother to the fetus seems to be negligible (Goslings, 1975), which is in agreement with the experience that hypothyroid mothers can give birth to normal infants.

On the other hand, it is well known that children born with congenital defects of the thyroid (congenital athyreosis, dystopic hypoplasia, or thyroid enzyme defects) reveal a varying degree of mental deficiency in a high percentage of cases. Normal thyroid function during the second and third trimester of pregnancy is therefore a prerequisite for normal mental development.

It is important, finally, to recognize what happens to the central nervous system after birth. Human brain cells as a total population continue multiplication well into the second postnatal year, and rapid myelination continues for even longer (Dobbing, 1975). It is against the background of these facts that we will discuss the effect of thyroid hormones on human mental development.

FORMS OF CRETINISM

Knowledge about the relationship of thyroid hormones to mental development has very practical significance. There are two important areas of health care where this problem is present, and which are currently being intensively studied. These relate, respectively, to two different models of pre- and postnatal development in the presence of an inadequate supply of thyroid hormones.

The first model is at present the concern of the industrially developed countries. Techniques have been developed for the recognition of *congenital hypothyroidism* at birth (sporadic cretinism), a condition which is known to be present in 1 out of 5000 babies. The aim here is to immediately institute adequate substitution therapy, the hope being to prevent irreversible mental retardation in these babies. Aside from humanitarian reasons, there is also the aspect that adequate prevention of mental retardation gives important economic benefits.

The second model is mainly the concern of the developing countries, and addresses itself to the problem of preventing *endemic goiter and cretinism* in regions of severe iodine deficiency (which is still widespread throughout the world). Also in this situation there are two aspects: viz. the humanitarian problem, and the creation of conditions which enable optimal socio-economic development in such countries. As indicated in Fig. 1, the two models present quite different conditions and problems.

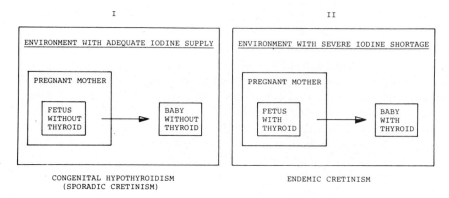

Fig. 1.

Both conditions have in common fetal hypothyroidism during pregnancy, as shown by Tilly et al. (1974) through umbilical cord blood analysis, and through analysis of bone development in severe endemic goiter. In both conditions, we also find evidence that thyroid hormones are needed for normal mental development, and for the prevention of neurological abnormalities as well. In severe congenital hypothyroidism, neurologic signs such as spasticity, tremor and hyperactive deep tendon reflexes are present. In endemic cretinism, besides these abnormalities, squinting, hearing loss and spastic paresis are also seen with high frequency.

SPORADIC CRETINISM

Let us focus first on congenital hypothyroidism. Since the classic article of Smith et al. (1957), early recognition of the syndrome and the administration of adequate thyroid substitution therapy, have been strongly advocated in order to achieve optimal prevention of mental retardation. From the results of their studies (see Fig. 2), it is clear that in 10 out of 22 severe hypothyroid cases, early treatment (before 6 months of age) achieved I.Q. values of 90 or greater. This is much better than in the large group of severe congenital hypothyroidism, where treatment was done between 6 months and 1 year of age, and in which only 15% reached the same favorable I.Q. score. Of 32 patients with *mild* hypothyroidism on the other hand, 41% achieved an I.Q. of 90 or greater despite the fact that the average age at the institution of therapy was 3 years. Similar results have been obtained by others (e.g. Van Gemund and Laurent de Angulo, 1971).

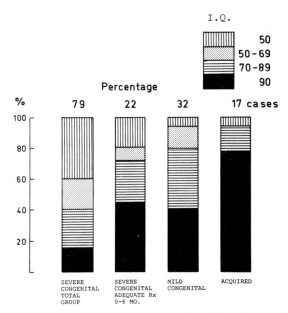

Fig. 2. The mental prognosis of the patients with severe cretinism, given adequate therapy before 6 months of age (second column), is contrasted with the total results in the three categories of hypothyroidism. (From Smith et al., 1957.)

From the above data it can be concluded that the prevention and reversibility of damage caused by thyroid deficiency depend upon the *degree* of hormone depletion, and also on the *time* of starting replacement therapy. The latter aspect is highly relevant for the great effort being presently developed to institute routine screening for hypothyroidism at birth. The idea behind this is that the frequency of congenital hypothyroidism is 1 per 5000 births, and that screening cost and effort (aside from the benefits to the affected children) has a very good cost-benefit ratio with regard to the prevention of institutionalization. It remains to be seen, however, whether treatment from *birth* onwards will increase the favorable results already attained.

ENDEMIC CRETINISM

The second model, that of endemic cretinism through iodine deficiency, is more complicated and far more difficult to study. It has in common with congenital hypothyroidism that the deficiency is present both prenatally and (in a great number of cases) also post-

340

natally. How serious the deficiency in both of these periods actually is, however, depends mainly upon environmental factors. In endemic cretinism, the final result depends upon the level of iodine supply because the thyroid is able to synthesize thyroid hormones. After birth, the infant depends directly upon the environment for its iodine supply. I have seen many places where 10% of the population is severely retarded because of iodine deficiency. Is this the result of prenatal damage, or of postnatal hypothyroidism? Technically, it is not feasible to study the *effect* of thyroid substitution therapy after birth, because areas which are recognized as being severely iodine deficient should receive adequate iodine prophylaxis, either through iodization of salt or (temporarily) with injections of iodized oil. The second aspect is the difficulty of adequately measuring intelligence performance; the great influence of socio-economic development for the expression and development of intelligence should also be taken into consideration (see Fig. 3).

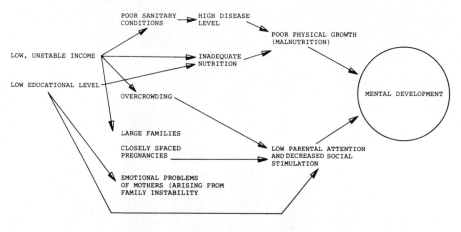

FACTORS WITH A POSSIBLE ADVERSE INFLUENCE ON MENTAL DEVELOPMENT

Fig. 3. Factors with a possible adverse influence on mental development. (From WHO chronicle, 1974.)

We have the privilege of an ongoing cooperation between the Leiden Medical Faculty and the Medical Faculty of Diponegoro University, in Semarang, for studies of the effect of severe iodine deficiency on populations in Central Java. In these severely iodine deficient areas, both endemic goiter and endemic cretinism are widespread. Endemic cretinism is characterized by abnormalities of the central nervous system, such as mental deficiency, squinting, deafness, neuromotor abnormalities and spasticity (for review see Querido, 1975). These abnormalities of the central nervous system are seen in different combinations, and to a different degree, in a relatively limited number of persons. However, *the entire population has been exposed to iodine deficiency during pregnancy and thereafter.* The question therefore rises whether in the so-called normal, non-cretinous, part of the population there exist a number of persons who are subnormal in mental development, but who escape observation because school education is not obligatory and social adaptation is rather easy. To study this problem, the Leiden Medical Faculty and the Diponegoro University in Semarang obtained the cooperation of the Psychology departments of the Free University of Amsterdam and the Universitas Indonesia in Djakarta.* Two villages were chosen for

* We gladly acknowledge the assistance and cooperation of the members of the project team in Djakarta: Drs. Saparinah Sadli, Sudirgo Wibono and Engelien Bonang.

comparison (Gowok and Lonjong). A number of characteristics of these villages relevant for the study are given in Table I.

TABLE I

PARAMETERS OF LONJONG (LONJONG) AND GOWOK (SENGI)

	Lonjong	Gowok
Inhabitants	489	411
Farmers	99%	100%
Distance Magelang	23 km	30 km
Altitude	600 m	600 m
Distance to main road	1 km	5 km
Schools	0	0
Primary school at distance	1 km	4 km
Goiter rate (OB up)	3%	58%
Protein-bound iodine μg%	4.9 ('76) (3.4–6.6)	3.4 (1.2–5.9)
Urinary excretion of iodine μg/g creatinine	41.5 ('73) 40.9 ('76)	18.9
TSH μU/ml	normal	18.4

Based on the experience of the Psychology departments of the Free University, Amsterdam, and of Unpad Bandung, a battery of tests was chosen, which can arbitrarily be divided into two sets. One is directed mainly towards the testing of factors of *general intelligence,* and is therefore strongly sensitive to educational experience. The second group of tests was directed more towards *non-intelligence factors* such as motor skills, concentration and perceptual capacity. The tests were tried out in small villages with test leaders who were M.A. students of the Psychological Faculty of Universitas Indonesia, and were especially trained for this project. After the try-out, a definite choice of tests was made for different age groups. Translation of the tests into Javanese had to be carried out, after which the battery was tried out in a rural area near the villages Gowok and Lonjong. Only after all of this were the definitive observations carried out.

In Table II and III an impression is given of the composition of the test battery.

TABLE II

TESTS USED IN GOWOK AND LONJONG (1976).
GENERAL INTELLIGENCE

Fluency	Form board
Visual memory	Memory span
Learning names	Progressive matrices
Exclusion	Hidden patterns
Quantity	Block design
Discs	Mazes
Verbal meaning	Exclusion B.
	Components

TABLE III

TESTS USED IN GOWOK AND LONJONG (1976). NON INTELLIGENCE FACTORS (MOTOR SKILLS, CONCENTRATION OR PERCEPTUAL CAPACITIES)

Pinboard (finger dexterity)
Throwing balls
Balance
Reaction time
Choice reaction time
Tapping
Figure comparison

The subjects in the two villages were divided into the following three age groups: 6–8 years, 9–12 years, and 13–20 years. In Gowok, the cretins were not included among the subjects to be tested. For their identification we used the presence of 2 out of 3 diagnostic characteristics: mental retardation, hearing loss, and neuromotor abnormalities.

In this report we will present only the *average* results obtained. We will first discuss the tests directed mainly towards general intelligence. In the youngest age group, that of 6–8 years, there was (to our astonishment!) no significant difference between the results attained in Gowok and in the control village. In the other age groups, most of the results in Gowok were below those attained in the control village. Close analysis of the educational background, however, revealed some essential differences between the population of the two villages in these age groups; we therefore are not inclined to attach any special meaning to these results (Table IV).

TABLE IV

NUMBER EXAMINED PERSONS, AVERAGE AGE AND AVERAGE EDUCATIONAL LEVEL FOR 3 AGE GROUPS

	Lonjong			Gowok		
	Number	*Age*	*Education*	*Number*	*Age*	*Education*
6–8 years	40	7.2	0.4	21	7.1	0.1
9–12 years	41	10.5	2.6	41	10.6	0.3
13–20 years	58	15.6	4.1	44	16.1	0.6
6–20 years	139	11.7	2.5	106	12.2	0.4

When it comes to the results of the second set of tests (more directed towards *non*-intelligence factors, such as motor skills, concentration and perceptual capacity — which we consider to be less dependent on educational background) we did find clearcut differences in all age groups, and usually at the 1% level of significance (Table V). Four of the tests (pinboard, tapping test, reaction time and choice reaction time) are considered to be 'perceptual-motor abilities'. Factors such as finger dexterity, manual dexterity and response orientation are also involved here. In the test of 'figure comparison' (which also showed differences in outcome) 'perceptual speed' was studied in addition.

Thus, we did indeed find significant differences in the second group of tests between the two communities, i.e. the severely iodine-deficient village, Gowok, and the control village, Lonjong. These results pose many questions: are such differences reversible; are the dif-

TABLE V

SUMMARY OF DIFFERENCES OF TEST RESULTS IN LONJONG AND GOWOK

Subtests	6–8 yr	9–12 yr	13–30 yr
16. Pinboard	**	**	
17. Throwing balls	–	**	–
18. Balance	–	**	–
19. Single reaction time	–	**	**
20. Choice reaction time	–	**	**
21. Tapping	*	**	**
22. Figure comparison		**	**

** Significant at 1% level.
* Significant at 5% level.
– Not significant.

ferences the consequence of prenatal or of postnatal conditions; is an anatomical substrate demonstrable (e.g. degree of dendritization or myelination, or number of cells)?

CONCLUSIONS

As was stated in the beginning, there are similarities between congenital hypothyroidism and endemic cretinism with respect to the periods during which the development of the central nervous system is exposed to hypothyroidism, prenatally as well as postnatally. Both conditions are subject, for instance, to a *variable* degree of hypothyroidism. The fact is recalled that the people with mild congenital hypothyroidism seen by Smith et al. (1957), and treated either early or late, end up in 41% of the cases with an I.Q. of 90 or better. We naturally ask ourselves whether cases of mild hypothyroidism which did *not* achieve an I.Q. of 90 or more, if seen in Gowok would all have been classified as cretins. If so (which we doubt), our observations on general intelligence in Gowok would be in line for the two conditions. If, however, this should *not* be the case, we are left with no explanation for the failure to find any instances of mild retardation in Gowok.

We are now in the process of analyzing individual results, in relation to the biochemical parameters of hypothyroidism. Unfortunately, to our knowledge no studies using differentiated tests comparable to those reported here have been made in congenital hypothyroidism. Such studies will be very necessary in the near future, because of the high hopes being placed on the early diagnosis of this condition.

ACKNOWLEDGEMENT

The support of the Netherlands Foundation for the Advancement of Tropical Research (WOTRO) Grant: W 94-31, is gratefully acknowledged.

REFERENCES

Balàzs, R. (1976) Hormones and brain development. In *Perspectives in Brain Research, Progress in Brain Research, Vol. 45,* M.A. Corner and D.F. Swaab (Eds.), Elsevier, Amsterdam, pp. 139–159.

344

Dobbing, J. (1974) The later development of the brain and its vulnerability. In *Scientific Foundations of Pediatrics,* J.A. Davis and J. Dobbing (Eds.), Heinemann Medical Books, London, pp. 565–577.

Dobbing, J. (1975) Normal brain development in human. In *Brain Development and Thyroid Deficiency,* A. Querido and D.F. Swaab (Eds.), North-Holland, Amsterdam, pp. 7–11.

Eayrs, J.T. (1971) Thyroid and the developing brain: anatomical and behavioural effects. In *Hormones in Development,* M. Hamburgh and E.J.W. Barrington (Eds.), Appleton-Century-Crofts, New York, pp. 345–355.

Gemund, J.J. van and Laurent de Angulo (1971) The effects of early hypothyroidism on I.Q., school performance, and electroencephalogram pattern in children. In *Normal and Abnormal Development of Brain and Behaviour,* G.B.A. Stoelinga and J.J. van der Werff ten Bosch (Eds.), Leiden University Press, pp. 299–313.

Holt, A.B., Cheek, D.B. and Kerr, G.R. (1973) Prenatal hypothyroidism and brain composition in a primate, *Nature (Lond.),* 243: 413–414.

Querido, A. (1975) Endemic cretinism – a continuous personal educational experience during 10 years, *Postgrad. med. J.,* 51: 591–599.

Smith, D.W., Blizzard, R.M. and Wilkins, L. (1957) The mental prognosis in hypothyroidism of infancy and childhood. A review of 128 cases, *Pediatrics,* 19: 1011–1022.

Thilly, C., DeLange, F., Camus, M., Berquist, H. and Ermans, A.M. (1974) Fetal hypothyroidism in endemic goitre: the probable pathogenic mechanism of endemic cretinism. In *Endemic Goiter and Cretinism: Continuing Threats to World Health,* Sci. Publ. No. 292, Pan American Health Organization, Washington, D.C., pp. 121–128.

W.H.O. Chronical (1974) *Malnutrition and Mental Development,* W.H.O., Geneva, pp. 95–102.

DISCUSSION

BALÁZS: I suppose that the basic question you are asking us is how reversible are the changes in the central nervous system when a metabolic insult, such as abnormal thyroid state or undernutrition, has been inflicted during development. The literature on animal experiments is quite confusing, so I am not at all surprised that the evaluation of the human situation is even more complicated. There is no unambiguous answer to the question. If brain maturation is assessed in terms of biochemical or structural parameters it is frequently observed that metabolic imbalance, including thyroid deficiency, results in a severe retardation. The emphasis here is on *retardation*, since most of the parameters are restored more or less to normal after proper treatment. For example, Eayrs (1971) has found that the structural changes in the thyroid deficient cerebral cortex are reversible to a great extent after implementing replacement therapy at different times after birth. However, unless animals are rehabilitated within a relatively short time after birth, the behavioral impairments persist. So it seems that there is a discrepancy between the reversibility of the physical and the behavioral changes: the plasticity of the system, in terms of structure and biochemistry, is greater than the plasticity of the system in terms of behavior. This leads us to an important question: what are the proper estimates for correlating the structure and biochemistry of the brain with behavior? Cragg has studied the effect of undernutrition and thyroid deficiency on the number of synapses per nerve cell in the cerebral cortex. In the current repertoire of neuroanatomy, this estimate is probably the nearest to 'higher nervous function'. However, Cragg has pointed out that, since there are about 10^4 synapses per neuron, it is very difficult to appreciate the implication of even a marked deficit. Thus we have real problems when we try to choose the proper physical correlates of behavior; the estimates we are presently using are far from ideal.

QUERIDO: In the beginning of this week Dr. Dobbing claimed that there is one insult for which you cannot compensate, and that is an early insult after birth in the human when cerebellar cell division is still going on. This would result in what they call 'clumsy people'. My question is whether, on the basis of our data, you would call the people from the village with endemic cretinism 'clumsy people', and whether you would expect a reduced cell number in the cerebellum.

BALÁZS: Well, the evidence is quite good that, even in man, neurogenesis *does* occur in the cerebellum in the postnatal period. However, the important question here is: how far will even a deficit of 10–30% in granule cell numbers influence the functioning of the neuronal circuits in the cerebellum? There is a real chance that the effect will be relatively small as a result of the great redundancy of cells and circuits in the CNS. I really don't think that deficit in cell number on its own could explain the impairment of behavioral performance.

SWAAB: But this is arguing the other way round. Dr. Querido has shown clumsiness, which presumably means that that the cerebellum must be affected seriously in one way or another.

BALÁZS: Yes, but the defect is not necessarily, or exclusively, due to a deficit in cell numbers. It may be something else, e.g. balance of neuronal circuits, and I would put my money on the 'something else' as the major factor.

SWAAB: One question about the set-up of this kind of experiment: I think the better you look at villages, the greater the chance that you will find a difference, for example in school distance or something else. It seems impossible to get two villages that are absolutely similar in all parameters except iodine intake. Would it not be easier to develop an experiment in such a way that performance of individuals is related to their TSH-levels, PBI, etc.?

QUERIDO: First of all, we are going to do that with the individual data we have now. I mean, in addition to calculating the average, we are going to study the individual correlations. The problem, however, is that the data on thyroid function give only a snapshot. A certain hormone level does not tell you how the thyroid gland was functioning some years ago.

BLOM: Were you giving iodine to the people in the affected village after the observations? And if so, are you doing a follow-up study on the results?

QUERIDO: Together with Dr. Djokomoeljanto we are carrying out prophylaxis in that area and we plan to come back in 5 years time for a follow-up study. However, it is not so simple to mobilize this effort again and to get the same cooperation. Moreover, the people would have to stay in the same village. Dr. Djokomoeljanto is currently doing the follow-up of our prophylaxis program in another village in Java, by measuring the correction of the iodine metabolism. It turned out that after 3 years part of the original population had moved to Sumatra. For an extensive follow-up we should, in addition, have a similar group of investigators again, and that will also be difficult. The doctoral students of the University of Indonesia were remarkable young men and women. They stayed in such villages for weeks, and they were playing and singing with these children when they had done a good job during the day. There was a very impressive relationship between the testing group and the population, and it would be difficult to get such a group again.

SWAAB: If there is indeed plasticity in the brain, such a relationship would influence your experiments!

QUERIDO: They did it in both the 'experimental' and the control villages.

BALÁZS: Your data give a very optimistic outlook. If iodine was the only crucial factor, one would also have expected a significant difference in the 6–8-year-old group. I suppose that the degree of education, probably even in the control village, was not very high. Nevertheless, it seems that education has influenced performance in the intelligence tests in a positive way. This means that, at least in man, the social environmental stimulation must have a very important role. This brings me back to the plasticity of the central nervous system, and to the different means with which one can try to rectify an abnormal situation. It would appear that, even if physical alterations lead to a handicap, there is a chance of correct behavioral performance, to some extent, by the proper intervention.

QUERIDO: Yes, I agree; it resembles the data of Davenport et al. (1976). He enriched the environment of rats exposed perinatally to thiouracil and changed in that way the behavior in a positive sense.

DE GROOT: I was wondering about another disadvantage in the village with iodine deficiency. One would expect that the parents too had a lower educational level because of the iodine deficiency, and that this would have also a negative influence on the next generation, since their possibility to stimulate the children would be less.

QUERIDO: Well, that is the general problem when measuring I.Q. everywhere in the world. It is, as you know, still a major issue at present.

REFERENCE

Davenport, J.W., Gonzalez, L.M., Carey, J.C., Bishop, S.B. and Hagquist, W.W. (1976) Environmental stimulation reduces learning deficits in experimental cretinism, *Science,* 191: 578–579.

SECTION VI

NEUROBEHAVIORAL ONTOGENY

Spontaneous Motor Rhythms in Early Life — Phenomenological and Neurophysiological Aspects

MICHAEL CORNER

Netherlands Institute for Brain Research, Amsterdam (The Netherlands)

INTRODUCTION

This paper will begin by reviewing the evidence and lines of thought which have led to the formulation of certain descriptive principles, potentially applicable to early spontaneous motility throughout the animal kingdom (Corner, 1977). The possibility will then be explored that the neural systems generating these most primitive of behavior patterns persist into later life, and that they again become manifestly active during sleep. Finally, what little is presently known about the physiological basis of embryonic, fetal and larval movements, and about their possible importance in development, will be briefly considered.

The factual material presented in the first two sections is admittedly too scanty to prove either of the propositions discussed there. Indeed, I am personally convinced that only a profound insight into the underlying neuronal organization and its embryonic origins can ever establish 'homologies' of behavior such as are suggested here. This implies that it is futile for that purpose to increase the range and accuracy of quantitative descriptive studies beyond a certain point. A demonstration of characteristic variations in behavior patterns among species or individuals would not necessarily mean that there were any qualitative differences in the neural mechanisms causing the different behaviors. Nor, on the other hand, would the most striking phenomenological similarities establish that the neuronal basis must be similar in the different organisms studied. Additional knowledge about the functional properties and interconnections of developing nerve cells may provide such answers, but the required information can probably be best obtained under the guidance of a challenging and reasonably convincing working hypothesis. The point of diminishing returns on a purely descriptive research investment, then, would appear to be when the *plausibility* of one or another unifying theory has been satisfactorily established. The following survey will perhaps persuade you that that point may now have been reached in the field of *'behavioral embryology'*.

UNIVERSALITY OF GENERALIZED MOTOR DISCHARGES IN EARLY DEVELOPMENT

Reflexive motility

In the 'classical' period of investigations into the beginnings of behavior in embyros, the emphasis centered upon movements which could be evoked in different species by somatic sensory (tactile) stimulation (for reviews see Carmichael, 1954; Corner and Bot, 1967;

Hamburger, 1963). An emphatic distinction was made at that time between localized and 'total-body' reflex movements; indeed, the competing candidates for a general theory of behavioral embryology were predicated upon the ontogenetic priority of, respectively, the one or the other of these two types of motor response. That controversy is now of little more than historical interest, what with our current realization that both classes of reflex, the *partial* and the *total,* are an equally fundamental aspect of the behavior of very immature nervous systems. It has proven possible to confirm this last point for groups as disparate as cephalopod molluscs, anuran amphibians and galliform birds (see Corner, 1977). The confusion turns out to have lain in technical limitations combined with biased theoretical expectations: at very early stages, − and in some species more than in others − it requires care to stimulate the organism without triggering a generalized bout of movements; on the other hand, *localized* activation of muscle groups is favored if the embryo becomes slightly hypoxic. A fortuitous combination between a particular experimental animal and set of physiological conditions could, therefore, easily lead to a spurious 'confirmation' of either one of the above-mentioned theories.

It is nonetheless striking that embryonic and larval behavior patterns lend themselves so readily to the local vs total dichotomy. This is due to the existence of a motor *response threshold,* in analogy with the 'all-or-none' law at the neuronal level: up to a certain intensity, tactile or electrical stimuli elicit graded (and usually short-lasting) contractions in the musculature near the site of stimulation but, beyond that point, a total response which long outlasts the stimulus is triggered instead. Such bursts commonly vary from a few hundred milliseconds up to 4−5 sec, but at certain times become highly regular in their timing. For many seconds following each of these generalized responses, increased stimulus intensities are required to elicit a second burst, which is not necessarily any weaker or shorter than the first one (see Corner et al., 1973). It is intriguing that motor bursts such as those described above occur not only early in ontogeny but also in phylogeny. In forms as primitive as coelenterates, bursting patterns are generated which (as at early stages of development in higher animals) are sometimes quite regular, but at other times are highly variable in their timing (Fig. 1).

Interestingly enough, the electrical activity of embryonic neural networks cultured in vitro reveals a very similar response pattern to brief shocks of increasing intensity, applied either directly to the central nervous tissue or to sensory ganglion cells connected with it. Thus, one usually sees only graded local responses up to a certain point, and then the triggering of a long-lasting stereotyped discharge which scarcely changes with the application of still stronger stimuli (see Crain, 1974, 1976). This sort of behavior has been observed in cultures of many different kinds of neural structures (cerebral cortex, hypothalamus, cerebellum, medulla oblongata, spinal cord) as well as in embryos of widely disparate taxonomic groups.

Spontaneous motility

Bursts of motor activity resembling those evoked by brief stimuli also occur 'spontaneously' in the embryos or larvae of many species (Corner, 1977; Corner et al., 1973). Periods of variability in the duration of successive motor bursts typically alternate with periods of great regularity (Fig. 2). Similarly, while these movements sometimes come in trains at quite consistent intervals, the successive intervals at other times in the same preparation may be highly inconsistent. Trains of generalized movement bursts have also been reported during the neonatal period in those mammals which are born relatively immature, such as the rat and the cat, and during the late fetal period in precocial species (see Corner, 1977). Intense spontaneous bursting was also found to occur in a high proportion of explants taken from

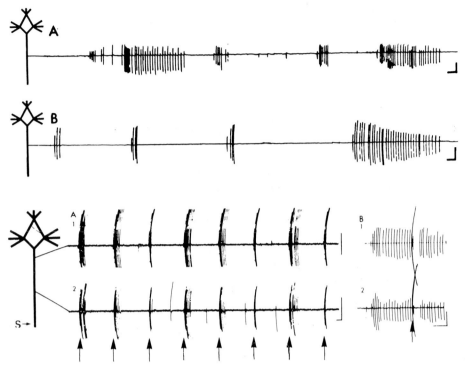

Fig. 1. Stalk motor bursting patterns recorded electrically in the coelenterate *Corymorpha palma*. Above: spontaneous activity in two specimens, A and B, showing intermittent highly regular discharges but also periods of great irregularity. (From Ball, 1973.) Calibrations: 500 μV and 5 sec. Below: A, bursts evoked by single brief (5 msec) shocks, as indicated by the arrows. B, inhibition of local background activity following a short generalized discharge. (From Ball and Case, 1973.) Calibrations: 100 μV and 5 sec.

different regions of the fetal CNS and cultured in vitro; it could be demonstrated in addition that the observed neuronal (and correlated muscular) discharges persist in the absence of afferent nerve input (Corner, 1964a; Corner and Crain, 1972). There is apparently an endogenous source of excitation present in such networks which summates with excitation introduced via the afferent nerve pathways (also Corner, 1964b). The presence of *inhibitory* mechanisms even at very early stages may be preventing much of this neural activity from expressing itself fully as overt motility in the intact organism (Crain, 1974, 1976; Provine, 1976; also see Sedláček, 1978).

Spontaneous total-body movements in early stages of ontogeny are (with the possible exception of crustacean embryos: Berrill, 1973) seldom stationary over extended periods of observation. Rather, the motility pattern alternates between epochs of relatively high activity and epochs in which activity is absent, or is at a low level (Fig. 3). Even when the frequency is maximal, the spontaneous movements rarely lose their more-or-less discrete burst-like character, so that fluctuations in the motility–time curves can best be described as comprising *clusters* of brief, 'phasic', discharges (Corner, 1977). The periodicity of spontaneous movements is quite clear at times, even though the length of the cycles often appears to be shifting over time (Figs. 4 and 5). In addition to rhythms of the order of 1–2 min. and/or 5–10 min, longer fluctuations sometimes appear in the motility records. These latter have not yet been well characterized for any species; they appear to vary from 20–30 min to upwards of an hour (also see Brodsky, 1975).

352

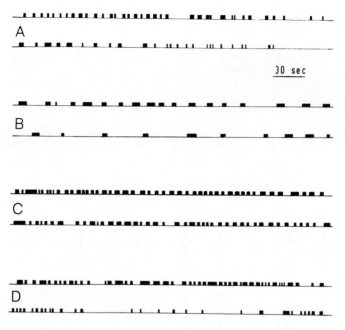

Fig. 2. Spontaneous swimming in four *Discoglossus pictus* frog tadpoles (A–D) at early larval stages, during phases of relatively high motility (continuous 10 min event-recordings: solid blocks represent bursts of swim movements). Note the large fluctuations in durations, intervals and degree of regularity of the bursts (T = 20 °C).

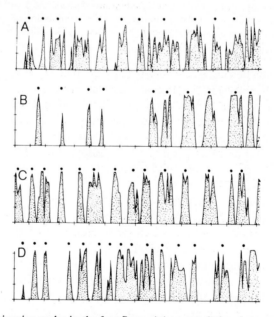

Fig. 3. Spontaneous swimming cycles in the frog *Rana pipiens* at early larval stages (T = 15 °C). The time spent swimming (ordinate: 3 sec/div) is given per 10 sec epoch in four different tadpoles (A–D), continuously over a 30 min recording period (abscissa: 100 sec/div). Each 'activity phase' in the motility cycle is indicated by a filled circle. (From Corner, 1977.)

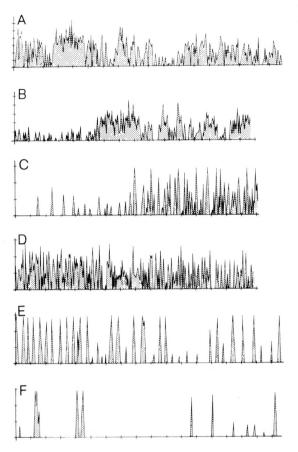

Fig. 4. Time-course of spontaneous swimming at early larval stages in the frog *Discoglossus pictus* (T = 20 °C). Six specimens (A–F), covering the range of observed individual variations, recorded continuously for about 1.5 hr (abscissa: 400 sec/div) and plotted as the amount of time spent swimming per consecutive 20 sec epoch (full-scale on the ordinate equals approximately 20 sec in all records). Different cycles of motility can be discerned with varying degrees of clarity.

The emphasis up till now has been only upon those features of early behavior which appear to be *similar* in all animals regardless of their taxonomic position. There presumably exists a primordial pattern of motility operative at early stages of development, one that in very primitive organisms continues to dominate behavior even into maturity. However, we should not fail to call attention to the differences among animals in the parameters defining their spontaneous movements. Some species, for instance, characteristically show shorter burst durations than do others, while also the frequency, periodicity and regularity of spontaneous motor activity cycles can vary considerably from one group of animals to the next (Figs. 3–5; also see Corner, 1977).

PERSISTENCE OF PRIMITIVE MOTILITY RHYTHMS IN LATER LIFE

Sleep in mammals

It was mentioned earlier that total-body movement bursts can still be observed during the neonatal period in some mammalian species (see Corner, 1977). In the rat, these movements

354

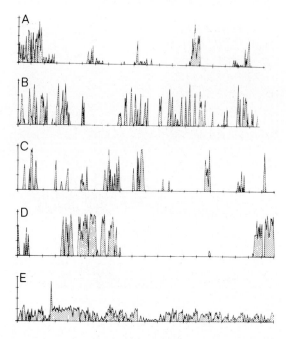

Fig. 5. Time-course of spontaneous swimming at early larval stages in the toad *Xenopus laevis* (T = 20 °C). Five specimens (A–E), showing the observed range of individual variations, recorded continuously for about 1.5 hr (abscissa: 400 sec/div) and plotted as the amount of time spent swimming per consecutive 20 sec epoch (full-scale on the ordinate equals about 20 sec in all records). The overall motility level is somewhat lower than in *D. pictus* (see Fig. 4) and the periodicity is usually more evident.

normally occur throughout the first two weeks after birth, thereafter becoming very infrequent. Simultaneous EEG and motility recordings reveal that the motor bursts sometimes occur during slow-wave sleep (SWS), but are most frequent during periods of *low* voltage EEG activity (during which time continuous theta waves – i.e. 4–8 cycles per sec – are usually visible; Fig. 6). The behavior itself consists of brief bouts of vigorous writhing movements or jerky twitching which occur while the animal is otherwise lying quietly on its side, and which are often preceded and/or followed by a few seconds of irregular breathing or of apnea. The EEG pattern, in combination with the repetitive bursts of gross body movements, is in vivid contrast with the picture seen when the animal is unmistakably awake. Such behavioral manifestations have therefore usually been regarded as being signs of PS (*paradoxical,* c.q. *REM,* sleep; i.e. the 'active' phase of Kleitman's 'basic-rest–activity-cycle': 1963) even at ages when no EEG or other physiological correlates of PS are as yet present (see Corner, 1977; Verley and Garma, 1975).

This point of view is supported by a series of experiments which we carried out in 2–3-week-old rat pups, restrained in a quasi-fetal position (Corner and Kwee, 1976). Under such conditions, a state of sleep is induced following a few minutes of intermittent struggling: the eyes close, the body relaxes, and large amplitude slow waves become predominant in the cortical EEG. After a variable time trains of total-body movements appear, closely resembling those described for younger pups. The eyes seldom or never open during these bursts (indeed, it is extremely difficult during such restraint to evoke eye-opening even with normally adequate sensory stimuli) and the movements are preceded and/or followed by irregular breathing, and sometimes also by complete muscular atonia. Some of this generalized motility

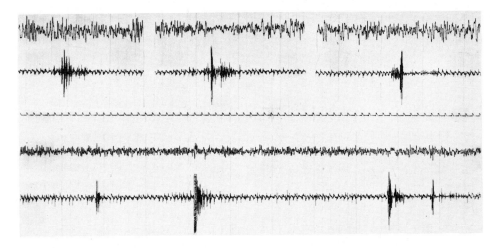

Fig. 6. Electrocorticogram (upper traces: R. fronto-occipital) in an unrestrained 12-day-old white rat pup, correlated with respiration and spontaneous gross body movements (lower traces). Above: during *slow-wave sleep*, the EEG sometimes desynchronizes for a few seconds during a burst of movements (middle) but at other times remains unchanged; associated respiratory irregularities are also quite variable in their occurrence. Below: during *paradoxical sleep*, continuous θ-wave activity is seen in the EEG, and motor bursts of variable intensity and duration occur frequently. (In both phases of the sleep cycle, total-body burst durations range from a fraction of a second to about 5 sec.) Time calibration: 1 sec per division.

occurs during SWS but it is much more frequent during the epochs of low voltage EEG activity (Fig. 7). It is not yet known if, and at what age, these 'rapid body-movements' eventually disappear from sleep under restraint in rats.

The chick as model system

A remarkably similar behavioral phenomenon was described by us many years ago in chicks (Corner et al., 1966) and, indeed, provided the basis both for subsequent experiments and for the working hypothesis being reviewed here (also see Corner et al., 1973; Corner, 1977). Thus, when properly restrained, chicks of up to about two weeks of age go into a state of sleep (as demonstrated by the usual polygraphic criteria) from which it is virtually impossible to arouse them, even by the application of what would normally be strongly suprathreshold sensory or electrical stimulation. Intermittent trains of movements resembling short bouts of struggling appear after a few minutes, sometimes during SWS but at other times associated with episodes of EEG flattening.

Subsequent research on newly hatched chicks in our laboratory (Bakhuis, 1977; Bour, 1977) has revealed an interesting new aspect of this phenomenon. In contrast to young rats, 'struggling' bursts in sleeping chicks take place predominantly during periods of continuous *high* voltage EEG activity, i.e. SWS (Fig. 8). Whenever the EEG amplitude is low, on the other hand, rapid eye movements interspersed with isolated jerky body muscle twitches (PS) dominate the registrations. This cannot be dismissed as being an avian peculiarity, since the absence of generalized movement bursts during PS has been reported for the sheep fetus too (Ruckebusch et al., 1977). When such bursts occur, however, it is usually either immediately prior to or just at the end of a period of REM activity. The picture also bears a certain resemblance to the episodic sleep movements characteristic of a condition in man called *nocturnal myoclonus,* or the 'restless-legs' syndrome, where bursts of gross body movements occur repetitively every 20–30 sec throughout much of the night (for the most part during

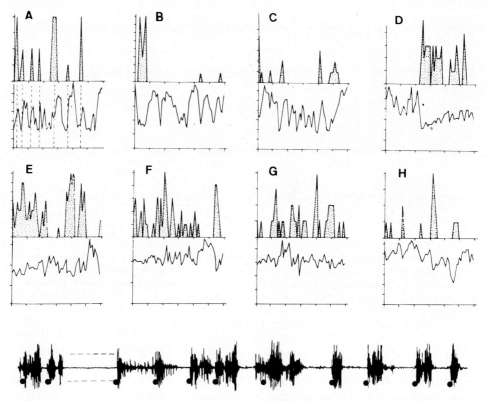

Fig. 7. The frequency of spontaneous gross body movements (upper traces: bursts/min, on the ordinate) as correlated with the EEG amplitude (lower traces: mean delta-wave intensity per min, on the ordinate) in 8 restrained rat pups, A–H, recorded continuously for 1 hr (10 min/div, on the abscissa). There is a highly significant inverse correlation between the spontaneous motility level and the amplitude of the cortical EEG. Underneath is a 1 min sample of the raw motility record, showing the amplitude criterion for defining the occurrence of a 'burst' (filled circles). (From Corner, 1977.)

light slow-wave sleep: Lugaresi et al., 1972). Suppression of pathological myoclonic discharges during stage-REM sleep (PS) has recently been noted in a child with hereditary hyperexplexia (see Fig. 9), and the similarity to the phenomenology in restrained chicks was explicitly mentioned (De Groen and Kamphuisen, 1977).

Physiological considerations

The resolution of the apparent discrepancy between neonatal rats and chicks may lie in the fact that paradoxical sleep is not only a time of intense motor excitation but of *inhibition* as well, with the former seeming to appear earlier in ontogeny (e.g. Jouvet, 1965; Prechtl, 1974; Roffwarg et al., 1966; Verley and Garma, 1975). For instance, while gross body movements occur primarily during REM-sleep in infants, they are largely absent from this phase in the adult. Dement and Kleitman (1959) showed, however, that the frequency of gross body movements in fact rises to a peak just before the onset of stage-REM, then falls abruptly but returns transiently to a high level upon termination of REM-sleep (PS). The *overall* level of muscular activity nevertheless remains quite high during PS (Fig. 10), bursts of rapid eye movements almost always being accompanied by diffuse twitching in muscles of the extremities (Aserinsky, 1967; Pompeiano, 1969). The intensity of the

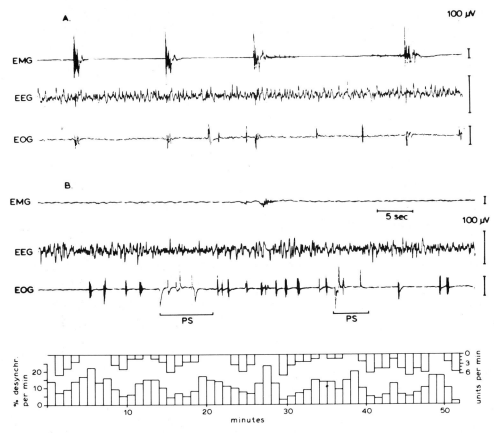

Fig. 8. Association of *body movements* (EMG), *eye movements* (EOG) and *cerebral EEG* in restrained chicks (*Gallus domesticus*) shortly after hatching, during periods of (A) continuous slow-wave sleep, and (B) sleep with 'paradoxical' EEG episodes. Underneath is shown the inverse correlation between the density of PS (lower bars) and the frequency of total-body motor bursts (upper bars). (Modified from Bour, 1977; also see Bakhuis, 1977.)

generalized bouts of movement during PS can be augmented by lesions of the cerebellum or, more dramatically, of the locus coeruleus (e.g. Jouvet, 1975). The inescapable conclusion must be that a tendency towards vigorous spontaneous movements persists during stage-REM in mammals, but normally becomes suppressed when a sufficient degree of maturity has been attained.

The chick being relatively mature at birth, it would not be too surprising if the periodic inhibitory mechanisms of PS were already operational at that time, thus damping the intensity of spontaneous body movements which occur during this phase of sleep. If, however, adequate *tonic* excitation from another source were to be fed into the same motor circuits throughout the entire sleep cycle, total-body bursts would be fully triggered during SWS even though expressed only weakly during PS (Fig. 11). This is what appears to happen in birds during hatching, where the anterior diencephalon facilitates stereotyped bursts of vigorous movements (Bakhuis, 1974) which actually are being generated in the lower brain stem (Corner and Bakhuis, 1969; Oppenheim, 1973). The descending excitation enables hatching to continue uninterrupted until the chick has succeeded in breaking out of the shell (at which point the hatch bursts become abruptly superseded by characteristic waking

358

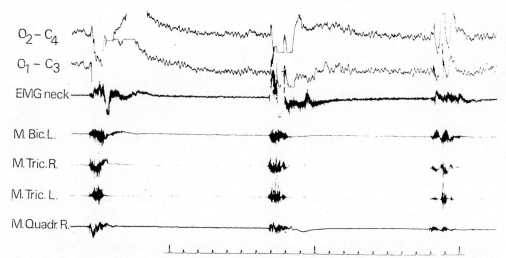

Fig. 9. Segment of polygraph record made during a prolonged train of bursts of generalized body movements, occurring throughout slow-wave sleep in a hyperexplectic child. The top two traces are, respectively, right and left contro-occipital EEGs, while the other traces are EMGs recorded from various muscles: biceps, triceps and quadriceps (time calibration: 1 sec/div). Courtesy of Dr. Hans de Groen, Neurological Clinic, Leiden University.

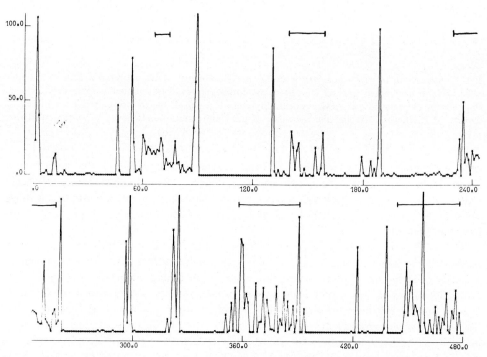

Fig. 10. Overall frequency of *body movements* (number/min, on the ordinate) occurring 'spontaneously' throughout 480 min of night-time sleep in a normal human adult; phases of stage-REM are indicated by the lines above the record. A 4–5 min motility cycle during REM-sleep (PS) can sometimes be seen quite clearly. (Courtesy of Dr. Alain Muzet; also in Corner, 1977.)

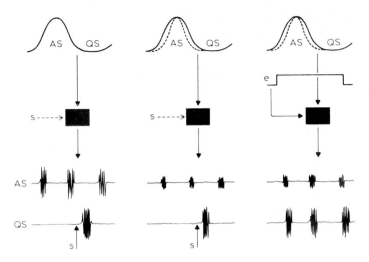

Fig. 11. Hypothetical schema to illustrate the relationship between phasic motility and the sleep cycle in three different situations. Left: *immature mammal:* total-body bursts are triggered repetitively during the active, c.q. 'paradoxical', phase of the cycle (AS), but can also be evoked by a sensory stimulus (S) presented during the quiet phase (QS), c.q. 'slow-wave' sleep. (The solid line represents a fluctuating *endogenous excitation* feeding into an output circuit of the CNS.) Middle: *mature mammal:* spontaneous motor bursts are reduced in intensity by the action of *concurrent inhibition* which is generated during AS (dashed line), whereas a full response (at S) is still typically evoked during QS. Right: *peri-hatch chick:* a forebrain (tonic) source of excitation (e) is strong enough to trigger typical total-body movements during QS, but usually not to overcome the inhibitory action which is present together with endogenous excitation during AS.

activity patterns: Corner et al., 1973). Hatching behavior is thus a fascinating example of the apparent adaptation of a primitive mode of central nervous functioning to the specific ecological requirements of a highly evolved class of animals.

Alternatively, the possibility that hatch behavior is a form of *arousal* (i.e. wakefulness) associated with struggling to escape from confinement has recently been argued by Bakhuis (1977). This is indeed the first impression anyone will get when watching these movements, or when listening to the loud vocalizations which usually accompany them. A number of curious features soon led us to question this interpretation, however (Corner et al., 1966; Corner and Bot, 1967).

(1) The eyes usually stay tightly shut and the EEG *synchronized* (i.e. as in SWS, slow waves of large amplitude are prominent) during the apparent struggling behavior; indeed, both of these criteria for arousal remain absent even if the chick is subjected to strong sensory stimulation. If the restraints are loosened a bit, on the other hand, typical signs of arousal reappear following external stimuli or 'startle' movements, as well as spontaneously from time to time.

(2) The struggling bursts have a mechanical quality, occurring as they do for a second or two at a time (and often at impressively regular intervals), which contrasts with the escape behavior of chicks which clearly are awake.

(3) The muscle tone invariably falls back almost immediately to the sleeping level – in fact there is sometimes complete atonia – following a stereotyped struggling burst (in contrast with the *gradual* loss of tonus always seen when a chick falls asleep after a clear arousal episode, however brief).

(4) Stereotyped struggling during sleep declines in frequency towards the end of the first

week of life, and has virtually disappeared by two weeks post-hatch (Corner and Bakhuis, 1969). This development parallels an increase in the amount of time spent awake by the maturing chick, and in its ability to be awakened even while tightly restrained.

(5) The generalized movement bursts during sleep in the peri-hatch chick look suspiciously like certain late embryonic motility patterns ('type III': see Oppenheim, 1973; also Corner et al., 1973). These are present long before the embryo begins to show behavior suggestive of wakefulness (such as head elevation, eye-opening or orientation movements) and they do *not* require that the animal be still inside the egg, or restrained in any other way.

This last point had originally led us to assume that sleep under restraint (by making arousal difficult or impossible) was merely a permissive condition which allowed the resurgence of a characteristically *fetal* behavior pattern, unrelated physiologically to either sleep or wakefulness (Corner et al., 1966). This even led to some words of caution (Corner et al., 1973) being addressed to sleep physiologists who were using similar movements in neonatal mammals as the chief, or even sole, criterion for the presence of PS ('sleep-with-jerks'). It was only later that the idea finally crystallized that normal sleep motility might indeed be intimately related to 'embryo-motor' mechanisms in the brain stem and spinal cord (see Corner, 1977). The answer, however, could of course turn out to be a combination of these possibilities, for they are not necessarily mutually exclusive. Furthermore, even the distinction between arousal and *PS* systems might not be quite so sharp, neurophysiologically speaking, as seems to be the case when viewing them at the behavioral level.

Returning now to the question of the origins of sleep motility, one can point to certain phenomenological similarities to the behavior patterns described in the first section of the paper for very early stages of development. For instance, rapid eye movements commonly occur as trains of short-lasting bursts, having durations and intervals which approximate those of the generalized motor bursts under consideration here (e.g. Aserinsky, 1967; Jouvet, 1975; Kryzincki, 1975; Pompeiano, 1969). Genetic analysis in mice (see Valatx, 1978) has shown that these parameters are strain specific, a finding reminiscent of the quantitative species difference noted earlier for spontaneous *total-body* motility. Finally, bodily movements are often clustered during PS epochs so as to define cycles with a period of several minutes (see Fig. 10), a phenomenon also seen in early development. These parallels suggest that motility rhythms seen during sleep could reflect the continuing operation of neurological mechanisms of great ontogenetic and phylogenetic antiquity.

NEUROLOGICAL FOUNDATIONS OF SPONTANEOUS MOTILITY CYCLES

Location of generator systems

A large number of experiments (reviewed in Hobson et al., 1976) have led to the strong suspicion that a generator system for phasic discharges during sleep, as well as for the alternation between active (PS) and quiet (SWS) sleep, is located within the brain stem at the level of rhombencephalon (hindbrain). The pontine reticular formation has been specifically implicated, but recent findings suggest that more caudal regions (medulla oblongata) are also involved (Netick et al., 1977). The precise nature of the structures and the circuitry comprising such a generator system is as yet poorly understood.

It is noteworthy that the hindbrain also plays a central role in the generation of the total-body motility cycles in early ontogeny. The 'type III' movement bursts seen in the late chick embryo (e.g. Oppenheim, 1973) are largely of lower brain stem origin, as are the spontaneous swimming bursts seen in larval fish and amphibians (see Corner, 1977; Corner et al., 1973).

These discharges are probably generated endogenously by the nervous tissue, rather than being triggered by afferent nerve impulses. The patterning into repetitive brief discharges is accomplished through a 'relaxation' oscillator, i.e. a gradually declining depression of excitability in the network, which lasts for 30 sec or more following each burst. Similar conclusions have also been reached using in vitro preparations of muscle tissue innervated by brain stem or spinal cord fragments, both with and without sensory nerves (see Crain, 1974, 1976). Such 'model system' experiments have established, moreover, that longer activity cycles (up to at least 10 min) need not be attributed to fluctuations in environmental variables, but can be intrinsic to the neural tissues themselves. Sensory input appears in all these preparations simply to add to the endogenous excitation level, and thus to trigger stereotyped responses identical to those which occur spontaneously.

Origins and significance of CNS generators

Following up on an approach pioneered by Paul Weiss (1950, 1977), it could be shown that the motor bursting pattern in amphibians is preferentially programmed into the prospective lower brain stem area (basal rhombencephalon) already at the early neurula stage of development (Corner, 1964a). Presumptive mesencephalon and spinal cord areas of the neural plate consistently gave rise to other patterns of spontaneous activity, but these differences could be shown to be only quantitative in kind. Under certain conditions of explantation, moreover, also spinal cord and midbrain motor regions showed stable 'medullary' type discharge patterns (and vice versa). This finding is of interest in view of the considerable part normally played by the spinal cord in the generation of larval and fetal motility, especially at early stages (see Corner, 1977; Hamburger, 1973; Provine, 1976). It is now well established, at least for the chick embryo, that this cord activity is mostly *non*-reflexogenic in nature, and that it declines drastically towards the end of the prenatal period (also see Sedláček, 1978). Several basic features of embryonic behavior patterns can be simulated by model neural networks composed exclusively of *randomly* interconnected units (e.g. Anninos and Elul, 1974; MacGregor, 1972; Okuda et al., 1974).

What could be the biological utility of this intense excitation being generated within the developing nervous system? Experiments with isolated neural tissues in which all bioelectric activity was suppressed during maturation showed that such activity is unnecessary for neuro- or synaptogenesis per se, either ultrastructurally or electrophysiologically speaking (see Crain, 1974, 1976). It has not been proven, however, that the fine details of functional organization are unaffected in such 'virgin' neural networks. The suggestion was made recently (Changeux and Danchin, 1976; Changeux and Mikoshiba, 1978) that the stabilization of synaptic connections, which initially are laid down in excess, requires that a network be electrically active during ontogenesis. REM sleep — a source of intense endogenous excitation which is present for a large proportion of the time in young organisms — has similarly been suspected of playing an important role in neural and behavioral development (Roffwarg et al., 1966; Jouvet, 1975).

Skeletal and muscular defects result when chick embryos have been paralyzed experimentally (see Hamburger, 1973; Changeux and Danchin, 1976), and the prevention of such abnormalities would certainly represent an important function for spontaneous motor activity in early life. Hormonal systems are known to be active early in development (e.g. Hughes, 1974), and it is surely not unreasonable to suppose that their secretions are already under some degree of neuronal control. Finally, we may also consider the variety of known direct effects of electric activity upon the functional properties of nervous tissue, ranging from 'kindling' of epileptic foci (e.g. Morell, 1973) to the still largely unknown mechanisms underlying learning and memory (Mark, 1974). Arguments for the existence of such effects in *immature* nervous systems are necessarily speculative, however, given the dearth of information on the subject (but see Changeux and Mikoshiba, 1978). Here is surely an important area for future investigations, not merely to find out if spontaneous bioelectric discharges are more than an epiphenomenon of functional neurogenesis but, more important, to contribute to the eventual assessment of different brain regions, cell types and periods of development in terms of their potential for undergoing 'experiential' modifications.

SUMMARY

A review has been made of some recent findings in *behavioral embryology,* and of related phenomena in the field of sleep research. Attention is called to a number of striking parallels which suggest that motor activity cycles during sleep may have as their antecedents the spontaneous motility rhythms typical of early stages in development and evolution. The neurological mechanisms underlying such primitive behavior patterns, and their possible significance for the maturation of the nervous system, are still virtually unknown. These appear to be potentially fruitful areas for further research.

ACKNOWLEDGEMENTS

Ton Richter carried out the observations on which Figs. 2—5 are based. Bob Scholte made the registrations used for Fig. 6, Harry Bour those for Fig. 8, Hans de Groen those for Fig. 9, and Alain Muzet those for Fig. 10. Jopie Sels saw to the typing of the manuscript. The constructive criticisms of Harry Bour, Herms Romijn, Dick Swaab, Harry Uylings and Nanne van de Poll were most useful in clarifying murky portions of the original text.

REFERENCES

Anninos, P.A. and Elul, R. (1974) Effect of structure on function in model nerve nets, *Biophys. J.,* 14: 8—19.

Aserinsky, E.L. (1967) Physiological activity associated with segments of the rapid eye movement period. In *Sleep and Altered States of Consciousness,* S.S. Kety, E. Evarts and H. Williams (Eds.), *Res. Publ. Ass. nerv. ment. Dis.,* 45: 338—350.

Bakhuis, W.L. (1974) Observations on hatching movements in the chick, *J. comp. physiol. Psychol.,* 87: 997—1003.

Bakhuis, W.L. (1977) *The Causal Organization of Climax (Hatching) Behavior in the Domestic Fowl (Gallus dom.),* Doctoral dissertation, University of Groningen.

Ball, E. (1973) Electrical activity and behavior in the solitary hydra *Corymorpha palma.* I. Spontaneous activity in whole animals and in isolated parts, *Biol. Bull.,* 145: 223—242.

Ball, E. and Case, J. (1973) Electrical activity and behavior in *Corymorpha palma.* II. Conducting systems, *Biol. Bull.,* 145: 243—264.

Berrill, M. (1973) The embryonic behavior of certain crustaceans. In *Behavioral Embryology,* G. Gottlieb (Ed.), Academic Press, New York, pp. 141—160.

Bour, H. (1977) *Vigilance States during Hatching Behavior in Chicks.* Masters dissertation, Municipal University of Amsterdam (in Dutch).

Brodsky, W.Y. (1975) Protein synthesis rhythm, *J. theoret. Biol.,* 55: 167—200.

Carmichael, L. (1954) The onset and early development of behavior. In *Manual of Child Development,* L. Carmichael (Ed.), Wiley, New York, pp. 60—185.

Changeux, J.P. and Danchin, A. (1976) Selective stabilisation of developing synapses as a mechanism for the specification of neural networks, *Nature (Lond.)*, 264: 705–712.

Changeux, J.P. and Mikoshiba, K. (1978) Genetic and 'epigenetic' factors regulating synapse formation in vertebrate cerebellum and neuromuscular junction, this volume.

Corner, M.A. (1964a) Localization of capacities for functional development in the neural plate of *Xenopus laevis, J. comp. Neurol.*, 123: 243–256.

Corner, M.A. (1964b) Rhythmicity in the early swimming of anuran larvae, *J. Embryol. exp. Morph.*, 12: 665–671.

Corner, M.A. (1977) Sleep and the beginnings of behavior in the animal kingdom – studies of ultradian motility cycles in early life, *Progr. Neurobiol.*, 8: 279–295.

Corner, M.A. and Bakhuis, W.L. (1969) Cerebral electrical activity, forebrain function and behavior in the chick at the time of hatching, *Brain Res.*, 13: 541–555.

Corner, M.A., Bakhuis, W.L. and Van Wingerden, C. (1973) Sleep and wakefulness during early life in the domestic chicken, and their relationship to hatching and embryonic motility. In *Behavioral Embryology*, G. Gottlieb (Ed.), Academic Press, New York, pp. 245–279.

Corner, M.A. and Bot, A.P.C. (1967) Somatic motility during the embryonic period in birds, and its relation to behavior after hatching. In *Developmental Neurology, Progress in Brain Research, Vol. 26*, C.G. Bernhard and J.P. Schadé (Eds.), Elsevier, Amsterdam, pp. 214–236.

Corner, M.A. and Crain, S.M. (1972) Patterns of spontaneous bioelectric activity during maturation in culture of fetal rodent medulla and spinal cord tissues, *J. Neurobiol.*, 3: 25–45.

Corner, M.A. and Kwee, P. (1976) Cyclic EEG and motility patterns during sleep in restrained infant rats, *Electroenceph. clin. Neurophysiol.*, 41: 64–72.

Corner, M.A., Peters, J.J. and Rutgers van der Loeff, P. (1966) Electrical activity patterns in the cerebral hemispheres of the chick during maturation, correlated with behavior in a test situation, *Brain Res.*, 2: 274–292.

Crain, S.M. (1974) Tissue culture models of developing brain functions. In *Aspects of Neurogenesis*, G. Gottlieb (Ed.), Academic Press, New York, pp. 69–114.

Crain, S.M. (1976) *Neurophysiologic Studies in Tissue Culture.* Raven Press, New York.

Dement, W.C. and Kleitman, N. (1957) Cyclic variations in EEG during sleep and their relation to eye movements, body motility and dreaming. *Electroenceph. clin. Neurophysiol.*, 9: 673–690.

Groen, J.H.M. de and Kamphuisen, H.A.C. (1977) Hyperexplexia (startle disease): the counterpart of the sleep apnoea syndrome? *Electroenceph. clin. Neurophysiol.*, 43: 492.

Hamburger, V. (1963) Some aspects of the embryology of behavior, *Quart. Rev. Biol.*, 38: 342–365.

Hamburger, V. (1973) Structural basis of embryonic motility in birds and mammals. In *Behavioral Embryology*, G. Gottlieb (Ed.), Academic Press, New York, pp. 52–76.

Hobson, J.A., McCarley, R.W. and McKenna, T.M. (1976) Cellular evidence bearing on the pontine brain-stem hypothesis of desynchronized sleep control, *Progr. Neurobiol.*, 6: 279–376.

Hughes, A.F.W. (1974) Endocrines, neural development, and behavior. In *Aspects of Neurogenesis*, G. Gottlieb (Ed.), Academic Press, New York, pp. 223–243.

Jouvet, M. (1965) Paradoxical sleep – a study of its nature and mechanisms. In *Sleep Mechanisms, Progress in Brain Research, Vol. 18*, K. Akert, C. Bally and J.P. Schadé (Eds.), Elsevier, Amsterdam, pp. 20–57.

Jouvet, M. (1975) The function of dreaming: a neurophysiologist's point of view. In *Handbook of Psychobiology*, M.S. Gazzaniga and C. Blakemore (Eds.), Academic Press, New York, pp. 499–527.

Kleitman, N. (1963) *Sleep and Wakefulness* (rev. ed.) University of Chicago Press.

Krynicki, V. (1975) Time trends and periodic cycles in REM sleep eye movements, *Electroenceph. clin. Neurophysiol.*, 39: 507–513.

Lugaresi, E., Coccagna, G., Mantovani, M. and Lebrun, R. (1972) Some periodic phenomena arising during drowsiness and sleep in man, *Electroenceph. clin. Neurophysiol.*, 32: 701–705.

MacGregor, R.G. (1972) A model for reticular-like networks: ladder nets, recruitment fuses and sustained responses, *Brain Res.*, 41: 345–363.

Mark, R.F. (1974) *Memory and Nerve Cell Connections.* Clarendon Press, Oxford.

Morrell, F. (1973) Goddard's kindling phenomenon: a new model of the 'mirror focus'. In *Chemical Modulation of Brain Function*, H.C. Sabells (Ed.), Raven Press, New York, pp. 207–223.

Netick, A., Orem, J. and Dement, W.C. (1977) Neuronal activity specific to REM sleep and its relationship to breathing, *Brain Res.*, 120: 197–207.

Okuda, M., Yoskida, A. and Takahashi, K. (1974) A dynamical behavior of active regions in randomly connected neural networks, *J. theoret. Biol.*, 45: 51–73.

364

Oppenheim, R.W. (1973) Prehatching and hatching behavior: a comparative and physiological consideration. In *Behavioral Embryology,* G. Gottlieb (Ed.), Academic Press, New York, pp. 163–244.

Pompeiano, O. (1969) Sleep mechanisms. In *Basic Mechanisms of the Epilepsies,* H. Jaspers, A. Ward and A. Pope (Eds.), Churchill, London, pp. 453–473.

Prechtl, H.F.R. (1974) The behavioral states of the newborn (a review), *Brain Res.,* 76: 185–212.

Provine, R.R. (1976) Development of function in nerve nets. In *Simpler Networks and Behavior,* J. Fentress (Ed.), Sinauer, Sunderland, Mass., pp. 203–220.

Roffwarg, H., Muzio, J. and Dement, W.C. (1966) Ontogenetic development of the human sleep–wakefulness cycle, *Science,* 152: 604–619.

Ruckebusch, Y., Graujoux, M. and Eghbali, B. (1977) Sleep cycles and kinesis in the foetal lamb, *Electroenceph. clin. Neurophysiol.,* 42: 226–237.

Sedláček, J. (1978) The development of supraspinal control of spontaneous motility in chick embryos, this volume.

Valatx, J.L. (1978) Possible embryonic origin of sleep interstrain differences in the mouse, this volume.

Verley, R. and Garma, L. (1975) The criteria of sleep stages during ontogeny in different animal species. In *Experimental Study of Human Sleep: Methodological Problems,* G.C. Lairy and P. Salzarulo (Eds.), Elsevier, Amsterdam pp. 109–125.

Weiss, P. (1950) Deplantation of fragments of the nervous system in amphibrains, *J. exp. Zool.,* 113: 317–462.

Weiss, P. (1977) Neurobiology in statu nascendi. In *Perspectives in Brain Research, Progress in Brain Research, Vol. 45,* M.A. Corner and D.F. Swaab (Eds.), Elsevier, Amsterdam, pp. 7–38.

DISCUSSION

AXELRAD: When a bird is hatching out of its egg, or even in the mammalian fetus (where there also are extensive spontaneous movements), can one really say that excitatory networks of randomly coupled units exist? I wouldn't suppose that the spinal cord in the chick at hatching constitutes a randomly coupled network of units.

CORNER: At later stages of evolution or development it is conceivable that the primitive core of the nervous system retains many of its early physiological characteristics, even though it is no longer completely randomly coupled. That would be the simplest assumption at the present time, and I think it is a lead which should be followed up, because some deviation from randomness of connections appears to be possible without compromising the behavioral patterns which have been described for random networks. Increasing structural order could then be merely refining the basic functional pattern, for example the threshold level for a burst to be triggered, the type of oscillations appearing during the burst, or the number of units which are recruited into it (e.g. Anninos, 1974).

ADRIEN: The idea of randomness in neuronal connectivity sounds plausible for the very immature animal, but how can you imagine that this kind of random network could persist and be responsible for paradoxical sleep in the adult, a system which is apparently highly organized?

CORNER: If you can accept the plausibility of a mechanism being present early in development, and there is a certain (albeit only phenomenological) similarity to behavior persisting into later life, should one begin by invoking a completely different mechanism to explain these later phenomena? Is it not more satisfactory to begin with the simpler working hypothesis that what we are seeing is the *persistence of the earlier mechanism,* which may be modified by later additions to the circuit without necessarily losing its basic character? Furthermore, one can easily imagine the appearance during ontogeny or phylogeny of new mechanisms which completely suppress the expression of the primordial motor system. However, if this suppression fluctuates daily and is withdrawn in certain periods (which we call 'sleep'), then perhaps the primitive mechanisms will again express themselves overtly, but in a form that is not detrimental to the animal. There must be a very good reason why, during sleep, you are not continuously going through the violent movements characteristic of the fetus or neonate! With a properly modulated expression such as rapid-eye-movements or weak bodily twitches, however, some freedom for such networks would surely be permissible during sleep.

MEETER: When one takes fetal spinal cord tissue, makes a suspension and plates it out in culture, one sees rich interconnections growing between isolated cells and small aggregates. You then often come across neurons which give beautiful bursts of action potentials at highly regular intervals, which go on for as long as you care to record from them. This is probably as near as possible to a random innervation pattern with living cells, and it does exactly what Dr. Corner would predict it would do.

LILIEN: Although it may be as near to random as you possibly can get in your tissue culture model, it is still probably not pure in that sense. We know that some neurons do innervate each other readily, while other neurons certainly don't do so in tissue culture (see Crain, 1976).

LYNCH: Do you have any idea about what function or value these spontaneous movements have for the organism?

CORNER: There is very little known about this but there are two broad areas in which one might pursue it. One relates to the possible survival value of the behaviour per se, for example the spontaneous movements one sees in animals such as fish and amphibians, which are hatched at a very early stage of development. The largely unpredictable gross motility that they display might be helpful in preventing a predator from synchronizing its attack upon the larvae. And we have another ecological example in terms of the hatching of a bird's egg, where a presumably similar behavioral mechanism is adapted to the specific requirements of this class of animals. But there is another dimension in which one can look at the problem, and that is: what role does the neuronal excitation underlying the movements play in the maturation of the network? Crain (1976) did some very interesting experiments a few years ago by exposing CNS tissue cultures (which were devoid of synapses at the time of explantation) for a long period of time to media which block synaptic transmission. He showed that the basic functional properties of nerve cells, as well as their ability to form synapses, did not depend upon bioelectric activity. Nevertheless, I think it would be premature to conclude that this is the whole story: that if you look at the fine details of organization of such a neural network, and at some of its quantitative features, there will be no abnormalities found to result when functional activity is interfered with.

CHANGEUX: You emphasized the fact that at later stages of development the rhythm or bursting activity was often quite similar to that seen in the very early stages. Do you suggest that it is the same *mechanism*, or rather the same *category* of neurons which is involved?

CORNER: I did not have a chance to go into the meagre neurology which is known about these things, but it certainly is true that the whole spinal cord is generating bursts in the chick embryo, and also in frog larvae. It is *not* true that at much later stages of development the spinal cord is still involved in the generation of spontaneous motility: the brain stem begins to dominate more and more motor rhythms in the chick embryo, as is known from Hamburger's work. And from our early frog work we could see that there was a gradient in the frequency of spontaneous bursts, with the hindbrain giving a very high level, and a progressive decline down along the spinal cord. So it could be that there is a primordial motor pattern which, under normal conditions, gradually disappears from most of the original substrate. And it would not be surprising that the portion of the CNS to which it becomes restricted is located at the head end of the original gradient (where the activity had always been the highest). But what is the *effect* of this activity on the generator network itself? Could it not be that it loses some of its initial randomness in interconnectivity under the influence of the very activity which, as a randomly coupled network, it was generating to begin with?

REFERENCE

Anninos, P.A. (1974) The usefulness of artificial neural nets as models for the normal and abnormal functioning of the mammalian CNS, *Progr. Neurobiol.*, 4: 59–77.

The Development of Supraspinal Control of Spontaneous Motility in Chick Embryos

J. SEDLÁČEK

Research Laboratory of Psychiatry, Charles University, Prague (Czechoslovakia)

INTRODUCTION

One of the most fascinating events of prenatal development is the onset, development and maturation of embryonic motility, which has attracted research attention ever since Harvey's observation that the 5-day-old chick embryo — in the brain of which nothing more was seen than transparent fluid enclosed in thin vesicles — performed spontaneous movements of the body and head (Harvey, 1651; for an excellent review, see Gottlieb, 1973).

Chick embryo behavior and its origins have since become the object not only of extensive experimentation but also of many theoretical conceptions and hypotheses. At the present time it is possible to state with confidence that the motility of the chick embryo is neurogenic from the start, and is primarily initiated by spontaneous discharges of spinal neurons (Hamburger, 1963, 1971; Provine, 1973). For this reason, the spontaneous motility of the chick embryo is a good measure of endogeneous central motor activity.

Another basic question in this field of research is the problem of the development of regulation of spontaneous spinal motor activity by successively maturing supraspinal regions of the central nervous system. The present paper was undertaken in order to give a short review of recent experimental results on the development of supraspinal motor control in chick embryos. Particular attention was directed at: (1) the onset of supraspinal influences upon the spontaneous activity of spinal motor output; (2) the development of inhibitory mechanisms, and (3) the possible participation of central aminergic systems in the supraspinal control.

DEVELOPMENT OF SUPRASPINAL CONTROL OF EMBRYONIC SPONTANEOUS MOTILITY

Windle and his collaborators (Windle and Orr, 1934; Orr and Windle, 1934; Windle and Austin, 1935; Windle and Baxter, 1936) concluded from their observations that motility until day 6 of incubation is realized without any integrative factors, the substrate of which would be later the descending reticulo-spinal tract. A different viewpoint is found in the work by Visintini and Levi-Montalcini (1939). They supposed that the chick embryo's motility is subject to supraspinal control from its onset at day 3—4 of incubation. Such regulating influences would be mediated via the descending pathways, even from the diencephalic level, and would travel in ventral and lateral bundles down to the lumbar segments. The authors based this conclusion upon observations in which the youngest embryos were motionless following spinal transection, whereas the same operation between days 4 and 7 of incubation provoked an increase of embryonic motility, and at day 8 a decrease. However, Rhines (1942) did not succeed in repeating the findings of the Italian authors, and questioned their basic conclusions.

The same question was later extensively studied in Hamburger's laboratory. Hamburger and Balaban (1963) found effects of chronic spinal transection upon spontaneous motility only after day 6 of incubation. They concluded from the reduction of spontaneous motility in operated embryos that, starting from this embryonic age, higher parts of the CNS exert an excitatory effect upon the functional activity of spinal neurons. In subsequent studies from the same laboratory this conclusion was modified, and the onset of supraspinal effects was set at day 9 of incubation (Hamburger et al., 1965; Decker and Hamburger, 1967; Oppenheim and Narayanan, 1968; Oppenheim, 1972). Oppenheim (1975) once more examined the results of spinal transection, and reached the conclusion that supraspinal control does not begin until day 10 of incubation. Changes take place at later stages in the periodicity of spontaneous motility in operated embryos, without there being any obvious effects upon the frequency and character of spontaneous movements.

In our own experiments, we found rather different consequences of decentralization of the embroyonic spinal cord (Sedláček and Doskočil, 1978). The only methodological difference in comparison with Hamburger's and with Oppenheim's approach consisted in full decapitation as opposed to a spinal gap. The decentralization was carried out at the highest cervical level, either as an acute transection at different embryonic stages, or as a chronic decapitation performed at stage 11–13 (Hamburger and Hamilton, 1951).

Acute transection

Acute decapitation produced an effect for the first time in 15-day-old embryos, consisting of a significant transient decrease in the frequency of spontaneous movements (but without full cessation of motility). The frequency of spontaneous movements decreased during the first 60 min after acute decapitation, from 21.4 ($\pm$ 1.77) per min to 2.8 ($\pm$ 0.42) per min, and 24 hr later had returned to 13.2 ($\pm$ 1.23) per min. From day 17 onwards, acute spinal transection evoked typical spinal shock with complete depression of spontaneous movements. During the postoperative period (up to 48 hr) the spontaneous motility in 17- and 19-day-old embryos gradually recovered, but remained below the control level (Fig. 1). In 19-day-old embryos, spinal shock depressed the normal frequency from 43.4 ($\pm$ 2.65) movements per min to 0.1 ($\pm$ 0.01) per min during the first 60 min, and to 15.4 ($\pm$ 1.76) per min within 24 hr after the decapitation.

The most evident sign of motility in decapitated embryos during restitution from spinal shock consisted of spontaneous paroxysmal movements. The development of paroxysms in the decentralized spinal cord can be regarded as evidence that disconnection of supraspinal control after day 15 alters the normal relationship between excitatory and inhibitory mechanisms in the spinal synaptic apparatus. This evaluation is supported by the findings that glycine and GABA, which normally produce inhibition of spontaneous motility at this age, produced a transient paroxysmal activation of spontaneous movements in the isolated cord preparation. The abnormal paroxysmal activity had two peaks in 19-day-old spinal embryos (n = 13; 24 hr after the decapitation). The first one occurred within the first 5 min after glycine application, when the frequency of spontaneous movements increased from 8.6 ($\pm$ 1.79) per min to 66.4 ($\pm$ 11.42) per min. In the second peak, which occurred 45 min after glycine application, the frequency rose from 8.9 ($\pm$ 1.59) to 45.1 ($\pm$ 4.80) movements per min.

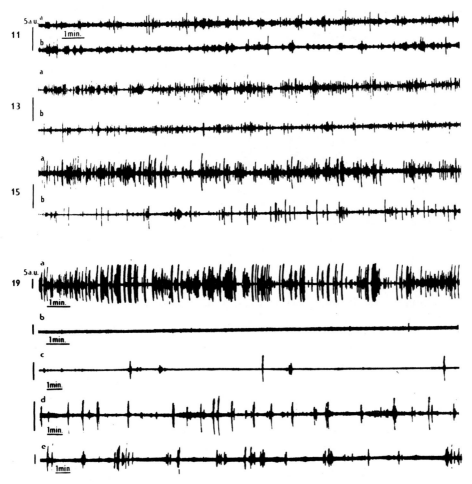

Fig. 1. The spontaneous motility in chick embryos after *acute* decapitation. a: the normal motility before operation. b–e: motility after decapitation: b, 25 min; c, 6 hr; d, 24 hr; e, 48 hr. Numbers in front of each group of records indicate the age of embryo in days of incubation; vertical bars indicate the amplitude calibration in arbitrary units.

The elevated motility usually lasted about 10 min. This paradoxical effect of the two putative inhibitory transmitters was never observed in chronically decapitated embryos, in which the spinal neurons had lost their connections with the brain long before the onset of supraspinal control (Sedláček, 1978a).

Chronic transection

Spontaneous motility in embryos after chronic decapitation did not significantly differ from the motility in control sham-operated embryos until day 15 of incubation. In 17-day-old embryos, the quantitative measure of spontaneous motility remained at the level reached prior to day 15 of incubation (Fig. 2).

The morphological findings in the spinal cord support the above interpretation of motility changes following chronic decapitation. It was shown (Sedláček and Doskočil, 1978) that chronic decapitation is followed by evident defects in the lateral and ventromedial columns – which contain the vestibulospinal and reticulospinal pathways (Donkelaar, 1975).

370

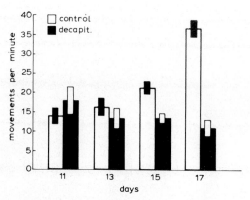

Fig. 2. The total frequency (mean ± S.E.M.) of spontaneous movements in normal (white columns) and spinal chick embryos (black columns) *chronically* decapitated at stage 11–13 (Hamburger and Hamilton, 1951). Abscissa: the age of embryos in days of incubation; ordinate: frequency of spontaneous movements per minute.

The fibers in this field were replaced by an exuberant glial overgrowth, such defects being found both in 12- and in 16-day-old embryos. Another result of chronic decapitation consisted of changes in the motoneurons of the ventral horns (cell necrosis to a varying degree, changes in cell staining from hypo- to hyperchromasy, and cellular debris with glial cleaning reactions) which were seen in 16-day-old but not in 12-day-old decapitated embryos (Fig. 3).

The following conclusions may be drawn from the age-dependent results of chronic decapitation.

(1) The descending pathways, which are the substrate of supraspinal control, are well developed even before day 15 of incubation, but are not yet effectively connected with the spinal motor networks. After day 15, their chronic absence manifests itself by transneuronal degeneration of spinal motoneurons (Gutmann, 1964; Hughes, 1965).

(2) The reduction of spontaneous motility after day 15 in chronically decapitated embryos may be caused, partly by the absence of supraspinal activatory influences, and partly by a reduction in the number or efficacy of active spinal motor units.

Further information on the development of supraspinal control has been obtained by studies in embryos with individual parts of the brain removed.

Brain defects

Decker and Hamburger (1967) showed that the motility in bulbar chick embryos was consistently lower, even from day 9 of incubation, and that the normal motility development in 15- and 17-day-old embryos stagnated. Oppenheim (1975) performed partial or total removals of individual parts of the brain at embryonic stages 10 and 11. He did not observe any quantitative changes in spontaneous motility until day 20, either after full removal of the telencephalon, plus anterior diencephalon, or in embryos with only the medulla intact. The defects produced by the absence of brain parts were limited to the development of pre-hatching and hatching behavior (Corner and Bakhuis, 1969; Oppenheim, 1972).

In contrast to these findings, we have observed quantitative changes in spontaneous motility which suggest a successive switching of individual brain parts into the system of supraspinal control. These experiments were based on the extirpation of brain vesicles at stage 11–13. The frequency of spontaneous movements following removal of the first brain vesicle (entire forebrain) developed as in control embryos until day 16 of incubation, and

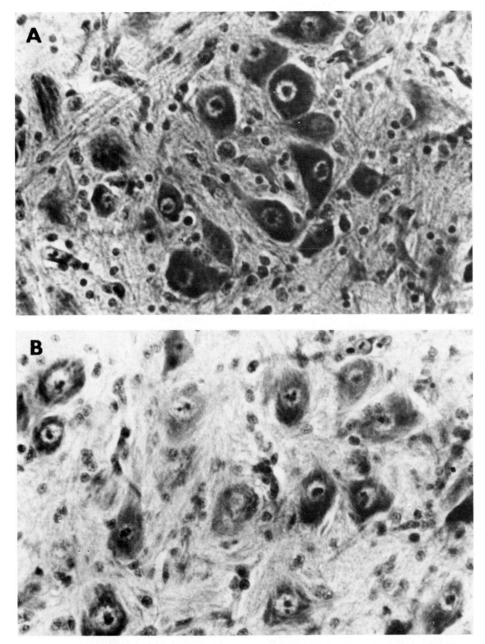

Fig. 3. Microphotographs of spinal motoneurons from lumbal cord in 16-day-old normal (A) and spinal embryos (B) decapitated at the stage 11–13. Fixation Bouin-Holland, hematoxylin-eosin.

thereafter became clearly reduced. In embryos developing without the first and second brain vesicles (forebrain plus midbrain), behavior was normal until day 15, after which a significant reduction of motility occurred. In embryos with extirpation of all 3 brain vesicles (chronic decapitation), the development of spontaneous motility was arrested at about day 14 of incubation (Table I).

TABLE I

THE TOTAL FREQUENCY (MOVEMENTS/MIN) OF SPONTANEOUS MOTILITY IN
NORMAL EMBRYOS (A) AND IN EMBRYOS AFTER EXTIRPATION OF BRAIN
VESICLES AT STAGE 11–13 (B–D)

A: control embryos (sham operated); B: embryos after extirpation of the first vesicle; C:
embryos after extirpation of the first and second brain vesicles; D: embryos after total decapitation. (N = 10 embryos at each day of incubation in all groups: A–D.)

Age in days of incubation	A Cerebrospinal activity	B Mes-rhomben-cephalospinal activity	C Rhombencephalo-spinal activity	D Spinal activity
11	15.6 ± 1.61*	14.9 ± 1.49	13.3 ± 0.61	17.9 ± 3.70
12	15.8 ± 1.82	14.8 ± 1.59	14.3 ± 1.05	13.2 ± 2.16
13	17.6 ± 2.65	15.4 ± 1.56	15.3 ± 0.86	13.4 ± 2.62
14	18.0 ± 2.12	17.1 ± 1.92	17.8 ± 0.82	15.8 ± 2.57
15	22.8 ± 1.92	22.0 ± 1.89	21.8 ± 1.65	12.6 ± 1.68**
16	27.5 ± 2.43	25.8 ± 2.58	16.9 ± 1.08**	12.8 ± 2.12**
17	38.3 ± 1.72	14.4 ± 2.42**	9.2 ± 1.24**	11.1 ± 2.11**
18	42.6 ± 3.28	11.6 ± 1.25**	8.7 ± 1.04**	
19	45.3 ± 3.12	9.2 ± 1.14**	8.1 ± 0.75**	

* Mean ± S.E.M.
** Indicates a statistically significant difference (Student's *t*-test: $P < 0.001$) in comparison
with cerebrospinal activity (A).

Comparison of spontaneous motility in normal and chronically decapitated embryos
permits the conclusion that spontaneous motility in 11- and 13-day-old embryos is in
essence *spinal* motility, without any noticeable supraspinal components. From 15 days of
incubation the motility begins to be composed of two components.

(a) *The spinal component,* i.e. the motility seen in chronically decapitated embryos,
amounting to about 60% of normal spontaneous motility and (b) the *supraspinal component,*
which accounts for the rest. In 17-day-old embryos the spinal component amounts to 33%
only, and the supraspinal component to 67% of the total motility (Sedláček, 1978a). The
following pattern of developing supraspinal control may be derived from these results: (1)
the major brain divisions become gradually recruited into the system of supraspinal control
of spinal motor output, in a caudorostral sequence beginning on day 15 of incubation; and
(2) the most recent brain part to mature takes over the leading position in supraspinal
control, only to be subsequently subordinated to the later maturing brain parts. Thus,
supraspinal control comes under the leading role of prosencephalon from day 17 of incubation.

From this brief presentation of our findings it is clear that more refined experimental
approaches are needed before definitive conclusions can be reached regarding the embryonic
development of supraspinal control over spontaneous spinal motor activity.

DEVELOPMENT OF SUPRASPINAL INFLUENCES IN OTHER EMBRYOS AND FETUSES

Little experimental information is available for comparison of chick embryos with other
species. The first and very important attempt was made by Babák (1903, 1907, 1909), who
studied the effects of spinal transection in young versus older larvae and in juvenile versus

adult frogs. In larval stages, no signs of spinal shock developed after a high cervical transection. The first signs of spinal shock occurred at early stages of metamorphosis (froglets still with tail), and was relatively severe following transection through the high cervical spinal segments. In young frogs the spinal shock was fully evident after transection at the upper segments, while in adult frogs severe signs of spinal shock developed even after transection at lower vertebral segments. The author concluded that sensitivity of the developing anuran CNS to spinal transection gradually increases, and spreads from rostral to caudal parts of the spinal cord. Spinal shock is an expression of the onset of inhibitory functions during ontogeny, and this inhibition matures differently in different parts of the CNS.

The development of the spinal shock phenomenon was confirmed by Hooker and Nicholas (1930), who observed an increase in the threshold to tactile stimulation following spinal transection in 13- and 17-day-old rat fetuses. There were no differences noted in overt embryonic motility following operation at this stage of maturation, however Barcroft and Barron (1937) found the first signs of depression of motility after brain transection between day 50 and 60 of gestation in sheep fetuses, and complete inactivity only after day 70 of gestation.

Another set of investigations provides evidence for the role of different brain regions in producing embryonic motility. Detwiler (1948) concluded from his observations on the salamander *Amblystoma* that the forebrain did not affect body movements at early tail bud stages, whereas midbrain structures were able to modify the duration of activity discharges in the spinal neuronal circuits generating spontaneous somatic motility. Corner (1964) confirmed the autonomy of spinal motility at different larval stages in developing anurans (*Rana pipiens, Xenopus laevis*). Transections at various brain levels resulted in abnormal motility patterns only if there was damage in the hindbrain region. The increasing importance of the brain for regulating spinal motility is also suggested by a comparison of the compensation process in young and adult animals following spinal transection (Dimitrijev, 1951). In young rabbits, cats and pigeons this process was 2—4-fold faster than in adults.

These experimental findings in embryos and fetuses other than the chick appear to signify a progressive encephalization (Oppenheim, 1975), which from a certain stage of embryonic development suppresses the early spinal autonomy, and thus gradually subordinates spinal activity to regulatory influences from higher parts of the CNS.

INHIBITORY MECHANISMS IN DEVELOPING SUPRASPINAL CONTROL OF EMBRYONIC SPONTANEOUS MOTILITY

For the further analysis of the ontogeny of supraspinal control, information concerning the morphology, function and biochemistry of the developing spinal synaptic organization are required.

Structural studies

The data on the morphologic development of spinal synapses are still incomplete, but there are 5 basic sources of present information about synaptogenesis in the chick embryo.

The first electron microscopical study in this area was made by Glees and Sheppard (1964). They concluded that the first sign of synaptic maturation — the membrane thickening — develops in axosomatic synapses of the spinal cord in 5-day-old embryos. Two days later, this event is seen also in axodendritic synapses. At day 10, mitochondria and synaptic vesicles are present in the nerve endings. The number of mitochondria increases gradually through day 16, and by day 18 most of the synapses appear to be fully developed.

Wechsler (1966) observed the maturation of embryonic chick spinal synapses in the following steps, starting from day 9: (1) thickening of pre- and postsynaptic membranes; (2) increase in number of round synaptic vesicles; and (3) development of mitochondria and specialized synaptic structures.

Stelzner et al. (1973) observed the first synapses at day 3–4, within the marginal zone near the motor area. On day 5 the number of synapses increases, and they occur also within the motor area. An apparent increase of the synaptic population develops in 8-day-old embryos, mostly in the spinal motor area. At this age some of the presynaptic elements contain flattened vesicles.

An extensive study of this problem was carried out by Oppenheim and his coworkers (Oppenheim and Foelix, 1972; Oppenheim et al., 1975). The first axodendritic synapses were observed in the spinal cord of 4-day-old embryos. They regularly contained spherical vesicles and were characterized by symmetrical membrane thickenings. There were more synapses in the white matter than in the motoneuron neuropil. By day 7 the uniformity of vesicles had given way in some synapses to a mixed vesicle population, and asymmetric synaptic membranes had made their appearance. The axosomatic synapses on spinal motoneurons were first identified at day 6 of incubation, at first with only spherical vesicles and symmetrical membrane thickenings. Flattened vesicles appeared in spinal synapses only at day 10.

From all the above-mentioned findings it may be concluded that, at the end of the first half of incubation, there are synaptic structures in the spinal cord which could mediate the transmission of supraspinal regulatory influences. The existence of developing synaptic elements in the embryonic spinal cord is a good enough reason to search for the chemical substances involved in synaptic transmission, being one of the important indications of actual synaptic function. Morphological indications of synaptic maturation in themselves, of course, do not provide more than indirect evidence for the physiological capacities of developing synaptic machinery in the spinal cord.

Functional studies

Stokes and Bignall (1974) observed that strychnine, which can block certain types of postsynaptic inhibition, caused an increase in the spontaneous bioelectric activity in the motor area of the lumbal cord from day 13 of incubation. They concluded from this that central inhibition influences the spontaneous discharges of spinal motoneurons only after day 12. Oppenheim and Reitzel (1975) found that rather high concentrations of strychnine (7–53 mg/kg, applied onto the chorioallantoic membrane in 7-day-old embryos) caused a marked depression of spontaneous motility, while there was no reaction with lower concentrations. On day 9, strychnine evoked a brief hyperactivity, the duration of which increased on subsequent days, but not until day 13 did this drug produce any signs of convulsions. Myoclonic convulsions first appeared (following a period of overall hyperactivity) in 16-day-old embryos. In older embryos, strychnine evoked the convulsive response without any preceding hyperactivity. The authors suggest that the first signs of strychnine-sensitive (presumably postsynaptic) inhibitory processes may occur as early as 8–9 days of incubation in chick spinal cord. They support this conclusion with evidence that glycine (400 mg/kg) evokes a statistically significant reduction of spontaneous motility both at 9 and at 13 days of incubation.

It is important to compare the behavioral observations with investigations of glycine metabolism in the spinal cord of chick embryos (Zukin et al., 1975). The [^{3}H] glycine up-take increased in two stages, the first one being completed at day 14, and the second one at day 19 of incubation. The receptor binding capacity for glycine gradually increased between day 11 and 14, while the main increase occurred between day 14 and 19.

Our own experiments on intact eggs (Sedláček, 1976) showed that *strychnine* (1 mg/kg egg weight) and *picrotoxin* (1 mg/kg) cause an increase in spontaneous motility at 11 and 13 days (from 16.4 ($\pm$ 2.21) movements/min to 24.4 ($\pm$ 2.22) per min) but no *motor paroxysms* were ever registered at this age. Paroxysmal activation of spontaneous motility occurred for the first time in 15-day-old embryos, and increased in intensity during subsequent days. In 17-day-old embryos, the frequency of motor activity increased by almost 300% during the first 5 min after strychnine application, from 36.4 ($\pm$ 2.14) movements/min to 144.3 ($\pm$ 8.31)

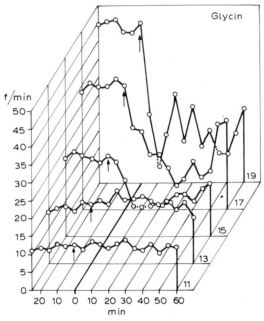

Fig. 4. The development of inhibitory effect of glycine (100 mg/kg egg weight) on the frequency of spontaneous motility in 11–19-day-old chick embryos. Axis x: time in minutes before and after application of glycine (arrows) on the chorioallantoic membrane of egg air space; axis y: total frequency of spontaneous movements per minutes; axis z: age of embryos in days of incubation.

per min – for further quantification, see Fig. 5. The strychnine paroxysms lasted 155.1 ($\pm$ 26.3) sec on the average, and were regularly followed by a resting period of 126.5 ($\pm$ 24.7) sec. The whole period of strychnine-evoked paroxysmal activity lasted about 35 min. In this, our results are consistent with the findings by Oppenheim and Reitzel (1975).

In contrast, the putative inhibitory amino acid transmitters, *glycine* (100 mg/kg egg weight) and *GABA* (100 mg/kg), both had an *inhibitory* effect upon spontaneous motility – for the first time in 15-day-old embryos, and with an apparent increase in this depression on subsequent days of incubation (Sedláček, 1977a; Fig. 4). This result is supported by the finding that the antagonisms between strychnine and glycine, and between picrotoxin and GABA, appeared in characteristic fashion only after day 15 of incubation. In younger embryos, glycine and GABA were unable to modify or to reverse the augmentation of spontaneous motility caused by the two excitatory drugs (Sedláček, 1977b).

376

The effectiveness of strychnine and picrotoxin, and the ineffectiveness of inhibitory amino acids before day 15 of incubation, raises questions about the effect of these drugs prior to the onset of sensitivity for glycine and GABA. One possibility for explaining the effects of strychnine and picrotoxin in the spinal cord before day 15 is a direct depolarizing action on the excitable membranes of spinal neurons (Li, 1959; Curtis, 1969). This mode of action could be mediated by direct changes of membrane permeability, which would be reflected in increased excitability — and even spontaneous discharges — of the motoneurons. In such a case, the effects of excitatory drugs would not require the presence (and sensitivity) of specific inhibitory receptors in the postsynaptic membranes. This means that the synaptically mediated inhibitory mechanisms in the spinal cord would develop relatively late, possibly in relation to the maturation of synaptic connections from supraspinal control mechanisms (Änggard et al., 1961; Bergström et al., 1962; Naka, 1964; Mellström, 1971).

There is some support for this viewpoint in analogy with the distinction made between spinal and supraspinal components of spontaneous motility, it is possible to characterize the effects of the excitatory drugs and the inhibitory amino acids in the same way. Thus, in 13-day-old embryos the excitatory effects of strychnine and picrotoxin were the same in normal as in spinal embryos, in agreement with the exclusively spinal origin of spontaneous motility at this age. In 17-day-old embryos, however, the spinal component of strychnine activation was only 30%, and the supraspinal component 70% (Fig. 5), i.e. the same developmental

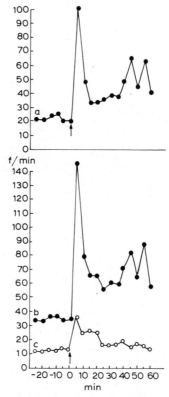

Fig. 5. Spinal and supraspinal components of strychnine activation of spontaneous motility in 17-day-old chick embryos. Abscissa: time in minutes before and after application (arrows) of strychnine (1 mg/kg egg weight); ordinate: frequency of spontaneous movements per minute. a: supraspinal component of total motility (= line b − c); b: cerebrospinal activity (i.e. motility in normal embryos); c: spinal component of motility (i.e. motility in chronically decapitated embryos).

pattern as that characterizing the excitatory effect of picrotoxin (Sedláček, 1978b). A similar comparison could be made with the glycine and GABA inhibitory effects in normal and spinal embryos (Sedláček, 1978a): in 15-day-old embryos the supraspinal component of the glycine effect was only 3% of the total effect, while in 17-day-old embryos it had increased to more than 40% (Fig. 6).

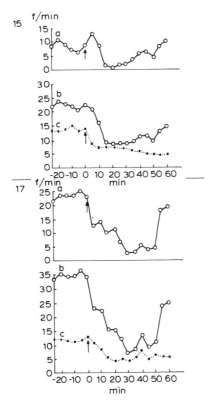

Fig. 6. Spinal and supraspinal components of glycine inhibition of spontaneous motility in 15- and 17-day-old chick embryos. Abscissa: time in minutes before and after application (arrows) of glycine (100 mg/kg egg weight); ordinate: frequency of spontaneous movements per minute. a: supraspinal component of motility (i.e. line b — line c); b: cerebrospinal activity (i.e. motility in normal embryos); c: spinal component of motility (i.e. motility in chronically decapitated embryos).

From these findings we derive the following working hypothesis.

(1) The excitatory effects of strychnine and picrotoxin, prior to the onset of supraspinal control at day 15 of incubation, are caused by a direct depolarizing effect upon the excitable membranes of spinal motoneurons, an effect which does not require the intervention of synaptic transmission.

(2) After the onset of supraspinal control, the major part of the excitatory effects of strychnine and picrotoxin upon spinal motor output is mediated by synaptic elements sensitive to the putative inhibitory transmitters glycine and GABA.

(3) The onset of supraspinal control over the motor activity of the cord is identical to the onset of active inhibition of spontaneous motoneuron output. The periodicity of spontaneous motility in chick embryos before this stage of development may reflect primarily the intrinsic cycles of excitability of spontaneously discharging spinal inter- and/or motoneurons.

The above viewpoint, derived from the present stage of our research, admittedly needs further experimental support, especially in view of the differences from other conceptions regarding the embryonic development of supraspinal control of spontaneous motility in the chick (see Oppenheim, 1975).

GENERAL DEVELOPMENT OF CENTRAL EXCITATORY AND INHIBITORY MECHANISMS

The results on chick embryos require comparison with other developmental studies about the maturation of central excitatory and inhibitory mechanisms. Attempting to answer this question at our present level of knowledge meets with considerable difficulty, due to numerous discrepancies among the reported experimental results. A fruitful approach, however, has been the study of fetal nervous tissue cultivated in vitro. Crain (1976) summarizes his extensive results on the appearance of sensitivity to excitatory and inhibitory drugs (in explants of several different regions of the fetal rodent CNS) by the following major conclusions.

(1) The excitatory activity of simple cell assemblies, which is the first to occur in the functional development of tissue explants, is quickly subjected to tonic inhibitory mechanisms during the early stages of synaptogenesis in vitro (Crain, 1976).

(2) Early tonic inhibition has the same neuropharmacological characteristics as do central inhibitory mechanisms in situ (i.e. sensitivity to picrotoxin, bicuculline, strychnine, chloride-free medium, etc.: Crain et al., 1975).

(3) Spinal cord sensitivity in culture to glycine and GABA provides evidence for the existence of inhibitory circuits in the spinal cord during early embryogenesis (Crain, 1976).

It is important to emphasize two points which have special significance for the evaluation of Crain's results. The first is that there are some indications that the excitatory effect of strychnine is not due solely to the blockage of glycine-sensitive inhibition. Straughan (1974) reported a strychnine-induced reduction of depressant effects evoked by glycine or various other drugs (GABA, dopamine, noradrenaline, and 5-hydroxytryptamine). In addition, strychnine has been shown to interfere with ionic movements across neuronal membranes (Araki, 1965), resulting in direct excitatory effects (Curtis et al., 1971). Secondly, Crain's conclusions were derived from experiments carried out on cultures of spinal cord and cerebral cortex from rodent fetuses (mouse and rat), explanted at 13—21 days of gestation, but with neuropharmacological analysis usually being started only some days afterwards. Rodent fetuses in situ, however, exhibit spontaneous motility as early as the 15th day of gestation (Angulo y Gonzales, 1932; Narayanan et al., 1971), and for this reason there is a problem in comparing the results obtained from tissue culture models of neural maturation to the normal step-by-step development of the intact nervous system.

This difficulty can be demonstrated by studies of spinal inhibition carried out on fetuses in situ. There are several indications that central inhibition develops only *after* the onset of excitatory nervous activity. Thus, simultaneous contractions of antagonistic muscles in the chick embryo were still observed at day 13, while reciprocal inhibition did not become fully evident until 19 days of incubation (Bekoff, 1976). Similarly, antagonistic motor inhibition in sheep fetuses develops after day 90 of gestation, whereas excitatory processes are evident 50—60 days earlier (Anggard et al., 1961). Essentially the same temporal relationship has been observed in fetal guinea pig (Bergström et al., 1961, 1962), rhesus monkey (Bodian, 1968), and human fetuses (Hooker, 1952; Humphrey, 1964, 1969). On the other hand, there is some experimental evidence indicating precocious development of inhibitory synaptic mechanisms in certain systems, perhaps even *before* the onset of excitatory ones (e.g. functional inhibitory synapses in the hippocampus of the newborn kitten: Purpura, 1971); sensitivity to picrotoxin and bicuculline occurs several days before the onset of sensitivity to strychnine in the chick embryo (Oppenheim and Reitzel, 1975).

It is evident from the presented material that the problem of development of central excitatory and inhibitory mechanisms is still open for further experimental research, and that no definitive conclusions can be formulated at the present time.

PARTICIPATION OF AMINERGIC MECHANISMS IN SUPRASPINAL CONTROL OF EMBRYONIC SPONTANEOUS MOTILITY

A large body of experimental information has been recently obtained about the importance of aminergic neural mechanisms for different forms of behavior in adult organisms, including man. These findings come from the fields of *behavioral* investigations, *biochemical* analysis, and *morphological* studies of aminergic neurons and systems within the CNS (Coyle and Axelrod, 1972; Coyle and Henry, 1973; Jacobowitz and Palkovits, 1974; Lindvall and Björklund, 1974; Gripois, 1975; Jacobs et al., 1975; Seiden et al., 1975; Watanabe and Watanabe, 1975). Furthermore, recent neuropharmacological research has corroborated the importance of aminergic synaptic mechanisms associated with different behaviors (Strömbom, 1975). This approach offers possibilities for detecting, at the cellular level, the participation of monoaminergic systems in specific behavioral patterns. Apomorphine and dopamine have been shown to inhibit neuronal firing in DA-neurons (Aghajanian and Bunney, 1973; Bunney et al., 1973). Similar inhibition was obtained after treatment with clonidine and noradrenaline in NA-neurons (Svensson et al., 1975) and in 5-HT-neurons after treatment with LSD or 5-hydroxytryptamine (Haigler and Aghajanian, 1974).

It is known from biochemical observations in chick embryos that the aminergic transmitters – noradrenaline, dopamine and 5-hydroxytryptamine – and their specific enzyme systems go through their main developmental changes only during the second half of incubation (Bourne, 1965; Sparber and Shideman, 1969, 1970; Lydiard and Sparber, 1972; Dolezalova et al., 1974; Suzuki and Yagi, 1975). The effects of systemic application of all 3 aminergic transmitters showed that spontaneous motility in chick embryos is not affected before day 15 of incubation. From day 15, all 3 transmitters caused a depression of spontaneous motility (Sedláček, 1977c; Fig. 7).

In accordance with these results are data concerning the development of sensitivity to several drugs which interfere with the metabolism, storage and liberation of aminergic transmitters (Seiden et al., 1975). Chloropromazine, reserpine and dehydrobenzperidol, all of which are ineffective in 11- and 13-day-old embryos, begin from day 15 to produce depression of spontaneous motility. In reserpinized chick embryos at 17 and 19 days in ovo, apomorphine produces 4 hr long activation of spontaneous motility, the characteristics of which depend upon both the embryonic age and the interval between administration of the two drugs. Whereas *reserpine* alone (2.5 mg/kg egg weight) depressed the motility in 19-day-old embryos from 43.3 (± 2.65) movements/min to 11.4 (± 1.29) per min, *apomorphine* (1 mg/kg) brought the frequency up to 34.0 (± 2.88) per min i.e. 78.5% of the normal value, and more than three times the reserpine-depressed value. The excitatory behavioral effect of apomorphine in the reserpinized chick embryo consisted mainly of an initial attack of large movements (already in the first few minutes after application) followed by a

380

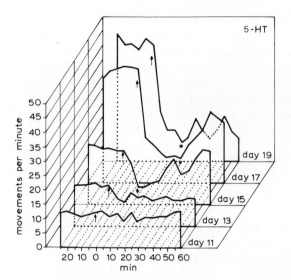

Fig. 7. Development of the effect of 5-hydroxytryptamine (5 mg/kg egg weight) on spontaneous motility in 11–19-day-old chick embryos. x axis: time in minutes before and after 5-HT application (arrows); y axis: total frequency of spontaneous movements per minute; z axis: age of embryos in days of incubation. Asterisks indicate the statistically significant minima of movement frequency.

continued augmentation of the spontaneous motility level. This effect is in striking contrast with the explicit *depressive* effect of apomorphine alone.

All these results are in good agreement with the known inhibitory effects of aminergic transmitters upon spinal activity (McLennan, 1961; Biscoe and Curtis, 1966; Biscoe et al., 1966; Engberg and Ryall, 1966; Weight and Salmoiraghi, 1966, 1967; Phillis et al., 1968). Further support follows from the results of biochemical and of fluorescent histochemical analysis, which have demonstrated the highest concentration of biogenic amines in the lateral and in the ventral spinal horn, especially surrounding the motoneurons (Ikeda and Gotoh, 1974; Zivin et al., 1975). The data cited provide a good basis for the further study of aminergic participation in the development of supraspinal control over spontaneous motility in the chick embryo.

SUMMARY AND CONCLUSIONS

There have been several different conceptions about the development of supraspinal control of spontaneous motility in chick embryos. The earliest view supposes the origin of supraspinal control to be at very early stages of embryonic development (Windle and Orr, 1934; Visintini and Levi-Montalcini, 1939). A later view places the onset of supraspinal influences about halfway through incubation, viz. just before day 10 (Hamburger et al., 1965; Oppenheim, 1975).

Our own viewpoint is based upon a common feature present in a variety of experimental findings (development of spinal shock, the effects of chronic decapitation, the development of inhibitory effects of glycine and GABA, and the development of sensitivity to aminergic transmitters and related drugs). All these events occur in chick embryos, at least for so far as they are manifested in the level of spontaneous motility, at about day 15 of incubation. We deduce from these correlations that prior to day 15 the spinal cord is a largely sovereign generator of the spontaneous motility. From day 15 onwards, however, the spinal motor system becomes gradually subordinated to effective supraspinal control, which maintains and modulates the activity of spinal motor output by both excitatory and inhibitory descending pathways.

The differences between our own experimental findings and conclusions, and those of other authors, indicate that an important task for developmental neurophysiology is to classify the relationship between intrinsic and extrinsic sources of spontaneous motor activity within the spinal cord.

REFERENCES

Aghajanian, G.K. and Bunney, B.S. (1973) Central dopaminergic neurons: neurophysiological identification and responses to drugs. In *Frontiers in Catecholamine Research*, E. Usdin and S. Snyder (Eds.), Pergamon Press, New York, pp. 643–648.

Anggard, L., Bergström, R. and Bernhard, V.G. (1965) Analysis of prenatal reflex activity in sheep, *Acta physiol. scand.*, 53: 128–136.

Angulo y Gonzales, A.W. (1932) The prenatal development of behavior in the albino rat, *J. comp. Neurol.*, 55: 395–442.

Araki, T. (1965) The effects of strychnine on the postsynaptic inhibitory action. In *Lectures and Symposia, XXIII Int. Congr. Physiol. Sci.*, Tokyo, pp. 96–97.

Babák, E. (1903) Ueber die Entwicklung der locomotorischen Coordinationsthätigkeit im Rückenmarke des Frosches, *Pflügers Arch. ges. Physiol.*, 93: 134–162.

Babák, E. (1907) Ueber die Shockwirkungen nach der Durchtrennung des Zentralnervensystems und ihre Beziehung zur ontogenetischen Entwicklung, *Zbl. Physiol.*, 21: 9–11.

Babák, E. (1909) Zur ontogenetischen und phylogenetischen Betrachtung der Funktionen des Zentralnervensystems, insbesonders des Rückenmarksshocks, *Zbl. Physiol.*, 23: 151–155.

Barcroft, J. and Barron, D.H. (1937) Movements in mid-foetal life in the sheep embryo, *J. Physiol. (Lond.)*, 91: 329–351.

Bekoff, A., (1976) Ontogeny of leg motor output in the chick embryo: a neural analysis, *Brain Res.*, 106: 271–291.

Bergström, R.M., Hellström P.E. and Stenberg, D. (1962) Studies in reflex irradiation in the foetal guinea pig, *Ann. Chir. Gynec. Fenn.*, 51: 171–178.

Biscoe, T.J. and Curtis, D.R. (1966) Noradrenaline and inhibition of Renshaw cells, *Science*, 151: 1230–1231.

Biscoe, T.J., Curtis, D.R. and Ryall, R.W. (1966) An investigation of catecholamine receptors of spinal interneurons, *Int. J. Neuropharmacol.*, 5: 429–434.

Bodian, D. (1968) Development of fine structure of the spinal cord in monkey fetuses. II. Pre-reflex period to period of long inter-segmental reflexes, *J. comp. Neurol.*, 133: 133–166.

Bourne, B.B. (1965) Metabolism of amines in the brain of the chick during embryonic development, *Life Sci.*, 4: 583–592.

Bunney, B.S., Aghajanian, G.K. and Roth, R.H. (1973) Comparison of effects of L-DOPA, amphetamine and apomorphine of firing rate of rat dopaminergic neurons, *Nature New Biol.*, 245: 123–125.

Corner, M.A. (1964) Rhythmicity in the early swimming of anuran larvae, *J. Embryol. exp. Morphol.*, 12: 665–671.

Corner, M.A. and Bakhuis, W.L. (1969) Developmental patterns in the central nervous system of birds. V. Cerebral electrical activity, forebrain function and behavior in the chick at the time of hatching, *Brain Res.*, 13: 541–555.

Coyle, J.T. and Axelrod, J. (1972) Dopamine-β-hydroxylase in the rat brain: developmental characteristics, *J. Neurochem.*, 19: 449–459.

Coyle, J.T. and Henry, D. (1973) Catecholamines in fetal and newborn rat brain, *J. Neurochem.*, 21: 61–67.

Crain, S.M. (1976) *Neurophysiologic Studies in Tissue Culture*, Raven Press, New York.

Crain, S.M., Raine, C.S. and Bornstein, M.B. (1975) Early formation of synaptic networks in culture of fetal mouse cerebral neocortex and hippocampus, *J. Neurobiol.*, 6: 329–336.

382

Curtis, D.R. (1969) The pharmacology of spinal postsynaptic inhibition. In *Mechanisms of Synaptic Transmission, Progress in Brain Research, Vol. 31,* K. Akert and P.G.Waser (Eds.), Elsevier, Amsterdam. pp. 171–189.

Curtis, D.R., Duggan, A.W. and Johnston, G.A.R. (1969) Glycine, strychnine, picrotoxin and spinal inhibition, *Brain Res.,* 14: 759–762.

Curtis, D.R., Duggan, A.W. and Johnston, G.A.R. (1971) The specificity of strychnine as a glycine antagonist in the mammalian spinal cord, *Exp. Brain Res.,* 12: 547–565.

Decker, J.D. and Hamburger, V. (1967) The influence of different brain regions on periodic motility of the chick embryo, *J. exp. Zool.,* 165: 371–384.

Detwiler, S.R. (1948) Quantitative studies on locomotor responses in *Amblystoma* larvae following surgical alterations in the nervous system, *Ann. N.Y. Acad. Sci.,* 49: 834–855.

Dmitrijev, V.D. (1951) *The Role of Brain Hemispheres in Compensatory Processes after Damage of the Spinal Cord.* Doctoral Dissertation, University of Leningrad (in Russian).

Dolezalova, H., Giacobini, E., Giacobini, G., Rossi, A. and Toschi, G. (1974) Developmental variations of choline acetyltransferase, dopamine-β-hydroxylase and monoaminooxidase in chicken embryo and chicken sympathetic ganglia, *Brain Res.,* 73: 309–320.

Donkelaar, H.J.ten (1975) *Descending Pathways from the Brain Stem to the Spinal Cord in Some Reptiles.* Doctoral Dissertation, University of Nijmegen.

Engberg, I. and Ryall, R.W. (1966) The inhibitory action of noradrenaline and other monoamines on spinal neurons, *J. Physiol. (Lond.),* 185: 298–322.

Glees, P. and Sheppard, B.L. (1964) Electron microscopical studies of the synapse in the developing spinal cord. *Z. Zellforsch.,* 62: 356–362.

Gottlieb, G. (1973) Introduction to behavioral embryology. In *Behavioral Embryology,* G. Gottlieb (Ed.), Academic Press, New York, pp. 3–45.

Gripois, D. (1975) Developmental characteristics of monoamineoxidase (review). *Comp. Biochem. Physiol.,* 51: 143–151.

Gutmann, E. (1964) Neurotrophic relations in the regeneration process. In *Mechanisms of Neural Regeneration, Progress in Brain Research, Vol. 13,* M. Singer and J.P. Schadé (Eds.), Elsevier, Amsterdam, pp. 72–112.

Haigler, H.J. and Aghajanian, G.K. (1974) Lysergic acid diethylamide and serotonin: a comparison of effects on serotonergic neurons and neurons receiving a serotonergic input, *J. Pharmacol. exp. Ther.,* 188: 688–699.

Hamburger, V. (1963) Some aspects of the embryology of behavior, *Quart. Rev. Biol.,* 38: 342–365.

Hamburger, V. (1971) Development of embryonic motility. In *The Biopsychology of Development,* E. Tobach, L.R. Aronson and E. Shaw (Eds.), Academic Press, New York, pp. 45–66.

Hamburger, V. and Balaban, M. (1963) Observations and experiments on spontaneous rhythmical behavior in the chick embryo, *Develop. Biol.,* 7: 533–545.

Hamburger, V., Balaban, M., Oppenheim, R.W. and Wenger, E. (1965) Periodic motility of normal and spinal chick embryos between 8 and 17 days of incubation, *J. exp. Zool.,* 159: 1–14.

Hamburger, V. and Hamilton, H.L. (1951) A series of normal stages in the development of the chick embryo, *J. Morph.,* 88: 49–92.

Harvey, W. (1651) *Exercitationes de Generatione Animalium,* London.

Hooker, D. (1952) *The Prenatal Origin of Behavior,* University of Kansas Press, Lawrence.

Hooker, D. and Nicholas, J.S. (1930) Spinal cord section in rat fetuses, *J. comp. Neurol.,* 50: 413–459.

Hughes, A. (1965) Some effects of de-afferentation on the developing amphibian nervous system, *J Embryol. exp. Morphol.,* 14: 75–87.

Humphrey, T. (1964) Some correlations between the appearance of human fetal reflexes and the development of the nervous system. In *Growth and Maturation of the Brain, Progress in Brain Research, Vol. 4,* D.P. Purpura and J.P. Schadé (Eds.), Elsevier, Amsterdam, pp. 93–133.

Humphrey, T. (1969) Postnatal repetition of human prenatal activity sequences with some suggestion of their neuroanatomical basis. In *Brain and Early Behaviour Development in the Fetus and Infant,* R.J. Robinson (Ed.), Academic Press, New York, pp. 43–84.

Ikeda, H. and Gotoh, J. (1974) Distribution of monoamine-containing terminals and fibers in the central nervous system of the chicken, *Jap. J. Pharmacol.,* 24: 831–841.

Jacobowitz, D.M. and Palkovits, M. (1974) Topographic atlas of catecholamine and acetylcholinesterase-containing neurons in the rat brain, *J. comp. Neurol.,* 157: 13–28.

Jacobs, B.L., Wise, W.D. and Taylor, K.M. (1975) Is there a catecholamine-serotonin interaction in the control of locomotor activity? *Neuropharmacology,* 14: 501–506.

Li, C.L. (1959) Cortical intracellular potentials and their responses to strychnine, *J. Neurophysiol.*, 22: 436–450.

Lindvall, O. and Björklund, A., (1974) The organization of the ascending catecholamine neuron systems in the rat brain as revealed by the glyoxylic acid fluorescence method, *Acta physiol. scand..* Suppl. 412.

Lydiard, R.B. and Sparber, S.B. (1972) Possible induction of tyrosine hydroxylase in chick embryo brain from reserpine administration prior to incubation. In *Proc. Int. Pect. Meet.,* San Francisco, California.

McLennan, H. (1961) The effect of some catecholamines upon a monosynaptic reflex pathway in the spinal cord, *J. Physiol. (Lond.),* 158: 411–425.

Mellström, A. (1971) Recurrent and antidromic effects on the monosynaptic reflex during postnatal development in the cat, *Acta physiol. scand.,* 82: 490–499.

Naka, K.I. (1964) Electrophysiology of the fetal spinal cord. II. Interaction among peripheral inputs and recurrent inhibition, *J. gen. Physiol.,* 47: 1023–1028.

Narayanan, C.H., Fox, M.W. and Hamburger, V. (1971) Prenatal development of spontaneous and evoked activity in the rat *(Rattus norvegicus albinus), Behaviour,* 40: 100–134.

Oppenheim, R.W. (1972) Experimental studies on hatching behavior in the chick. III. The role of the midbrain and forebrain, *J. comp. Neurol.,* 146: 479–505.

Oppenheim, R.W. (1975) The role of supraspinal input in embryonic motility: a re-examination in the chick, *J. comp. Neurol.,* 160: 37–50.

Oppenheim, R.W., Chu-Wang, I. and Foelix, R.F. (1975) Some aspects of synaptogenesis in the spinal cord of the chick embryo: a quantitative electron microscopic study, *J. comp. Neurol.,* 161: 383–418.

Oppenheim, R.W. and Foelix, R.F. (1972) Synaptogenesis in the chick embryo spinal cord, *Nature (Lond.),* 235: 126–128.

Oppenheim, R.W. and Narayanan, C.H. (1968) Experimental studies on hatching behavior in the chick. I. Thoracic spinal gaps, *J. exp. Zool.,* 168: 387–394.

Oppenheim, R.W. and Reitzel, J. (1975) Ontogeny of behavioral sensitivity to strychnine in the chick embryo: evidence for the early onset of CNS inhibition, *Brain Behav. Evol.,* 11: 130–159.

Orr, D.W. and Windle, W.F. (1934) The development of behavior in chick embryos: the appearance of somatic movements, *J. comp. Neurol.,* 60: 271–285.

Phillis, J.W., Tebecis, A.K. and York, D.H. (1968) Depression of spinal motoneurons by noradrenaline, 5-hydroxytryptamine and histamine, *Europ. J. Pharmacol.,* 4: 471–475.

Provine, R.R. (1973) Neurophysiological aspects of behavior development in the chick embryo. In *Behavioral Embryology,* G. Gottlieb (Ed.), Academic Press, New York, pp. 77–102.

Purpura, D.P. (1971) Synaptogenesis in mammalian cortex: problems and perspectives. In *Brain Development and Behavior,* M.B. Sterman, D.J. McGinty and A.M. Adinolfi (Eds.), Academic Press, New York, pp. 23–41.

Rhines, R. (1943) An experimental study of development of the medial longitudinal fasciculus in the chick, *J. comp. Neurol.,* 79: 107–127.

Sedláček, J. (1976) Development of spontaneous motility in chick embryos. Normal development and activatory effects of strychnine and picrotoxin, *Physiol. bohemoslov.,* 25: 505–510.

Sedláček, J. (1977a) Development of spontaneous motility in chick embryos. Inhibitory effect of glycine and γ-aminobutyric acid, *Physiol. bohemoslov.,* 26: 9–12.

Sedláček, J. (1977b) Development of spontaneous motility in chick embryos. Interaction of strychnine, glycine and GABA, *Physiol. bohemoslov.,* 26: 111–114.

Sedláček, J. (1977c) Development of spontaneous motility in chick embryos. The possible role of aminergic transmission, *Physiol. bohemoslov.,* 26: 425–433.

Sedláček, J. (1978a) Development of spontaneous motility in chick embryos. Spinal and supraspinal components of inhibitory effects of glycine and GABA, *Physiol. bohemoslov.,* 27: 105–115.

Sedláček, J. (1978b) Development of spontaneous motility in chick embryos. Spinal and supraspinal components of strychnine and picrotoxin activation, *Physiol. bohemoslov.,* 27: 97–103.

Sedláček, J. and Doskočil, M. (1978) Development of spontaneous motility in chick embryos. The role of supraspinal control, *Physiol. bohemoslov,* 27: 7–14.

Seiden, L.S., McPhail, R.C. and Oglesby, M.W. (1975) Catecholamines and drug-behavior interactions, *Fed. Proc.,* 34: 1823–1831.

Sparber, S.B. and Shideman, F.E. (1969) Estimation of catecholamines in the brains of embryonic and newly hatched chickens and the effect of reserpine, *Develop. Psychobiol.,* 2: 115–119.

384

Sparber, S.B. and Shideman, F.E. (1970) Elevated catecholamines in thirty-day-old chicken brain after depletion during embryogenesis, *Develop. Psychobiol.*, 3: 123–129.

Stelzner, D.J., Martin, A.H. and Scott, G.L. (1973) Early stages of synaptogenesis in the cervical spinal cord of the chick embryo, *Z. Zellforsch.*, 138: 475–488.

Stokes, B.T. and Bignall, K.E. (1974) The emergence of inhibition in the chick embryo spinal cord, *Brain Res.*, 77: 231–242.

Straughan, D.W. (1974) Convulsant drugs: amino acid antagonism and central inhibition, *Neuropharmacology*, 13: 495–508.

Strömbom, U. (1975) On the functional role of pre- and postsynaptic catecholamine receptors in brain, *Acta physiol. scand.*, Suppl. 431.

Suzuki, O. and Yagi, K. (1975) 5-Hydroxytryptamine and monoamine-oxidase in developing chick spinal cord, *J. Neurochem.*, 25: 189–190.

Svensson, T.H., Bunney, B.S. and Aghajanian, G.K. (1975) Inhibition of both noradrenergic and serotonergic neurons in brain by the α-adrenergic agonist clonidine, *Brain Res.*, 92: 291–306.

Visintini, F., e Levi-Montalcini, R. (1939) Relazione tra differenziazione strutturale e funzionale dei centri e delle vie nervose nell'embrione di pollo, *Arch. Suiss Neurol. Psychiat.*, 43: 1–45.

Watanabe, H.Y. and Watanabe, K. (1975) The effect of lowering the serotonin content of rat brain on spontaneous locomotor activity, *Chem. Pharmacol. Bull.*, 23: 1192–1196.

Wechsler, W. (1966) Elektronmikroskopischer Beitrag zur Nervenzell-differenzierung und Histogenese der grauen Substanz des Rückenmarkes von Hühnenembryonen, *Z. Zellforsch.*, 74: 401–422.

Weight, F.F. and Salmoiraghi, G.C. (1966) Responses of spinal cord interneurons to acetylcholine, norepinephrine and serotonin administered by microelectrophoresis, *J. Pharmacol. exp. Ther.*, 153: 420–427.

Weight, F.F. and Salmoiraghi, G.C. (1967) Motoneurone depression by norepinephrine, *Nature (Lond.)*, 213: 1229–1230.

Windle, W.F. and Austin, M.F. (1936) Neurofibrillar development in the central nervous system of chick embryos up to 5-days incubation, *J. comp. Neurol.*, 63: 431–463.

Windle, W.F. and Baxter, R.E. (1936) Development of reflex mechanisms in the spinal cord of albino rat embryos. Correlations between structure and function and comparisons with the cat and chick, *J. comp. Neurol.*, 63: 189–209.

Windle, W.F. and Orr, D.W. (1934) The development of behavior in chick embryos: spinal cord structure correlated with early somatic activity, *J. comp. Neurol.*, 60: 287–308.

Zivin, J.A., Reid, J.L., Saavedra, J.M. and Kopin, I.S. (1975) Quantitative localization of biogenic amines in the spinal cord, *Brain Res.*, 99: 293–301.

Zukin, S.R., Young, A.B. and Snyder, S.H. (1975) Development of the synaptic glycine receptors in chick embryo spinal cord, *Brain Res.*, 83: 525–530.

Possible Embryonic Origin
of Sleep Interstrain Differences
in the Mouse

J.L. VALATX

Laboratoire de Médecine Expérimentale, Université Claude Bernard, 69373 Lyon Cedex 2 (France)

INTRODUCTION

This paper reviews data about the relationships between genetics and sleep, that is to say, about the hereditary transmission of sleep traits in animals. For 20 years, the phenomenology and biochemical mechanisms of sleep have been described in many different mammals (Allison and Van Twyver, 1974; Jouvet, 1972, 1973; Zepelin and Rechtshaffen, 1974). In each species, results have been obtained in randomly selected individuals representing the average of non-homogenous populations. In spite of considerable intraspecific variability, significant differences have been shown to exist among different species. Are these differences due to environmental factors, or to the results of alterations in the functioning of the central nervous system? To answer this question a genetic approach can be a good model. However, in genetics the choice of animal is a very important point.

In animals, *Escherichia coli* and the fruit fly, *Drosophila,* are well known in genetic research but are not suitable models for sleep because, as far as we know, these two types of living beings do not 'dream' at all. It is necessary to take a mammal having both slow wave sleep (SWS) and paradoxical sleep (PS), and with many different available strains and mutants. For these reasons, the mouse (*Mus musculus*), used in genetic research since 1910, has been chosen. The mouse is not the only animal that can be used in this approach. Indeed, many different mammals could in principle be employed for genetic studies of sleep, such as cats or monkeys, but the speed of reproduction is often a very serious limitation.

Almost all the hereditary neurological diseases described in man exist also in mice: epilepsia, many dysgeneses, and atrophias of different parts of the brain (Sidman et al., 1965). Numerous inbred strains have been isolated by brother-sister matings for at least 20 generations. As a consequence, all the subjects from a given strain are almost completely homozygous for all of their genes. The laboratory mouse now can be used as a prototype in behavioral genetics to separate the different components of a given behavior, and to determine the respective influence of environmental and hereditary factors (Green, 1966; Friedman, 1974; Oliverio, 1974; Valatx and Bugat, 1974; Valatx et al., 1977). The combination of relatively low intrastrain variability and high interstrain variability in sleep patterns allows the approach of 'genetic dissection' of the sleep-waking cycle, in order to attempt to understand the neurophysiological mechanisms of the observed variations.

The results to be presented here suggest that the origin of these sleep variations might be traced back 'in utero' to the moment of the formation of the nervous system. The proposed model also allows for the study of fetal development and eventual alterations of nervous structures involved in the production and regulation of the sleep-waking cycle, as well as of their role in the development of the central nervous system.

EXPERIMENTAL FINDINGS IN MOUSE SLEEP STUDIES

Selection of animals

All the subjects were male, 12–15-week-old, mice from four inbred strains: C57BR/cd/Orl(BR), C57BL/6/Orl (B6), Balb/c/Orl (C), CBA/Orl, F1 hybrids: BRxCBA and BRxC. To study eventual linkages with the histocompatibility genes (H loci) used as markers, *Recombinant Inbred Strains* (RI) of Bailey were studied. Production of these strains is described by Bailey (1975): "The RI strains were derived from the cross of two unrelated and highly inbred progenitor strains, C and B6, and then maintained independently from the F2 generation under a full-sib mating regimen. This procedure progressively fixed the chance recombination of alleles as inbreeding proceeded and as full homozygosis was approached. The resulting battery of strains can be looked upon as a finite but replicable recombinant population". For each H locus, a characteristic strain distribution pattern (SDP) is established by determining which of the alleles (B6 or C) is present in these RI strains. We have studied parental strains: C57BL/6By, Balb/c By, F1 hybrids and 7 RI strains: CxBD, CxBE, CxBG, CxBH, CxBI, CxBJ, CxBK.

Methods for sleep recordings

Under Nembutal anesthesia, at least 8 mice from each strain were chronically implanted with cortical and muscular electrodes. Each mouse was put on synthetic litter in a glass jar with standard food and tap water ad libitum. Environmental conditions were constant as far as possible: ambient temperature was 24 ± 1 °C, on a lighting schedule consisting of 12 hr light (7.00–19.00) and 12 hr darkness (19.00–7.00). After a 10-day period of adaptation to recording conditions, continuous recording (24 hr per day) for a week was carried out. By visual analysis, all the recordings were scored by 30-sec epochs. Statistical analysis described elsewhere (Kan et al., 1976; Valatx and Chouvet, 1975) was performed on the sleep data from 5 consecutive days after the adaptation period, in order to give an estimation of rhythmicity using the method of sine-wave harmonic decomposition. Statistical analysis of Bailey strains (variance and Student-Newman-Keuls multiple range test) was performed at the Jackson Laboratory, Bar Harbor, U.S.A.

Genetics of EEG sleep parameters

During SWS, the EEG activity consists of characteristic spindle activity (8–10 Hz, 800 μV) associated with slow waves (SWS) in CBA and C mice. In B6 mice, the spindle activity is more rapid (12–15 Hz, 400 μV), while in BR mice only SWS without any spindles have been registered (Valatx and Bugat, 1974). During PS, the EEG activity consists of a very regular theta activity, the frequency of which varies according to the strains: 7.22 ± 0.4 Hz in C mice and 8.33 ± 0.2 Hz ($P < 0.001$) in BR mice. In F1 hybrids, the theta frequency was intermediate (7.5 ± 0.3 Hz).

Genetics of sleep durations

Results in inbred strains can be summarized as follows: (1) total, night and day sleep durations differed significantly from strain to strain; (2) day-night variations were a good parameter for discriminating the strains. Both of the C57 strains show the greatest difference, while in C mice there is no significant difference between day and night sleep duration. (Table I).

TABLE I

SLEEP PATTERNS IN INBRED STRAINS AND F1 HYBRIDS

Duration: minutes ± standard error of the mean.

	Slow wave sleep duration			Paradoxical sleep duration			PS/SWS		
	24 Hr	Night	Day	24 Hr	Night	Day	24 Hr	Night	Day
CBA	746 ± 7.10	322 ± 5.14	424 ± 3.75	66.5 ± 1.62	24.0 ± 0.77	42.5 ± 1.24	08.91	07.91	10.03
CBA.BR F1	741 ± 10.7	331 ± 2.25	410 ± 6.97	65.0 ± 2.10	26.5 ± 1.40	38.5 ± 1.84	08.77	08.00	09.39
BR.CBA F1	754 ± 11.9	316 ± 9.76	438 ± 6.76	65.5 ± 2.26	23.0 ± 1.56	42.5 ± 2.01	08.68	07.27	09.70
BR	672 ± 7.70	213 ± 8.72	459 ± 3.20	73.0 ± 2.50	19.0 ± 1.35	54.0 ± 1.49	10.85	08.92	11.76
BR.C F1	692 ± 8.65	277 ± 3.50	415 ± 3.60	67.0 ± 2.0	20.0 ± 1.20	47.0 ± 1.40	09.68	07.22	11.32
C.BR F1	735 ± 7.42	342 ± 4.34	393 ± 3.32	80.0 ± 2.5	36.0 ± 1.3	44.0 ± 1.20	10.88	10.52	11.19
C	744 ± 9.34	339 ± 6.49	405 ± 8.74	56.0 ± 1.8	29.0 ± 1.5	27.0 ± 1.15	07.52	08.55	06.66

In F1 hybrids, the results differed according to the type of crossings. In CBAxBR hybrids, animals from reciprocal crosses (CBAxBR and BRxCBA) are identical for all sleep parameters (night, day, PS and SWS durations) and do not differ significantly from the CBA strain. In CxBR hybrids, the reciprocal crosses (BRxC and CxBR) were not statistically different from one another for total PS and SWS durations. However, PS duration in the hybrids was not different from BR mice, while SWS duration was not different from C mice. For day-night differences, maternal effects seemed to be important in CxBR hybrids but not in CBAxBR hybrids.

Sleep-waking cycle in RI strains

Variance analysis and Student-Newman-Keuls multiple range test allowed the RI strains to be rank-ordered with regard to parental strains and F1 hybrids. We have observed the most reliable differences for the PS duration: a SDP could be established for total and night durations. Comparison with H loci SDP indicated that total and night PS durations were possibly linked to H-2 and non H-2 loci, respectively (Valatx et al., 1977) (Table II).

TABLE II

STAIN DISTRIBUTION PATTERN OF SLEEP IN RECOMBINANT INBRED STRAINS OF MICE, COMPARED TO STRAIN DISTRIBUTION PATTERN OF THREE HISTOCOMPATIBILITY GENES

Brackets indicate intermediate duration between B6 and C mice. Thus, there are least two possibilities of linkage for night PS duration (H-37 and H-38).

	CxBD	CxBE	CxBG	CxBH	CxBI	CxBJ	CxBK
24 hr PS duration	( )	B6	B6	C	B6	C	B6
H-2	B6	B6	B6	C	B6	B6	B6
Night PS duration	B6	C	C	( )	C	B6	C
H-37	B6	C	C	B6	C	B6	C
H-38	B6	C	C	C	C	B6	C

Circadian rhythm of sleep

Sleep rhythmicity of mice from two widely different strains (BR and C) and their F1 hybrids has been studied.

Slow wave sleep. In both strains, the best fitting sine wave had a 24 hr period but the maximum of sleep occurred earlier in C mice (8:40 a.m.) than in BR mice (11:50 a.m.). The daily mean level of 'hourly duration' (i.e. minutes spent sleeping per hour) was only slightly lower in the BR strain than in the C strain (28 vs 31 min). The amplitude of variation around the mean value was much higher in BR mice (± 15.50 min) than in C mice (± 9.00 min). In the C strain, the small difference between day and night durations can be explained by the fact that sleep duration progressively increases throughout the night until 8.40 a.m. and then decreases during the light period, whereas in the BR strain the sleep duration dramatically increases at the end of the night, and declines again only at the end of the light period. In both of the reciprocal crosses (F1 hybrids), the amplitude of variations around the mean level closely resembled that in C mice. In BRxC hybrids, the maximum of sleep was not noticeably different from BR parental mice, while in CxBR hybrids it was not different from the C parental mice.

Paradoxical sleep. The results are quite similar to those for SWS: the amplitude of variations around the mean level was twice as high in the BR than in the C strain, but in the latter the maximum of PS duration occurred during the period of darkness (4.32 a.m.).

Genetics of phasic activity. Cespuglio et al. (1975) have shown that eye movements during PS represent the best peripheral criterion for PGO activity. The analysis of the EOG demonstrated that the total number and pattern of REM are different in BR and C mice. The study of the EOG from F1 hybrids and backcrosses (F1xBR and F1xC) are in progress.

POSSIBLE SIGNIFICANCE OF THE RESULTS

These results from inbred and recombinant strains give some new insights into sleep physiology. Sleep behavior may now be considered as a complex somatic trait which can be subdivided into several units: duration of each stage of sleep, circadian rhythm and phasic activity.

The strain distribution pattern (SDP) of RI strains indicates that the interstrain differences for the total PS duration might be linked to H-2 locus, the major histocompatibility complex of the mouse. Only further studies with specific congenic lines will be able to confirm or disprove this linkage. This is an important point, because the H-2 locus has been located on chromosome 17 next to the T locus region, the genes of which specify cell surface structure in embryos. Several recessive mutations at the T locus are known to provoke selective defects in the neural tube during embryonic development (Bennett, 1975). The observed differences in sleep pattern could be the consequence of alterations in discrete parts of the brain which are directly or indirectly involved in the production of sleep (raphe nuclei, locus coeruleus complex, etc.), or else in the regulation of the sleep-waking cycle (pineal gland, suprachiasmatic nucleus, etc.). If this is the case, it becomes possible to predict what alterations are capable of inducing such differences: (1) changes in the number of neurons in a given part of the brain; (2) alterations of neuron surface affecting the number of receptors, number of connections, etc.; (3) changes in metabolic activity: quantity or substrate affinity of a given enzyme involved in neurotransmitter synthesis (Ross et al., 1976).

Knowing the nervous structures supposed to be related to sleep mechanisms, and using mice bearing mutations at the T-H2 complex, it will be possible to refine genetic dissection and go further into the understanding of biological mechanisms controlling this complex behavior. This last is an important point because paradoxical sleep is virtually the only stage of sleep 'in utero' and at birth (see Adrien, 1978; Corner, 1978). A hypothetical function of PS during ontogenic development would be to participate in the setting up of neuronal circuitry responsible for primary motor automatisms, a function different from that in the adult, where the importance of PS would be more in the area of adaptation to the 'milieu extérieur' (Astic, 1976; Greenberg and Pearlman, 1974; Jouvet, 1973; Jouvet-Mounier et al., 1970; Kitahama et al., 1976; Valatx et al., 1964; Valatx et Nowaczyk, 1977; Valatx et al., 1977).

SUMMARY

The genetic approach provides a good model for studying sleep mechanisms, not only in adults but also in pre- and post-natal maturation. Using several inbred strains of mice, their F1 hybrids and backcrosses, it was possible to show that SWS duration was determined independently of PS duration. Furthermore, using histocompatibility genes as markers, a sleep study of recombinant inbred strains of Bailey indicated that: (1) several genes are directly or indirectly involved in the determination of total PS duration; (2) these genes seem to be linked to H-2, the major histocompatibility complex of the mouse; and (3) they are different from the genes which determine night-time PS duration. Further studies with specific congenic lines of mice will most likely allow us to demonstrate these linkages. The major histocompatibility complex has been located on chromosome 17, next to the T locus which specifies cell surface structure in embryos. In the future, this model ought to prove useful in studying the overall development of brain structures involved in the production and regulation of the sleep cycle.

ACKNOWLEDGEMENT

This work has been supported by INSERM (U 52), CNRS (LA 162, ATP 2378) and DRME (74232).

REFERENCES

Adrien, J. (1978) Ontogenesis of some sleep regulations: early postnatal impairment of the monoaminergic systems, this volume.

Allison, T. and van Twyver, H. (1974) The evolution of sleep, *Nat. Hist.,* 79: 169–175.

Astic, L. (1976) *Le Sommeil Avant et Après la Naissance.* Thèse de Doctorat d'Etat es Sciences, Lyon.

Bailey, D.W. (1975) Genetics of histocompatibility in mice. I. New loci and congenic lines, *Immunogenetics,* 2: 249–256.

Bennett, D. (1975) The T-locus of the mouse, *Cell,* 6: 441–454.

Cespuglio, R., Musolino, R., Debilly, G., Jouvet, M. et Valatx, J.L. (1975) Organisation différente des mouvements oculaires rapides du sommeil paradoxal chez deux souches de souris, *C.R. Acad. Sci. (Paris),* 280: 2681–2684.

Corner, M.A. (1978) Spontaneous motor rhythms in early life – phenomenological and neurophysiological aspects, this volume.

Friedman, J.K. (1974) A diallele analysis of the genetic underpinnings of mouse sleep, *Physiol. Behav.,* 12: 169–175.

Green, E.L. (1966) *Biology of the Laboratory Mouse,* 2nd ed. McGraw-Hill, New York.

Greenberg, R. and Pearlman, C. (1974) Cutting the REM nerve: an approach to the adaptive role of REM sleep, *Perspect. Biol. Med.,* 17: 513–521.

Jouvet, M. (1972) The role of monoamine and acetylcholine containing neurons in the regulation of the sleep-waking cycle, *Ergebn. Physiol.,* 64: 165–307.

Jouvet, M. (1973) Essai sur le rêve, *Arch. ital. Biol.,* 111: 564–576.

Jouvet-Mounier, D., Astic, L. and Lacote, D. (1970) Ontogenesis of the states of sleep in rat, cat, and guinea pig during the first post natal month, *Develop. Psychobiol.,* 2: 216–239.

Kan, J.P., Chouvet, G., Hery, F., Debilly, G., Mermet, A. and Pujol, J.F. (1977) Daily variations of tryptophan 5-hydroxylase in the raphé nuclei and the striatum of the rat brain, *Brain Res.,* 123: 125–136.

Kitahama, K., Valatx, J.L. et Jouvet, M. (1976) Apprentissage d'un labyrinthe en Y chez deux souches de souris. Effets de la privation instrumentale et pharmacologique du sommeil, *Brain Res.,* 108: 75–86.

Oliverio, A. (1974) Genetic and biochemical analysis of behaviour in mice, *Progr. Neurobiol.,* 3: 193–215.

Ross, R.A., Judd, A.B., Pickel, V.M., Joh, T.H. and Reis, D.J. (1976) Strain dependent variations in number of midbrain dopaminergic neurons, *Nature (Lond.),* 264: 654–656.

Sidman, R.L., Green, M.C. and Appel, S.M. (1965) *Catalog of the Neurological Mutants of the Mouse,* Harvard University Press, Boston.

Valatx, J.L. et Bugat, R. (1974) Facteurs génétiques dans le déterminisme du cycle veille-sommeil chez la souris, *Brain Res.,* 69: 315–330.

Valatx, J.L. and Chouvet, G. (1975) Genetics of the sleep-waking cycle. In *Sleep 1974,* P. Levin and W.P. Koella (Eds.), Karger, Basel, pp. 19–24.

Valatx, J.L., Chouvet, G. and Kitahama, K. (1977) Genetics of sleep and learning processes: possible relationships. In *Genetics, Environment and Intelligence,* A. Oliverio (Ed.), Elsevier, Amsterdam, pp. 133–146.

Valatx, J.L., Jouvet, D. et Jouvet, M. (1964) Evolution électroencéphalographique des différents états de sommeil chez le chaton, *Electroenceph. clin. Neurophysiol.,* 17: 218–233.

Valatx, J.L. et Nowaczyk, T. (1977) Essai de suppression pharmacologique du sommeil paradoxal chez le rat nouveau-né, *Rev. E.E.G. Neurophysiol.,* in press.

Zepelin, H. and Rechtshaffen, A. (1974) Mammalian sleep, longevity and energy metabolism, *Brain Behav. Evol.,* 10: 425.

DISCUSSION

CHANGEUX: In your back-crossing experiments, are you sure that there is a linkage between the H-locus and the parameters you measured? Are you measuring a single gene or are there several genes within this locus?

VALATX: The putative linkage between the genes involved in the PS duration and genes of the histo-compatibility system (H-system) used as marker genes is suggested, not by back-crossing experiments (F1 × parental strains), but by the results from the recombinant inbred strains (RI) derived from C57BL/6 and BALB/c strains. Study of congenic lines (identical to C57BL/6 except for one gene, or a set of genes, coming from the BALB/c strain) could prove or disprove this linkage. From back-crossing experiments and RI strains, the presence of intermediate pattern of sleep duration leads to the hypothesis that several genes (more than one) are involved in the determination of PS duration. Other experiments are necessary to go further in the 'genetic dissection' of sleep physiology.

STIRLING: I was interested in the differences between C57 and Balb/c; that they are also quite different in their learning abilities. What happens when you do the back-crossing: is there a relationship between sleep and learning?

VALATX: We have studied learning ability (active avoidance response) in (1) Balb/c and C57BR mice, which have different patterns of sleep and of learning, and (2) C57BR and C57BL/6 mice, which have the same sleep patterns but different learning abilities. The second experiment is thus a good model for studying the relationship between sleep and learning processes. Briefly, BR mice learn faster than do B6 mice. Only BR mice present an increase of PS duration after the two first learning sessions. Moreover, after PS deprivation both strains are able to learn, but acquisition is very slow. In my opinion, only the *rapid* integration of new information requires paradoxical sleep (see Valatx et al., 1977).

Ontogenesis of Some Sleep Regulations: Early Postnatal Impairment of the Monoaminergic Systems

JOËLLE ADRIEN

Physiologie, CHU Pitié Salpètrière, 75013 Paris (France)

INTRODUCTION

The monoaminergic systems appear to play a role in several complex regulations such as: sleep states (Jouvet, 1969, 1972), thermoregulation (Roussel et al., 1976), feeding behavior (Smith et al., 1973; Ungerstedt, 1971), learning (Anlezark et al., 1973; Smith et al., 1973), analgesia (Akil and Liebeskind, 1975), synaptic plasticity in the central nervous system (Kasamatsu and Pettigrew, 1976) and phasic events of 'paradoxical' sleep (Jouvet, 1969, 1972). The developmental aspects of these regulations have not yet been widely studied, however (Kasamatsu and Pettigrew, 1976; Maeda et al., 1974; Smith et al., 1973). In the sleep field, even though numerous experiments have been performed in the adult animal, there have been only a few attempts to impair the monoaminergic systems in the developing animal (Adrien, 1976, 1977; Adrien et al., 1977; Saucier 1976). We shall present here the effects of lesioning the monoaminergic systems, at different stages of development, upon the subsequent sleep polygram of the newborn rat and kitten.

The postnatal ontogenesis of the monoaminergic systems has been described morphologically in the rat (Loizou, 1970) and in the kitten (Loup and Cadilhac, 1970; Maeda and Gerebtzoff, 1969). Both catecholaminergic (CA) and serotoninergic (5-HT) cell bodies are present at birth, and the pathways and terminals achieve their maturation only at two months of age. During postnatal maturation, these systems appear to be biochemically functional (Bourgoin, 1976; Loizou, 1972), and the question here is to test their possible role in the sleep regulation processes during this period, especially in the very early stages of development.

The sleep states undergo well-known modifications during the first postnatal month (Jouvet-Mounier et al., 1970; Shimizu and Himwich, 1968). Schematically, the state of *active sleep* (AS) is present at birth in the rat pup and in the kitten. It appears to be the ontogenetic precursor of *paradoxical sleep* (PS), a state which will meet all of the accepted criteria by the third or fourth postnatal week in both species (Bowe-Anders et al., 1974). Meanwhile, the state of *quiet sleep* (QS) emerges clearly during the second postnatal week. It then becomes quantitatively more and more important, and by the third week dominant cortical slow waves are observed during that state. At this time, all the criteria of *slow-wave sleep* (SWS) are met, and the sleep polygram resembles that of the adult in its qualitative aspects.

We have carried out lesion experiments on the newborn cat and rat according to the following logic: if a system is functional in terms of sleep regulation at one point in development, then any major impairment of this system ought to induce (at least temporarily) a modification in the sleep pattern. In the *opposite* case, i.e. where the definitive control system is not yet functional, sleep patterns will not be modified whatever the injury to the system. Even though we are currently investigating the long-term effects of this type of lesions, we shall restrict this report mostly to the short-term level of analysis, in order not to enter the complex field of functional recovery and compensatory plasticity. The following experiments will demonstrate that the monoaminergic systems are not decisive in terms of sleep regulation in the newborn animal, or during the early postnatal period, and that their functional maturation occurs in the course of the first postnatal month.

METHODOLOGICAL CONSIDERATIONS IN PERFORMING BRAIN LESION STUDIES

Two means of lesioning the monoaminergic systems have been employed: (a) electrolytic lesion of the cell bodies, which induces a complete degeneration of all the terminals, and (b) chemical destruction of the monoaminergic terminals by the injection of specific neurotoxins for the CA or 5-HT systems. One method is complementary to the other because the electrolytic lesion also destroys non-monoaminergic cells (as well as damaging the vascularization), and the results obtained might be due in part to these uncontrolled factors. In this sense, the chemical destruction of the terminals represents a good control for the specificity of the results. On the other hand, chemical lesions do not destroy all of the cell somas, and consequently there is always the possibility of local sprouting (Nygren et al., 1974) — which could then account for any transient effect of the lesion observed in the immature organism. In this regard, electrolytic lesions constitute a control for the specificity of chemical lesions.

Electrolytic lesions

Under general anesthesia, the anterior raphe nuclei and the locus coeruleus complex were stereotaxically destroyed by electrolytic lesioning, according to a method already described (Adrien, 1976; Adrien et al., 1977). These lesions were performed in the young rat at 5 days and at 4 weeks after birth, and in the kitten at one week and at 3 weeks of life. A set of 6 electrodes was implanted for recording the conventional sleep parameters (Adrien, op cit.; Bowe-Anders et al., 1974; Jouvet-Mounier et al., 1970). In all instances, the early-lesioned group will be referred to as the E group, and the juvenile-lesioned one as the J group. The rats were separated from their mother at the time of the recording sessions, since the mother rats were inclined to chew on the recording cables. In contrast, kittens stayed with their mother at all times. The recording period lasted from 8 days to 3 weeks, after which the animals were sacrificed. The forebrain was saved for biochemical analysis of the endogenous monoamine content, while the posterior part was used for histological verification of the lesion placement and extent.

Chemical lesions

These experiments were performed only in the kitten. Bilateral intraventricular cannulae were stereotaxically implanted under general anesthesia. During the same surgical procedure, a set of 6 recording electrodes were implanted according to a method already described (Adrien, 1976; Bowe-Anders et al., 1974). After control recordings had been obtained, we injected either 6-OHDA or 5,7-HT, (or else the vehicle alone, by way of control) through the cannulae into the brain ventricles. The doses were respectively: 1 mg 6-OHDA per 6 g of brain weight (Laguzzi et al., 1972; Petitjean et al., 1972), and 0.7 mg 5,7-HT per 10 g of brain weight (Baumgarten et al., 1972; Froment et al., 1974). The injections were given while gently holding the kitten by wrapping it in a towel. The animals were subsequently recorded for 8–15 days post-injection, and then sacrificed for biochemical brain analysis.

EXPERIMENTAL FINDING FOLLOWING EARLY LESIONING IN MAMMALS

Lesions in the 5-HT system

(1) Electrolytic lesion of the anterior raphe nuclei

(a) In the rat (Adrien et al., 1977). In the E group, several animals could not perform efficient suckling, because of ataxia consecutive to the lesion, so that they had to be fed by means of intraesophageal tubing. Those which did not recover suckling activity after 3 days either died, or else were so underweight that they had to be discarded from the data. Furthermore, only the animals for which the histology revealed an extensive and specific lesion of the anterior raphe nuclei were included in the experimental groups. In these conditions, we had a total of 10 pups in the E group (6 lesioned and 4 control pups). The animals did not exhibit any motor defects other than inability for suckling in some cases. At one month of age, however, it was obvious that the early lesioned animals gave a more intense startle reaction in response to tactile or auditory stimuli. The J group exhibited the behavior pattern already described in the adult (Kotowski et al., 1968; Lorens et al., 1971; Mouret et al., 1968): the rats were very active, and were running around the cage. Half of them died within 4 days postlesion and were discarded from the data, leaving a total of 5 lesioned and 5 control animals in the J group.

The polygraphic recordings indicated that, in the E group, all the electrophysiological characteristics of sleep were unchanged after lesioning. Quantitatively, we could observe no modifications in the sleep cycles for any state of sleep and for any time postlesion, as indicated in Fig. 1. In the J group, however, the lesion led to an immediate decrease in both sleep states as has been described in the adult (Kotowski et al., 1968; Lorens et al., 1971; Mouret et al., 1968) (Fig. 1). There was no recovery trend of the sleep quantities during the period of investigation (3 weeks).

(b) In the cat (Adrien, 1976). The same type of raphe lesions were performed in the kitten at the first week of life (E group), and after 3 weeks of age (J group). The behavioral effects of the lesions were the same as those described earlier for the rat. A considerable number of kittens died within 8 days after the lesion because of undernutrition. There was a total of 13 kittens in the E group, with lesions of the anterior raphe nuclei estimated to range from 20 to 100% of the total area (Jouvet, 1969, 1972) (Fig. 2). In this group the polygraphic characteristics of sleep were not affected by the lesion, either qualitatively or quantitatively, even in animals with a 100% lesion (Fig. 3).

In the J group, on the other hand, for all 5 experimental animals the lesion induced a degree of insomnia in both sleep states, even when the lesion was not as extensive as the ones in the E group (Fig. 3). For these juvenile animals, our results correlating the amount of sleep with the extent of raphe destruction are in agreement with the data obtained in the adult cat (Jouvet op. cit.; Pujol et al., 1971). However, we do find that PS is more affected by such lesions than in SWS, which is not the case in the adult cat where, under the same conditions, PS amounts are not modified.

(c) Biochemical data. Since we are dealing with developing systems, their morphology is continually undergoing change during maturation. It is consequently important to test the

396

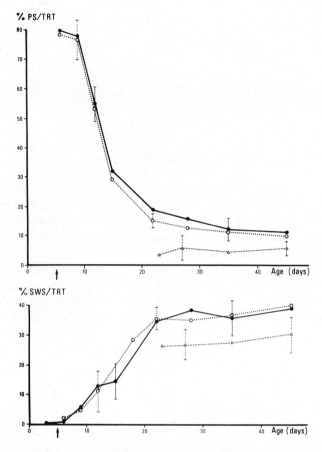

Fig. 1. Lower graph: development of QS (up to 20 days) and SWS (from 20 days on) in the rat. The arrow indicates the time when the *early* lesion was performed, and the open circles represent the mean evolution of sleep in that group. The graph is superimposable with that of the control group (filled circles), whereas *late* lesions (after 3 weeks) induce a significant SWS reduction (open triangles). Sleep quantities are expressed in per cent of total recording time, and vertical bars indicate the values of the standard deviation. Upper graph: development of AS (up to the third week) and PS (from the third week on) in the rat. Note that there is no difference between the early-lesioned (open circles) and control (filled circles) animals, whereas a significant reduction of PS appears when the lesion is performed after the third week of life (open triangles). (From Adrien et al., 1977.)

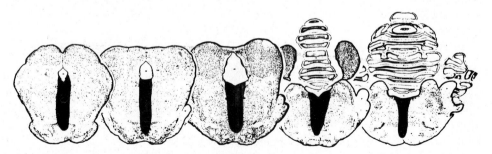

Fig. 2. Drawings obtained from frontal sections of the brain of a kitten lesioned at 3 days of age and sacrificed at 12 days of age. The black area represents the extent of the lesion. This is an example of the largest lesion which did not induce major sleep disturbances. (From Adrien, 1977.)

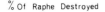

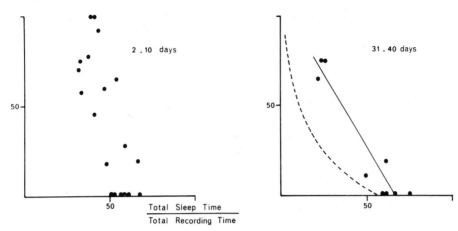

Fig. 3. Correlation graph between the proportion of total sleep time and the amount of raphe destroyed, in the two different age groups. On the right, the dotted curve represents the data obtained from the adult cat. (From Adrien, 1976.)

efficacy of our lesions with regard to the actual impairment of the 5-HT system. A good means for this purpose is to have a biochemical index of the injury to the 5-HT system, e.g. the concentration of 5-HT in the brain after the lesion. Biochemical analysis performed on rats of the E group (Bourgoin et al., 1977) indicated a rapid (2–5 days postlesion) and permanent (9 month postlesion) reduction of the endogenous 5-HT and 5-HIAA levels in the forebrain, to 75–95% of control values (Fig. 4). The decrease of 5-HT after the lesion is most extreme in the J group, ranging from 60 to 83% of control values (not shown).

We have less data for the cat, but they are in agreement with those for the rat. In the E group, the forebrain 5-HT and 5-HIAA content was reduced to 50–65% of control values (in 4 animals sacrificed at 1–2 months of age). In both rat and cat, the ratio of 5-HIAA to 5-HT was not modified as compared to controls, and in the rat no hypersensitivity of the 5-HT receptors linked to adenylate cyclase activity could be found as a consequence of the early lesion.

(2) Chemical lesions in the 5-HT system

We used 5,7-HT, injected intracisternally in the kitten, as a means of selectively destroying the 5-HT terminals in the entire brain. Our results are necessarily preliminary, considering the small number of animals which have so far been submitted to this treatment. These experiments, however, support the data obtained with electrolytic lesions of the 5-HT cell bodies.

Lesions in the CA system

(1) Electrolytic lesion of the CA system

Bilateral electrolytic lesions of the locus coeruleus and nucleus subcoeruleus were performed in the kitten at the first week of age for the E group, and after 3 weeks of age for the J group (Adrien, 1976). The extent of the lesion was verified after sacrifice, using the histological method of Glenner. Only animals with a lesion estimated at 60% or more were

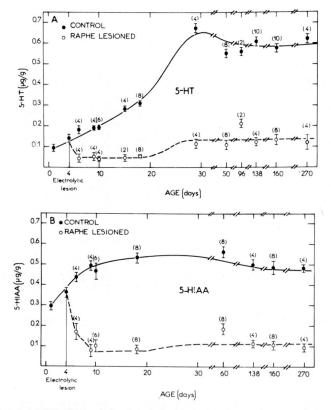

Fig. 4. 5-HT (A) and 5-HIAA (B) levels in the whole forebrain of rats at various times after electrolytic lesion of B7 and B8 nuclei. Electrolytic lesion was performed on the fourth postnatal day. Each point corresponds to the mean ± S.E.M. of 4—10 determinations. Number in parenthesis indicates the number of animals used in each case. (From Bourgoin et al., 1977.)

taken into account. The kittens in the E group exhibited severe ataxia after the lesion. For this reason, it became very difficult for them to nurse, and many of these animals had to be discarded from the data. In total, we had 4 lesioned kittens in the E group, and 4 in the J group, for which all the symptoms described for the adult cat were present (adypsia, hypothermia, hypertonia) (Carli and Zanchetti, 1965; Henley and Morrison, 1974; Jones et al., 1969).

In the E group, however, the qualitative characteristics of the sleep polygram were not modified after the lesion. In particular, we never obtained the lack of atonia during PS which was so typical in the case of an adult lesion (see below). Neither were the quantitative characteristics of the sleep states severely impaired by the lesions, even the most extensive ones (Fig. 5). In some cases, a slight sleep deficit appeared in the first few days postlesion, but from our observations of the kitten's behavior (attempting to catch the nipple, failing to do so, and then crying) it seems to be an unspecific effect of the lesion due to difficulty in nursing, rather than to an alteration of sleep regulation itself.

In the J group, on the other hand, the data are in complete agreement with those obtained in the adult cat. The animals exhibited normal SWS, but never showed any PS when the lesion was extensive (Fig. 5). When the lesion had spared the anterior part of the locus coeruleus, which occurred in two kittens, one could observe at the time of the PS phases the

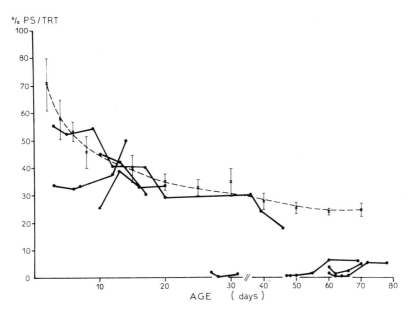

Fig. 5. Evolution of PS quantities with age in control kittens (crosses: mean of 6 animals) and in coeruleus-lesioned kittens (filled circles: individual tracings). Left: 4 kittens lesioned at 1 and 8 days of age (E group). Right: 4 kittens lesioned at 26, 45 and 59 days of age (J group). The two kittens in the E group which exhibited relative sleep loss had very large pontine lesions and severe ataxia.

spectacular 'pseudo-hallucinatory' behaviors which have been described in the adult cat (Carli and Zanchetti, 1965; Henley and Morrison, 1974; Jones et al., 1969), and which appear when the animal cannot achieve atonia during PS as a consequence of the lesion.

(2) Chemical lesion of the CA system

The details of the experiments involving 6-OHDA injection, with or without previous treatment with chlorimipramine, are described elsewhere (Laguzzi and Adrien, 1978). In this paper we will consider only the injections of 6-OHDA alone, performed at 5 days of age (n = 2) and at 3 weeks of age (n = 3).

(a) *Behavioral and polygraphical aspects.* In the E group, the kittens cry for 1–2 hr after the injection. This effect might be due to sudden release of noradrenaline (NA) at the level of the terminals before they are destroyed. AS returned to normal 1–2 hr post-injection in the E group, while in the J group PS returned on the second day postinjection, but stayed at a relatively low level throughout the recording period. As shown in Fig. 6, the E group exhibited no deficits in quiet sleep or active sleep during the 8 days postinject-tion, while the J group showed the same sleep deficit as the one described in the adult cat under the same condition (Laguzzi et al., 1972).

(b) The biochemical data indicated that in both groups 6-OHDA had been very efficient in destroying the NA terminals (Fig. 6): the NA levels were drastically reduced in all fore-brain areas (Petitjean et al., 1972). In the brain stem there appeared to be an increase of endogenous NA in the E group. This phenomenon, which could be due to local sprouting of the brain stem cells, is now being investigated. In any case, a hypothetical sprouting at the brain stem level could not by itself explain the lack of sleep deficit in the E group, because *at no time* postinjection did the animals show any such deficit. In other words,

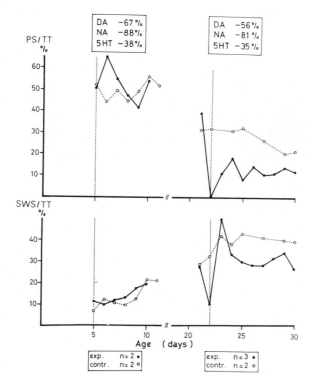

Fig. 6. Effects of intraventricular injection on sleep in the kitten, for two age groups. The E group was injected at 5 days of age, and the J group at 22 days of age (time of injection is represented by the vertical dotted line). PS and SWS durations have been calculated for the 6-OHDA-injected, and for the vehicle-injected animals. Note the lack of sleep deficit in the E group as compared to control animals. Contrarily, notice the drastic reduction of PS in the J group following the 6-OHDA injection. The biochemical data are expressed in per cent drop from control values (TT = total recording time).

sprouting could at most account for a *recovery* phenomenon, but not for a complete lack of effect from the very beginning.

THEORETICAL CONSIDERATIONS

The data presented above demonstrate that a sub-total electrolytic or chemical lesion of the monoaminergic systems has no disruptive effect on sleep when performed early in life. If the same lesion is made later in life, when the sleep characteristics are almost mature, it induces a partial or complete insomnia. The latter results confirm the findings of other authors, i.e. that the monoaminergic systems are somehow involved in sleep regulation in adult and juvenile mammals (cat and rat) (Jouvet, 1969, 1972). There are, however, recent controversial findings that the 5-HT system is *not* implicated in sleep regulation in the rat (Ross et al., 1976). Such data are difficult to interpret, because most of the lesion work related to sleep has been done in the cat, and there could be crucial species differences affecting this kind of experiment. In our experimental conditions, however, juvenile-lesioned rats did exhibit the expected sleep deficits following the operation, whereas the early-lesioned ones did not do so. Consequently, whatever the extent and the nature of its involvement in sleep regulation, the 5-HT system achieves functional maturity only a few weeks after birth in the rat.

More generally, our data provide strong evidence that the sleep regulations mediated by the monoaminergic systems are not functional at birth, either in the cat or in the rat. These regulations apparently come into being during the course of the first postnatal month. This implies that in no case can the newborn be considered simply as a miniature adult. This statement is well known in other fields (see Hamburger, 1970) but for some reason has never been seriously considered in the sleep area, where the newborn has always been forced into the adult model. From the ontogenetic point of view, one would expect that the impairment of the 5-HT system would have little, or no, effect on sleep in the early postnatal period, in view of the small amount of QS in the sleep cycles (QS being considered as the precursor of SWS, which is regulated mainly by the 5-HT system: Jouvet, op cit.). The puzzling result, then, concerns the CA system, which has been implicated in the control of PS. Since active sleep is considered to be the ontogenetic precursor of PS, one might have expected that early postnatal impairment of the CA system would have seriously disrupted AS. Since we failed to obtain such an effect, it might be that the immature mammal uses sleep regulation mechanisms other than the monoaminergic ones, which mechanisms would be most worthwhile to investigate. Furthermore, the developing mammal provides a good model for studying the manner in which the monoaminergic systems enter into the sleep regulation process during maturation.

In the immediate postnatal period, and furthermore in utero, AS would seem to be very different — even in terms of underlying mechanisms — from what we know of the sleep phenomenon in the adult (Jouvet, op. cit.). Immature sleep appears as a rather loosely organized constellation of parameters, probably owing to the immaturity of the neuronal networks which have been implicated in sleep regulation processes in the adult, particularly at the lower brain stem and midbrain levels. Only when these neuronal networks develop all of their interconnections, do the regulatory systems presumably become anatomically and functionally established according to the adult model.

ACKNOWLEDGEMENT

We are grateful to Mrs. A. Sicard for her technical assistance. This work was supported in part by Grant 75-5-148-6. CRL. INSERM.

REFERENCES

Adrien, J.A. (1976) Lesion of the anterior raphe nuclei in the newborn kitten and the effects on sleep, *Brain Res.,* 103: 579–583.

Adrien, J. (1977) Organisation du sommeil chez le chaton après lésions précoces des structures impliquées dans la régulation des états de vigilance, *Rev. Electroenceph. Neurophysiol. Clin.,* 3: 278–283.

Adrien, J., Bourgoin, S. and Hamon, M. (1977) Midbrain raphe lesion in the newborn rat. I. Neurophysiological aspects of sleep, *Brain Res.,* 127: 99–100.

Akil, H. and Liebeskind, J.C. (1975) Monoaminergic mechanisms of stimulation-produced analgesia, *Brain Res.,* 94: 279–296.

Anlezark, G.M., Crow, T.J. and Greenway, A.P. (1973) Impaired learning and decreased cortical norepinephrine after bilateral locus coeruleus lesions, *Science,* 181: 628–634.

402

Baumgarten, H.G., Evetts, K.D., Holman, R.B., Iversen, L.L., Vogt, M. and Wilson, G. (1972) Effects of 5-6HT on monoaminergic neurons in the central nervous system, *J. Neurochem.*, 19: 1587–1597.

Bourgoin, S. (1976) *Evolution du métabolisme de la sérotonine chez le rat au cours du developpement*, Doctorat d'Etat es-Sciences, Univ. de Paris-VII.

Bourgoin, S., Enjalbert, A., Adrien, J., Hery, F. and Hamon, M. (1977) Midbrain raphe lesion in the newborn rat. II. Biochemical alterations in serotoninergic innervation, *Brain Res.*, 127: 111–126.

Bowe-Anders, C., Adrien, J. and Roffwarg, H.P. (1974) Ontogenesis of ponto-geniculo-occipital activity in the lateral geniculate nucleus of the kitten, *Exp. Neurol.*, 43: 242–260.

Carli, G. and Zanchetti, A. (1965) A study of pontine lesions suppressing deep sleep in the cat, *Arch. ital. Biol.*, 103: 752–788.

Froment, J.L., Petitjean, F., Bertrand, N., Cointy, C. et Jouvet, M. (1974) Effets de l'injection intracérébrale de 5,6-dihydroxytryptamine sur les monoamines cérébrales et les états de sommeil du chat, *Brain Res.*, 67: 405–417.

Hamburger, V. (1970) Embryonic motility in vertebrates. In *The Neurosciences, Vol. II*, Schmitt, F.O. (Ed.), The Rockefeller Univ. Press, New York, pp. 141–151.

Henley, K., and Morrison, A.R. (1974) A re-evaluation of the effects of lesions of the pontine tegmentum and locus coeruleus on phenomena of paradoxical sleep in the cat, *Acta neurobiol. exp.*, 34: 215–232.

Jones, B.E., Bobillier, P. et Jouvet, M. (1969) Effet de la destruction des neurones contenant les catécolamines du mésencéphale sur le cycle veille-sommeil du chat, *C.R. Soc. Biol. (Paris)* 163: 176–180.

Jouvet, M. (1969) Biogenic amines and the states of sleep, *Science*, 163: 32–41.

Jouvet, M. (1972) The role of monoamine and acetylcholine-containing neurons in the regulation of sleep-waking cycle, *Ergebn. Physiol.*, 64: 165–307.

Jouvet, M., Bobillier, P., Pujol, J.F. et Renault, J. (1966) Effets des lésions du système du raphé sur le sommeil et la sérotonine cérébrale, *C.R. Soc. Biol. (Paris)*, 160: 2343–2346.

Jouvet-Mounier, D., Astic, L. and Lacote, D. (1970) Ontogenesis of the states of sleep in the rat, cat, and guinea pig during the first postnatal month, *Develop. Psychobiol.*, 2: 216–239.

Kasamatsu, T. and Pettigrew, J.D. (1976) Depletion of brain catecholamines: Failure of ocular dominance shift after monocular occlusion in kittens, *Science*, 194: 206–209.

Kotowski, W., Giacalone, E., Garattini, S. and Valzelli, L. (1968) Studies on behavioral and biochemical changes in rats after lesion of midbrain raphe, *Europ. J. Pharmacol.*, 4: 371–376.

Laguzzi, R. et Adrien, J. (1978) Effets de l'injection intraventriculaire de 6-hydroxydopamine sur le sommeil du chaton au cours du développement, *C.R. Acad. Sci. (Paris)*, 285: 1061–1063.

Laguzzi, R., Petitjean, F., Pujol, J.F. et Jouvet, M. (1972) Effets de l'injection intraventriculaire de 6-hydroxydopamine. II. Sur le cycle velle-sommeils du chat, *Brain Res.*, 48: 295–310.

Loizou, L. (1970) Uptake of monoamines into central neurones and the blood brain barrier in the infant rat, *Brit. J. Pharmacol.*, 40: 800–813.

Loizou, L.A. (1972) The postnatal ontogeny of monoamine-containing neurons in the central nervous system of the albino rat, *Brain Res.*, 40: 300–311.

Lorens, S.A., Sorensen, J.P. and Yunger, L.M. (1971) Behavioral and neurochemical effects of lesions in the raphe system of the rat, *J. comp. Physiol.*, 77: 48–52.

Loup, M. et Cadilhac, J. (1970) Le développement des neurones à monoamines du cerveau chez le chaton, *C.R. Soc. Biol. (Paris)*, 164: 1582–1587.

Maeda, T. et Gerebtzoff, M.A. (1969) Recherches sur le développement du locus coeruleus du rat. *Acta. neurol. psychol. belg.*, 69: 11–19.

Maeda, T., Tohyama, M. and Shimizu, N. (1974) Modification of postnatal development of neocortex in rat brain with experimental deprivation of locus coeruleus, *Brain Res.*, 70: 515–520.

Mouret, J., Bobillier, P. and Jouvet, M. (1968) Insomnia following parachlorophenylalanine in the rat, *Europ. J. Pharmacol.*, 5: 17–22.

Nygren, L.G., Fuxe, K., Jonsson, G. and Olson, L. (1974) Functional regeneration of 5-hydroxytryptamine nerve terminals in the rat spinal cord following 5-6-dihydroxytryptamine induced degeneration, *Brain Res.*, 78: 377–394.

Petitjean, F., Laguzzi, R., Sordet, F., Jouvet, M. et Pujol, J.F. (1972) Effets de l'injection intraventriculaire de 6-hydroxydopamine. I. Sur les monoamines cérébrales du chat, *Brain Res.*, 48: 281–293.

Pujol, J.F., Buguet, A., Froment, J.L., Jones, B. and Jouvet, M. (1971) The central metabolism of serotonin in the cat during insomnia. A neurophysiological and biochemical study after administration of p-chlorophenylalanine or destruction of the raphe system, *Brain Res.*, 29: 195–212.

Roussel, B., Pujol, J.F. et Jouvet, M. (1976) Effets des lésions du tegmentum pontique sur les états de sommeil chez le rat, *Arch. ital. Biol.*, 114: 188–209.

Ross, C.A., Trulson, M.E. and Jacobs, B.L. (1976) Depletion of brain serotonin following intraventricular 5-7-dihydroxytryptamine fails to disrupt sleep in the rat, *Brain Res.*, 114: 517–523.

Saucier, D. (1976) *Recherche sur les Fonctions due Sommeil Paradoxal au cours de l'Ontogenèse.* Thèse d'Université., Univ. Cl. Bernard, Lyon.

Shimizu, A. and Himwich, H.E. (1968) The ontogeny of sleep in kittens and young rabbits, *Electroenceph. clin. Neurophysiol.*, 24: 307–318.

Smith, R.D., Cooper, B.R. and Breese, G.R. (1973) Growth and behavioral changes in developing rats treated intracisternally with 6-hydroxydopamine: evidence for involvement of brain dopamine, *J. Pharmacol. exp. Ther.*, 185: 609–619.

Ungerstedt, U. (1971) Adipsia and aphagia after 6-hydroxydopamine induced degeneration of the nigro striatal dopamine system, *Acta physiol. scand.*, 82, Suppl. 367: 95–122.

DISCUSSION

SOTELO: As you know, there are many papers now on destroying the locus coeruleus in newborn animals. You have observed that from a single injection of 6-hydroxydopamine you have a decrease in the forebrain concentration of monoamines, but an increase in the brain stem. My question is: what happens to the brain stem concentration of noradrenaline in your animals?

ADRIEN: The increase of noradrenaline in the brain stem is not immediate. We have recently performed a study on the kinetics of the phenomena occurring in the brain stem after 6-OHDA treatment: it seems that there is an initial drop in the monoamine concentration in the brain stem, just as there is in other parts of the brain. And, at 8 days post-injection, we could observe an increase in the quantity of endogenous noradrenaline in the brain stem and *exclusively* in the brain stem. The other monoamines remained at a very low level in *all* brain areas.

CHANGEUX: My first question concerns the pattern of electrical activity: is it your basic idea that you are looking at the same phenomenon in both early stages of development and in later stages? The second question concerns the fact that, as you said, you still have some neurons remaining (about 5%) which are responsible for some kind of recovery. If, when they reach adulthood, you again add 6-OHDA to animals which have been treated with it at early stages, can you produce an insomnia?

ADRIEN: We have not performed a second 6-OHDA injection in grown-up animals which had already received one at early stages of development, but we certainly should do it. However, you do get insomnia when you pharmacologically inhibit the synthesis of serotonin in the early raphe-lesioned animals when they are one month old. So it seems that the serotonergic system is still playing some kind of regulatory role upon sleep, even in these animals. As concerns the first question, the problem is that it is difficult to know if it is the same phenomenon, especially because we were demonstrating that the structures in question do not have the same regulatory role on the sleep behavior. So we may only state that it is not the same phenomenon in the sense that it is not being regulated by exactly the same *mechanism*.

CHANGEUX: You said that, in ontogenesis, there is first a generalized motor activity, and only later more localized mechanisms. The pacemakers you see first expressed are widespread in the whole nervous system (see Corner, this volume) whereas the pacemakers for sleep cycles in the adult appear to be localized in certain brain stem structure. Are there any areas of the brain stem where bursting activity is found in the newborn?

ADRIEN: I think that it is the whole circuitry at the brain stem level which is not fully developed in the immature animal. In the adult the brain stem has taken over the control of all the phasic motor events, but if you do a spinal transection in a newborn rat, perfectly normal appearing twitching of the limbs will persist (also see Sedláček, this volume). Therefore, it is certainly not the case that early sleep-like motor activity is being triggered at the brain stem level, as it is in the adult animal. Nothing is yet known, however, about the neuronal sources of spontaneous bursting in immature animals.

CORNER: To the extent that your interpretations are correct about sleep truly persisting after chemical lesions in young animals, the whole monoamine circuitry would only be exerting *modulatory* influences in the control of sleep, i.e. facilitatory and inhibitory actions which permit the real generator systems to express themselves. And if you knock them out at early stages, the basic sleep-generating systems may develop with less dependence upon these secondary influences than they would have had in the course of normal maturation.

AXELRAD: Could not one explanation be that triggering sleep depends upon different thresholds to the influence of the monoaminergic systems? In none of the experiments does the biochemical level of the transmitters fall down to zero, so that in the immature animal the sensitivity might conceivable be much greater than later on in life.

ADRIEN: What I am trying to say is that the monoamine system has only a regulatory role in sleep. And I think that there is no longer much disagreement on this point. It may be that, if one were to quantify it, one could say that the role of the monoaminergic systems in immature sleep regulation is worth 2% while in the adult it is worth 100%. If you wish to express it this way, I would agree.

VALATX: But when you raphe-lesioned the kittens, did you try to inject PCPA? Because in the adult the relationship between the level of serotonin in the forebrain and the insomnia is only true during the first 3 weeks after raphe lesion.. After 3 weeks, there is a sleep recovery in the adult cat, but if you inject PCPA at this moment you get an insomnia with a lower dose than in a normal cat.

ADRIEN: Yes, we have done this, not only in the cat but also in the rat, and it is the long-term study which I was talking about. In the early-lesioned kitten or rat pup the injection of PCPA at one month of age produces insomnia. But now if you want to reverse this insomnia with 5-HTP – and this is interesting because it has been said to be the actual crucial step for establishing a causal relationship between serotonin and sleep control – you see that the lesioned animals are in fact *less* sensitive than are the controls when you do a dose response study. This would mean that, if such an animal uses the serotonergic system at all, it uses it less efficiently than do the control animals.

LYNCH: I have a simple question. Is the pharmacology of sleep in the very young rat or kitten similar to the pharmacology in the adult with regard to catecholamines, looking at reserpine for example?

ADRIEN: There has been very little pharmacology of sleep done in the newborn, and the problem in such experiments is that one has to use very high doses to be able to get adult-like effects. This is probably because the current pharmacological model is not the correct one. For example, when you are able to demonstrate that the monoaminergic systems play little or no role in the regulation of sleep in the newborn, and then you use a drug which depletes or prevents the synthesis of serotonin, for example, and you think you will get an insomnia: well, you are obviously using the wrong model for your pharmacology.

The Development of Motivational Systems

R.F. DREWETT

Department of Psychology, University of Durham, Durham (Great Britain)

INTRODUCTION

Newborn mammals, like adults, survive only if their water balance, energy stores and body temperature are maintained within narrow limits. Unlike adults, however, they do not mate. The perinatal processes of sexual differentiation are part of the development of motivational systems used only later, by the adult. The water balance, energy stores and body temperature of the infant, however, are regulated from birth, although the behavioral mechanisms used in this regulation are different from those used in the adult. In dealing with the development of these systems, therefore, we are dealing not with the setting up of a system that is used only later by the adult, but rather with the transition between different solutions to the problems of homeostasis at different stages of life.

This review therefore concentrates on two different but related topics: on the features of milk intake that are specific and unique, and on the way in which the controls of milk intake in the infant relate to the controls of food and water intake in the adult.

FEEDING BEHAVIOR AND MILK INTAKE

Unlike food and water intake in the adult, milk intake in the infant always involves a social interaction, viz. that between the mother and the infant. In this respect it is like sexual behavior in the adult, though in other respects it is more like feeding or drinking. Because the mechanisms of hunger and thirst in the adult are best understood in the rat, this review concentrates primarily on the controls of milk intake in the same species.

The feeding interactions between mother and pups can be divided for convenience into the following three phases:

Initiation

The feeding patterns of infant mammals are very varied, ranging from the more or less continual access to the mother's nipple allowed in many apes and monkeys, to the 48 hourly feed of the tree shrew (Blurton-Jones, 1972). The contribution of the mother to the initiation of the feeding interaction is important but it will not be dealt with here since the main focus of this review is on the motivational development of the infant.

It is possible to study some aspects of the approach of the pup to the mother by using anesthetized mothers (Drewett et al., 1974). Both rats and rabbits suck readily on anesthetized

408

mothers, and do not in any obvious way distinguish them from conscious mothers. The latency with which pups attach to the mother's nipple is hunger sensitive, being much longer in satiated pups than in pups separated from their mothers overnight (Drewett et al., 1974). In these experiments the pups were held by hand close to the nipple. Others (Teicher and Blass, 1976) have shown that simply placing the pup on the mother and leaving it to root for itself is equally suitable; these authors compared the two testing methods directly, and showed that they gave identical results.

There is now a great deal of evidence that olfactory stimuli are critical at this stage of the nursing interaction. Eliminating olfactory cues by washing the nipple prevents attachment of the pups, whereas painting the washed nipple with rat pup saliva reinstates it (Hofer et al., 1976; Teicher and Blass, 1976). There is evidence that human babies respond differentially to their own and other mothers' smells by the age of six weeks (Macfarlane, 1975; Russel, 1976) though there is currently no evidence that rats do.

Sucking, and the stimulation of milk ejection

Sucking patterns are species specific. In rate they vary from about 4 sucks/sec in goats, to the 1 suck/sec characteristic of great apes. Human infants change their sucking rate and pattern when milk flow from the nipple is stopped. This switching of rates in response to changes in milk flow appears, however, to be unique to humans; it is not found in other mammals (Wolff, 1968).

By means of a cannulation of the nipple from within the mammary gland, Wakerley and Drewett (1975) showed that rat pups suck in bursts, with a mean of 2.7 sucks in each burst and a mean interval of 13.7 sec between bursts. The sucking of the pups stimulates milk ejection in the mother. The milk ejection is a rise in the pressure in the mammary glands resulting from the contraction of myoepithelial cells under the influence of oxytocin. The oxytocin is secreted by nerve terminals in the posterior pituitary gland, projecting from neurons in the supraoptic and paraventricular nuclei of the hypothalamus. The release of oxytocin is intermittent, and occurs only once every few minutes. It is not, however, stimulated by changes in the sucking patterns of the pups, but is a gated response to an essentially constant stimulus (Wakerley and Drewett, 1975).

Rat pups respond to the milk ejection with a characteristic sequence of behavior. It was first noted by Vorherr et al. (1967) and Lincoln et al. (1973) and analyzed in more detail by Drewett et al. (1974). The pups' first response at milk ejection is a vigorous 'treading' on the mammary gland. This lasts about 3 sec and is followed by 'stretching' in which the pups stretch out while pushing against the nipple with their snout. The treading response and the burst of sucking that accompanies it are not responses to milk flow itself, but to some correlated stimulus; this is shown by the fact that both occur even if the flow of milk from the nipple is prevented by a ligature (Drewett et al. 1974). The stretching, however, is eliminated if milk flow is prevented. As a last reaction to milk ejection, many pups leave the nipple. Why they do this is not known. They do not leave as a result of satiation, since they generally immediately reattach themselves to another nipple. Nor is the probability of leaving the nipple affected by the rate of milk flow (Drewett and Trew, 1978).

Termination of suckling

Little is known about the termination of suckling in the rat. We do not even know whether the feed is terminated by the mother or the pups. One thing that is clear, however, is that rat pups feeding freely on their mothers are not usually satiated. The limit on their milk intake is set by the milk production of the mother, not by their own motivational state.

It is for this reason that rats in smaller litters grow at a much faster rate than those in larger litters (Kennedy, 1967). And increasing the supply of milk available to the pups increases their growth rate (Heggeress et al., 1961).

METHODS OF MOTIVATIONAL ANALYSIS

Two types of measure have dominated work on the control of milk intake in the newborn rat. The first is a *latency* measure, generally the latency with which pups seize the nipple of an anesthetized mother. This is hunger sensitive (Drewett et al., 1974) and has its uses (e.g. Hall et al., 1975; Teicher and Blass, 1976; Drewett and Cordall, 1976). Its main limitation is that it does not give any measure of the amount of intake. Part of the interest of motivational analysis in the adult is in its quantitative aspects; for example, rats given a salt load, and lacking kidneys (and so lacking any renal modification of the load) drink enough to reduce the load to isotonicity (Fitzsimons, 1971); similarly rats loaded with foodstuffs reduce their subsequent intake calorie for calorie in response to the load (Booth, 1972). Latency measures do not give information of this sort.

For this reason, we have been interested in the use of weight gain as a measure of milk intake. There is a temptation to think that a rat pup suckled by its mother is roughly comparable with an adult feeding from a food hopper, but nothing could be further from the truth. There are a number of special problems — biological problems and problems of experimental design — to be borne in mind if milk intake is to be used as a measure of motivational state:

Limitations on milk supply

The fact that the mother's milk supply sets the upper limit on the intake of the pups has two obvious consequences. One is that pups taken from their mother are not necessarily satiated. This needs bearing in mind in relation to experiments that find no difference between deprived and 'satiated' animals (e.g. Hall et al., 1975). The second is that tests of milk intake do not necessarily provide information on the pups own preferred level of intake, unless special precautions are taken to ensure a milk supply adequate for this purpose. Friedman (1975) has shown directly that the milk supply of a single mother previously deprived of pups is not enough to satiate a litter of young in a short (90 min) test. Placing the young with two or three milk-loaded mothers in succession is necessary.

Urine loss

Rat pups do not urinate spontaneously, but store urine until elimination is stimulated by the mother. A 10-day-old pup deprived of its mother overnight can store 0.5 ml of urine, and lose this amount during a subsequent feeding test. This may be a third of the weight of milk taken in (depending, of course, on the exact circumstances of the test). Urine loss is therefore potentially a major source of error in studies of milk intake in the infant. The error is obviously compounded if treatments are given which affect urine formation differentially across experimental groups. Although it is true that very young rats do not increase their urine output in response to water loads (Heller, 1947), they do decrease it when they are milk deprived (Heller, 1949), and 10-day-old rats decrease their urine output in response to hypovolemia induced by polyethylene glycol (Drewett and Trew, unpublished). To infer directly from weight gain to milk intake is therefore dubious, unless one also has information on urine loss. This is a central problem for work in this area, and a number of approaches have been taken to it.

An initial investigation of the validity of weight gain as a measure of food intake is reported by Houpt and Epstein (1973). They weighed suckling rats and then infused them intragastrically with a liquid diet for one hour using a peristaltic pump. The pups were then reweighed. They showed that there was a high correlation between the weight of liquid diet infused and the weight gain of the rats, and concluded that "weight gain is therefore a valid technique for measuring intake of mothers milk in the suckling rat" (Houpt and Epstein, 1973, p. 60). What this correlation demonstrates is that the milk intake of pups fed intragastrically is reflected in their weight gain. Since rat pups separated from their mothers do not urinate spontaneously, this is what one would indeed expect. But as Houpt and Epstein point out, pups suckling on a mother are stimulated to urinate by her, and their weight gain is therefore a resultant of their milk intake and urine loss (principally; obviously there are other possibilities still). It is not, therefore, valid to use the correlation established by Houpt and Epstein as if it provided a general validation of the use of weight gain as a measure of intake when pups are feeding on their mother (Houpt and Houpt, 1975).

A second attempt to deal with this problem has been reported by Friedman (1975). His strategy was to look at urine loss in a separate group of pups, treated as the experimental group except that they were kept with a non-lactating foster mother rather than a lactating mother. All the urine formed was removed, either by the mother or by bladder puncture, at the end of the test period; the weight loss of the pups gives a measure of urine formation and loss. The limitation on this method is that the rates of urine formation in pups left with non-lactating mothers are not necessarily going to be the same as those in the experimental pups fed on lactating foster mothers, since milk intake itself affects rate of urine formation (Heller, 1949).

A third and simple solution to this problem that we have found of value is to seal the external urethra of the pup with colloidon before the feeding test. This obviously is a method that can only be used during brief tests. With urine loss prevented the urine is stored in the bladder, as it is when the pups are separated from the mother. Weight gain is then a simple measure of milk intake, and we have shown directly that this sealing of the urethra itself has no effect on milk intake. If, in addition to weighing the pups one also measures the urine content of the bladder at the end of the experiment, one can work out what the weight change of the pups would be if the experiment were run without this necessary control procedure; thereby reconciling some inevitable discrepancies.

Experimental designs

A very common design used in research in this area involves splitting a litter (i.e. 6—10 pups) into halves (or other fractions) at random and comparing milk intake of the groups when the pups are replaced on the same mother. This is a valuable design since it means that differences in the milk supply (or, for example, nursing behavior) of the mothers are balanced across the experimental groups.

A recent paper (Lincoln et al., 1973) looks somewhat disquieting in this context. These authors were concerned with the stimulation of milk ejection in rats. They showed that when the mothers were anesthetized, the occurrence of milk ejection was dependent on the number of pups suckled: milk ejection was usually not stimulated unless at least six pups were sucking. The milk ejection is essential if milk in any quantity is to be available to the pups. If milk ejection failed because some of the pups were not sucking, then very little milk would be available even to those pups that were sucking. The possibility that this interdependence of the milk available to the experimental and control groups might wreak havoc on quantitative work in this area led us (Drewett and Trew, 1978) to examine this possibility with some care. In the event, the results were reassuring. Using the same conditions as Lincoln et al. (1973), we were able to replicate their results exactly. Fortunately, however, the loss of milk ejection when the number of pups suckled was reduced was found only when the mother was anesthetized. When the mother was conscious, the milk obtained by individual pups was quite independent of the number suckled. This was so whether the sucking stimulus was varied by varying the number of pups suckled (over a range of 1−12) or by satiating half the pups completely before the feeding test began.

A second problem is statistical in nature, and affects the kind of inference one can properly make from experimental results. Experiments of this nature can generally be analyzed using a two-way analysis of variance, with litters as one factor and experimental conditions as another. In this type of analysis, the error term used in the analysis of the difference between groups can be either the litter X treatment mean square or the residual mean square. The important difference is that the use of the first error term treats litters as a random factor, and allows a generalization to the whole population from which the litters were a sample; the second treats litters as a fixed factor, and does not allow a generalization beyond the litters actually used in the experiment. The same logic, of course, applies to the use of other (for example, non-parametric) analyses. What matters in practice is that one uses sufficient *litters,* as well as sufficient individual *animals,* to ensure that the result can be generalized across litters. A simple test for this is that if the data from the pups of each experimental group in each litter are pooled, so that each litter contributes only one data point to the results, the difference between the results (across experimental groups) should still be significant.

The considerations raised in this section should make it clear why experiments in this area are not always easy to interpret correctly. With that in mind, we turn now to a consideration of some experiments concerned with the factors that control milk intake.

CONTROL OF MILK INTAKE

Effects of milk deprivation

A number of studies have examined the effects of milk deprivation on the subsequent feeding behavior and milk intake of rat pups.

Separation of the mother and pups leads the pups, on reuniting with the mother, to attach to the nipples more rapidly at least by the tenth day of life (Drewett et al., 1974; Hall et al., 1975). Deprived pups also drink more milk (as assessed from weight gain; Houpt and Espstein, 1973). As regards a finer control, there is some doubt. Houpt and Epstein (1973) found no difference in weight gain among pups deprived for 3, 4 and 5 hr, while Houpt and Houpt (1975) found no difference between the intake of 6, 7 and 8 hr deprived pups. One might, perhaps, not expect such small differences in deprivation time to affect subsequent intake. Another possibility is raised by Friedman (1975). He showed a significant difference in intake between pups deprived for 2 hr and pups deprived for 8 hr. This difference was not found, however, if the pups were tested for intake on a single mother (as in the experiments of Houpt et al.). It was found only when the pups were fed on three mothers in succession, the difference in intake being found on the second and third mothers. This, then, may be one of the situations in which the limited milk supply of a single mother is an important consideration. In future quantitative work on this topic using weight gain as a measure of milk intake, it also needs to be borne in mind that urine loss is itself affected by milk deprivation. Deprived animals form less urine than satiated animals (Heller, 1949).

412

Hunger stimuli

Surprisingly, it is not yet entirely clear whether the distension of the stomach by a feed affects subsequent intake of milk. The problem is not a simple one. It is easy to find a load that gives no energy (e.g. water) or one that does not, like water, change plasma osmolality (e.g. saline isotonic with plasma), but even a load isotonic with plasma expands plasma volume, and it is important to remember that these postingestive consequences might affect milk intake via a thirst mechanism.

Houpt and Epstein (1973) showed that weight gain of 3–7-day-old rats in a subsequent feeding test was reduced by a preload of 1:3 kaolin in water. Kaolin is insoluble in water, so this is a hypotonic load. Although some of the water could have been absorbed, a load of water alone of the same size had no significant inhibitory effect on milk intake, so the effects of water after absorption are not likely to have been important, and one can probably attribute the inhibition found with the kaolin load to gastric distention. A similar conclusion comes from the experiment of Drewett and Cordall (1976). In this a load of water given by stomach tube was found to produce a small but significant increase in latency to attach to the nipple in 10-day-old pups. The inhibition was present 5 min after the load, but absent 1 hr later when most of the water would have been absorbed. The inference therefore seems justifiable that it was a gastric, and not a postingestional, effect of the water that was important.

As regards isotonic loads there is some disagreement. Houpt and Houpt (1975) found that a gastric load of isotonic saline (4% of body weight) decreased subsequent intake in 3–7-day-old rats, while Friedman (1975) found that a similar isotonic load had no significant effect in 10-day-old rats. His load was slightly smaller (3% of body weight) and it is worth noting that in both cases these loads are quite small in relation to normal intake – a 3% load in a 20 g, 10-day-old rat is only 0.6 ml, and one quite often finds twice that volume of milk in the stomach of pups feeding ad libitum.

In the adult, the energy yield of feeds is a major determinant of satiation, independent of gastric stretch effects. Foods given via the stomach to normally fed rats inhibit subsequent intake in proportion to the metabolizable energy they yield, roughly calorie for calorie. Although there are glucose-sensitive nerves in the liver (Niijima, 1969), with relays into the lateral hypothalamus, it is doubtful that these can be the sole monitoring system, as the inhibition is independent of the form in which the food is given (carbohydrate, fat or protein) (Booth, 1972b). The demonstration of such an inhibition has depended upon methods by which the effects of the energy yield of the food could be analyzed independently of its osmotic effects, and its effects on stomach volume. One method has been to load the stomach and test after the food has been wholly absorbed by the small intestine (Booth and Jarman, 1976); another is to compare the effect of an energy-yielding load with a load that yields no energy but empties from the stomach at the same rate.

As regards the infant, depriving rat pups of their mothers for one night reduces their blood glucose levels by about 20%. According to Drewett and Cordall (1976) a 1 ml load of 5.3% glucose raises their blood glucose levels back to, or above, the levels of undeprived controls for several hours after the load, but it does not reduce the speed with which the pups attach to the nipple. Houpt and Houpt (1975), on the other hand, found that water was less effective than 5% glucose in suppressing milk intake. Neither of these experiments is entirely satisfactory, since the correct control load is not water but a non-nutritive solution that leaves the stomach at the same rate.

The rate control of gastric emptying in the adult (human) is mainly inhibitory. Sugars and salts inhibit gastric emptying in proportion to their osmolality, while fats also slow gastric emptying by an action on fatty acid receptors (Hunt and Knox, 1968). Such evidence as is available suggests similar controls of gastric emptying in the newborn rat. Salt solutions of increasing osmolality empty from the stomach at a decreasing rate (Houpt and Houpt, 1975) while salt and glucose loads of the same osmolality empty at the same rate (Drewett and Trew, unpublished). It is therefore possible to match loads of sugars with control loads that empty at the same rate on the osmotic basis. Using loads of glucose and saline isotonic with one another and with plasma, Klauss et al. (1976) found that rat pups inhibited their milk intake differentially to glucose by the 14th day of life, but not before.

In the adult rat, feeding can be induced by treatment with the glucose-analogue, 2-deoxy-D-glucose, a drug which produces cellular glucose privation (Smith and Epstein, 1969). In addition to stimulating feeding, it causes a pronounced hyperglycemia, mainly due to the release of catecholamines from the adrenal medulla. Treatment of infant rats with 2-deoxy-D-glucose, however, did not stimulate milk intake (3—7-day-old rats: Houpt and Epstein, 1973) or reduce sucking latencies (10-day-old rats: Drewett and Cordall, 1976). This is in spite of its demonstrated effectiveness in raising blood glucose levels (although even this response is less marked than that found in adults: Gil-ad et al., 1975).

As regards the role of fats, there is less evidence. In the adult fats inhibit feeding by a specific mechanism, the release of the gut hormone cholecystokinin (Gibbs et al., 1973), and this hormone is an effective satiater immediately after weaning (Bernstein et al., 1976). Rat milk is high in fat and relatively low in sugar (Luckey et al., 1954) and ketone body utilization is much more important in the brain of the suckling (relative to glucose utilization) than in the adult (Moore et al., 1971; Page et al., 1971). The possibility that fats might have specific inhibitory effects on milk intake in the suckling is therefore an attractive one. Although corn oil (Houpt and Houpt, 1975) and oleic acid (Drewett and Trew, 1977) do strongly inhibit feeding, there is no evidence yet available which shows whether this inhibition is due to gastric distention, maintained over a long period by the inhibitory effects of fats on gastric emptying, or by effects of the fat after it has left the stomach, and mediated hormonally or otherwise.

Thirst stimuli

In the adult rat, two internal stimuli increase drinking — increased plasma osmolality and decreased plasma volume. Water deprivation produces both stimuli, and there is evidence that the increased water intake found after water deprivation is a result of combined stimuli from the extracellular and intracellular fluid compartments (Ramsey et al., 1977).

Milk deprivation in the suckling rat, although it increases subsequent milk intake, does not increase plasma osmolality (Drewett and Cordall, 1976; Wirth and Epstein, 1976). Loads of salt that produce an increase in osmolality greater than the 1—3% (Fitzsimons, 1971) necessary to stimulate drinking in adults, do not make 10-day-old pups attach to their mothers nipples more rapidly (Drewett and Cordall, 1976), nor do they increase milk intake when given either subcutaneously (Friedman, 1975) or via the stomach (Houpt and Houpt, 1975).

In the adult, an isotonic reduction in plasma volume stimulates drinking by a different mechanism from the osmotic induction of thirst. This volumetric stimulus to thirst is probably mediated partly by direct neural links from the stretch receptors in the low pressure circulation, and partly via the release of renin from the kidney. Renin so released acts on plasma substrates to produce angiotensin-1 followed by angiotensin-2, and there is evidence that this hormone can act directly on the brain to stimulate drinking. Although there is no doubt that hypovolemia does stimulate water intake, the exact role of the kidney hormone in this response is currently much argued (see, for example, Abraham et al., 1975; Malvin et al., 1977).

The renin-angiotensin system is certainly functional and responsive to reduced blood volume from birth in mammals (Mott, 1975). Since separation from the mother causes a reduction in plasma volume in 10-day-old rats (Friedman, 1975), it is possible that this reduction acts as a stimulus to milk intake. Friedman (1975) examined the effect of poly-ethylene glycol (a hyperoncotic colloid that reduces plasma volume), and found that pups treated with this substance gained more weight than controls during a feeding session.

We (Drewett and Trew, unpublished) have recently re-examined this effect in pups treated in exactly the same way, except that the loss of urine from their bladders was prevented by sealing the external urethra at the urinary papilla. What we found was that weight gain was identical in the two groups, but urine formation was greater in the controls than in the hypovolemic group. Had the urethras been unsealed, as in Friedman's experiment, this would presumably have meant that the hypovolemic group would have gained more weight — not as a result of greater intake, but as a resultant of the same intake and a smaller urine loss.

Overall, therefore, we can provisionally conclude that the milk intake of pups suckled naturally on their mother is unaffected by thirst stimuli, whether volumetric or osmotic.

MILK INTAKE, WATER INTAKE AND FOOD INTAKE

The conclusion of the last section was that milk intake in the suckling is not affected by stimuli to thirst that are effective in the adult. There is now good evidence, however, that this is not because the thirst system is immature and develops later in ontogeny; Wirth and Epstein (1976) have shown that *water* intake is responsive to osmotic stimulation as early as the second day of life, although the testing conditions must be carefully controlled. What Wirth and Epstein did was to hold the pup onto a water spout, so that only the minimal ingestive behavior was necessary for water to be drunk. Using this method, they found that osmotic stimuli increase water intake from the second day of life, and hypovolemia induced by colloid dialysis from the fourth day of life. The response induced was not sucking but licking — a response, in other words, related to drinking in the adult rather than milk intake in the suckling. The implication seems to be that the thirst system is responsive to the normal adult stimuli from the first few days of life, but that the system controlling milk intake is dissociated from it. They are, in other words, different systems.

The data on hunger are much less clear, but there are shreds of evidence that a picture similar in its implications may be found of the relationship between hunger and milk intake. It might seem at first sight that the development of glucose sensitivity in the system control-ling milk intake indicates its continuity and homology with the adult hunger system. But the hunger system of rats is actually *insensitive* to the energy yield of foods when it first comes into operation after weaning (Booth and Jarman, 1975), and remains insensitive until they reach 200 g in weight. The implication may be that the development of glucose sensitivity in the system controlling milk intake does not imply a corresponding development in the hunger system, which again implies that they are separate systems. That both milk intake and food intake can be inhibited by gastric distention is probably irrelevant, since any system controlling intake will have to protect the animal against overloading. There is other evidence that also points to milk intake and food intake being controlled by different systems. Adult rats with lateral hypothalamic lesions, for example, which otherwise starve to death, will suck milk from nipples (Teitelbaum, 1971) suggesting that their milk intake system is still intact.

It is also worth remembering in this context how very unusual, by mammalian standards, are those human beings who regularly drink milk as adults. Milk is a substance generally consumed only by infant mammals. Even in humans it is only restricted groups who drink milk (the Northern Europeans and their descendents happen to be one of them: McCracken, 1971). Other human groups are unable to drink milk for the same reason that other adult mammals are – they lack the enzymes that break down lactose. That some human adults are accustomed to treat milk as a food should not blind us to the fact that most adult mammals are not so accustomed.

When all these considerations are taken into account, it seems possible that we should cease to think of the system controlling milk intake as homologous and continuous with those controlling food or water intake in the adult. The stimulus conditions leading to feeding in the infant are unique to suckling. The motor aspects of suckling – the species typical sucking rates, and so on – are also unique to it. And as detailed above, there is good evidence that the internal stimuli to thirst do not affect milk intake, and some much more tentative evidence that the controls of food intake and milk intake may also dissociate. Attention has been drawn to the problems of interpretation of many experiments in this area, and it is too early to draw any conclusion. As things stand, however, it seems a defensible initial hypothesis that the system controlling milk intake in infant mammals is neither hunger nor thirst, but a motivational system sui generis.

ACKNOWLEDGEMENT

The author's work in this area is supported by the Medical Research Council.

REFERENCES

Abraham, S.F., Baker, R.M., Blaine, E.H., Denton, D.A. and McKinley, M.J., (1975) Water drinking induced in sheep by angiotensin – a physiological or pharmacological effect? *J. comp. physiol. Psychol.,* 88: 503–518.

Berstein, I.L., Lotter, E.C. and Zimmerman, J.C. (1976) Cholecystokinin-induced satiety in weaning rats, *Physiol. Behav.,* 17: 541–543.

Blurton-Jones, N. (1972) Comparative aspects of mother-child contact. In *Ethological Studies of Child Behaviour,* N. Blurton-Jones (Ed.), Cambridge University Press, pp. 305–328.

Booth, D.A. (1972a) Satiety and behavioural caloric compensation following intragastric glucose loads in the rat, *J. comp. physiol. Psychol.,* 78: 412–432.

Booth, D.A. (1972b) Postabsorptively induced suppression of appetite and the control of feeding, *Physiol. Behav.,* 7: 199–202.

Booth, D.A. and Jarman, S.P. (1975) Ontogeny and insulin-dependence of the satiation which follows carbohydrate absorption in the rat, *Behav. Biol.,* 15: 159–172.

Booth, D.A. and Jarman, S.P. (1976) Inhibition of food intake in the rat following complete absorption of glucose delivered into the stomach, intestine or liver, *J. Physiol. (Lond.),* 259: 501–522.

Drewett, R.F., Statham, C. and Wakerley, J.B. (1974) A quantitative analysis of the feeding behaviour of suckling rats, *Anim. Behav.,* 22: 907–913.

Drewett, R.F. and Cordall, K.M. (1976) Control of feeding in suckling rats: effects of glucose and of osmotic stimuli, *Physiol. Behav.,* 16: 711–717.

Drewett, R.F. and Trew, A.M. (1978) The milk ejection of the rat, as a stimulus and a response to the litter, *Anim. Behav.,* in press.

Fitzsimons, J.T. (1971) The physiology of thirst: a review of the extraneural aspects of the mechanisms of drinking. In *Progress in Physiological Psychology, Vol. 4,* E. Stellar and J.M. Sprague (Eds.), Academic Press, New York, pp. 119–194.

Friedman, M.I. (1975) Some determinants of milk ingestion in suckling rats, *J. comp. physiol. Psychol.,* 89: 636–647.

Gibbs, J., Young, R.C. and Smith, G.P. (1973) Cholecystokinin elicits satiety in rats with open gastric fistulas, *Nature (Lond.),* 245: 323–325.

Gil-Ad, I., Udeschini, G., Cocchi, D. and Muller, E.O. (1975) Hyporesponsiveness to glucoprivation during postnatal period in the rat, *Amer. J. Physiol.,* 229: 512–517.

Hall, W.G., Cramer, C.P. and Blass, E.M. (1975) Developmental changes in suckling of rat pups, *Nature (Lond.),* 258: 318–320.

Heggeress, F.W., Bindschadler, D., Chadwick, J., Conklin, P., Hulnick, S. and Oaks, M. (1961) Weight gain of overnourished and undernourished preweanling rats, *J. Nutr.,* 75: 39–44.

Heller, H. (1947) The response of newborn rats to administration of water by the stomach, *J. Physiol. (Lond.),* 106: 245–255.

Heller, H. (1949) Effects of dehydration on adult and newborn rats, *J. Physiol. (Lond.),* 108: 303–314.

Hofer, M.A., Shair, H. and Singh, P. (1976) Evidence that maternal ventral skin substances promote suckling in infant rats, *Physiol. Behav.,* 17: 131–136.

Houpt, K.A. and Epstein, A.N. (1973) Ontogeny of controls of food intake in the rat: GI fill and glucoprivation, *Amer. J. Physiol.,* 225: 58–66.

Houpt, K.A. and Houpt, T.R. (1975) Effects of gastric loads and food deprivation on subsequent food intake in suckling rats, *J. comp. physiol. Psychol.,* 88: 764–772.

Hunt, J.N. and Knox, M.T. (1968) Regulation of gastric emptying. In *Handbook of Physiology: Section 6 – Alimentary Canal, Vol. IV,* Charles F. Code (Ed.), American Physiological Society, Wash., D.C., pp. 1917–1935.

Kennedy, G.C. (1967) Ontogeny of mechanisms controlling food and water intake. In *Handbook of Physiology: Section 6 – Alimentary Canal, Vol. I,* Charles F. Code (Ed.), American Physiology Society, Wash., D.C., pp. 337–351.

Klauss, S.D., Mooney, E.G., Ewing, A.T. and Vandeweele, D.A. (1976) Comparative aspects of the development of glucostatic mechanisms in infant rats and guinea pigs, *Neurosci. Abstr.,* 2: 431.

Lincoln, D.W., Hill, A. and Wakerley, J.B. (1973) The milk ejection reflex of the rat: an intermittent function not abolished by surgical levels of anaesthesia, *J. Endocr.,* 57: 459–476.

Luckey, T.D., Mende, T.J. and Pleasants, J. (1954) The physical and chemical characterization of rat's milk, *J. Nutr.,* 54: 345–359.

MacFarlane, A. (1975) Olfaction in the development of social preferences in the human neonate. In *The Human Neonate in Parent-Infant Interaction, Ciba Found. Symp. 33,* Amsterdam, pp. 103–117.

Malvin, R.L., Mouw, D. and Vander, A.J. (1977) Angiotensin: physiological role in water-deprivation-induced thirst of rats, *Science,* 197: 171–173.

McCracken, R.D. (1971) Lactase deficiency: an example of dietary evolution, *Curr. Anthropol.,* 12: 479–500.

Moore, T.J., Lione, A.P., Regen, D.M., Tarpley, H.L. and Raines, P.L. (1971) Brain glucose metabolism in the newborn rat, *Amer. J. Physiol.,* 221: 1746–1753.

Mott, J.C. (1975) Place of the renin-angiotensin system before and after birth, *Brit. med. Bull.,* 31-1 (Perinatal Research): 44–50.

Niijima, A. (1969) Afferent impulse discharge from glucoreceptors in the liver of guinea pig, *Ann. N.Y. Acad. Sci.,* 157: 690–700.

Page, M.A., Krebs, H.A. and Williamson, D.H. (1971) Activities of enzymes of ketone-body utilization in brain and other tissues of suckling rats, *Biochem. J.,* 121: 49–53.

Ramsay, D.J., Rolls, B.J. and Wood, R.J. (1977) Body fluid changes which influence drinking in the water deprived rat, *J. Physiol. (Lond.),* 266: 453–469.

Russell, M.J. (1976) Human olfactory communication, *Nature (Lond.),* 260: 520–522.

Smith, G.P. and Epstein, A.N. (1969) Increased feeding in response to decreased glucose utilization in the rat and monkey, *Amer. J. Physiol.,* 217: 1083–1087.

Teicher, M.H. and Blass, E.M. (1976) Suckling in newborn rats: eliminated by nipple lavage, reinstated by pup saliva, *Science,* 193: 422–424.

Teitelbaum, P. (1971) The encephalization of hunger. In *Progress in Physiological Psychology,* E. Stellar and J.M. Sprague (Eds.), Academic Press, New York, pp. 319–346.

Vorherr, H., Kleeman, C.R. and Lehman, E. (1967) Oxytocin induced stretch reaction in suckling mice and rats: a semi-quantitative bio-assay for oxytocin, *Endocrinology,* 81: 711–715.

Wakerley, J.B. and Drewett, R.F. (1975) Pattern of sucking in the infant rat during spontaneous milk ejection, *Physiol. Behav.,* 15: 277–281.

Wirth, J.B. and Epstein, A.N. (1976) Ontogeny of thirst in the infant rat, *Amer. J. Physiol.,* 230: 188–198.

Wolff, P.H. (1968) Sucking patterns of infant mammals, *Brain Behav. Evol.,* 1: 353–367.

DISCUSSION

BERRY: At some stage or other, the control of milk drinking is presumably taken over by the *thirst* mechanism. Or can the two motivational systems live on independently in the rat? Presumably there must be a merging of these two behaviors as the animal matures and needs an adult amount of nourishment.

DREWETT: I am not so sure that there is. The stimulus that attracts the pup to the mother when it needs milk could not possibly take it to water. Obviously there is an unspecific aspect to the motor behavior used, for example, in approaching the mother; but attaching to the nipple and sucking are behavior patterns unrelated to anything needed for the drinking of water. So I suspect that the two systems do live on independently. Teitelbaum (1971) cites Cheng as showing that adult rats with lateral hypothalamic lesions — these animals that will neither eat nor drink — will, nonetheless, take in milk if they are allowed to suck reflexly from a nipple.

D'UDINE: Is there olfactory motivation working immediately after birth?

DREWETT: There is evidence that the rat pup is attracted to the nipple by the odor of saliva. And that leads one to wonder how the pup first gets onto the nipple when it is born. It is an interesting feature of the maternal behavior of the rat that she spends a lot of time licking down the nipple line before birth. This might serve to provide the saliva for the initial attraction. Mother rabbits do not, as far as I know, lick down the nipple line, and we are trying to find out whether the attachment of the rabbit kitten to the nipple is controlled in a different way, i.e. other than by saliva.

BLOM: You said something about the olfactory stimulus which starts the drinking. I wonder whether olfactory stimuli are involved in the process of weaning. There must be a point in the life of a rat where the original stimulus does not work any more.

DREWETT: It is a very interesting time, weaning. There is a completely different olfactory stimulus that attracts the rat pup to its mother, one that only becomes effective at about 14 days. This is derived from cecotrophe, which is fecal in origin. It doesn't attract rat pups to their mothers before 14 days, but it does between about 14 and 30 days.

Subject Index

420